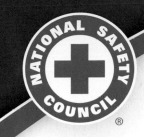

NATIONAL SAFETY COUNCIL

Advanced First Aid, CPR & AED

3.1M0117

NSC–in it for life

NATIONAL SAFETY COUNCIL MISSION STATEMENT
The National Safety Council saves lives by preventing injuries and deaths at work, in homes and communities, and on the roads through leadership, research, education and advocacy.

nsc.org

NSC promotes April as Distracted Driving Awareness Month and June as National Safety Month.

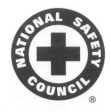

Welcome...

to a training course of the National Safety Council

The nation's leading safety advocate for more than 100 years, the National Safety Council is a nonprofit organization with the mission to save lives by preventing injuries and deaths at work, in homes and communities, and on the roads through leadership, research, education and advocacy. Working to make the world measurably safer, NSC advances this mission by engaging businesses, government agencies, elected officials and the public to help prevent the fourth leading cause of death in the United States – unintentional injuries.

The Council is data driven, relying on research to inform best-practice solutions to safety issues. To make the greatest impact, NSC focuses on where the most preventable injuries and deaths occur – cell phone use while driving, teen driving, workplace safety, prescription painkiller use and safety in the community. As a catalyst for behavior change, NSC promotes April as Distracted Driving Awareness Month and June as National Safety Month.

Acknowledged as the go-to source for safety, NSC provides a variety of educational opportunities – many through NSC University – including First Aid, Workplace Safety and Driver Safety courses, and is a leading source of occupational safety information through Safety+Health® magazine. The NSC Congress & Expo brings together the world's largest annual gathering of safety professionals. Through the Safe Communities America program, NSC certifies communities with rigorous safety initiatives.

The Campbell Institute at NSC is the global center of excellence for environmental, health and safety management, and collaborates with top-performing organizations to share research and best practices widely across industries. The Council recognizes organizations that have focused on safety as a critical part of their operations with the prestigious Robert W. Campbell Award®.

Celebrating significant safety achievements, NSC presents the Green Cross for Safety® award for safety excellence, innovation and advocacy. The highest safety recognition for individuals is the Council's Distinguished Service to Safety Awards, given annually.

NSC uses the concept of the Journey to Safety Excellence® as a roadmap for organizations to continually improve their safety practice to ensure zero harm. A 501c3 nonprofit, chartered by Congress with local chapters and global networks, and more than 50,000 members, NSC is committed to helping keep people safe wherever they are.

Author Acknowledgments

Many National Safety Council staff and affiliates have contributed to the production of this book, and we would like to acknowledge the following people for their assistance:

Paul Satterlee MD, for reviewing and providing oversight of content

Tom Lochhaas, Editorial Services, for providing technical writing services

Donna M. Siegfried, Senior Director, First Aid Programs, for providing vision and support

Robb Rehberg, PhD, ATC, NREMT, Director, Program Development and Training, for providing oversight of content, development and production

Donna Fredenhagen, Product Manager, for providing marketing support

David A. Middlemas, EdD, ATC, Subject Matter Expert, for assistance with technical review

Joanne Ploch, MEd, ATC, Subject Matter Expert, for assistance with technical review

Michael A. Prybicien, MA, ATC, Subject Matter Expert, for assistance with technical review

Barbara Caracci, NREMT

Envision Group Consulting, Inc.

The Council also recognizes with appreciation the many other NSC employees who devoted time to this project.

Reviewer Acknowledgments

Rebecca Gribben, BS, EMT
Instructor/Instructor Trainer
Medical Emergency Response Training
Houston, TX

James M. Howson, CEM, NRP
Unit Chief
Operational Medicine Unit
United States Department of State
Bureau of Diplomatic Security

J. Timothy Sensor, ATC, LAT
Director
Safe Sports Training Consultants
Scotch Plains, NJ

Bob Ward, MEd, ATC, LAT
Assistant Athletic Director
Head Athletic Trainer
Moravian College
Bethlehem, PA

Table of Contents

Chapter 1 • Preparing to Act 1

Chapter 2 • Acting in an Emergency 16

Chapter 3 • The Human Body 34

Chapter 4 • Assessing the Victim 49

Chapter 5 • Cardiopulmonary Emergencies
and Cardiopulmonary Rescuscitation 62

Chapter 6 • Automated External Defibrillators (AEDs) 85

Chapter 7 • Airway Obstructions 97

Chapter 8 • Controlling Bleeding 107

Chapter 9 • Shock 119

Chapter 10 • Wounds and Soft Tissue Injuries 129

Chapter 11 • Burns 149

Chapter 12 • Head and Spinal Injuries 168

Chapter 13 • Chest, Abdominal and Pelvic Injuries 183

Chapter 14 • Bone, Joint and Muscle Injuries 194

Chapter 15 • Extremity Injuries and Splinting 211

Chapter 16 • Sudden Illness 227

Chapter 17 • Poisoning 248

Chapter 18 • Substance Misuse and Abuse 260

Chapter 19 • Bites and Stings 273

Chapter 20 • Cold and Heat Emergencies 292

Chapter 21 • Behavioral Emergencies 306

Chapter 22 • Pregnancy and Childbirth 325

Chapter 23 • Remote Location First Aid 337

Chapter 24 • Rescuing and Moving Victims 359

Chapter 25 • Are You Prepared? 377

Chapter 26 • Moving Forward 385

Appendix A • Advanced Rescuscitation Techniques 389

Appendix B • Performance Checklists for Skills 408

Appendix C • Natural Disasters: Earthquakes 443

Appendix D • Natural Disasters: Floods 453

Appendix E • Natural Disasters: Hurricanes 459

Appendix F • Natural Disasters: Tornadoes 465

Appendix G • Answers to Learning Checkpoints and Review Questions 473

Glossary 493

Index 504

CHAPTER 1

Preparing to Act

LESSON OBJECTIVES

- List the 4 primary goals of first aid.

- Explain why there is a need for first aid training.

- Decide to help in an emergency.

- Describe how to stay prepared for emergencies.

- Describe the EMS system and the different types of EMS professionals.

- Explain when to call 9-1-1 and what information to give the dispatcher.

- Explain what first aiders need to understand about legal issues related to first aid.

You are staying late at work to catch up on a project, when a coworker returns to the office to pick up something she forgot. While she is in her office, her young son, whom she left in the reception area, is running around. He falls and hurts his arm, and you hear him crying and come out to see if you can help. His mother calms him while you get a first aid kit.

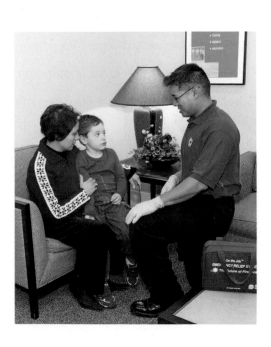

First aid training is important because injuries and sudden illness occur frequently. People of all ages, in all places, may experience an injury or sudden illness requiring immediate attention when a doctor or medical professional is not present. Oftentimes, the person needing first aid is a family member or loved one. In many cases, the victim's life or well-being depends on actions that first aiders take during the first few minutes before emergency responders take over.

This chapter will help you become prepared to act in an emergency. It explains the need for first aid and how to decide to help when you recognize an emergency. You will also learn what it means to be prepared, your role in the Emergency Medical Services (EMS) system and relevant legal issues in first aid.

What Is First Aid?

First aid is the immediate help given to a victim of injury or sudden illness until appropriate medical help arrives or the victim is seen by a health care provider. First aid is typically given by a friend or family member, a coworker or a bystander at the scene with minimal or no medical equipment. First aid is generally not all the treatment the person needs, but it helps the victim for the usually short time until advanced care begins. First aid can also be simple care given when medical attention is not needed, such as caring for a small wound.

The primary goals of first aid are to:

• Keep the victim alive until he or she receives medical care.

• Prevent the victim's condition from getting worse.

• Help promote early recovery from the injury or illness.

• Ensure the victim receives appropriate medical care.

Other goals include reassuring the victim and providing comfort until medical care is provided.

Most first aid does not require extensive training or equipment. With the first aid training in this course and a basic first aid kit, you can perform first aid in most situations.

The Need for First Aid

Heart attack is the single most common cause of death in emergency situations, followed by strokes and injuries. According to the American Heart Association's 2015 Heart Disease and Stroke Statistics Update,[1] each year in the United States:

• More than 735,000 heart attacks occur, resulting in 120,000 deaths.

• More than 326,000 people experience out-of-hospital cardiac arrests.

• Strokes result in about 129,000 deaths.

Additionally, unintentional injuries account for over 29 million emergency department visits and 130,800 deaths each year in the United States.[2]

[1]*American Heart Association. heart.org/idc/groups/ahamah-public/@wcm/@sop/@smd/documents/downloadable/ucm_470704.pdf Accessed January 2016.*

[2]*National Safety Council. (2015). Injury Facts®, 2015 Edition. Itasca, IL: Author.*

Table 1-1 lists the most common causes of injuries for which the victim went to a hospital emergency department in the most recent year for which data are available. Table 1-2 lists the deaths resulting from the most common types of injuries in the most recent year for which data are available.

TABLE 1-1	
Unintentional Injuries Treated in Hospital Emergency Departments in 2012	
Falls	8,974,762
Struck by or against object	4,533,417
Overexertion	3,385,127
Motor vehicle occupants	2,564,003
Cut or pierced by object	2,145,927
Other specified*	1,580,574
Bites and stings (other than dog bites)	1,250,916
Poisoning (includes drug overdose)	972,923
Unknown/unspecified	734,164
Foreign body	588,322

Source: National Safety Council, "Injury Facts", 2015; data from NEISS All Injury Program, Office of Statistics and Programming, National Center for Injury Prevention and Control, the Centers for Disease Control and Consumer Product Safety Commission.

*Includes electric current, explosions, fireworks, radiation, animal scratch, etc.; excludes all causes listed in the table and bb/pellet gunshot, drowning and near drowning, firearm gunshot, suffocation, machinery, natural and environmental conditions, pedestrians and motorcyclists.

TABLE 1-2

Deaths Due to Unintentional Injuries in 2013

Poisoning (includes drug overdose)	38,800
Motor vehicle incidents	35,500
Falls	30,300
Choking	4,800
Drowning	3,700
Fires, flames and smoke	2,400
Mechanical suffocation	1,800
All other unintentional injuries*	13,500

Source: National Safety Council, Injury Facts 2015; National Safety Council analysis of National Center for Health Statistics mortality data and Bureau of the Census population data.

*Includes natural heat and cold, firearms, struck by or against object, machinery, electric current and air, water and rail transport.

These tables present unintentional injury data for the general population. In addition, workplace injuries take a major toll, as shown in Figures 1-1 and 1-2. About 60 million worker-days are lost each year to work-related injuries.

FIGURE 1-2

Workers' on- and off-the-job injuries, United States, 2013.

Source: National Safety Council. Injury Facts®, 2015 Edition.

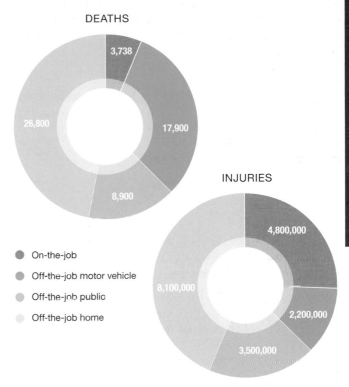

DEATHS

3,738

17,900

26,800

8,900

- On-the-job
- Off-the-job motor vehicle
- Off-the-job public
- Off-the-job home

INJURIES

4,800,000

8,100,000

2,200,000

3,500,000

FIGURE 1-1

Occupational unintentional-injury-related deaths and death rates by industry, United States, 2013.

Source: National Safety Council. Injury Facts®, 2015 Edition.

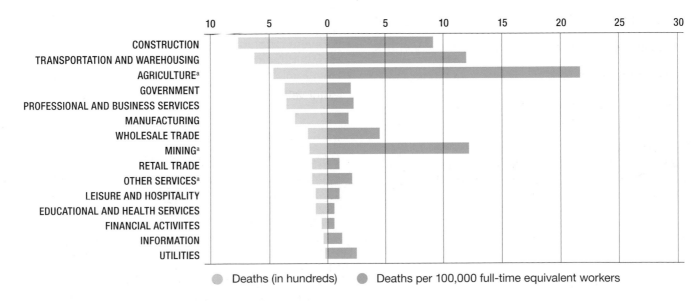

- Deaths (in hundreds)
- Deaths per 100,000 full-time equivalent workers

ª Agriculture includes forestry fishing and hunting. Mining includes oil and gas extraction. "Other services" excludes public administration.

In many cases, these deaths could have been prevented. In other cases, the victim might have lived if a trained first aider had been present to give help until medical help arrived. This text describes both injury and illness prevention and the care to give until help arrives. With what you learn in this first aid course, you can help make a difference and perhaps save a life.

 LEARNING CHECKPOINT 1

Circle **True** or **False** for each of the following statements:

1. When first aid is given, the victim does not need further medical attention.

    True   False

2. First aid given promptly can save lives and reduce the severity of injuries.

    True   False

Deciding to Help

Recognizing the need for first aid and knowing what first aid to give are the first steps in preparedness, but you also need to make the conscious decision to help in an emergency. This is not always an easy decision. You may hesitate to act because of any of the following common concerns:

- **You may be worried about not doing the right thing.** Remember that you have first aid training. This course will teach you all you need to know to be able to help. Once you call for help, professionals will arrive very soon. Usually, you are needed to help only for a few minutes.

- **You may think someone else would provide better care.** Do not delay giving first aid because you hope someone else will do it. Many people are naturally shy about stepping forward in an emergency, but unless someone else has already begun to help the victim and is obviously trained in what to do, it is up to you to help the victim. People without first aid training can assist you, such as by calling 9-1-1, going to get first aid supplies or helping calm a victim they know. But do not let precious minutes pass while waiting to see if someone else will help.

- **You may not be sure it is an emergency.** This first aid course will teach you the signs of an emergency when an injured or suddenly ill person needs help right away. When in doubt, call 9-1-1 and tell the dispatcher what you see. It is better to make the call and find out later the victim's condition was not serious after all, than to not call and allow a victim's condition to deteriorate before seeking care for the victim.

- **You may be upset by the sight of blood or the injury.** Some injuries can be very upsetting, especially those involving blood, badly burned skin, vomiting and other factors. You may have to muster your self-control. Try to focus on the immediate tasks at hand to prevent the experience from overwhelming you. You may need to look away and take a deep breath. You may need to ask others to help. People who are easily upset may gain from learning stress-reduction techniques along with first aid to stay in control in an emergency. If you react strongly to photographs of severe injuries such as those in this text, and if you believe you might have difficulty acting in an emergency because of such factors, talk with your instructor about relaxation techniques that may be appropriate for you.

- **You may be worried about catching a disease from the victim.** Most of us would not worry about helping a family member or friend because of a fear of disease, but we may be reluctant to touch a stranger. Because some diseases can be transmitted through contact with another person's blood or other body fluids, this is – and should be – a concern. As discussed in **Chapter 2**, you should take steps in any emergency to prevent disease transmission. When you give first aid using the precautions you will learn in this course, you will not face a higher risk of contracting a disease.

Stay Prepared to Help

An emergency can occur at any time in any place, and most emergencies occur without warning. One moment you are enjoying dinner with friends, and the next moment someone at the table is choking on food and unable to breathe. A child is running through a playground and falls on broken glass, and suddenly, is bleeding severely. A coworker abruptly clutches his chest and collapses. In each of these cases, you need to act immediately, for the victim may have only minutes to live unless you give first aid. Therefore, it is essential to always be prepared to act as needed.

Being prepared means knowing what to do – but it also means feeling ready and taking steps to ensure you do not lose precious time when responding to an emergency:

- **Know the appropriate first aid techniques.** This first aid course will teach you what to do in all emergencies involving injury or sudden illness.

- **Be confident in your skills.** Sometimes, people at the scene of an emergency are hesitant to help. Remember that you have first aid training, however, and you should feel confident that you can help the victim. Never hesitate or wait for others to act – remember that the victim's life may depend on acting quickly.

- **Have a personal first aid kit at home and in your car.** Be sure first aid kits are well stocked with the right supplies. Keep emergency phone numbers, such as EMS, the Poison Control Center and other emergency agencies, in a handy place.

- **Know whether your community uses 9-1-1 or a different emergency telephone number.** Note that this text says "Call 9-1-1" throughout. If your community does not use the 9-1-1 system, call your local emergency number instead. Some companies have an internal emergency number employees are expected to call (that department will then call EMS).

- **When teaching children to call 9-1-1, say "nine-one-one" and never "nine-eleven."** Young children are known to lose valuable time searching for an "eleven" button on the telephone keypad.

- **If you or your significant others have a medical condition, be sure that information is available to others in an emergency.** Information should include the telephone numbers of healthcare providers, allergies and any prescription medications. People with certain medical conditions such as diabetes, epilepsy and severe allergies are advised to wear a medical alert bracelet or necklace to alert others in an emergency **(Figure 1-3)**.

People with certain illnesses or conditions may also carry medications for emergency use. For example, people with severe allergies may carry an epinephrine auto-injector such as an EpiPen, and some people with heart conditions may carry nitroglycerine tablets.

FIGURE 1-3

Medical alert jewelry.

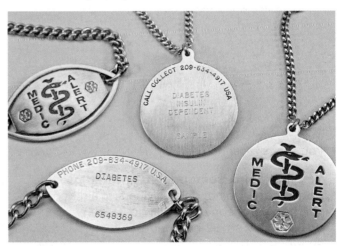

Accidental injury deaths vary according to the age of the person involved, as shown in **Figure 1-4**. **Table 1-3** presents a breakdown of injury episodes by the victim's age and activity at the time of the injury. When you put all this data together, you realize that first aiders need to be prepared to give first aid in any place at any time.

FIGURE 1-4

Leading causes of fatal, unintentional injuries by age group, United States, 2011.

Source: National Safety Council. Injury Facts®, 2015 Edition.

KEY — Poisoning · Falls · Motor vehicle traffic/occupant · Suffocation · Drowning · Overexertion · Struck by/against · Cut/pierce

Rank	All ages	Younger than 1	1-4	5-9	10-14	15-24	25-34	35-44	45-54	55-64	65 or older
1	Poisoning 36,280	Suffocation 896	Drowning 438	Motor vehicle traffic 350	Motor vehicle traffic 437	Motor vehicle traffic 6,926	Poisoning 7,652	Poisoning 8,075	Poisoning 10,379	Poisoning 5,048	Falls 22,901
2	Motor vehicle traffic 33,783	Motor vehicle traffic 93	Motor vehicle traffic 330	Drowning 128	Drowning 107	Poisoning 3,440	Motor vehicle traffic 5,569	Motor vehicle traffic 4,425	Motor vehicle traffic 5,240	Motor vehicle traffic 4,184	Motor vehicle traffic 6,225
3	Falls 27,483	Drowning 52	Suffocation 144	Fire/burn 91	Other land transport 47	Drowning 543	Drowning 442	Falls 542	Falls 1,368	Falls 2,141	Unspecified 4,360
4	Suffocation 6,242	Unspecified 28	Fire/burn 130	Suffocation 34	Suffocation 43	Falls 205	Falls 279	Drowning 414	Suffocation 536	Suffocation 644	Suffocation 3,402
5	Unspecified 5,871	Fire/burn 24	Pedestrian, other 98	Other land transport 91	Fire/burn 42	Other land transport 177	Other specified 212	Suffocation 240	Drowning 479	Fire/burn 522	Poisoning 1,581
6	Drowning 3,556	Natural/ environment 21	Struck by/ against 56	Natural/ environment 28	Poisoning 35	Fire/burn 138	Suffocation 176	Other specified 209	Fire/burn 425	Unspecified 496	Fire/burn 1,073
7	Fire/burn 2,813	Poisoning 15	Natural/ environment 40	Firearms 16	Other transport 32	Firearms 130	Fire/burn 175	Fire/burn 201	Natural/ environment 401	Natural/ environment 424	Natural/ environment 825
8	Natural/ environment 2,193	Falls 11	Poisoning 34	Pedestrian, other 16	Firearms 29	Suffocation 127	Other land transport 173	Natural/ environment 182	Other specified 345	Drowning 412	Other specified n.e.c.* 604
9	Other specified 1,409	Other specified 10	Firearms 25	Other transport 15	Natural/ environment 21	Other specified 122	Natural/ environment 155	Unspecified 175	Unspecified 336	Other specified 240	Drowning 540
10	Other land transport 1,301	Struck by/ against 6	Falls 24	Poisoning 15	Falls 19	Pedestrian, other 109	Other transport 152	Other land transport 166	Other land transport 232	Other transport 181	Other land transport 285

All causes of fatal, unintentional injury

	All ages	Younger than 1	1-4	5-9	10-14	15-24	25-34	35-44	45-54	55-64	65 or older
#	126,438	1,163	1,377	761	874	12,330	15,518	15,230	20,479	15,158	43,278[b]
Per 100,000 population	39.0	29.3	8.5	3.7	4.2	28.1	37.1	37.5	46.4	39.8	104.6[b]

Source: Center for Disease Prevention and Control, National Center for Injury Prevention and Control. Web-based Injury Statistics Query and Reporting System (WISQARS), data accessed July 16, 2014 at cdc.gov/injury/wisqars/index.html.

[a] "n.e.c." means not elsewhere classified.

[b] Includes 20 cases with age unknown.

TABLE 1-3

Number of injury episodes by age and activity at time of injury, United States, 2012

	Total episodes[a] (000)	Activity at time of injury[b] (number in thousands)						
		Driving[c]	Working at paid job	Working around house or yard	Attending school	Sports	Leisure activities	Other[d]
All ages	37,401	2,576	4,247	5,401	1,043	6,062	7,263	10,849
Younger than 12	4,976	203[f]	0	(e)	465	978	2,006	1,301
12-17 years	4,540	(e)	(e)	(e)	441	2,268	874	609
18-44 years	11,413	899	2,342	1,639	(e)	1,939	1,802	2,579
45-64 years	10,621	1,065	1,775	2,257	0	653	1,461	3,439
65-74 years	3,074	191[f]	(e)	664	0	(e)	610	1,314
75 or older	2,777	(e)	0	649	0	0	510	1,607

Source: Adams, P.F., Kirzinger W.K., & Martinez, M.E. (2013, December). Summary of health statistics for the U.S. population: National health interview survey, 2012. National Center for Health Statistics. Vital and Health Statistics, Series 10 (No. 259).

[a] Numbers may not sum to respective totals due to rounding and unknowns.

[b] Activity at time of injury and poisoning episodes is based on the question, "What was [person] doing when the injury/poisoning happened?" Respondents could indicate up to 2 activities.

[c] Driving includes both drivers and passengers.

[d] "Other" includes unpaid work such as housework, shopping, volunteer work, sleeping, resting, eating, drinking, cooking, hands-on care from another person and other unspecified activities.

[e] Estimate is not shown because it does not meet standard of reliability or precision.

[f] Estimate does not meet standard of reliability or precision and should be used with caution.

YOUR FIRST AID KIT

Keep a well-stocked first aid kit in your home and vehicle, and know where one is kept at work or at school. Take one with you on recreational activities. A cell phone is also helpful in most emergencies.

Make sure your first aid kit includes the items shown in **Figure 1-5**. Note that you may not necessarily use all items in a kit.

FIGURE 1-5

Components of a first aid kit (*denotes minimum requirements for workplace first aid kits). Include optional supplies based on specific hazards in a particular work environment.

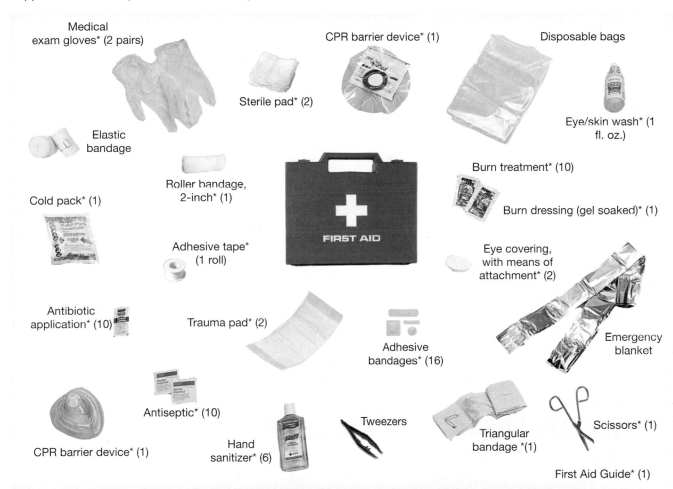

Medical exam gloves* (2 pairs)

Sterile pad* (2)

CPR barrier device* (1)

Disposable bags

Eye/skin wash* (1 fl. oz.)

Elastic bandage

Cold pack* (1)

Roller bandage, 2-inch* (1)

Burn treatment* (10)

Burn dressing (gel soaked)* (1)

Adhesive tape* (1 roll)

FIRST AID

Eye covering, with means of attachment* (2)

Antibiotic application* (10)

Trauma pad* (2)

Adhesive bandages* (16)

Emergency blanket

Antiseptic* (10)

CPR barrier device* (1)

Hand sanitizer* (6)

Tweezers

Triangular bandage *(1)

Scissors* (1)

First Aid Guide* (1)

Minimum requirements for workplace Class A first aid kits used for the most common types of workplace injuries. Class B kits contain a broader range and quantity of supplies for use in more complex or high-risk locations. Supplement these supplies with additional items or additional quantities of required supplies based on specific hazards in your particular work environment. For more information on the minimum requirements standard, consult the American National Standards Institute (ANSI) website at ansi.org/news_publications/news_story.aspx?menuid=7&articleid=b4472a01-f4ac-4466-afd5-77559633a5f8

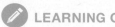

1. Select the best answer. Being prepared for an emergency means –

    a.   knowing what to do.

    b.   being ready to act any time, anywhere.

    c.   knowing how to get medical care for a victim.

    d.   All of the above

2. Select the best answer. It is a good idea to have a first aid kit –

    a.   in your home.

    b.   in your car.

    c.   on recreational outings.

    d.   All of the above

Emergency Medical Service System

People trained in first aid are the first link in the **Emergency Medical Service (EMS)** system. The EMS system in the United States is a comprehensive network of professionals linked together to provide appropriate levels of medical care for victims of injury or sudden illness.[1] As a first aider, your role in the system, in addition to giving the victim first aid until he or she is seen by advanced caregivers, is to make sure the EMS system responds as quickly as possible to help the victim, by calling 9-1-1. In most communities, help will arrive within minutes.

The EMS system includes a number of different professionals with different levels of training and responsibilities **(Box 1-1)**.

[1]*The term **sudden illness** is generally used to describe medical conditions that occur suddenly and require first aid until the person can be seen by a medical professional. This term will be used throughout this text. "Sudden" illness is generally different from other illness situations in which the sick person is already under the care of a healthcare professional or has time to see a healthcare professional for a nonemergency condition. Note that in some cases, a person with a nonemergency chronic illness, such as diabetes or asthma, may suddenly experience an emergency situation as a result of that illness. If so, that immediate emergency situation, such as a person with asthma having an attack and not being able to breathe, is then called sudden illness.*

WHEN TO CALL EMS

Call 9-1-1 immediately if you recognize a life-threatening injury or illness. A life-threatening emergency is one in which a problem threatens the victim's breathing or circulation of blood (i.e., cardiac arrest or severe bleeding), as described in later chapters. If you are alone with the victim and not near a telephone, shout for help and ask someone to call 9-1-1. Do not try to transport a victim to the emergency department yourself. Movement may worsen his or her condition, or the victim may suddenly need additional care on the way. An ambulance can also usually reach the emergency department faster than you can, and the EMTs can provide care as needed on the way. If you are not sure whether a situation is serious enough to call, do not hesitate – call 9-1-1. It is better to be safe than sorry.

If the victim is responsive and may not be seriously injured or ill, go on to the next step and check the victim further before calling 9-1-1, and then call 9-1-1 or a healthcare provider if needed.

Always call 9-1-1 when:

• The victim may have a life-threatening condition.

• The victim is unresponsive (not talking, moving or responding to you).

• The victim's condition may become life threatening.

• Moving the victim could make his or her condition worse.

Box 1-2 lists serious conditions for which to call 9-1-1. Later chapters also describe when to call 9-1-1 for other specific problems.

Note that victims may say their condition is not all that serious. For example, heart attack victims often say they have "indigestion" even when they have clear heart attack signs and symptoms. You should call 9-1-1 anyway and let the dispatcher decide if the situation is an emergency.

In addition to calling 9-1-1 for injury or illness, call in these situations:

• Fire or explosion

• Vehicle crash

• Downed electrical wire

• Chemical spill, gas leak or the presence of any unknown substances

• Swiftly moving or rapidly rising water

BOX 1-1: EMS PROFESSIONALS

DISPATCHER

A 9-1-1 call for help is usually received by an EMS dispatcher. This person is trained in obtaining information and determining what emergency personnel and equipment will likely be needed. The EMS dispatcher then sends the appropriate EMS unit to the scene.

EMERGENCY MEDICAL RESPONDER (EMR)

The first professional with BLS training to arrive at the scene of a medical emergency is often an emergency medical responder (formerly called a first responder). You may be the first professional rescuer if you are close to the scene. The EMR generally takes over care of the victim from a lay person who may be giving first aid or from anyone with less training. The EMR also gathers any information concerning the victim, may control the scene or direct others to do so and in some instances, prepares for the arrival of an ambulance. In a healthcare setting, a professional rescuer may provide emergency care until a physician, nurse or other health care professional with a higher level of training takes over. In an out-of-hospital setting, emergency care may be given until emergency medical technicians arrive with an ambulance.

EMERGENCY MEDICAL TECHNICIANS (EMT) AND PARAMEDICS

In an out-of-hospital emergency, EMTs and/or advanced EMTs and paramedics usually arrive in an ambulance. They take over the medical care of the victim, give necessary medical care at the scene, and transport the victim for advanced medical care. EMTs with different levels of training perform different medical treatments. Paramedics have the highest level of training.

MEDICAL DIRECTOR

The medical director is a physician within the EMS system who oversees the care given by EMTs and some EMRs. The medical director establishes protocols for medical care to be given to victims at the scene, and is available for consultation by radio or telephone to EMTs giving care.

HOSPITALS AND SPECIALIZED CENTERS

EMRs and EMTs provide prehospital care before and during the transport of the victim to a hospital. Depending on the medical care needed and facilities in the area, the victim receives care from physicians in a hospital emergency department or a specialized center such as a trauma center, burn center or pediatric center.

BOX 1-2: WHEN TO CALL 9-1-1

- Unresponsiveness or altered mental status (dizzy, confused, disoriented, etc.)
- Not breathing normally, difficulty breathing
- Chest pain or pressure that does not go away
- Severe bleeding
- Head or spine injuries
- Poisoning, drug overdose
- Vomiting blood
- Seizures
- Severe burn
- Drowning or near drowning
- Threatened suicide
- Imminent childbirth
- When you are not sure

WHEN YOU CALL EMS

When you call 9-1-1 or your local emergency number, be ready to give the following information. (If, however, this information is not readily available, do not delay making the call.)

- Your name
- The phone number you are using
- The location and number of victims – specific enough for the arriving crew to be able to find them
- What happened to the victim(s) and any special circumstances or conditions that may require special rescue or medical equipment
- The victim's condition. For example, is the victim responsive? Breathing? Bleeding?
- The victim's approximate age and sex
- What is being done for the victim(s)? For example, is anyone on the scene able and willing to give CPR, is an AED present, etc.

It is important to not hang up until the dispatcher instructs you to do so, because you may be given advice on how to care for the victim.

If another responsible person is present, tell him or her to call 9-1-1 while you go on to check the victim and give first aid **(Figure 1-6)**. Tell the other person to give the dispatcher the information listed previously.

Many communities have an **enhanced 9-1-1** system that automatically provides the dispatcher with the caller's phone number and the location of landlines. This information can be lifesaving if the call is interrupted, but do not depend on the dispatcher already knowing your location. The exact location of a cell phone may not be known, and even when using a landline, you may need to specify where you are (such as to say you are with the victim in the yard behind the house), to prevent the loss of precious time while EMTs knock at the front door.

If 9-1-1 is not used as the emergency number in your community, post your local emergency telephone number by all telephones and keep the number with you if you travel with a cell phone. Having to find a telephone directory to look up a number will consume critical time. **Box 1-3** describes other issues you may encounter with telephones.

In some remote locations, you may not be near a telephone. In these cases, you may need to care for the victim for a longer time until the victim receives medical assistance. **Chapter 23** discusses common first aid situations in remote areas. In most other areas, however, your shouts for help will likely attract someone who can reach a telephone quickly to call 9-1-1.

FIGURE 1-6

Call 9-1-1 to get emergency help on its way.

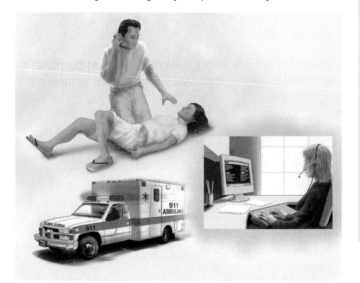

BOX 1-3: 9-1-1 AND TELEPHONE ISSUES

Internet telephone services, commonly called VoIP (Voice Over Internet Protocol) services, have become increasingly popular for computer users with broadband Internet service. In 2005, after incidents in which people were unable to call 9-1-1 on their computer phones, the FCC ruled that all VoIP telephone services must allow a connection to EMS through the 9-1-1 number. The FCC warns, however, that in some situations, a 9-1-1 call over VoIP may still not be properly routed, and urges anyone depending on VoIP telephone service to contact their provider to ensure reliability of this service.[1] Many VoIP telephone users do not realize, in addition, that their telephone will work only as long as their computer and Internet connection are functioning. In a power outage, for example, a VoIP telephone connected to a computer without an independent power source may stop working, potentially leaving the user with no way to call 9-1-1.

Similarly, many people do not realize that most cordless telephones also require electrical power – not just a charged battery in the handset. In a power failure, a wired land telephone should still work, being powered by the telephone line rather than the power circuit, but most cordless telephones will not, even if connected to a land telephone line. Cell phones are not affected by local power outages, but may not have a strong signal in all locales.

By one method or another, it is important to ensure that you can always call 9-1-1 in an emergency, even when the power is off.

Note that cell phone users have been encouraged to put a personal contact in their phone directory under the name "ICE" or "In Case of Emergency" so that emergency responders can learn who to call if needed. As a first aider, you would not check a victim's telephone or try to contact family members, but you may want to carry your own "in case of emergency" phone number.

[1]*fcc.gov/consumers/guides/voip-and-911-service Accessed January 2016.*

LEARNING CHECKPOINT 3

1. What number should you call to access EMS? Select the best answer.

   a. 9-1-1 (if your community uses that number)

   b. The local emergency number (if not 9-1-1)

   c. Your employer's emergency number (when company policy)

   d. All of the above

2. Select the best answer. Call 9-1-1 for –

   a. medical problems only.

   b. police and fire services only.

   c. medical problems and fires only.

   d. medical problems and all emergencies.

3. Who usually arrives first at the scene after you have called 9-1-1?

   _____

4. List 7 things you should be prepared to tell the EMS dispatcher when you call.

   _____

   _____

   _____

   _____

   _____

   _____

Legal Concepts in First Aid

The United States is often said to be a litigious society because lawsuits are common. We hear so much in the media about people being sued that often we are afraid to act – even to help one another – because we worry we might be sued if something goes wrong. Although legal problems very seldom arise in first aid situations, certain legal concepts are important when you interact with another person to give first aid. If you follow certain simple guidelines, you need not be concerned about being sued for giving first aid. If you give first aid as you are trained

to do in this course, and do your best, there is little chance of being found legally liable even if the victim does not recover.

To protect yourself, follow these general guidelines:

- Act only as you are trained to act.

- Get a victim's consent before giving first aid.

- Do not move a victim unnecessarily.

- Call for professional help.

- Keep giving care until help arrives.

GOOD SAMARITAN LAWS

Most states have **Good Samaritan laws** designed to encourage people to help others in an emergency without having to worry about being sued. These laws vary somewhat from state to state, but in general, they are designed to protect people who give first aid in an emergency.

These laws do not provide blanket protection, however, regardless of the person's actions. In general, first aiders are legally protected only:

- when acting in an emergency, voluntarily and without compensation.

- when acting as a reasonable, prudent person with the same training would act.

- when performing first aid techniques as trained.

- when not doing something outside their training.

- when not abandoning a victim after starting to give care.

Ask your instructor about the specific Good Samaritan laws in your area. Remember, however, that regardless of specific laws, first aiders who act with good intentions and as they have been trained will very rarely face any legal issues.

MUST YOU GIVE FIRST AID?

In most places, private citizens or bystanders at the scene of an emergency have no legal obligation to give first aid. Many people feel an ethical or moral obligation to help others in need, but this is different from a legal obligation.

Because laws do vary in different areas, however, ask your instructor about the law in your area.

There are 3 important exceptions to the principle that you are not legally required to give first aid. First, once you begin giving first aid in an emergency, you are obligated to continue giving care if you can and to remain with the victim. By beginning to give care, you accept and take on an obligation to continue giving care in an emergency. Abandoning a victim in this situation could lead to the worsening of an injury or illness, disability or death.

The second exception is that some people are required to give first aid as a job responsibility. As a paid employee with this job requirement, you then are legally obligated. This is called a **duty to act**, and you may be held liable for failing to act or for acting inappropriately. Off the job, however, depending on your state's laws, you are usually not legally required to give first aid except in special cases.

The final exception is a parent or guardian who is responsible for a child, who has the duty to give the child adequate care. Federal and state laws against child abuse and neglect require parents and guardians to prevent harm and provide medical treatment (see **Chapter 21**).

CONSENT

Before you give first aid, you must have the victim's **consent**. This means the victim gives you permission to help him or her by using first aid techniques. Touching another person without consent is a criminal action called battery. Consent may be either expressed or implied.

Expressed consent means the victim explicitly gives you permission to give first aid. To ask for consent, first tell the victim who you are and that you have had first aid training, and say what you want to do to help. The victim should understand that you are asking for consent, not stating what you plan to do regardless of what the victim wishes. A victim who is responsive (awake and alert) and able to communicate must give you expressed consent before you can give first aid. The victim may give consent by telling you it is okay or by nodding in agreement. With an injured or ill child, a parent or guardian present must give expressed consent **(Figure 1-7)**.

If an adult is unresponsive, however, or a child's parent or guardian is not present and cannot be reached quickly enough for consent, then you have **implied consent** to give first aid in an emergency. In this case, you can assume, unless there is some evidence to the contrary, that the person would, if able, consent to receiving care for a life-threatening condition. Similarly, if a person who initially refused consent becomes unresponsive, consent for care is now implied.

FIGURE 1-7

A parent or guardian present at the scene must give consent for first aid for a child.

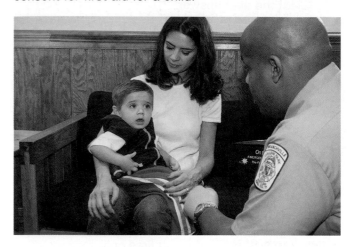

REFUSING CONSENT

Most competent victims of a medical emergency will give consent for first aid when they understand the importance of this first aid. **Competent** means the person is able to understand what is happening and the implications of his or her decision about receiving first aid. A victim may not be competent because of intoxication, the influence of a drug or altered mental status caused by a severe injury or a diabetic emergency.

Rarely, however, a competent victim may refuse your care when you seek consent. The person may have religious reasons, may be afraid, may not trust you or may have some other reason. A competent adult has the right to refuse medical care, even care that has already begun, and you must not try to force care on this person. Refusal may be expressed through words, by shaking the head or signaling you to stop or by trying to push you away. If this happens, follow these guidelines:

- Make sure 9-1-1 has been called even though the victim may seem to refuse all care. The victim may accept treatment from a medical professional.

- Do not try to argue with the victim, especially about personal beliefs. Keep talking to the victim, who may change his or her mind. Explain that you respect his or her right to refuse care, but ask the person to reconsider. Explain what may happen if the victim does not receive care.

- To protect yourself legally, make sure someone else at the scene sees or hears the victim's refusal to accept your care.

SCOPE OF CARE

As noted earlier, first aiders should perform first aid only as they have been trained. The set of first aid techniques one learns in a first aid course is called the **scope of care**. Acting outside your scope of care as a first aider, such as trying to do something you have heard about but have not been trained to do, may make you legally liable for the results of your actions.

STANDARD OF CARE

While scope of care refers to what you do, **standard of care** refers generally to how you perform first aid. Standard of care refers to what others with the same training would do in a similar situation. It is important to give first aid only as you are trained. Any other actions could result in the injury or illness becoming worse.

NEGLIGENCE

Legally, you may be liable for the results of your actions if you do not follow accepted standards of care when providing first aid; this is called **negligence**. If you are negligent, an injured party may sue you to recover financial damages for the result of your actions. For you to be found guilty of negligence, three conditions must be met:

1. You had a duty to act (for example, first aid is your job responsibility).

2. You breached that duty (by not acting or by acting incorrectly).

3. Your actions or inaction caused injury or damages (including such things as physical injury or pain).

Examples of negligent actions could include moving a victim unnecessarily, doing something you have not been trained to do n or failing to give first aid as you have been trained.

ABANDONMENT

Once you begin giving first aid in an emergency, do not stop until another trained person takes over. Stay with the victim until help arrives or someone with the same or a higher level of training takes over. If you leave the victim and the injury or illness becomes worse, this is called **abandonment**, a type of negligence. Note that abandonment is different from justified instances of stopping care, such as if you are exhausted and unable to continue, or you are in imminent danger because of hazards at the scene.

CONFIDENTIALITY

When giving first aid, you may learn private information about the victim. That information should not be shared with anyone other than EMS professionals arriving at the scene to take over care of the victim. Although laws vary in terms of precise definitions regarding violation of privacy, **confidentiality** is the general principle that you should not give out any private information about a victim to anyone except for those caring for him or her.

 LEARNING CHECKPOINT 4

Circle **True** or **False** for the following statement:

1. The best thing to do in any emergency is to move the victim to your car and rush to an emergency department. | True | False |

2. Select the best answer. You have a duty to act when –

    a. you stop at the scene of an emergency.

    b. you have taken a first aid course.

    c. you have a first aid kit with you.

    d. your job requires you to give first aid when needed.

3. To which of the following victims do you have consent to give first aid? (Check all that apply.)

    ☐ An unresponsive adult victim

    ☐ A child without parent or guardian present

    ☐ All victims, all of the time

    ☐ A victim who nods when you ask if it is okay to give him or her first aid

    ☐ A child whose parent or guardian gives consent for him or her

4. Check off things you should always do when giving first aid.

    ☐ Move the victim.

    ☐ Do what you have been trained to do.

    ☐ Try any first aid technique you have read or heard about.

    ☐ Ask for the victim's consent.

    ☐ Stay with the victim until another trained person takes over.

    ☐ Transport all victims to the emergency department in your vehicle.

CONCLUDING THOUGHTS

How often have you heard people say something like "It can't happen to me?" No one ever expects to be injured seriously or experience a sudden crisis of illness, yet it happens to tens of millions of us every year. In fact, it is almost inevitable that eventually, you or someone close to you will need first aid – and you can be the one who makes the difference. The following chapters will help you to be prepared.

 CRITICAL THINKING CHALLENGE QUESTIONS

SCENARIO 1

Driving along a quiet residential street, you come upon a car that apparently has just collided with a tree. You stop behind the car and realize the driver is still in the car, seemingly alone. You have a cell phone with you and your first impulse is to call 9-1-1. What should you do before you call 9-1-1? What information should you have ready to give the emergency dispatcher who answers?

_____

_____

_____

_____

SCENARIO 2

As you are leaving work, you encounter a man in the parking lot who has cut himself badly on a piece of broken glass. You are not sure if you are still considered to be at work, and you are concerned that if you give him first aid, he may later sue you if he has any complications from the injury. What 5 things can you do to protect yourself and prevent future legal problems?

_____

_____

_____

_____

SCENARIO 3

On a very hot day, you see a woman who has been working outdoors suddenly fall to her knees. You rush to her, determine that she is responsive and ask what's wrong. Before she answers, she collapses and seems to have passed out. You did not have a chance to ask for her consent to help. What should you do?

_____

_____

_____

_____

ADDITIONAL ACTIVITIES AND RESOURCES

As of this writing, Internet-based telephones (VoIP) were required to access 9-1-1, although some companies still had technical issues. For a special project, research the current status of VoIP telephones in your state and consider other issues related to power outages and cell phone signal strength.

Research trends in injuries based on statistics for different types of injuries. Much information is available on the Internet, including from these sites:

• Bureau of Labor Statistics, United States Department of Labor: **bls.gov/iif/**

• National Center for Health Statistics: **cdc.gov/ nchs/fastats/injury.htm**

• You may also research analyses that attempt to explain the trends you observe in the statistics.

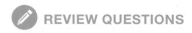

REVIEW QUESTIONS

Select the best answers.

1. The goals of first aid include –

   a. keeping the victim alive until he or she receives medical care.

   b. preventing the victim's condition from getting worse.

   c. ensuring the victim receives appropriate medical care.

   d. All of the above

2. If you are in a crowd of people when someone is suddenly injured, it is best to –

   a. wait to see if someone steps forward to help the victim.

   b. be confident and do not hesitate to offer your help.

   c. offer your cell phone to anyone who wants to call for help.

   d. stay nearby and wait to see if the victim asks for help.

3. Most nonfatal injuries occur in –

   a. workplaces.

   b. homes.

   c. public places.

   d. schools.

4. Your primary role in the EMS system is to –

   a. call 9-1-1 in an emergency.

   b. assist the EMS crew in caring for a victim.

   c. diagnose the victim's condition to determine which EMS personnel should come.

   d. advise the dispatcher on how many emergency responders to send.

5. Before calling 9-1-1, you should know –

   a. where you are.

   b. the telephone number you are calling from.

   c. whether the victim is responsive.

   d. All of the above

6. For which conditions should you call 9-1-1?

   a. Not breathing normally or difficulty breathing

   b. Poisoning, drug overdose

   c. Vomiting blood or having seizures

   d. All of the above

7. You are obligated to give first aid when –

   a. any person who is alone needs it.

   b. the victim is seriously injured.

   c. you have already begun voluntarily giving it.

   d. All of the above

8. You usually have automatic consent to give first aid to –

   a. all victims.

   b. all responsive victims.

   c. all unresponsive adults.

   d. all child victims.

9. If a responsive, competent adult refuses your first aid, what should you do?

   a. Give first aid anyway.

   b. Ask the person's spouse for consent to give first aid.

   c. Walk away.

   d. Call 9-1-1 and keep talking to the victim.

10. Standard of care refers to –

    a. what others with your training would do in a similar situation.

    b. the standard duty to act.

    c. having a written authorization to give first aid.

    d. guidelines published by the government.

CHAPTER 2

Acting in an Emergency

LESSON OBJECTIVES

- Explain how bloodborne pathogens may be transmitted from an infected person to someone else.

- List common serious bloodborne diseases.

- Describe standard precautions to take to prevent disease transmission when giving first aid.

- Describe the step-by-step actions to take whenever you recognize an emergency.

- List 8-10 types of dangerous emergency scenes you should not enter.

- List signs of stress that may occur after an emergency, and describe how one can get help if needed.

You are driving home from work when you see a vehicle swerve off the road. It strikes a telephone pole, which breaks off, and a power line falls down on top of the vehicle. You pull to a stop some distance back. You can see the driver inside, and he is not moving. What should you do?

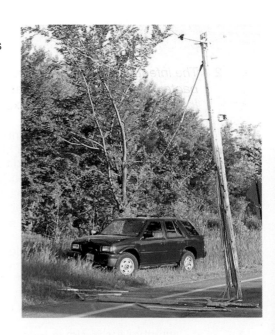

A medical emergency caused by injury or sudden illness can occur at any time in any place. Emergencies vary in many different ways. These may include:

- The nature of the injury or illness

- The severity of the injury or illness

- The presence of other injuries or factors affecting the victim's well-being

- The scene of the emergency (indoors, outdoors, potential hazards present, etc.)

- The victim (child, adult, elderly person, friend, stranger, etc.)

Because of these and other factors, no 2 emergency situations are identical. Yet certain key principles apply to all emergencies. In all emergencies involving injury or illness, you should always follow the same basic steps outlined in this chapter.

Preventing Disease Transmission

In any emergency situation, there is some risk of a first aider contracting an infectious disease from a victim who has a disease. That risk is very low, however, and taking steps to avoid being infected greatly reduces that risk.

HOW ARE INFECTIOUS DISEASES TRANSMITTED?

The transmission of infectious disease occurs through a process involving 4 stages **(Figure 2-1)**:

1. The process begins with *someone or something having the infection.*

2. *The infectious pathogen (disease-causing bacteria, virus, fungus or parasite) leaves the infected person's body.* For example:

   - The person may bleed from a cut, and the pathogen is in that person's blood.

   - The person may sneeze or cough out little droplets carrying the pathogen.

3. *The infectious pathogen reaches another person and enters his or her body.* This can happen in a number of ways:

   1. The person may come into contact with the infected person's blood, other body fluid, or infectious material in a way that allows the pathogen to enter his or her body through mucous membranes or non-intact skin (**bloodborne transmission**).

   2. The person may inhale the pathogen in tiny droplets from the air (**airborne transmission**).

   3. The person may be bitten by an insect, such as a tick or mosquito, carrying the pathogen (**vector transmission** of bloodborne pathogen).

   4. The transmission of a pathogen from one person to another is said to occur through direct or indirect contact:

      - **Direct contact** occurs from contact with an infected person or with fluids or substances from that person.

      - **Indirect contact** occurs from contact with contaminated objects, food or drink, droplets in the air or vectors such as insects.

4. *The second person develops the infection.* Simply having the pathogen enter the body does not automatically mean a person will become ill. If vaccinated against the disease, the body will kill the pathogen before it can cause disease. A person's immune system may be able to kill some pathogens and thereby prevent illness. If it does not, a person may become infected. The process then starts all over again.

FIGURE 2-1

Different modes of disease transmission.

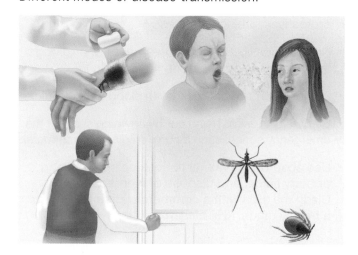

BLOODBORNE DISEASE

Several serious diseases can be transmitted from one person to another through contact with the infected person's blood. These are called **bloodborne diseases**. Bacteria or viruses that cause such diseases, called pathogens, are also present in other body fluids, such as semen, vaginal secretions, and bloody saliva or vomit. Body fluids such as nasal secretions, sweat, tears and urine do not normally transmit pathogens. Three serious bloodborne infections are HIV, hepatitis B and hepatitis C **(Table 2-1)**.

PROTECTION AGAINST BLOODBORNE DISEASE

Because these bloodborne diseases cannot be cured, they should be prevented. The best prevention is to avoid contact with all victims' blood and body fluids. You cannot know whether a victim (even a close friend) is infected, as oftentimes these diseases do not produce signs and symptoms. Even victims may not know that they are infected.

The Centers for Disease Control and Prevention (CDC) recommends taking **standard precautions** whenever you give first aid. The term **universal precautions** is also used to describe measures to prevent infection **(Box 2-1)**. Take these precautions for all victims, all the time, and always assume that blood and other body fluids may be infected. Follow these recommendations to avoid coming into contact with a victim's blood or body fluids:

- Use personal protective equipment.

- If you do not have medical exam gloves with you, put your hands in plastic bags or have the victim dress his or her own wound.

- Wash your hands with soap and water before and after giving first aid.

- Keep a barrier (such as gloves or a dry cloth) between body fluids and yourself.

- Cover any cuts or scrapes on your skin with protective clothing or gloves.

- Do not touch your mouth, nose or eyes when giving first aid (e.g., do not eat, drink or smoke).

- Do not touch objects soiled with blood or body fluids.

- Be careful to avoid being cut by anything sharp at the emergency scene, such as broken glass or torn metal.

- Use absorbent material to soak up spilled blood or body fluids, and dispose of it appropriately. Clean the area with a commercial **disinfectant** or a freshly made 10% bleach solution.

- If you are exposed to a victim's blood or body fluid, wash immediately with soap and water and call your health care provider. At work, report the situation to your supervisor.

Hand Washing

Effective hand washing is essential for preventing disease transmission. Follow these guidelines (see Skill "Hand Washing"):

- Wash any exposed skin with soap and water as soon as possible after an exposure.

- While washing, be gentle with any scabs or sores.

- Wash all surfaces, including the backs of hands and wrists, between the fingers, and under fingernails.

- Wash hands immediately after removing gloves or other personal protective equipment.

- Before handling any potentially infectious materials, know where the nearest hand-washing facility is. You can use facilities such as restrooms, janitor closets and laboratory sinks, as long as soap is available.

- Do not use sinks in areas where food is prepared.

- Merely wetting the hands will not prevent infection.

- If antiseptic towelettes or antibacterial hand-washing liquid is used without water for the initial cleaning after an exposure, a thorough scrubbing with soap and water is still needed as soon as possible **(Figure 2-2)**.

FIGURE 2-2

Waterless antibacterial hand-washing liquid.

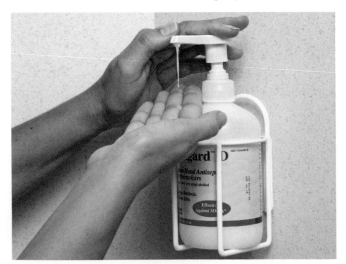

BOX 2-1: INFECTION CONTROL TERMINOLOGY

Because of changes in infection control terminology over the last 2 decades, there has been some confusion about the exact meanings and applications of the terms "universal precautions," "standard precautions" and "body substance isolation."

Universal precautions is the term the Centers for Disease Control and Prevention (CDC) originally promoted in 1987 for actions to protect providers of first aid and health care from exposure to bloodborne pathogens. Universal precautions apply to all people's blood, semen, vaginal secretions and other body fluids containing visible blood, or to any objects potentially contaminated with any of these. In its 1991 Bloodborne Pathogens Standard, the Occupational Safety and Health Administration (OSHA) required the use of universal precautions, which it defined as an approach to infection control.* According to the concept of Universal Precautions, all human blood and certain human body fluids are treated as if known to be infectious for HIV, HBV and other bloodborne pathogens. Many health care and first aid providers continue to use the term universal precautions, in part because this is the term used in federal and many state laws.

At the same time, many health care institutions were following principles of **body substance isolation**

(BSI), an infection control concept that originated in efforts to control all infections (not just bloodborne pathogens) that occur within health care facilities. BSI precautions assume that any body fluid or moist body tissue is potentially infectious.

In 1996, the CDC published new guidelines called **standard precautions** intended primarily for infectious disease control within health care facilities. Standard precautions combine the major features of universal precautions and BSI precautions. Although some providers believe that standard precautions have replaced universal precautions, the CDC states: "Standard precautions were developed for use in hospitals and may not necessarily be indicated in other settings where universal precautions are used, such as child care settings and schools." (Source: cdc.gov/HAI/settings/outpatient/basic-infection-control-prevention-plan-2011/fundamental-of-infection-prevention.html)

Because standard precautions are more rigorous than universal precautions, this text will use the term "standard precautions." Recognize, however, that in many first aid situations, universal precautions are appropriate.

*View the OSHA Bloodborne Pathogens Standard (1910.1030) at osha.gov/pls/oshaweb/owadisp.show_document?p_table=STANDARDS&p_id=10051.

STEP 1

Remove any jewelry and your watch. Use a paper towel to turn on water, and adjust the temperature to warm.

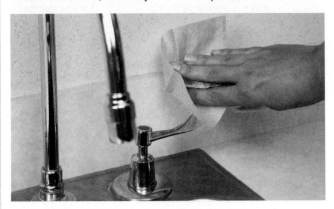

STEP 2

Wet your hands to above the wrists and lather up with soap. Keep your hands below your elbows throughout the hand-washing process.

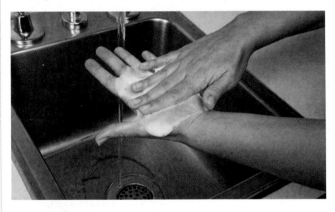

STEP 3

Wash all areas of your hands and wrists. Interlace fingers to scrub between them. If your hands were exposed to infectious material, scrub beneath fingernails with a nail brush or nail stick.

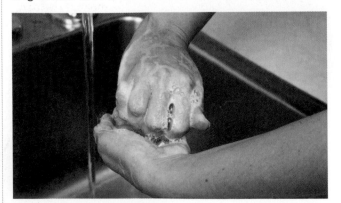

STEP 4

Rinse wrists and hands well. (Repeat soaping and washing if your hands were exposed to infectious material.)

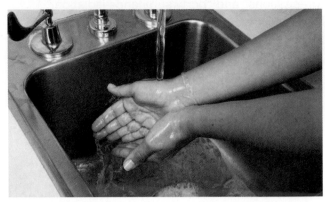

STEP 5

Dry hands thoroughly with paper towel, and dispose of it properly. Use a new, dry paper towel to turn off the water faucet and open the door, and dispose of it properly.

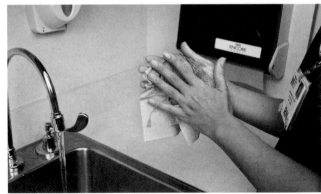

TABLE 2-1

Bloodborne Disease

Disease	Prevalence	Modes of Transmission	Signs and Symptoms	Testing	Prevention
Acquired immunodeficiency syndrome (AIDS). Caused by human immunodeficiency virus (HIV). Eventually fatal.	About 1.2 million HIV-positive people in the United States, 12.8% of whom are unaware of their infection.	Through infected person's body fluids, including: - Blood - Semen - Vaginal secretions - Breast milk - Other body fluids if blood is present HIV is not transmitted by casual contact.	HIV often has no symptoms. AIDS symptoms may include: - Loss of appetite - Weight loss - Fever - Skin rashes - Swollen lymph nodes - Diarrhea - Fatigue - Night sweats - Inability to fight off infections	Blood test recommended after a potential exposure. Generally positive 2-8 weeks after exposure. Confirmation test recommended 3-6 months after an exposure.	No vaccine currently available. Antiretroviral treatment may be begun immediately following a known exposure. Safe first aid practices significantly reduce the risk of contracting HIV or other infectious diseases. - Regular hand-washing - Use of barriers - Standard precautions
Hepatitis B (serum hepatitis). Caused by the hepatitis B virus (HBV). Major cause of liver damage, cirrhosis and liver cancer.	Over 30,000 new infections yearly. Between 700,000 and 1.4 million chronic carriers. Almost 2,000 people die of liver problems associated with HBV infection every year.	Transmitted by blood and materials contaminated with blood or body fluids. Blood and semen are the most infectious. - By injection (needlestick or puncture wound) Through mucous membranes (blood contamination through eye or mouth) and non-intact skin - Through sexual activity - From infected mother to newborn at birth The virus may survive for several days in dried body fluids on surfaces.	Often no symptoms. Symptoms usually appear gradually: - Loss of appetite - Nausea - Fatigue - Muscle or joint aches - Mild fever - Stomach pain - Occasional jaundice (yellow tint to whites of eyes or skin)	Blood test.	Use same precautions as with HIV. Vaccine is available and recommended for health care workers and professional rescuers. Employees at risk must be offered free vaccinations by employer. Vaccine also recommended for: - Those having unprotected sex with a partner with HBV or with multiple partners - Those having anal sex - Those using intravenous drugs - Those with hemophilia - Those who frequently work in countries where HBV is common - Those who live with someone with chronic HBV

2 · Acting in an Emergency

TABLE 2-1

Bloodborne Disease (continued)

Disease	Prevalence	Modes of Transmission	Signs and Symptoms	Testing	Prevention
Hepatitis C. Caused by the hepatitis C virus (HCV). Causes liver disease; may result in eventual liver failure.	Almost 30,000 new infections annually. 2.7 to 3.9 million people in the United States have chronic HCV infection. Over 19,000 people die of liver problems associated with HCV infection every year.	Spread most often through drug injections with contaminated needles. May result from unclean tattoo or body piercing tools, or from any item contaminated with blood. Spread through any direct contact with infectious blood.	Usually no symptoms. Occasionally one or more of the following symptoms: - Fatigue - Loss of appetite - Nausea - Anxiety - Weight loss - Alcohol intolerance - Abdominal pain - Loss of concentration - Jaundice	Blood test. Anyone testing positive should have follow-up test. Testing recommended for: - Health care workers exposed to HCV-positive blood - Anyone who has used intravenous recreational drugs - Anyone receiving a blood transfusion, organ transplant or kidney dialysis before 1992 - Anyone treated with a blood product prior to 1987 - Anyone with signs of liver disease	No vaccine available. Use same precautions as with HIV: - Follow barrier practices to prevent contact with blood. - Avoid recreational intravenous drug use. - Do not share toothbrushes, razors or other items that may be contaminated with blood. - Remember health risks associated with tattoos and body piercings if sanitary practices are not followed.

Source: Centers for Disease Control and Prevention, cdc.gov./DiseasesConditions/ and cdc.gov/hepatitis/statistics/index.htm Accessed January 2016.

PERSONAL PROTECTIVE EQUIPMENT

Personal protective equipment (PPE) is any equipment used to protect yourself from contact with blood or other body fluids. PPE includes gloves, barrier devices and other devices.

Gloves

Most important, keep **medical exam gloves** in your first aid kit and wear them in most first aid situations **(Figure 2-3)**. Gloves are a type of barrier; like other barriers, they separate you from potentially infectious materials (see Skill: "Putting on Gloves" and Skill: "Removing Contaminated Gloves"). Medical exam gloves suitable for protection from bloodborne pathogens are made of nitrile, vinyl, **latex** or other waterproof materials **(Box 2-2)**. For added barrier protection, 2 pairs of gloves may be worn together in some situations.

FIGURE 2-3

Wear gloves to protect yourself from contact with blood or other body fluids.

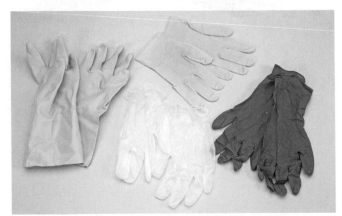

When using gloves, it is important to remember the following:

- **Check that your gloves are intact.** Check before you put them on and periodically afterward. If a hole or tear is present, replace the glove immediately with a new one.

- **Do not use petroleum-based hand lotions.** These lotions may cause latex gloves to disintegrate.

- **Remove contaminated gloves carefully.** Do not touch any part of the contaminated exterior of the gloves.

- **Dispose of gloves properly.** After working with any material that may be infected by bloodborne pathogens, dispose of your gloves in a container clearly marked for biohazardous waste.

- **Handle sharp objects carefully.** Gloves protect against infectious substances but not against sharp objects, such as needles, that may also transmit infection.

⚙ SKILL: PUTTING ON GLOVES

STEP 1
Pull glove onto one hand.

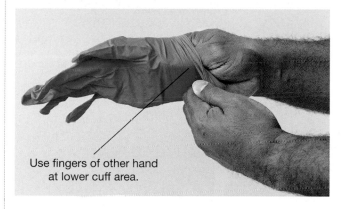

Use fingers of other hand at lower cuff area.

STEP 2
Pull glove tight.

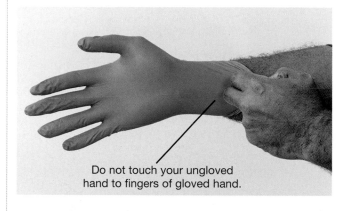

Do not touch your ungloved hand to fingers of gloved hand.

STEP 3
Put on other glove.

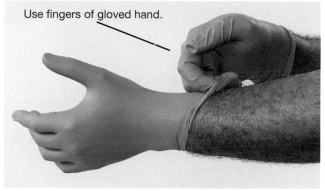

Use fingers of gloved hand.

STEP 1

Hold your hands away from your body, with fingers pointing down.

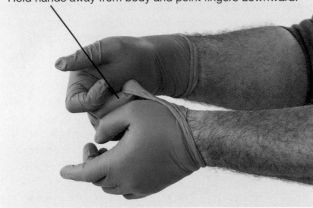

Hold hands away from body and point fingers downward.

STEP 2

With one hand, grasp your other glove at the wrist or palm, and pull it away from your hand. Then, pull the glove the rest of the way off.

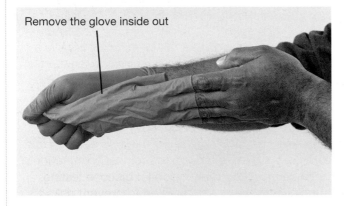

Remove the glove inside out

STEP 3

Holding the removed glove balled up in the palm of your gloved hand, insert 2 fingers under the cuff of the remaining glove.

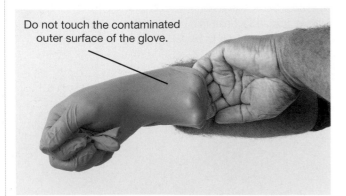

Do not touch the contaminated outer surface of the glove.

STEP 4

Remove the glove by stretching it up and away from the hand and turning it inside out as you pull it off.

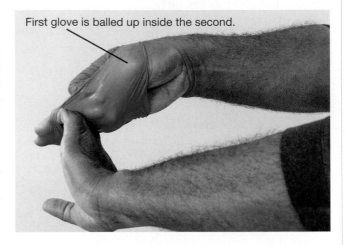

First glove is balled up inside the second.

STEP 5

Dispose of gloves safely (in a biohazard container if possible) and wash your hands.

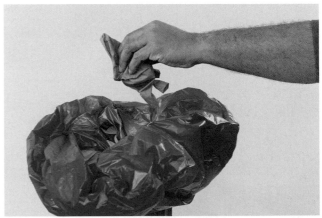

BOX 2-2: LATEX GLOVE ALLERGY

Medical exam gloves are often made of latex rubber, to which some people are allergic. Signs and symptoms of latex allergy may include skin rashes, hives, itching eyes or skin, flushing, watery or swollen eyes, runny nose or an asthmatic reaction. Use gloves made of vinyl or other material if you have any of these symptoms, or if you work with patients who may have a latex allergy.

BARRIER DEVICES

A **barrier device** is a pocket face mask or face shield used when giving rescue breaths during CPR. This device should be in the first aid kit, and you should always use it for added protection. Because giving rescue breaths with a barrier device can greatly reduce the chance of an infectious disease being transmitted from or to a victim, the use of a barrier device is always recommended **(Figure 2-4)**. **Chapter 5** discusses uses of airway barrier devices more fully.

FIGURE 2-4

A variety of barrier devices.

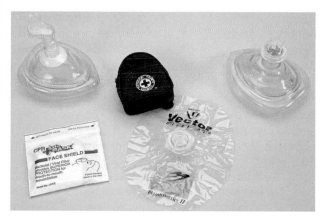

OTHER PPE

Other PPE devices include eye protection, masks, and gowns or aprons. These are not required in most first aid situations, although OSHA requires such protections to be available in some workplaces. In such cases, OSHA requires employees to be trained in the use of this PPE. Health care workers, for example, are required to wear masks and protective eyewear or face shields during procedures that are likely to generate droplets of blood or body fluids, and gowns or aprons when blood or body fluid may be splashed.

DISPOSAL AND DISINFECTION OF SUPPLIES AND EQUIPMENT

Preventing disease transmission also involves correct disposal or disinfection of used first aid supplies and equipment after caring for a victim. First aid kits include many disposable supplies, such as dressings and bandages, that may become soiled by a victim's blood or other body fluids. These must be appropriately disposed of because such items may remain infectious for some time after use. Never reuse any equipment or supplies that are meant to be disposable. Other equipment, such as tweezers used to remove debris from a wound, require disinfection after use.

If EMS personnel arrive to care for a victim of an emergency, they will usually manage the disposal of any soiled or infectious materials resulting from first aid care you have given. When professional rescuers are not involved, however, you need to ensure that soiled materials do not come into contact with other people. Many workplaces have a system in place for disposing of hazardous wastes; follow your company's policy. In the home, soiled supplies should be sealed inside a heavy plastic bag that is then sealed inside a second bag before being put in the trash. Make sure others do not come into contact with this trash. For contaminated sharps, such as needles used for insulin injections or lancets used to draw blood for glucose testing, special containers are required to prevent risks to those handling the trash. Talk with your health care provider about how to properly dispose of these objects.

To disinfect equipment or surfaces that are soiled by blood or other body fluids, use a commercial body fluid disposal kit, or a 10% solution of household bleach in water. Wear gloves and clean the items or area thoroughly. If clothing or other fabrics are soiled, wash them by themselves in hot, soapy water for at least 25 minutes. Be sure to take a shower and wash well, because your skin may have been contaminated through the clothing.

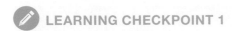

Circle **True** or **False** for each of the following statements:

1. Bloodborne diseases are transmitted only through contact with an infected person's blood.   True   False

2. The risk of contracting a serious infectious disease by giving first aid is greatly reduced when you take precautions.   True   False

3. Select the best answer. Standard precautions include:

   a. Treat all victims as if their body fluids are infected.

   b. Always wear gloves if blood may be present.

   c. Do not touch your mouth, nose or eyes when giving first aid.

   d. All of the above

4. Check off which of the following situations could lead to your getting an infectious disease.

   ☐ Touching a bloody bandage in a trash can

   ☐ Shaking hands with a person infected with HIV

   ☐ Receiving a hepatitis B vaccination

   ☐ Not wearing gloves and giving first aid if you have a cut on your finger

   ☐ Being near a person with hepatitis C who is coughing

   ☐ Contact with an unresponsive victim's urine

5. List at least 3 symptoms of a latex glove allergy.

   _____

   _____

   _____

Responding to Emergencies

There are 6 basic actions to take in any emergency:

1. Recognize the emergency.

2. Check the scene.

3. Check the victim.

4. Call 9-1-1 (when appropriate).

5. Give first aid.

6. Have the victim seek medical attention (when appropriate).

RECOGNIZE THE EMERGENCY

You usually recognize an emergency when you see one. You see an injured or ill victim, or someone acting strangely. You may hear sounds of an emergency and realize that someone may be hurt. For example, you might look in the door of a coworker's office and see a coffee cup overturned on the desk and the telephone receiver off the hook – and then see the man collapsed on the other side of the desk. You may see a crushed bicycle unattended alongside the road – and after checking further, see a child lying in the ditch. In situations like this one, the victim's life may depend on someone recognizing the signs that something is wrong and taking the time to investigate.

CHECK THE SCENE

Once you realize there is an emergency and someone is injured or ill, before going to the victim, look to see if there may be other victims. You may need to call immediately for help for multiple victims. Look for any clues that may help you to determine what happened and what first aid may be needed. Also, look for bystanders who may be able to help give first aid or to go call 9-1-1.

When we see that someone needs our help, our first tendency is often to rush in. In many emergency situations, however, hazards may be present at the scene. For example, if you saw smoke coming out of a window of a house where you know an elderly man lives, your first thought might be to rush inside to rescue him. Consider, however, that you also might be overcome by smoke. Not only would you not have helped the original victim, but you would have become a second victim yourself for others to rescue and care for.

Therefore it is important, when you recognize that an emergency has occurred, to always check the scene before approaching a victim. Remember that you must be safe yourself if you are to help another. Look for any hazards, such as the following:

• Smoke or flames

• Spilled gasoline or chemicals, fumes

• Downed electrical wires

• Risk of explosion or building collapse

• Roadside dangers or high-speed traffic

• Deep water or ice

• Potential for violence from someone present at the scene

If the scene is dangerous and you cannot safely approach the victim, *stay away and call for help*. Remember that help is usually only minutes away. The 9-1-1 dispatcher will send a crew with the appropriate training and equipment to safely reach and care for the victim. You may be able to monitor the scene from a safe distance and provide responding EMS personnel with critical information, such as the location of the victim. **Box 2-3** describes some specific examples of hazardous situations.

Scene safety also includes protecting yourself from exposure to potentially infectious body fluids or other materials. As you approach a victim, for example, consider the need for using PPE as discussed earlier in this chapter.

CHECK THE VICTIM

When you reach the victim, first check for life-threatening conditions requiring immediate first aid. These include being unresponsive, not breathing normally or severe bleeding. If the victim does not have a life-threatening condition, you then go on to look for lesser conditions requiring first aid. **Chapter 4** describes in detail both of these assessments. Unless the scene is dangerous or it is necessary to care for a life-threatening problem, do not move the victim. **Chapter 24** describes how to move a victim when necessary.

CALL 9-1-1

Call 9-1-1 (or your local or company emergency number) immediately if you recognize a life-threatening injury or illness. Do not try to transport a victim to the emergency department yourself in such cases. In some exceptional circumstances, you may give about 2 minutes of care before calling 9-1-1.

If the victim is responsive and may not be seriously injured or ill, go on to the next step to check the victim further before calling 9-1-1 – and then call 9-1-1 or a health care provider if needed.

GIVE FIRST AID

Give first aid once you have checked the victim and know his or her condition. Later chapters describe the first aid for the conditions you are likely to find. **Basic life support (BLS)** is first aid given to a victim with a life-threatening problem involving breathing or circulation. Generally, you provide basic life support to keep the victim alive until advanced help arrives. In most cases, however, the victim's condition is not life threatening, and your first aid consists of simple actions you can take to help the victim.

Note that first aiders do not administer medications to victims because of the risks of allergy or other complications. In some cases, first aiders may help victims to take their own medications if needed.

BOX 2-3: HAZARDOUS SCENES

TRAFFIC COLLISIONS

Vehicle crash scenes can be extremely dangerous for rescuers because of the risks from passing vehicles, downed electrical wires, fire or explosion, vehicle instability or other conditions. Rescuers have also been injured by unintentionally setting off an automatic airbag when attempting to reach a victim pinned inside a vehicle. For all of these reasons, it is crucial to ensure that the scene is safe before approaching the vehicle. Do not try to stabilize the vehicle unless you have special training. Never try to remove a victim trapped inside a vehicle, but wait for professional rescuers. You may be able to provide some first aid through an open window or from the back seat.

FIRE SCENES

Never enter a burning or smoky building unless you have special training and are functioning as part of a fire department. Firefighters are highly trained and use special equipment that protects against fire and smoke. Do not let others enter or approach a fire scene. Make sure 9-1-1 has been called, and then try to gather information for responding fire and EMS units, such as the possible number and location of victims, the cause of the fire, the presence of any explosives or chemicals, and other relevant facts.

ELECTRICITY HAZARDS

Downed electrical lines at an emergency scene are a major hazard to both the victim and rescuers. Never try to move downed wires; instead, call 9-1-1 immediately. If downed wires are across a vehicle, do not touch the vehicle. If victims are in the vehicle, tell them to remain still and not exit

BOX 2-3: HAZARDOUS SCENES (CONTINUED)

the vehicle. Never attempt to remove a victim from a vehicle with a downed wire across it, no matter how seriously injured the victim may be. If downed wires are across a chain link fence, metal structure or body of water, do not approach the scene.

WATER AND ICE HAZARDS

Water and ice create several hazards. Never enter deep water to reach a victim unless you have been properly trained, and then do so only as a last resort. Instead, try to get a flotation device or rope to the victim (see **Chapter 24**). Fast-flowing water is a common hazard following natural disasters such as floods and hurricanes. Never enter moving water; instead, wait for trained rescue personnel. A fast-water rescue requires careful planning, proper equipment and training. Ice is also treacherous. Cold-water immersion is very serious and can quickly doom even the best swimmers. Ice rescue should be left for specially trained personnel who have the necessary safety equipment.

NATURAL DISASTERS

Natural disasters include such events as tornadoes, hurricanes, earthquakes, forest and range fires, and floods. Rescue efforts after a natural disaster are usually coordinated through a federal or state emergency management agency. If you find yourself in a natural disaster, make personal safety your highest priority. Natural disasters often involve more hazards than you might think, including electrical risks, hazardous materials and fast-moving water (see **Appendices C, D, E and F**).

HAZARDOUS MATERIALS

A hazardous material is any substance, liquid or solid, that is highly flammable, explosive, caustic, toxic, radioactive or otherwise dangerous. Hazardous materials are usually marked with warning placards **(Figure 2-5)**, but treat any unknown substance as a hazard until proven otherwise. Avoid any spilled liquid or powder as well as possible fumes. Especially dangerous is a vehicular collision involving a truck carrying hazardous materials. Stay well out of the area of a hazardous material spill and keep bystanders away. Call 9-1-1 and let trained HAZMAT professionals handle the emergency.

FiGURE 2-5

A variety of hazardous materials placards.

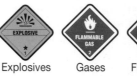

Explosives Gases Flammable liquids Flammable solids Oxidizers/ organic peroxides

Toxic materials Radioactive materials Corrosive materials Dangerous goods

Hazardous materials are not limited to industrial sites and transportation. There are many potential hazards in the home, including natural gas, gasoline, kerosene, pesticides and others. Many hazardous materials are odorless and not easily detected. Some hazardous materials, such as natural gas, are explosion hazards. A seemingly harmless action such as turning on a light switch or using a cell phone may create a spark and set off an explosion.

UNSAFE BUILDINGS/STRUCTURES

Buildings and other structures may be unsafe because of fire, an explosion, a natural disaster or deterioration. Never enter an unsafe building alone because of the risk of collapsing structures, hazardous materials, fire, and so on. Call 9-1-1 and let properly trained and equipped professionals manage the rescue.

WRECKAGE

Wreckage from an automobile, aircraft or machinery is hazardous because of the presence of sharp pieces of metal, glass, fuel and moving parts. The wreckage may also be unstable. Stay away from the scene and call 9-1-1.

SUICIDE

If a person is threatening suicide and has a weapon, do not enter the scene; call 9-1-1 or law enforcement personnel. **Chapter 21** discusses behavioral emergencies such as suicidal or potentially violent victims.

BOX 2-3: HAZARDOUS SCENES (CONTINUED)

HOSTILE VICTIM/FAMILY

Occasionally, a victim or family member may be hostile when you approach or offer first aid. Rage or hostility in a victim may be due to the injury or illness, or to emotional factors. Many emergency victims are afraid of losing control, and their fear may become anger. Drug or alcohol abuse may also cause hostile behavior. If a victim seems hostile, first try to quietly explain who you are and that you are there to help. Oftentimes, after the victim realizes that you are not a threat but are there to help, the hostility will dissipate. But if the victim refuses your care or threatens you, retreat from the scene and call 9-1-1. Never try to restrain, argue with or force care upon a victim. **Chapter 21** discusses how to deal with behavioral emergencies such as violent people.

Hostile family members can also be a problem, usually because they are fearful. Listen to what they have to say and act accordingly. If the situation remains hostile, retreat to a safe distance and wait for police officers and other EMS personnel. If at any time your personal safety appears threatened, leave the scene immediately.

HAVE THE VICTIM SEEK MEDICAL ATTENTION

As noted earlier, call 9-1-1 immediately for any emergency (life-threatening) condition. In many cases, the injury or sudden illness is not an emergency and you do not need to call 9-1-1, but the victim still needs to see a health care provider. For example, a victim may have a serious cut on the arm that stops bleeding quickly when you give first aid. Because of the risk of infection, or because the cut may need stitches to heal well, the victim needs medical attention and should be transported to a hospital emergency department or his or her health care provider. Later chapters about specific injuries and problems describe when a victim needs to go to the emergency department or see a health care provider. When in doubt, call a health care provider to see if medical care may be needed.

After an Emergency

Arriving EMS professionals will take over the care of the victim **(Figure 2-6)**. Continue giving first aid until EMS personnel ask you to stop, as it may take a few minutes for emergency responders to prepare equipment and take over. Then, you may still assist with crowd control, obtaining information from bystanders or assisting the emergency responders in other ways. Depending on the situation, you may have other follow-up activities. If the emergency was traumatic or especially stressful, you may also need help coping with the effects of stress.

After giving first aid, be sure to wash your hands and clean the area well. If the emergency involved bleeding or contamination of the area with other body fluids, disinfect surfaces using a 10% bleach solution or other approved disinfectant. Dispose of all potentially contaminated materials appropriately. If you were in contact with any of the victim's body fluids, report this to the emergency responders so they can take appropriate action.

FIGURE 2-6

EMS personnel with advanced training will take over care of an injured or ill victim after 9-1-1 is called.

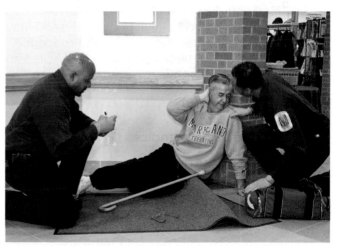

FOLLOW-UP ACTIVITIES

Arriving EMS professionals who take over the care of the victim will ask you questions about what happened, what you observed about the victim, and what first aid you gave. Answer as fully as you can, because the details you provide may be important for the victim's medical care. Review the entire experience in your mind to make sure you have not forgotten to relay some important piece of information. For example, a victim who became unresponsive while you were giving him first aid may have experienced a poisoning, and anything the victim said or did when you first saw him may offer medical workers a clue about his condition.

Your descriptions to EMS personnel of what happened and what you did may be, in some situations, a form of legal documentation of actions. If you have any reason to think you may be questioned in the future about your actions, it may be helpful to write down what happened and exactly what you did.

Some emergencies may be related to a crime, such as injuries resulting from an assault or abuse. In such cases, the first responders to the scene should help ensure that possible evidence is not destroyed or altered. When law enforcement officials arrive they will preserve and investigate the scene. If you gave first aid to the victim of a crime, your descriptions of what you witnessed may become legal evidence. It is important to cooperate fully with police officers and, again, be as detailed as possible in recounting your observations.

COPING WITH A TRAUMATIC EVENT

Emergencies are stressful, especially when the victim does not survive. Not even medical professionals can save every victim. Injuries, illness or circumstances are often beyond our control. Particularly stressful emergencies include those that involve multiple victims, children, victims of abuse or neglect, and death or injury of a coworker or friend.

It is normal to have a strong emotional reaction during and immediately after a stressful emergency. Oftentimes this reaction diminishes with time, but in some cases, the stress remains and problems may result. Stress can cause irritability when interacting with others, difficulty sleeping, problems concentrating, general anxiety or depression, and even physical symptoms. If you recognize that you are feeling or behaving differently after experiencing a traumatic emergency, you may need help coping.

- Talk to others: family members, coworkers, local emergency responders or your own health care provider (without breaching the confidentiality of the victim).

- Remind yourself that your reaction is normal, and that we all need help sometimes.

- Do not be afraid or reluctant to seek professional help. Students should ask at the student health center, and workers should check with their human resources department about an employee assistance program or member assistance program. Your health care provider can also make a referral.

 LEARNING CHECKPOINT 2

Circle **True** or **False** for the following statement:

1. If you see someone injured in an emergency, the first thing to do is get to him or her quickly and check his or her condition.   True   False

2. Select the best answer. When you encounter an injured victim, you should –

   a. give first aid until help arrives

   b. help a victim only if the scene is safe

   c. call 9-1-1 for life-threatening injuries

   d. all of the above

3. Which of the following scenes are unsafe?

   ☐ Spilled hazardous materials

   ☐ Structure fires

   ☐ Downed electrical wires

   ☐ Hostile person with a weapon

CONCLUDING THOUGHTS

Emergency situations vary widely, but in all cases, you respond to the emergency in the same basic way: Make sure the scene is safe, check the victim for life-threatening conditions and call 9-1-1, and give the appropriate first aid using standard precautions to minimize your exposure to infectious disease. These principles for acting in an emergency not only guide your response, but also ensure your safety while you give the most effective care to someone in need.

ACTING IN AN EMERGENCY

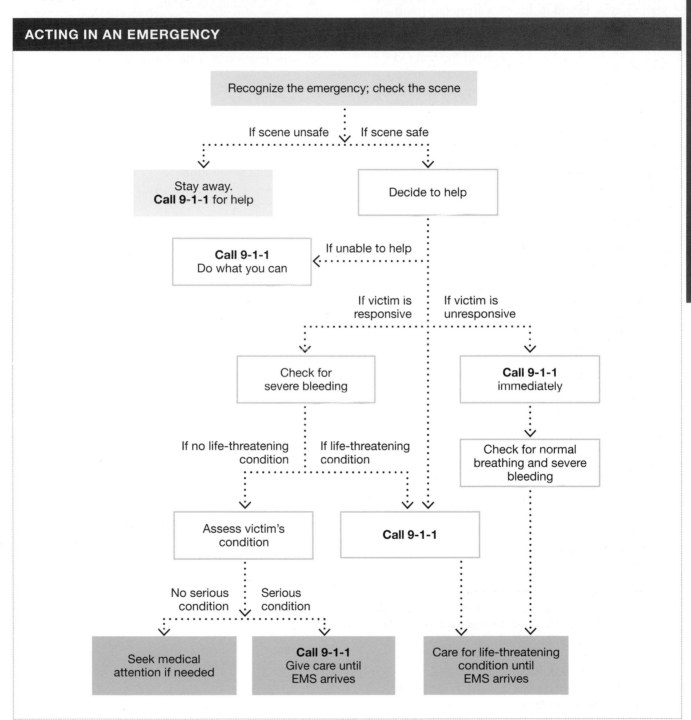

CRITICAL THINKING CHALLENGE QUESTIONS

 REVIEW QUESTIONS

SCENARIO 1

While you are at a meeting at work, another employee cuts herself on a shard from a broken water glass. Blood is spurting from her hand. You're not sure where the nearest first aid kit is and you know it is important to stop the bleeding as quickly as possible. But without the first aid kit, you have no gloves to wear to help stop her bleeding. What are 2 possible ways to handle this situation without risking contact with her blood?

_____

_____

 ADDITIONAL ACTIVITIES AND RESOURCES

1. If you are in a field of study leading to a health care career, you may benefit from a fuller understanding of the OSHA Bloodborne Pathogens Standard. You can research specific topics at OSHA's website: **osha.gov**. For example, you may want to learn more about these specific topics:

    • Hepatitis B vaccine

    • Workplace "engineering controls" to prevent exposure

    • Recommendations for "work practice controls"

    • Additional types of personal protective equipment

    • Required exposure control plans

2. The Centers for Disease Control and Prevention (CDC) website **(cdc.gov)** has a wealth of information about current trends in infectious disease. There, you may research any infectious disease of current interest.

Select the best answers.

1. A bloodborne pathogen can easily enter your body through –

    a. any break in your skin.

    b. food cooked by someone else.

    c. the municipal water supply.

    d. any physical touching of the victim's skin.

2. Bloodborne pathogens may also be transmitted in –

    a. semen.

    b. vaginal secretions.

    c. bloody vomit.

    d. All of the above

3. HIV infection can be prevented when giving first aid by –

    a. avoiding all contact with known HIV-positive individuals.

    b. following standard precautions.

    c. getting vaccinated.

    d. wearing a face mask.

4. An effective way to avoid becoming infected when giving first aid is to –

    a. ask the victim what diseases he or she may have before giving first aid.

    b. check an unresponsive victim for a medical alert bracelet or necklace.

    c. use barriers to prevent contact with any blood or body fluid.

    d. never touch the victim.

5. Standard precautions include –

    a. wearing a face mask at all times.

    b. using personal protective equipment.

    c. asking a victim about any communicable diseases before giving first aid.

    d. checking a victim's medical record after giving first aid.

6. If you believe someone may be inside a house where you see smoke coming from a window, you should –

    a. enter only the first floor if you see smoke from an upstairs window.

    b. take a deep breath and hold it while you run inside to look; try not to breathe once inside.

    c. search the house, staying low to the floor on hands and knees.

    d. not go inside but call 9-1-1 immediately.

7. You witness a low-speed car crash into a telephone pole. The driver has no obvious wounds and says he is okay. But he has not moved from behind the wheel, and he looks pale and shaky. What should you do?

    a. Call 9-1-1 and let the dispatcher decide what help may be needed.

    b. Call 9-1-1 only if the driver first gives his consent for you to call.

    c. Ask the driver to get into your vehicle so you can drive him to the nearest hospital.

    d. Wait for a police car to stop; the officer will decide whether help is needed.

8. When you have given first aid to a victim, you should tell arriving EMS personnel –

    a. what happened

    b. what you observed about the victim

    c. what first aid you gave

    d. All of the above

CHAPTER 3
The Human Body

LESSON OBJECTIVES

- Describe the primary areas of the body.

- List the 10 body systems and explain a key function of each.

- For each body system, describe at least 1 injury or illness that affects the functioning of that system.

You are called to the storage area at the back of the warehouse where an employee has just been found lying on the floor. As you approach, you believe she may have fallen from the stepladder or a higher shelf, but you do not immediately see what is wrong.

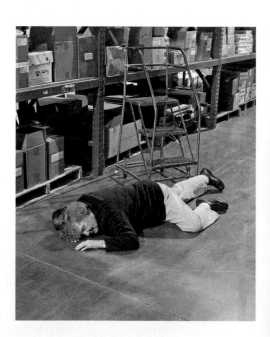

The human body is composed of many different organs and tissues, all working together to sustain life and allow for activity. In health, each organ performs its functions in concert with other body parts and organs. With injury or illness, however, one or more parts of the body are damaged or functioning less effectively. A minor injury may damage only a specific body part or function, but a serious injury or sudden illness can threaten body functions that are necessary for life. Understanding the human body will help you recognize the effects of injuries and illnesses and give effective first aid until the victim receives medical attention.

Primary Areas of the Body

A detailed understanding of medical language is not necessary for giving first aid and communicating with medical professionals or when speaking with the 9-1-1 dispatcher. It is helpful, however, to understand the general areas of the body when describing an injury or the victim's signs and symptoms of illness. Following are key terms referring to major body areas **(Figure 3-1):**

- *Extremities.* This refers to both the arms and the legs. Many first aid principles are the same for all the extremities, so this term is often used rather than saying "arms and legs."

- *Thorax.* This refers to the chest area enclosed by the ribs (including the back of the body). The thoracic cavity is the area inside the chest where the heart and lungs are located.

- *Abdomen.* This refers to the area immediately below the thoracic cavity. The stomach, intestines and other organs are located in the abdominal cavity. For the purposes of describing the location of injuries or signs and symptoms, the abdomen is often divided into quadrants based on the body's midline and an imaginary horizontal line through the umbilicus (navel) **(Figure 3-2)**. The **diaphragm,** the primary muscle used in breathing, is located between the thoracic cavity and the abdominal cavity.

- *Pelvis.* This refers generally to the area below the abdomen and specifically to the pelvic bones between the hip and the lower spine. The bladder and reproductive organs are located in the pelvic cavity.

FIGURE 3-1

Major areas of the body.

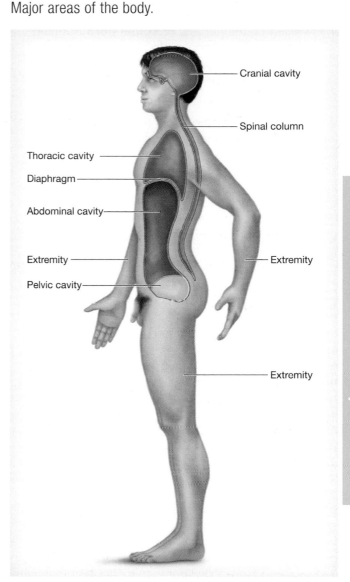

FIGURE 3-2

Abdominal quadrants.

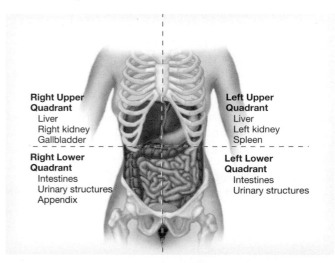

Right Upper Quadrant
Liver
Right kidney
Gallbladder

Left Upper Quadrant
Liver
Left kidney
Spleen

Right Lower Quadrant
Intestines
Urinary structures
Appendix

Left Lower Quadrant
Intestines
Urinary structures

- *Spine (spinal column).* This refers to the bones **(vertebrae)** of the back and neck extending from the base of the brain to the tailbone, as well as to the nerves, or **spinal cord,** running through the vertebrae. *Spine* is generally used in first aid to refer to injuries to these bones or nerves rather than the less specific words *neck* or *back.*

With these terms, you can generally describe the location of injuries and symptoms. Although health care professionals use a variety of directional and spatial terms to pinpoint exact locations in the body, first aiders can successfully communicate locations with general words, such as *above* or *below, left* and *right* and so on. Remember that *left* and *right* refer to the victim's left and right sides – not yours when facing the victim.

Body Systems

Life depends on the body carrying out a number of important functions, such as taking oxygen from the air and transporting it to all body cells, extracting nutrients from food, removing waste and managing the growth and repair of injured cells. An **organ** is a body part that accomplishes one or more specific functions. In most cases, several organs work together to achieve a larger body function. For example, the stomach and intestines accomplish much of the digestive process, but the gallbladder, pancreas and liver also play important roles. The combination of organs that work together to perform a major body function is called a **body system.** Following are brief descriptions of some of the primary functions of the different body systems. Each is described more fully later in this chapter along with its relevance to first aid.

- *Respiratory system.* Provides the oxygen needed by body cells and removes the waste product (carbon dioxide).

- *Cardiovascular system.* Moves the blood, which transports both oxygen and nutrients, throughout the body to supply cells and remove waste.

- *Nervous system.* Controls all body functions and movement and allows for sensory perception and consciousness.

- *Musculoskeletal system.* Gives the body shape and strength and makes movement possible.

- *Integumentary system (skin and related structures).* Protects the body from the environment and germs and helps regulate body temperature.

- *Gastrointestinal system.* Extracts nutrients from food to meet the body's need for energy and eliminates solid waste.

- *Immune system.* Helps fight disease.

- *Endocrine system.* Produces hormones that help regulate many body functions.

- *Urinary system.* Removes liquid wastes from the body and helps maintain the body's water balance.

- *Reproductive system.* Makes human reproduction possible.

Although we sometimes talk about each system as if it were separate from the others, body systems are closely interrelated and work together to perform many functions. For example, blood is part of the cardiovascular system, which pumps it to all areas of the body. Blood carries oxygen from the lungs (respiratory system) to the body cells, all of which need a continuous supply of oxygen to stay alive. Nerve sensors (nervous system) detect the amount of oxygen and carbon dioxide in the blood and speed up or slow down the heartbeat and breathing rate to control the oxygen level. If body temperature drops, muscles of the extremities (musculoskeletal system) may start shivering to produce heat, which is carried by the blood to vital organs. The kidneys (urinary system) filter the blood to remove waste products, which leave the body through the urine. These are just a few examples of the many complex ways body systems work together.

As you learn about different kinds of first aid throughout this text, remember that different parts of the body are often closely related. This will help you understand what is happening in the body during periods of injury and illness so you can provide first aid most effectively. For example, in someone with asthma, inhaling a substance, such as smoke may cause muscles in the airway to spasm and swell, making breathing difficult. As oxygen levels in the blood reaching the brain drop, the person feels dizzy. Changes then occur in the respiratory, cardiovascular and nervous systems. In this case, understanding how a breathing problem can affect a victim's mental status (responsiveness) can help you focus on correcting the cause.

As you will learn in later chapters, life-threatening injuries and illnesses most often affect the respiratory, circulatory and nervous systems. Problems affecting these systems may impair the essential delivery of oxygen to body tissues, leading to death. First aiders, therefore, must first assess a victim for problems related to breathing and circulation and then assess problems related to other body systems.

Respiratory System

The primary organs of the respiratory system are the structures of the airway and the lungs **(Figure 3-3)**. The **airway** is the path air takes from the nose and mouth to the lungs. Air entering the nose or mouth passes through the **pharynx** (throat) to the **trachea** (windpipe). The trachea branches into the left and right **bronchi** (singular: bronchus), the passageways into the lungs. The bronchi branch into smaller tubular passages in the lungs and eventually end in the **alveoli,** the tiny air sacs where oxygen and carbon dioxide pass into and out of small blood vessels called capillaries.

FIGURE 3-3

The respiratory system.

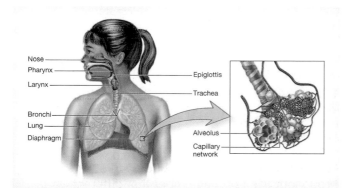

Because the pharynx also leads to the **esophagus,** the tube that carries food to the stomach, another structure, called the epiglottis, is very important for breathing. The **epiglottis** is a tissue flap that prevents solids and liquids from entering the trachea and blocking the airway or reaching the lungs. The epiglottis directs food and drink to pass from the throat to the esophagus and stomach.

Breathing depends on muscular movements that are under the control of the nervous system. When the **diaphragm** (the large muscle below the lungs) contracts, the thoracic cavity and lungs expand, pulling air into the lungs from which oxygen can move into the blood. When the diaphragm relaxes, the size

of the thoracic cavity is reduced, and air carrying out carbon dioxide flows back out of the lungs. **Table 3-1** provides some normal reference values for breathing.

TABLE 3-1	
Normal Reference Values for Breathing Rate	
	Breaths per minute
Adult	12-20
Child	15-30
Infant	25-50

The main function of the respiratory system is to allow oxygen to enter the blood from air that is breathed in (inhaled) and to remove carbon dioxide, a waste product of respiration, from the blood into air that is breathed out (exhaled). This is called **external respiration. Internal respiration** is the process of oxygen and carbon dioxide moving into and out of the blood within internal body tissues.

EMERGENCIES RELATED TO THE RESPIRATORY SYSTEM

Respiration is one of the most vital functions in the body, and many different injuries and illnesses can affect it. Any factor that impedes the flow of air into and out of the lungs can affect respiration and become life threatening. An **airway obstruction** is a physical blockage of the airway that prevents the flow of air. For example, a person who is eating may have a piece of food lodged in the pharynx, a condition called **choking.** In an unconscious person lying on his or her back, the tongue may block the opening into the pharynx. An injury to the head or neck may also cause the soft tissues of the upper airway to swell and obstruct the airway. All of these are life-threatening situations.

Another potential problem with the airway is a failure of the epiglottis to prevent substances from entering the trachea. The swallowing reflex normally prevents this, but in an unconscious person, this reflex may not be functioning. This can result in liquids or solids entering the trachea and lungs. For example, an unconscious person lying on his or her back may vomit, and the vomit may flow back down the throat and into the trachea and lungs, impeding respiration and possibly causing a severe lung infection. This is one reason why an unresponsive victim is never given anything to drink – the fluid may flow into the lungs.

Chest injuries may also affect respiration. A broken rib may puncture a lung, making breathing ineffective. A penetrating injury into the lungs from the outside, such as that caused by a bullet or sharp object, may alter the lung pressures needed for inhaling and keep the lungs from filling with air.

Because breathing is controlled by the brain, other factors that affect the nervous system may also cause respiratory emergencies. A poisoning or drug overdose, for example, may severely depress nervous system functions, slowing breathing to the point where the body is not getting enough oxygen. An electric shock may interrupt the normal nervous system control of respiration and cause breathing to stop.

Finally, some illnesses also cause breathing difficulties. Asthma is a common condition, especially in children, in which airway tissues swell and make it hard for the person to breathe. Chronic lung diseases, more common in the elderly and in smokers, may reduce lung functioning so much that the person struggles to catch a breath.

If the body is not receiving enough oxygen, other organs will begin to fail. The heart will soon stop, and brain cells will begin to die within minutes. In **Chapter 5,** you will learn how to recognize breathing emergencies and the appropriate first aid to give victims depending on the cause.

Cardiovascular System

The cardiovascular system consists of the heart, blood and blood vessels **(Figure 3-4)**.

The heart has four chambers: the left and right atria and the left and right ventricles. The **ventricles** pump the blood through two loops, or cycles, in the body. First, blood is pumped to the lungs to pick up oxygen and release carbon dioxide. The blood returns to the heart, which pumps it to all areas of the body, releasing oxygen for use by body cells and picking up carbon dioxide for removal. The term **cardiac** refers to the heart. The heart is also part of the body's muscular system, as the heart is composed of a unique kind of muscle **(myocardium)** that contracts to make the pumping action. This pumping action, called **contraction** is controlled by electrical signals that are in turn controlled by the nervous system.

FIGURE 3-4

The heart.

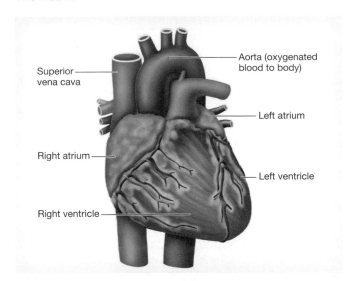

The blood flows from the heart to body areas through an extensive network of **arteries (Figure 3-5).** With the heartbeat, pulsing **blood pressure** changes occur in the arteries that can be felt in certain body locations as the **pulse.** Arteries progressively branch into smaller vessels that eventually reach **capillaries,** which are very small blood vessels with thin walls where oxygen and carbon dioxide are exchanged with body cells. From the capillaries, the blood drains back to the heart through an equally extensive system of **veins.** Blood flows more evenly through veins, which do not have a pulse. Arteries are generally deeper in the body than veins and are therefore more protected and less likely to be damaged by injuries.

The heart rate, which can be measured as the pulse, is affected by many factors. With exercise, fever or emotional excitement, the heart rate increases to meet the body's greater need for oxygen. Various injuries and illnesses may either increase or decrease the heart rate. **Table 3-2** provides some normal reference values for heart rate.

FIGURE 3-5

Major arteries of the body.

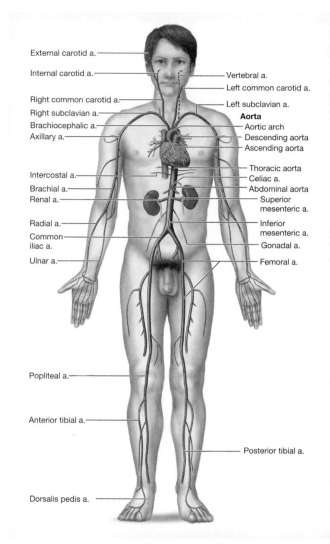

External carotid a.
Internal carotid a.
Right common carotid a.
Right subclavian a.
Brachiocephalic a.
Axillary a.
Intercostal a.
Brachial a.
Renal a.
Radial a.
Common iliac a.
Ulnar a.
Popliteal a.
Anterior tibial a.
Dorsalis pedis a.

Vertebral a.
Left common carotid a.
Left subclavian a.
Aorta
Aortic arch
Descending aorta
Ascending aorta
Thoracic aorta
Celiac a.
Abdominal aorta
Superior mesenteric a.
Inferior mesenteric a.
Gonadal a.
Femoral a.
Posterior tibial a.

The primary functions of the cardiovascular system are to transport oxygen and nutrients in the blood to all parts of the body and to remove carbon dioxide and other waste from tissues. Other functions include transporting hormones that regulate other body functions, helping regulate body temperature, transporting cells and substances that fight infection and helping maintain the body's fluid balance.

TABLE 3-2	
Normal Reference Values for Heart Rate	
	Beats per minute
Adult	60-100
Child	60-150
Infant	120-150

EMERGENCIES RELATED TO THE CARDIOVASCULAR SYSTEM

As with the respiratory system, the cardiovascular system's functions are vital for life, health and well-being. The most vital function is carrying oxygen to the body's tissues. As noted earlier, cells begin to die in vital organs, such as the brain, after only a few minutes without oxygen. Any injury or illness that affects respiration, therefore, also diminishes the ability of the cardiovascular system to deliver oxygen to the body.

Blood vessel problems may also affect cardiovascular functioning. Bleeding, which often occurs with injuries, may be so severe that not enough blood is left in circulation to adequately provide the oxygen the body needs.

Arterial bleeding is most severe because the blood may spurt out under pressure, leading within minutes to the life-threatening condition called **shock.** Shock occurs when vital body organs are not receiving enough oxygen (see **Chapter 9**).

Bleeding from veins is generally slower, but can still be serious or life threatening if it continues. Capillary bleeding is generally minor and usually stops by itself as the blood clots. **Chapter 8** describes the first aid techniques for controlling bleeding.

Stroke is another type of blood vessel problem involving arteries in the brain. A blood clot or bleeding in the brain may reduce circulation to a part of the brain, causing mental and physical impairments. **Chapter 16** describes first aid for stroke.

Problems involving the heart can also affect tissue oxygenation. Some conditions, such as congestive heart failure, reduce the heart's ability to pump to effectively meet the body's needs. If the heart muscle itself does not receive enough oxygenated blood because of blocked cardiac arteries, part of the heart muscle may die. This is called a heart attack, or **myocardial infarction.** The heart may also stop **(cardiac arrest),** in which case the person needs CPR, as described in **Chapter 5. Arrhythmia,** or an abnormal heartbeat, is another type of heart problem that may reduce the heart's pumping effectiveness.

1. Name two organs inside the thoracic cavity.

   _____

   _____

2. Which of the following is a function of the respiratory system? Select the best answer.

   a. Inhaling and exhaling

   b. Moving oxygen into the blood

   c. Moving carbon dioxide out of body tissues

   d. All of the above

3. At what structure is an airway obstruction most likely to occur?

   _____

   _____

4. The heart pumps blood to all body tissues through which blood vessels? Select the best answer.

   a. Arteries

   b. Veins

   c. Capillaries

   d. All of the above

5. Check off which cardiac problems can affect tissue oxygenation.

   ☐ Cardiac arrest

   ☐ Kidney failure

   ☐ Asthma

   ☐ Arrhythmia

   ☐ Diabetes

   ☐ Myocardial infarction

   ☐ Tetanus infection

Nervous System

The primary organs of the nervous system are the brain, spinal cord, sensory receptors and nerves throughout the body. The brain controls the nervous system **(Figure 3-6).** Specific areas in the brain control different functions, such as controlling heart rate, storing memories, creating visual images and directing muscle movements. The brain connects directly to the spinal cord, the pathway to and from nerves throughout the body. The brain and spinal cord form the **central nervous system.** After leaving the skull, the spinal cord is encased inside vertebrae, the bones of the spine **(Figure 3-7).** Nerves project out from the spinal cord between the vertebrae of the neck and back and extend throughout the body. Generally, nerves exiting the spinal cord nearer the top control movement and other functions higher in the body, and nerves from the spinal cord nearer the bottom control functions lower in the body.

FIGURE 3-6

The nervous system.

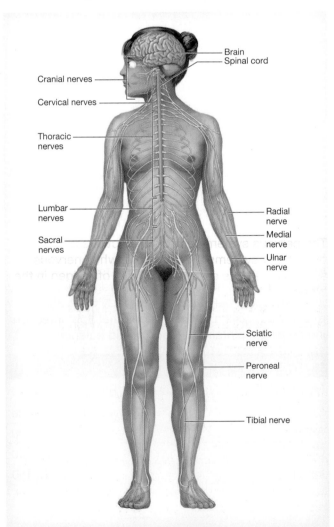

The nervous system has three general sets of functions:

1. Sensory receptors in the skin, eyes, ears, nose and mouth, as well as throughout the body, gather information about the internal and external environment and send this information to the brain.

2. The brain integrates and analyzes information, both consciously and automatically, for immediate and future use.

3. Nerve signals from the brain lead to movements and other actions throughout the body to accomplish specific tasks or to maintain **homeostasis,** a balanced state within the body necessary for effective functioning.

FIGURE 3-7

The spinal cord.

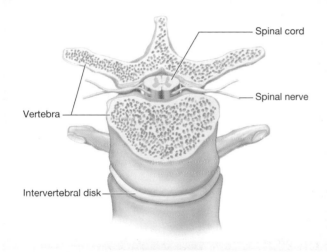

The nervous system controls the actions of most other body systems. For example, when nervous system receptors detect a low level of oxygen in the blood, the brain directs the muscles of breathing to speed up the respiratory rate and the heart to beat faster to ensure that the body gets enough oxygen.

EMERGENCIES RELATED TO THE NERVOUS SYSTEM

Injury or illness affecting the nervous system can have general or very specific effects on the body. Head and spinal injuries can have serious or life-threatening effects. An injury to a part of the brain, or a disease process, such as a stroke, that damages a particular brain area, may destroy or impair the function of that brain tissue. If the respiratory center in the brain is damaged, the person may stop breathing. If a muscle control center is damaged, a part of the body may be paralyzed. Head injuries may also cause bleeding or swelling of the brain. Because the brain is tightly encased in the skull, bleeding or swelling puts pressure on the brain and may cause more widespread effects.

Brain functions can also be more generally affected by injury or illness. **Altered mental status** is a phrase used to describe changes in a person's responsiveness, such as becoming confused, disoriented, lethargic or comatose. Altered mental status may result from such things as head injuries; any injury causing reduced oxygenation; or sudden illness, such as stroke, seizure, diabetic emergencies, severe infection, high fever, poisoning or drug overdose. **Chapter 16** describes first aid for such emergencies.

Damage to the spinal cord may occur at any level between the base of the skull and the lower back. Significant damage to the cord, such as complete severing caused by a neck or back fracture, often results in a complete loss of function in body areas controlled by nerves exiting the spine below that level. A lower back injury may result in a loss of feeling in the legs and inability to move the legs **(paralysis).** A similar injury to the spinal cord in the neck area may result in paralysis and loss of feeling in the entire body below the neck. The neck is a particularly vulnerable area because any trauma to the head, such as the head being snapped forward in a vehicle crash or striking a hard object after diving in shallow water, may injure neck vertebrae and the spinal cord. **Chapter 12** describes how to assess an injured victim for a possible head or spine injury and how to protect the spinal cord from additional injury caused by movement.

In addition to head and spinal injuries, injuries elsewhere in the body, as well as some illnesses, also affect the nervous system. Pain will result from damage to nerve fibers in many areas of the body, and therefore pain is always assessed as a symptom that may reveal something about a victim's injury or illness. The pain caused by injured nerves in a cut finger is obvious, but pain within the body is not always so clear cut. A crushing pain in the chest that extends into the left arm may be caused by a heart attack. Abdominal pain that begins in the area of the umbilicus (navel) and then settles into the lower abdomen on the right side may be a sign of appendicitis. Although pain is not always present with serious conditions, pain should be taken seriously whenever it occurs. The level of pain, however, should not be taken as an indicator of the severity of an injury or illness.

Musculoskeletal System

The musculoskeletal system combines two closely related body systems and is composed of bones, muscles and the structures that join them (ligaments and tendons). The bones of the body have several functions **(Figure 3-8)**:

- The skeleton provides shape and support for the body as a whole.

- Groups of bones protect vital internal organs (e.g., the ribs protect the heart and lungs, the skull protects the brain, the vertebrae protect the spinal cord).

- Bone marrow inside certain bones produces blood cells.

- Bones store calcium for use by the rest of the body when needed.

- Bones act as levers to allow movement at joints when muscles act on them.

FIGURE 3-8

Major bones of the body.

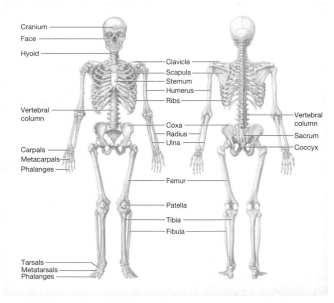

Skeletal muscles attach to bones to create body movements **(Figure 3-9)**. Another function is to produce body heat through movement or shivering. The phrase *musculoskeletal* usually refers to skeletal (voluntary) muscles, but the body also has other kinds of muscle tissue with special functions (called involuntary muscle tissue). As noted earlier, the heart's muscle tissue provides its beating force.

The esophagus is a muscular tube with special movements that aid in swallowing and moving food to the stomach. Muscle tissue throughout the gastrointestinal system keeps the products of digestion moving through the digestive tract. The diaphragm is a thin muscle below the lungs that does the primary work of breathing. Muscle tissue inside blood vessels helps keep blood moving through the body. All muscle activity is controlled by the nervous system.

Tendons are fibrous tissues that connect muscles to bones. **Ligaments** are tough bands of tissue that join bones together at joints.

FIGURE 3-9

Major muscles of the body.

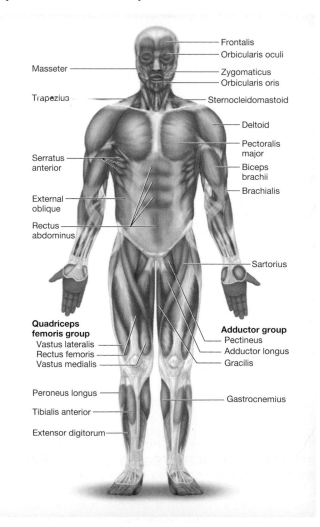

EMERGENCIES RELATED TO THE MUSCULOSKELETAL SYSTEM

Musculoskeletal injuries include fractures, dislocations, sprains and strains. A **fracture** is a broken bone. Although fractures can be serious injuries, particularly when nearby organs or blood vessels are damaged by the broken bone ends, most fractures are not life threatening. Dislocations and sprains are both joint injuries. In a **dislocation,** one or more bones move out of their normal position in a joint, preventing the joint from functioning as usual. Finger and shoulder dislocations are among the most common dislocations. A **sprain** is damage to ligaments and other structures in a joint; the ankle and wrist are commonly sprained by forces on these joints. A **strain** is a tearing of muscle or tendon tissue usually caused by overexertion of the muscle. All of these injuries require first aid as you will learn in **Chapter 14.**

Musculoskeletal injuries are often associated with other injuries. Vertebral fractures are likely to injure the spinal cord and cause nervous system damage. Fractures of the **femur,** the long bone in the thigh, often cause much soft tissue damage and bleeding. A fracture of the pelvis may damage the bladder or other organs in the pelvic cavity. A skull fracture may cause brain damage.

The musculoskeletal system is also affected by illnesses, although most of these do not occur suddenly and therefore seldom require first aid. Arthritis (chronic joint inflammation causing pain and restricted motion), muscular dystrophy (disorders of progressive degeneration of muscles), and osteoarthritis (weakening of bones, usually with aging) are all common musculoskeletal system diseases.

Integumentary System

The integumentary system consists of the skin, nails, hair and accessory structures, such as sweat and oil glands **(Figure 3-10).** The primary function of the skin is to protect the body from the external environment (temperature extremes, pathogens and other substances). Other functions include:

- *Regulating body temperature.* When the body is hot, blood vessels in the skin widen to bring heat to the surface to dissipate; sweating also helps cool the skin. When the body is cold, blood vessels constrict to conserve heat, and muscle movements occur, such as shivering and "goose bumps" (tiny muscle reactions in the hair follicles).

- *Preventing water loss from the body.* The skin acts as a barrier to prevent water loss.

- *Waste removal.* Through sweating, the skin removes some body waste.

- *Vitamin production.* Skin cells produce vitamin D.

- *Sensation.* Nerve sensors in the skin react to touch, pressure, pain and temperature.

FIGURE 3-10

Anatomy of the skin.

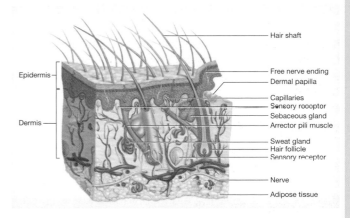

Labels: Hair shaft, Free nerve ending, Dermal papilla, Capillaries, Sensory receptor, Sebaceous gland, Arrector pili muscle, Sweat gland, Hair follicle, Sensory receptor, Nerve, Adipose tissue, Epidermis, Dermis

EMERGENCIES RELATED TO THE INTEGUMENTARY SYSTEM

Because skin is the organ most exposed to the environment, it is frequently damaged by traumatic injuries. Cuts and scrapes are common causes of bleeding. The blood vessels in the skin are relatively small, and bleeding from the skin seldom involves as much blood loss as from deeper blood vessels. Any openings in the skin, however, may allow pathogens into the body. As described in **Chapter 2, pathogens** are germs capable of causing disease, including bloodborne pathogens that can cause serious illnesses. Take precautions if you will be exposed to a victim's body fluids.

Exposure to temperature extremes can damage the skin. Skin exposed to freezing temperatures may get **frostbite,** a condition in which tissue freezes and dies. Very high temperatures and many chemicals cause skin **burns,** which destroy tissue and may allow loss of body heat and body fluid (see **Chapter 11**). Because sunburn damages skin in a way that makes skin cancer more likely later on, precautions should be taken to protect the skin from sun exposure.

Although skin functions help regulate body temperature, when a person is exposed to cold or heat, regulatory mechanisms may not be able to keep the body at its normal temperature. The skin of a victim of hypothermia (whole body cooling) often looks pale and cool. In heat stroke, a life-threatening condition in which the body becomes overheated, sweating stops and the skin is flushed and very hot to the touch. **Chapter 20** describes first aid for heat and cold emergencies.

The skin often reveals important information about the condition of the body. For example, when blood oxygen levels are low, the skin may look bluish, especially at the lips, under the nails and around mucous membranes. This skin color is called cyanosis. The skin of a victim in shock is often cool, clammy or sweating, and pale or bluish. Sweating and pale skin are also signs of a possible heart attack. Many sudden illnesses also cause sweating and skin color changes (flushed or pale). In dark-skinned individuals, the skin color generally becomes ashen rather than pale.

Because skin condition is a sensitive indicator of circulatory status, the skin can also help you monitor the effects of some first aid techniques. For example, when a victim's fractured arm or leg is splinted, the skin of the fingers or toes is periodically checked to ensure that circulation to the extremity has not been cut off.

 LEARNING CHECKPOINT 2

1. Check off injuries and illnesses that may cause altered mental status.

   ☐ Head injuries

   ☐ Seizure

   ☐ High fever

   ☐ Drug overdose

   ☐ Stroke

   ☐ Diabetic emergencies

   ☐ Poisoning

   ☐ Severe infection

2. Select the best answer. A spinal injury may result in –

   a. a myocardial infarction.

   b. lung infection.

   c. paralysis.

   d. All of the above

3. Define a dislocation.

   _____

   _____

   _____

4. Why might a fractured femur be life threatening? Select the best answer.

   a. Loss of calcium stored in the bone

   b. Severe bleeding

   c. Injury to soft tissues of the leg

   d. All of the above

5. In what situation can even a small skin cut be very serious?

   _____

   _____

   _____

   _____

Gastrointestinal System

The primary function of the gastrointestinal system is to digest food and extract nutrients to meet the body's needs for energy and specific dietary substances. Food and fluids pass through the esophagus to the stomach and then to the small and large intestines, where nutrients are absorbed into the blood to be transported to body cells **(Figure 3-11).** Waste is eliminated through the anus.

Accessory organs of digestion include the pancreas and liver, which produce substances that aid in digestion, and the gallbladder, which stores bile made by the liver. The liver has several other important functions.

FIGURE 3-11

The gastrointestinal system.

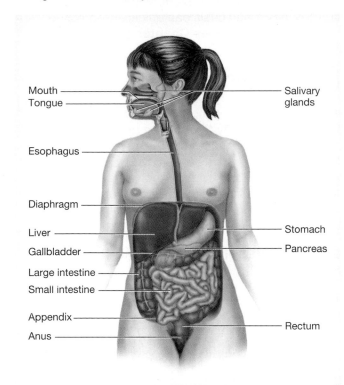

- Mouth
- Tongue
- Salivary glands
- Esophagus
- Diaphragm
- Liver
- Gallbladder
- Large intestine
- Small intestine
- Appendix
- Anus
- Stomach
- Pancreas
- Rectum

EMERGENCIES RELATED TO THE GASTROINTESTINAL SYSTEM

Because the abdominal cavity is not protected by bones, gastrointestinal organs can be easily injured by traumatic forces. In a closed abdominal injury, the skin is not broken, but pain or tenderness along with a swollen or rigid abdomen may suggest an internal injury. In an open abdominal wound, internal organs may be exposed to the outside, raising the risk of infection. **Chapter 13** describes first aid for abdominal injuries.

The gastrointestinal system may also be involved in a number of sudden illnesses and conditions. An ingested poison is absorbed in the same manner as nutrients from food, and once in the blood, can affect the entire body.

Various illnesses can cause vomiting or diarrhea. If either continues for a prolonged period, the victim may become dehydrated, a serious condition in which the body loses needed water. Infants, especially, can lose significant amounts of body fluid from diarrhea, which quickly becomes a medical emergency. Vomiting blood is likely a sign of serious illness.

The liver is also affected by many illnesses as well as by chronic alcohol use. As noted in **Chapter 2,** hepatitis is a bloodborne disease that frequently causes liver damage. Because the liver is a vital organ whose functions are necessary for life, it is critical to take appropriate precautions to prevent the transmission of hepatitis in first aid situations.

Lymphatic and Immune Systems

The lymphatic system consists of the lymph nodes and lymphatic vessels located throughout the body, along with other organs **(Figure 3-12).**

The lymphatic system helps the body absorb fats and maintain a fluid balance, but its primary function is to help defend against disease as part of the immune system. Lymphocytes, a type of white blood cell, help fight infection. Other organs and the cells of the immune system work together with the lymphatic system to provide defense mechanisms against pathogens and foreign substances that enter the body.

FIGURE 3-12

The lymphatic system.

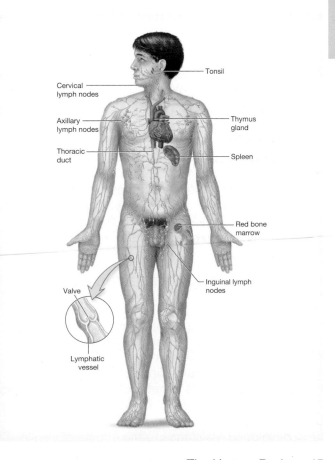

- Cervical lymph nodes
- Axillary lymph nodes
- Thoracic duct
- Tonsil
- Thymus gland
- Spleen
- Red bone marrow
- Inguinal lymph nodes
- Valve
- Lymphatic vessel

3 • The Human Body

The Human Body • 45

EMERGENCIES RELATED TO THE IMMUNE SYSTEM

Although many illnesses and other health problems may result from problems in the immune system, seldom do these occur suddenly and require first aid or immediate treatment. A wound that is not properly cared for, however, may develop an infection if the body's immune system does not eliminate pathogens that may enter the body through the wound. As described in **Chapter 2**, HIV, an infection attacking the immune system and causing AIDS, may also enter the first aid provider's body as a result of exposure to an infected victim's body fluids. Taking precautions against infection is necessary in all emergencies.

The related concept of **immunity** is also important in first aid. A **vaccine** is a form of preventive care that bolsters the body's immune system to prevent the vaccinated person from becoming infected by a specific pathogen. A vaccine is available for hepatitis B, for example, which health care workers and professional rescuers often receive because of the risk of acquiring this bloodborne infection when caring for victims of injury. The tetanus vaccine similarly gives protection against wounds being infected by the deadly tetanus bacterium, which is commonly present in the environment.

Endocrine System

The endocrine system includes a series of glands in various body areas that produce hormones. **Hormones** are chemical messengers that are carried in the blood and affect the functioning of organs throughout the body. More than two dozen hormones are produced in the body, each with specific functions and effects. For example, the thyroid gland produces hormones that regulate growth and development. The gonads (testes in men, ovaries in women) produce steroid hormones that stimulate the development of male and female sex characteristics and allow reproductive functions. The pancreas secretes a hormone called **insulin** that helps regulate blood sugar levels.

EMERGENCIES RELATED TO THE ENDOCRINE SYSTEM

All hormones affect a person's health, and the over- or underproduction of each can cause disease. Most of these problems develop more slowly, however, and are seldom issues for first aid – with one major exception. **Diabetes** is a metabolic disorder affecting more than 16 million people in the United States. Diabetics either do not produce enough insulin or have developed resistance to the effects of insulin.

A person with diabetes may suddenly become very ill because of very high or very low blood sugar levels related to this insulin problem. Without treatment or first aid, a diabetic crisis can quickly progress to a medical emergency (see **Chapter 16**).

Urinary System

The urinary system removes dissolved metabolic waste from the body through the urine and helps the body maintain fluid and electrolyte balances. Metabolic waste results from cellular functions within the body. The blood transports this waste to the **kidneys,** which filter them out and produce urine **(Figure 3-13).** Urine is transported to the **bladder,** which stores urine until it is passed to the outside.

EMERGENCIES RELATED TO THE URINARY SYSTEM

Traumatic injury may damage the bladder or kidneys, possibly resulting in blood in the urine. Blood in the urine is always a sign of a problem requiring medical attention.

Many medical problems affecting the urinary system do not develop suddenly and therefore are usually not first aid issues.

Because the frequency and amount of urine passed depends in part on how much water is present in the body, changes in urination may indicate the presence of a health problem. A long period without urination in an infant, for example, may be a sign of dehydration, which is a medical emergency.

FIGURE 3-13

The urinary system.

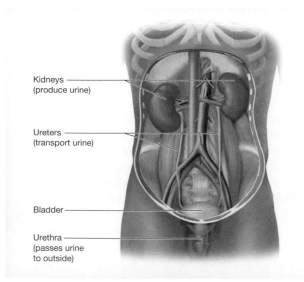

Kidneys
(produce urine)

Ureters
(transport urine)

Bladder

Urethra
(passes urine
to outside)

Reproductive System

Unlike other body systems that are identical or similar in males and females, the reproductive system involves different organs in males and females. The reproductive system in males produces sperm, the male reproductive cell, and transports the sperm for delivery into the female vagina. In females, the reproductive system produces eggs, the female reproductive cells, and supports and nurtures an egg fertilized by sperm as it develops into a fetus in the uterus; other functions relate to childbirth and lactation (producing milk for breastfeeding an infant). The term **genitals** refers to the male and female sex organs (penis and testicles in males; the labia, clitoris and vagina in females).

EMERGENCIES RELATED TO THE REPRODUCTIVE SYSTEM

Abdominal injuries may damage the genitals or reproductive organs, and such wounds may require special first aid (see **Chapter 10**). Because our culture views the genitals as a very private body area, care for these injuries should include concern for the victim's privacy and be performed with sensitivity.

In rare situations, a pregnant woman may develop complications. Occasionally, childbirth may occur without the pregnant woman being attended to by a doctor, midwife or other person trained in childbirth. In such cases, a first aider may need to assist the pregnant woman. Childbirth is usually a normal, natural process that takes place without problems or complications. Sometimes, however, a medical emergency may occur. **Chapter 22** describes first aid for pregnancy and childbirth.

 LEARNING CHECKPOINT 3

1. What is important about vomiting? Select the best answer.

   a. It can lead to dehydration.

   b. It may be a sign of serious illness.

   c. Vomiting blood often indicates a serious illness.

   d. All of the above

2. Name a vaccination *all* people should have periodically throughout their lives.

3. Diabetes involves a problem in the body with which hormone? Select the best answer.

   a. Insulin

   b. Bile

   c. Steroids

   d. Any of the above

4. Select the best answer. Blood present in the urine always means –

   a. a sexually transmitted disease is present.

   b. the person has a yeast infection.

   c. the person should seek medical attention.

   d. the person needs to restore electrolyte balance.

 CONCLUDING THOUGHTS

When you encounter a victim in need of first aid, the nature of the problem may be obvious or it may be difficult to judge. A simple cut that is bleeding, for example, does not require knowledge of the cardiovascular system before you can give first aid. With many injuries and illnesses, however, understanding what is going on in the body will help you assess the problem and remember what first aid to give. Understanding how a breathing problem can cause altered mental status, for example, or how a person with diabetes may experience a sudden emergency, can help you know what actions to take. The general principles described in this chapter will become more meaningful as you learn about specific injuries and illnesses throughout the rest of this text.

 ADDITIONAL ACTIVITIES AND RESOURCES

As you read the following chapters and learn about various specific problems caused by injuries or sudden illness, try to stay attuned to what is going on inside the body – how the specific functions of key body systems are affected. This broader understanding will help you remember key principles about steps to take in an emergency.

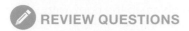

Select the best answers.

1. The main function of the respiratory system is to –

   a. filter the blood.

   b. transport nutrients to body tissues.

   c. protect the body from pathogens.

   d. provide oxygen for body tissues.

2. A problem in one body system –

   a. can also affect the functioning of other body systems.

   b. affects only that system.

   c. affects only that system plus the nervous system.

   d. affects every system in the body.

3. A person who is choking is said to have –

   a. altered mental status.

   b. an airway obstruction.

   c. an arrhythmia.

   d. a metabolic disorder.

4. What life-threatening problem occurs when vital organs are not receiving enough oxygen?

   a. Diabetes

   b. Hypothermia

   c. Shock

   d. Seizures

5. Inside the vertebrae is the –

   a. central nervous system.

   b. spinal cord.

   c. spinal ligament.

   d. peripheral nervous system.

6. Heart attack may cause –

   a. crushing pain in the chest.

   b. severe bleeding.

   c. seizures.

   d. airway obstruction.

7. The functions of the musculoskeletal system include –

   a. protecting internal organs.

   b. producing lymph.

   c. circulating blood.

   d. regulating hormones.

8. Skin changes may help you determine when a victim has –

   a. hypothermia.

   b. heat stroke.

   c. sudden illness.

   d. All of the above

9. A sign of an internal abdominal injury is –

   a. sweating.

   b. seizures.

   c. a swollen or rigid abdomen.

   d. All of the above

10. A person with diabetes may have an emergency caused by –

    a. very high blood sugar levels.

    b. very low blood sugar levels.

    c. either very high or very low blood sugar levels.

    d. a fluid balance problem.

CHAPTER 4

Assessing the Victim

LESSON OBJECTIVES

- Explain how to check the victim's responsiveness and normal breathing.

- Demonstrate how to move a victim into the recovery position and explain when this is done.

- Explain the importance of each element in the SAMPLE history.

- Demonstrate how to perform a physical examination of a responsive victim without a life-threatening problem.

Late in the afternoon, you stop by your supervisor's office to drop off a report. When you knock on the door, it swings open. You look inside and see him slumped over his desk. You call his name as you approach, but he doesn't respond, so you tap him on the shoulder and shout, "Are you OK?" He still does not respond. What do you do now?

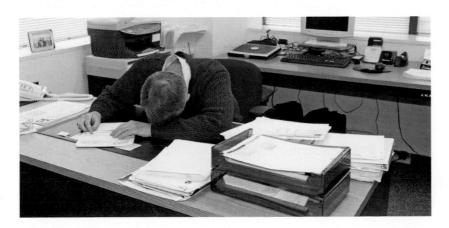

As described in **Chapter 2,** after you recognize the emergency and check the scene for safety, you then check the victim to see what problems may need emergency care or first aid. This check, called an **assessment,** has two primary steps:

1. In the **initial assessment,** check for immediate life-threatening conditions. Check for responsiveness, normal breathing and severe bleeding. Give immediate care for any life-threatening condition found.

2. In the **secondary assessment,** get the victim's history (find out what happened and what may have contributed to the emergency), and perform a physical examination of a responsive victim to check for any injuries or other signs of sudden illness.

   Then, while giving first aid for any injuries you find and while waiting for help to arrive, continue with a third step:

3. Monitor the victim for any changes.

Always perform these steps in this order. If you find a life-threatening problem, such as the absence of normal breathing, the victim needs immediate help. This victim could die if you first spend time looking for broken bones or asking bystanders what happened. **Always remember to conduct the initial assessment first.**

Initial Assessment

In the initial assessment, you check the victim for life-threatening conditions. As you come up to the victim, immediately look for responsiveness, normal breathing and severe bleeding. The entire initial assessment should take just a few seconds.

Because of the risk of aggravating a spinal injury, do not move the victim to perform this assessment, except when absolutely necessary in two circumstances:

1. The patient faces an immediate danger if not moved, because:

   • Fire is present or likely to occur.

   • Explosives are present or there is a danger of explosion (e.g., a natural gas leak).

   • The patient cannot be protected from other hazards at the scene.

   • You are unable to gain access to other patients who need lifesaving care.

   • You cannot make the scene safe (e.g., a structure is about to collapse).

2. You cannot give lifesaving care because of the patient's location or position (e.g., a victim who needs CPR is slumped in a chair or lying on a bed).

CHECK FOR RESPONSIVENESS

As you approach, you may notice immediately whether the victim is responsive. Responsive means a person is conscious and awake. A victim who is speaking, coughing, crying or moving is responsive. Even if the victim cannot talk because of an injury, he or she may be able to move and thereby signal responsiveness. A victim who cannot talk or move may be paralyzed but may still be able to respond through purposeful eye movements or other signs. This is why we say *responsive* rather than conscious: We cannot always know whether a person is conscious or unconscious, but we do know whether that person responds to us.

Just knowing the victim is responsive is not enough, however. Any victim who can talk is obviously responsive and is able to breathe – but the victim may have severe bleeding, which is a life-threatening condition. A victim who is awake and moving is responsive but if this person is not speaking, crying or coughing, the victim may be unable to breathe because of an obstructed airway (choking) or other breathing problem. Therefore, even with a responsive victim, you must still continue to check for normal breathing and severe bleeding – the next steps, described below.

If the victim is not speaking, making other sounds or moving, tap the person on the shoulder and shout, "Are you OK?" **(Figure 4-1).** Be careful not to move the victim in any way when assessing responsiveness. Do not shake the victim's shoulder or touch the head or neck, because the victim may have a spinal injury that any movement could worsen. If the victim still does not respond to your touch and voice, this is a life-threatening emergency, and you must act quickly. If someone else is present, have that person call 9-1-1, and get an automated external defibrillator after (AED) immediately (as described in **Chapter 6**) while you continue to check the unresponsive victim.

Unresponsiveness may be a sign of an urgent, life-threatening problem (such as not breathing) or it may result from a less urgent problem – you cannot know that. Regardless of its cause, and regardless of whether other life-threatening problems are present, *unresponsiveness in itself is considered an emergency.* For example, if the victim is on his or her back, the tongue may move back in the throat and block the airway, preventing breathing.

The degree of a victim's responsiveness is frequently assessed using the AVPU scale **(Box 4-1).** This scale is useful for noting changes in a victim's responsiveness during the time you are providing care and for communicating this information to arriving EMS professionals.

FIGURE 4-1

Check the victim for responsiveness by tapping the shoulder and asking, "Are you OK?"

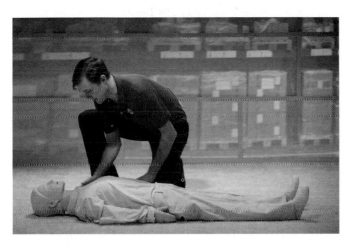

	BOX 4-1: THE AVPU SCALE
A	**Alert.** The victim is aware of the time and where he or she is.
V	Responds to **Verbal** stimuli. The victim is not clearly oriented to time and place but responds when spoken to.
P	Responds to **Painful** stimuli. The victim does not respond when spoken to but moves or responds to pain, as when pinched between the neck and shoulder.
U	**Unresponsive** to all stimuli. The victim's eyes are closed, and there is no movement or other response to painful stimuli.

CHECK FOR NORMAL BREATHING

At the same time you are checking for responsiveness, look for normal breathing. An unresponsive victim who is only gasping is not breathing normally and needs basic life support. If the victim can speak or cough, then he or she is breathing.

If you find an unresponsive person in a position other than lying on his or her back, do not immediately roll the victim onto his or her back to begin providing care. Moving a victim unnecessarily may cause additional injury, especially if the victim may have a spinal injury. If the victim is seen to be breathing normally, leave him or her in the position found while continuing your assessment.

Remember, if an unresponsive victim is not breathing normally, you must immediately start CPR as described in **Chapter 5.**

CHECK FOR SEVERE BLEEDING

After ensuring that the victim is breathing normally, check for severe bleeding. If the victim is bleeding profusely, vital organs are not receiving enough oxygen to sustain life.

Check for severe bleeding by quickly looking over the victim's body for obvious blood. Check for blood-saturated clothing or blood pooled under the body. Control any severe bleeding with direct pressure (see **Chapter 8**).

This step completes the initial assessment (see Skill: "Initial Assessment"). As described in the following chapters on basic life support, if the initial assessment reveals a life-threatening condition, you immediately begin to provide care for it. Only if it is clear that the victim is breathing normally and not bleeding severely, do you move on to the secondary assessment to check for additional injuries or signs of a sudden illness requiring care. An unresponsive victim who is breathing should be positioned (except in cases of trauma suggesting a neck, back, hip or pelvic injury) on his or her side in the recovery position following the initial assessment.

STEP 1
Ensure scene safety.

STEP 2
Check the victim for responsiveness.

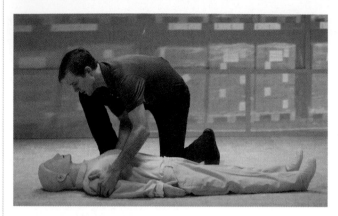

For a responsive victim:

STEP 3
Ask the victim what happened and about his or her condition.

STEP 4
Have someone call 9-1-1. If alone, correct any life-threatening conditions you see first (such as severe bleeding) before calling 9-1-1 and continuing to check the victim and providing other care.

For a unresponsive victim:

STEP 3
Call for help:

a. Shout for someone to call 9-1-1 and get an AED. Keep the phone at the victim's side.

b. If alone, call 9-1-1 from your mobile device, if you have one, and follow the dispatcher's instructions.

STEP 4
If alone without a mobile device, find a phone and call 9-1-1, and get an AED if available.*

*Correct any immediate life threats (such as opening the airway or controlling severe bleeding) before leaving an adult victim to call 9-1-1.

BOX 4-2: HELMET REMOVAL

Helmets are worn by people in a variety of activities: bicycle riders, motorcycle riders, athletes playing sports, such as football, and construction site workers. If an injured victim is wearing a helmet, it should be removed only if absolutely necessary to care for a life-threatening condition, because removal involves the risk of moving the victim's head or neck and possibly worsening a spinal or head injury. Leave the helmet in place for arriving EMS professionals, unless a full-face helmet absolutely must be removed to perform CPR. With many sports helmets, the face guard can be removed so that the helmet can be left on while CPR is given.

Recovery Position

An unresponsive victim who is breathing normally, and who is not suspected of having a spinal injury, should be put in the **recovery position** (see Skill: "Recovery Position"). This position is used for several reasons:

- It helps keep the airway open.

- It allows fluids to drain from the mouth so that the victim does not choke on blood, vomit or other fluids.

- It prevents the victim from inhaling stomach contents if the victim vomits.

For an unresponsive, breathing infant, hold the infant's face down over your arm with his or her head slightly lower than the body **(Figure 4-2).** Support the head and neck with your hand and keep the nose and mouth clear.

Once the victim is in the recovery position, continue to monitor breathing while waiting for advanced help to arrive, and observe the victim for bleeding, medical alert bracelets or insignia and any deformities that may indicate a serious injury. Give this information to responding EMS professionals.

FIGURE 4-2

Infant recovery position.

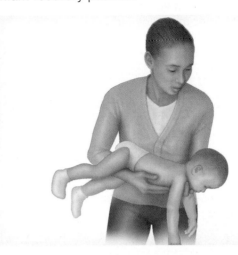

🧠 SKILL: RECOVERY POSITION

STEP 1
Position the victim's arm farthest from you across the victim's body.

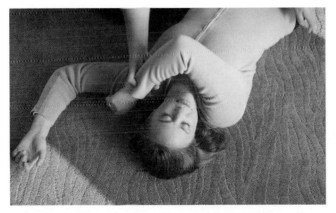

STEP 2
Grasp the victim at the shoulder and hips, and roll them toward you.

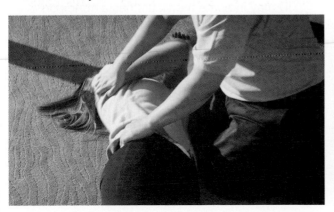

STEP 3
Bend both legs so the victim's position is stabilized.

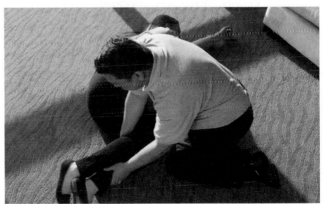

STEP 4
With the victim now in position, check the airway and open the mouth to allow drainage.

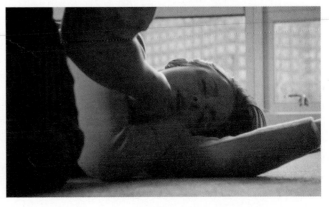

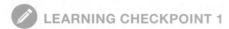

1. You first encounter a victim lying quietly on the floor. Number the following actions in the correct order.

   _____ Look around his body for a pool of blood.

   _____ Check to see if victim responds to your voice or touch.

   _____ Look for normal breathing.

2. Describe when you should *not* immediately proceed to the secondary assessment from the initial assessment.

   _____

Circle **True** or **False** for the following statement:

3. If you hear a victim coughing, you can assume he or she is breathing.   True   False

Secondary Assessment

Remember that the secondary assessment is performed only for victims without life-threatening conditions. Do not interrupt care for a serious problem in order to carry out a secondary assessment. But if the victim's condition seems stable and no threats to life require your attention, then the secondary assessment can provide additional information about the injury or illness. That information may help you care for the victim and may be of value to arriving EMS professionals. The secondary assessment can usually be performed with responsive victims of injury or sudden illness who are not experiencing a breathing problem. Some aspects of the secondary assessment may be performed with unresponsive victims.

The secondary assessment has two primary parts: the history and the physical examination. In both parts, focus your attention primarily on the injured area, taking into account the cause and nature of the injury (often called the "mechanism of injury").

GET THE VICTIM'S HISTORY

After the initial assessment, get the victim's **history** to try to find out more about what happened and the victim's condition. Talk to a responsive victim. With an unresponsive victim, ask bystanders what they know or saw. With a potentially serious injury, try to assess the forces involved. For example, a victim who fell from a height or was struck in the head by a heavy object is at greater risk of having a spinal injury, and you must be careful not to move this victim during your assessment or when giving first aid.

When taking the history of a responsive victim of sudden illness, ask fully about the victim's situation to learn possible causes. For example, in a case of poisoning, the victim may not immediately associate present symptoms with something ingested an hour or more ago. Or a victim could be experiencing the effects of breathing in carbon monoxide inside a building, even though you encountered the victim outside.

Use the **SAMPLE** format to ensure that you cover the victim's full history:

S	**Signs and symptoms.** What can you observe about the victim **(signs)?** Ask the victim how he or she feels **(symptoms),** and ask for a description of any pain felt.
A	**Allergies.** Ask the victim if he or she has any allergies to foods, medicines, insect stings or other substances. Look for a medical alert ID.
M	**Medications.** Ask the victim if he or she is taking any prescribed medications or over-the-counter products, including vitamins, supplements and herbal remedies.
P	**Previous problems.** Ask the victim if he or she has had anything like this before or if he or she has any other illnesses. Again, a medical alert ID may indicate the victim has a condition, such as diabetes or epilepsy.
L	**Last food or drink.** Ask the victim what he or she last ate and when.
E	**Events.** Ask the victim what happened, and try to identify the events that led to the current situation. When did the victim first begin to experience the problem?

If the victim is unresponsive, ask family members or bystanders whether they know the answers to these questions. Also check the scene for clues to what may have happened. The victim may have just taken a medication, for example, or you may see something like a syringe that could indicate possible drug abuse. A nearby container of a poisonous household product could indicate a possible poisoning. Consider the environment: a very cold or hot environment may produce a temperature-related emergency or contribute to sudden illness. Finally, consider the victim's age. A younger person who slips on ice and falls may have only a bruise, whereas an elderly woman who falls is more likely to have broken her hip.

The information from the SAMPLE history may help you give the right first aid. Even if information gained does not seem of immediate value to you, it may be important for the victim's medical care later, especially if the victim becomes unresponsive and cannot give that information again. When help arrives, give the information you gathered to the EMS professionals. It will help them to provide the appropriate medical care.

PHYSICAL EXAMINATION

The secondary assessment of an injured or ill victim who is responsive also includes a **physical examination.** With this examination you may find other injuries that need first aid or additional clues to the victim's condition. Remember that you do not stop giving first aid for a serious condition just to perform or complete this examination. Instead, keep the victim still and calm and wait for EMS professionals.

Remember that an unresponsive victim without a possible spinal injury should be kept in the recovery position until EMS professionals arrive. Continue to monitor the victim's breathing, and observe the victim for bleeding and other signs of serious injury.

Allow a responsive victim to remain in the position he or she finds most comfortable while conducting the physical examination. The victim does not need to be moved to lie on his or her back as shown later in the illustrations.

Ask a responsive victim for consent to do a physical examination, as with any other first aid, and describe what you are about to do before touching the victim. Keep away from any body area the victim tells you is very painful. Watch for a victim's facial expression or stiffening of a body part, which may reveal pain or tenderness the victim does not tell you about.

Focus on the area the victim knows is injured. You do not need to touch every body area, for example, if the victim has an injured arm and the nature of the injury does not suggest other body areas may be injured.

The physical examination of a responsive adult includes examining the victim from head to toe looking for anything out of the ordinary **(Box 4-3).** You begin at the head because injuries here are more likely to be serious than injuries in the extremities or lower in the body. As a general rule, look for the following signs and symptoms of injury or illness throughout the body, comparing one side of the body to the other:

- Pain when an area moves or is touched

- Bleeding or other wounds

- An area that is swollen or deformed

- Skin color (flushed, pale or ashen); temperature (hot or cold); and moisture (dry, sweating or clammy)

- Abnormal sensation or inability to move the area

While performing the examination, also watch for changes in the victim's condition. For example, the victim may at first be fully responsive and alert, but as you continue to check different body areas, the victim may become disoriented or dizzy, suggesting a changing mental status. The victim's breathing may change or stop. Call 9-1-1 if the victim's condition becomes more serious and the call was not made earlier.

You may have to remove some of the victim's clothing to examine an injured body area. Remove clothing or shoes only when necessary, such as to apply pressure on a wound to control bleeding, because moving the body part could cause additional injury. Protect the victim's privacy and prevent exposure to the cold. Follow these guidelines for removing clothing:

- Carefully roll or fold up a sleeve to expose an arm.

- To remove a jacket or shirt when an arm is injured, remove the uninjured arm from its sleeve first and then carefully work the jacket or shirt around the body and down off the injured arm while supporting it.

- Gently pull up a pants leg to expose the calf or knee. With scissors, carefully cut along the seam to expose the thigh.

BOX 4-3: SIGNS AND SYMPTOMS OF INJURY AND ILLNESS

The victim may tell you about:

- Pain, tenderness

- Dizziness, feeling faint

- Nausea

- Tingling or abnormal sensation, no sensation

- Thirst

- Hot, cold

You may see:

- Painful expression, guarding against movement

- Bleeding, wound, bruise, swelling

- Abnormal skin color

- Deformity, inability to move body part

- Unusual chest movement

- Vomit, incontinence

You may feel:

- Damp skin

- Hot or cold skin

- Swelling

- Deformity

You may hear:

- Noisy breathing

- Groaning, sounds of pain

- Stress in victim's voice

- Sucking chest wound

You may smell:

- Odor of a drug used

- Odor of poisonous or hazardous substance

- Fruity smelling breath (diabetic emergency)

- Support the victim's ankle when removing a shoe. Leave long boots on.

- If you cannot easily slide off a tight sock, lift it gently with your fingers and cut it open with scissors.

The acronym **DOTS** is often used as a reminder of what to look for in the physical examination of an injured victim:

D = Deformities

O = Open injuries

T = Tenderness (pain)

S = Swelling

Check the Head and Neck

Do not move the head or neck during the examination. Gently feel the skull for bleeding, bumps or depressions. Check the ears and nose for blood or a clear fluid. Check the pupils of both eyes, which should be of equal size and should respond to light when you cover and uncover the eyes with your hand. Check the victim's breathing for ease of breathing and regularity, and note any unusual breath odor. Check the mouth for burned areas. Check the neck for a medical alert necklace, deformity or swelling, bleeding and pain. Observe the skin of the head and neck for color, temperature and moisture.

Check the Chest and Abdomen

Check the chest and sides, feeling for deformity, wounds or tender areas. Look for blood in any area. Ask the victim to take a deep breath, and feel and look for easy, symmetrical expansion of the chest with breathing or for signs of pain while breathing. Gently feel along the collarbones and shoulders for deformity, swelling or pain.

If you suspect a problem in the abdominal or pelvic areas, gently check the abdomen for rigidity, pain or bleeding and gently feel both sides of the hips and pelvis to check for pain or deformity.

Check the Extremities

Check the arms for bleeding, deformity and pain. Ask the victim to bend his or her elbows, wrists and fingers. Look for a medical alert bracelet. Touch the fingers and ask if the sensation feels normal to the victim. Check the skin color and temperature of the hand to detect impaired circulation. Ask the victim to shrug the shoulders.

Check the legs for bleeding, deformity and pain. Unless you suspect a back, abdomen or pelvic injury, ask the victim to point and wiggle the toes. Check the

skin temperature and color of the feet. Touch the feet, and ask if the sensation feels normal to the victim.

If you find anything unusual in the extremities, compare that extremity with the opposite side and note differences (see Skill: "Physical Examination").

🧠 SKILL: PHYSICAL EXAMINATION

If you find any problems in any body area, do not let the victim move. Wait for help.

STEP 1
Being careful not to move the victim's head or neck, check the head.

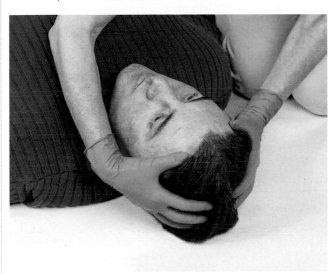

STEP 2
Check neck area for a medical alert necklace, deformity or swelling and pain. Do not move the neck.

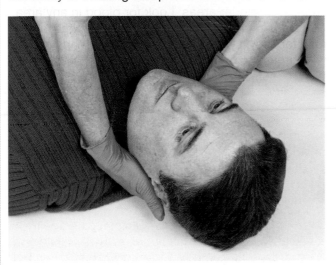

STEP 3
Check skin appearance, temperature and moisture.

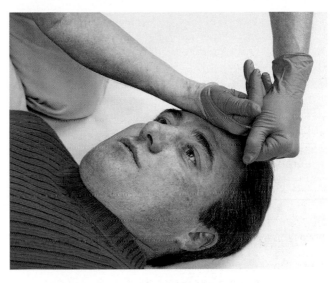

STEP 4
Check chest. Ask victim to breathe deeply.

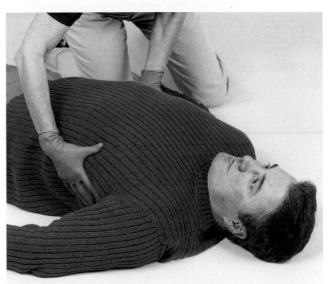

STEP 5
Check abdomen.

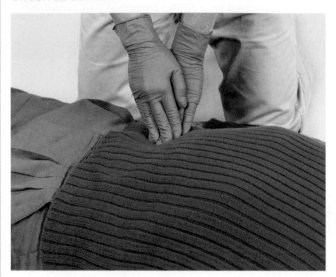

STEP 6
Check pelvis and hips.

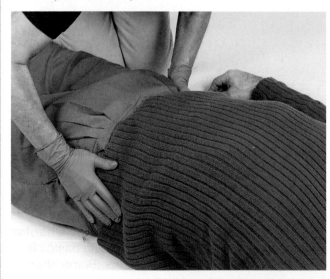

STEP 7
Check upper extremities. Look for medical alert bracelet.

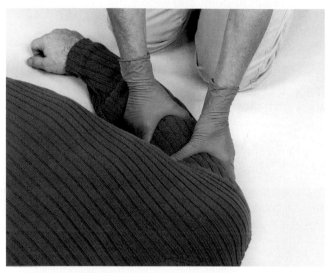

STEP 8
Check lower extremities.

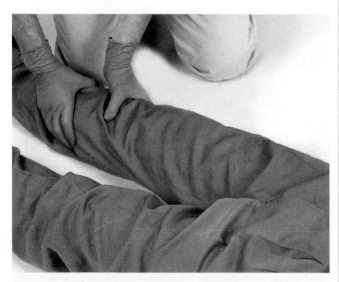

EXAMINING A CHILD OR INFANT

The assessment of a child or infant is similar to that of an adult, taking into account physical differences and the child's different language skills and emotional state. Use simple questions to gather the history, such as, "Where does it hurt?" Talk with the child's parents or guardians, if possible, and involve them in the physical examination **(Figure 4-3).** Allow a parent or guardian holding an infant or young child to continue to hold the victim during the examination. With a young child it is often better to perform the physical examination from toe to head rather than from the head first, to allow the child to get used to you. Because a child is more likely to become upset or anxious, talk to him or her calmly and soothingly before starting the examination, and look for signs of anything unusual before touching the child. A child who is upset often reacts with physical changes that may mask or confuse the signs of injury.

FIGURE 4-3

Involve the child's parent or guardian in the history and physical examination.

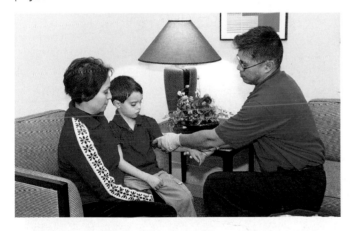

Monitor the Victim

Give first aid for injuries or illness you discover in your assessment, as described in the following chapters. With very minor conditions, the victim may need no more than your first aid. In other situations, the victim may need to see a health care provider or go to the emergency department. With all life-threatening or serious conditions, you should have called 9-1-1 and will now be awaiting the arrival of help.

While waiting, monitor the victim to make sure his or her condition does not worsen. With an unresponsive victim or a victim with a serious injury, repeat your assessment of breathing at least every 5 minutes.

1. When is the secondary assessment performed? Select the best answer.

   a. Immediately before giving CPR when needed

   b. In all victims, right after the initial assessment

   c. After checking for responsiveness

   d. After determining that there are no life-threatening conditions

2. Write what each letter in the SAMPLE history stands for:

   S =_____

   A =_____

   M =_____

   P =_____

   L =_____

   E =_____

3. Describe what signs and symptoms of injury you are looking for as you examine each part of a victim's body.

⏱ CONCLUDING THOUGHTS

You can see why a victim of injury or sudden illness is assessed in two stages: If the initial assessment reveals a life-threatening problem, then you must provide basic life support immediately without going on to the history and physical examination. **Chapter 5** is the first of three chapters describing basic life support for life-threatening problems. Remember: A breathing problem is an *immediate* threat to life, requiring action within seconds, because body tissues will begin to die within minutes.

4 • Assessing the Victim

SCENARIO 1

You are driving a coworker home after work when, without warning, he suddenly slumps forward in the seat beside you. As you brake and pull over onto the shoulder, you try to rouse him, but he seems unresponsive. As soon as you have safely stopped your car, how should you first check this victim?

_____

_____

_____

_____

SCENARIO 2

On the job, you encounter a coworker who is lying on the ground on his back, unresponsive, because of an unknown injury or illness. You see that he is breathing normally. After calling 9-1-1 for help, how should you position this victim? Why?

_____

_____

_____

_____

SCENARIO 3

You arrive at work and find a man lying on the ground in the parking lot, surrounded by several other workers and the man's wife, who had just dropped him off at work. He is unresponsive but breathing evenly and has no obvious signs of injury or illness. Someone has already called 9-1-1. While you are waiting, you ask his wife about what happened. She says he just seemed to suddenly collapse. What are other questions you could ask to gather more information about the man's history to give the professional rescuers when they arrive?

_____

_____

_____

_____

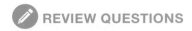 **REVIEW QUESTIONS**

Select the best answers.

1. The initial assessment checks the victim for –
   a. bone fractures.
   b. severe bleeding.
   c. severe allergies.
   d. spinal injuries.

2. Assess an adult or child victim for responsiveness by –
   a. tapping the shoulder and asking if he or she is OK.
   b. pinching the cheek between thumb and forefinger.
   c. checking for pupil reactions to light.
   d. checking skin for normal color and temperature.

3. If a victim can talk to you, you can be sure he or she –
   a. does not have a life-threatening condition.
   b. does not have a spinal injury.
   c. is breathing.
   d. All of the above

4. At what point do you begin providing care for a victim who is not breathing normally?
   a. Immediately
   b. As soon as the 9-1-1 dispatcher tells you to
   c. As soon as you complete the secondary assessment
   d. Right after positioning the victim in the recovery position

5. Advantages of the recovery position include which of the following?
   a. It lowers the victim's blood pressure.
   b. It allows fluids to drain from the mouth.
   c. It helps reduce shock.
   d. It helps ensure that the brain receives sufficient oxygen.

6. When gathering a SAMPLE history from a suddenly ill victim, which should you ask about?
   a. Allergies and medications taken
   b. Age and weight
   c. Favorite foods
   d. Most recent annual physical exam

7. During the physical examination, what are you looking for?
   a. Bleeding or wounds
   b. A swollen area
   c. Pain upon being touched
   d. All of the above

CHAPTER 5

Cardiovascular Emergencies and Cardiopulmonary Resuscitation

LESSON OBJECTIVES

- List the risk factors for cardiovascular disease.

- Explain general principles for maintaining cardiovascular health and preventing cardiovascular disease.

- Describe the age categories for adults, children and infants related to differences in basic life support skills.

- List the steps in the Cardiac Chain of Survival.

- Describe when to call 9-1-1 before starting CPR and when to give 2 minutes of CPR before calling 9-1-1.

- Demonstrate the procedures for giving CPR.

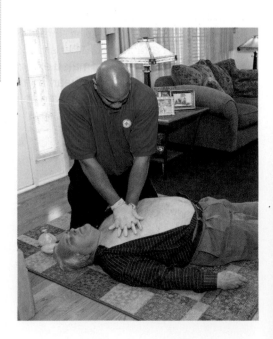

You are walking past your neighbor's house when you hear a scream for help. You knock on the door and offer to help. Your neighbor lets you in and you find her husband unresponsive on the floor. "He just collapsed," she tells you. You send her to call 9-1-1 and quickly check to see whether he is breathing normally. He is not breathing. How do you handle this situation?

Cardiac and respiratory emergencies are among the most serious threats to life. Basic life support is needed for a victim whose heartbeat or breathing has stopped. If the victim's heart has stopped beating normally, chest compressions are needed to circulate blood to vital organs. Rescue breaths are also given to oxygenate the blood.

Chest compressions combined with rescue breaths is called **cardiopulmonary resuscitation (CPR).** The chapter discusses cardiac and respiratory emergencies and the basic life support care given to victims with these threats to life.

Overview of Basic Life Support

Basic life support (BLS) refers to first aid given if the victim's breathing or heart stops. Many things can cause breathing or the heart to stop. Whenever either breathing or the heart stops, the other also stops very soon. BLS is often needed for victims of:

- Heart attack

- Drowning

- Choking

- Other injuries or conditions that affect breathing or the heart

Basic life support consists of several first aid skills, often called **resuscitation.**

A victim who is not breathing normally needs CPR to circulate blood in the body to keep vital organs alive to move oxygen into the body. A victim whose heart is in a condition called ventricular fibrillation, which is common after heart attacks and other situations, needs an electric shock given by an automated external defibrillator (AED) to restore a more normal heart rhythm. A victim who is choking also needs first aid to clear the airway to allow either natural breathing or rescue breaths.

This chapter focuses on cardiovascular and respiratory emergencies and the use of CPR. The additional skills for using an AED and giving choking care are described in the following two chapters.

DIFFERENCES AMONG ADULTS, CHILDREN AND INFANTS

Because of size and other differences, there are some distinctions in how BLS skills are used with adults, children and infants. These differences result from anatomical and physiological differences in the human body at different ages. The standard age groups for BLS are defined in the following way. Remember these age categories in reference to CPR and the use of an AED:

- An *infant* is up to 1 year of age.

- A *child* for purposes of CPR and choking care is 1 year up to the onset of adolescence or puberty (as determined by the occurrence of secondary sex characteristics, such as the presence of armpit hair in boys or breast development in girls); *for AED only*, a child means ages 1-8.

- An *adult* for all BLS skills except for AED means at or past puberty; *for AED only*, adult means older than 8.

 LEARNING CHECKPOINT 1

Fill in the correct answers:

1. Basic life support helps keep a victim alive when _____ or _____ _____ stops.

2. For purposes of using an AED, a child is defined as someone between the ages of _____ and _____ .

Cardiovascular Illness and Emergencies

CPR is most commonly needed by victims in cardiac arrest as a result of a heart attack. Because a heart attack is usually caused by cardiovascular disease, preventing cardiovascular illnesses by maintaining a healthy lifestyle is the most effective way to prevent heart attacks and other cardiovascular emergencies, such as stroke.

The term *cardiovascular illness* refers to several different diseases involving the heart and blood vessels **(Table 5-1).** Cardiovascular disease becomes more common as a person ages, as shown in **Table 5-2, becoming the number one cause of death in adults older than age 65.** But these diseases are also surprisingly common even in young adults. The three most common cardiovascular diseases are:

TABLE 5-1

Prevalence of Cardiovascular Diseases, United States

CVD	82,600,000
Hypertension	76,400,000
CHD	16,300,000
Acute Myocardial Infarction (AMI)	7,900,000
Angina Pectoris	9,000,000
Stroke	7,000,000
Heart Failure	5,700,000
Congenital Heart Defects	1,000,000
Atrial Fibrillation	2,200,000
Peripheral Arterial Disease	8,500,000

*Data from National Institutes of Health at
www.nhlbi.nih.gov/files/docs/research/2012_ChartBook.pdf
Accessed January 2016.*

- Heart disease, such as **coronary heart disease** (blockage of vessels supplying heart muscle with blood, often leading to heart attack)

- **Stroke** (sudden impairment of blood circulation in a part of the brain)

- **Hypertension** (high blood pressure, a very common condition that can lead to both heart attack and stroke)

Heart disease remains the most common cause of death in Americans, resulting in about 600,000 deaths a year.[1] Coronary heart disease kills over 370,000 people in the United States every year, and about 525,000 first-time heart attacks occur each year, plus another 210,000 repeat heart attacks.[2]

Stroke has been and remains the number three cause of death overall. About 795,000 people a year have a stroke, resulting in about 130,000 deaths.[3]

[1]*National Safety Council. (2015). Injury Facts®, 2015 Edition. Itasca, IL: Author.*

[2]*Centers for Disease Control and Prevention. http://www.cdc. gov/heartdiseasc/facts.htm Accessed January 2016.*

[3]*Centers for Disease Control and Prevention. www.cdc.gov/ dhdsp/data_statistics/fact_sheets/fs_stroke.htm Accessed January 2016.*

TABLE 5-2

Leading Causes of Death by Age and Rank, United States

Cause of Death	Age (Years)			
	1-24	25-44	45-64	≥65
Heart disease	5	3	2	1
Cancer	4	2	1	2
Cerebrovascular disease (stroke)	8	8	7	4
Accidents	1	1	3	9
Chronic lower respiratory disease	9	—	4	3
Influenza and pneumonia	7	10	—	7
Diabetes mellitus	—	9	5	6
Suicide	3	4	8	—
Chronic liver disease	—	7	6	—
Nephritis and nephrosis	—	—	10	8
Homicide	2	5	—	—
Septicemia	10	—	9	10
Congentital malformations	6	—	—	—
HIV disease	—	6	—	—
Alzheimer's disease	—	—	—	5

*Data from National Institutes of Health at www.nhlbi.nih.gov/files/docs/research/2012_ChartBook.pdf
Accessed January 2016.*

More than five million people are living with the effects of stroke, which often include severe disability. Stroke is discussed in **Chapter 16.**

Almost one-third of adults in the United States have high blood pressure – over 70 million people. More than 360,000 deaths a year involve high blood pressure as a primary or contributing cause. [4]

Taken together, these three cardiovascular diseases along with the others shown in **Table 5-1** constitute the number one health problem in the United States today. Yet many of the risk factors leading to these diseases can be prevented.

[4]*Centers for Disease Control and Prevention. http://www.cdc. gov/bloodpressure/facts.htm Accessed January 2016.*

CARDIOVASCULAR RISK FACTORS

A **risk factor** is anything that makes it more likely that a person will develop a particular disease. Some risk factors are beyond our control, but others are lifestyle factors that a person can avoid or change. Following are the known risk factors for cardiovascular disease:

Risk Factors That Cannot Be Changed

• Increasing age

• Gender

• Race

• Hereditary factors

Preventable Risk Factors

• Smoking

• High cholesterol levels

• High blood pressure

• Physical inactivity

• Obesity and being overweight

• Uncontrolled diabetes

• Stress

Even though some risk factors cannot be changed, it is important to be aware of them when they increase your risk of cardiovascular disease. In general, the risks of these diseases rise with increasing age. At some ages men are more likely to have cardiovascular disease than women, while at other ages the prevalence is higher in women; neither gender should feel immune to heart attacks and other problems. African-Americans generally have a higher prevalence of high blood pressure than Caucasians, and therefore have a greater risk for cardiovascular disease. Hereditary factors, such as a family history of heart disease, also can increase one's risk.

If you know your risk for cardiovascular disease is high because of risk factors beyond your control, it is all the more important to focus on those risk factors you *can* control. Risk factors often have an additive effect: the more risk factors you have, the higher your danger overall for developing disease.

Prevention of cardiovascular disease, therefore, involves eliminating risk factors by living a healthy lifestyle. In general, this means:

• Not using tobacco

• Eating healthy foods to prevent being overweight, to help lower cholesterol levels and blood pressure, and to help prevent diabetes

• Maintaining low cholesterol levels, with medication when appropriate

• Controlling high blood pressure with diet, exercise, weight control and medication if needed

• Getting sufficient regular exercise to help prevent being overweight, high blood pressure, diabetes and stress

• Preventing or managing stress

You should notice how these risk factors are interrelated. For example, inactivity puts one at risk for being overweight, and weight control helps prevent hypertension as well as helping one manage stress. Eating well also helps prevent being overweight and helps to control blood pressure. These interrelated risk factors are sometimes referred to as a *constellation* of factors. To maintain good cardiovascular health, we should focus not on one or two factors but on a whole constellation of healthy choices that together result in a healthy lifestyle.

PREVENTION OF CARDIOVASCULAR DISEASE

Cardiovascular health can be attained and maintained with a lifestyle that includes good diet, exercise, weight and blood pressure control and stress management.

All of these factors involve behavioral habits that typically begin in childhood, although they may also develop later in life. Adults who understand that they need to eat healthily and get exercise, for example, may have difficulty doing so if they have habitually behaved otherwise. The following sections, therefore, focus on establishing good habits early in childhood as well as developing them later in life when needed.

In recent years more media attention has been given to the cardiovascular health of children. The problems of childhood obesity, high cholesterol levels, poor diet, and lack of exercise are now recognized. Although few children actually experience heart disease other than rare congenital problems, from a very early age they form habits that often stay with them for life.

Smoking

Smoking and other uses of tobacco contribute to poor cardiovascular health as well as cancer. Smokers have a risk that is 2-4 times higher for cardiovascular disease than nonsmokers. Children learn about smoking at a very early age by observing adults. Nearly 4,000 children under age 18 try their first cigarette every day, or almost 1.5 million youth a year. Nearly 9 out of 10 smokers start smoking by age 18, and 99% start by age 26. On any given day, more than 2,500 youth and young adults who have been occasional smokers will become regular smokers.[1] Do not smoke around children, both because of the risks of secondhand smoke and because you as an adult caregiver are a role model and would be implicitly teaching children it is OK to smoke. Support the efforts of schools and other organizations to teach children that all tobacco use is unhealthy.

[1]Centers for Disease Control and Prevention. cdc.gov/tobacco/data_statistics/sgr/2012/consumer_booklet/pdfs/consumer.pdf Accessed January 2016.

Most adults who smoke know that it is an unhealthy habit yet still have difficulty quitting. About 40 million Americans still smoke (about 19% of men, 15% of women).[2] Many smoking cessation programs have been developed and have proved effective when one is motivated to stop. For information, contact the American Cancer Society, American Lung Association or American Heart Association. The American Cancer Society provides much information about different aspects of smoking cessation, including[3]:

- The immediate rewards of quitting smoking

- Getting help with the mental part of addiction

- Getting help with the physical part of addiction

- Nicotine replacement therapy

- Prescription drugs to help quit smoking

- Other methods of quitting smoking

- Steps for long-term success

- Making the decision to quit smoking

- Setting a quit smoking date and making a plan

- Dealing with smoking withdrawal

[2]Centers for Disease Control and Prevention. cdc.gov/tobacco/data_statistics/fact_sheets/adult_data/cig_smoking/index.htm Accessed January 2016.

[3]American Cancer Society. cancer.org/healthy/stayawayfromtobacco/guidetoquittingsmoking/index Accessed January 2016.

Admittedly, it is not easy to quit smoking, as nicotine is a highly addictive substance. But a commitment to quitting along with a realistic attitude and plan has led to millions of adults successfully breaking the habit. Your cardiovascular health and risk for cancer begin to improve the day you quit.

Diet

Good nutrition affects a child's health in the present and influences habits that will affect cardiovascular health later on. Children's food preferences are influenced by many factors, such as what the family eats at home, what they see other children eat at child care or at school, and what television commercials "teach" them to eat. You cannot counteract all of these influences, of course, but encouraging good eating habits is the responsibility of all adult caregivers.

Most current nutritional research continues to support what we have known for some time: High-fat and high-sugar foods are unhealthy, and eating a variety of foods with an emphasis on fruits, vegetables and whole grains and cereals is healthy and promotes a normal weight. The federal government's 2015-2020 Dietary Guidelines for Americans are outlined in **Box 5-1.** In addition, certain dietary changes are recommended for specific population groups, such as older adults, pregnant women, overweight adults and others. Talk to your health care provider about changes that may be important for you.

In almost all instances, healthy alternatives to unhealthy foods and snacks are available that taste just as good. Choose low-fat frozen yogurt or frozen fruit bars rather than ice cream, skim or low-fat milk rather than whole milk, whole wheat bread rather than white bread and so on. This will help you set the stage for a lifetime of cardiovascular health.

Cholesterol

Cholesterol is a fatty substance the body needs to carry out important functions. Cholesterol is taken into the body from the diet, especially from foods high in animal fats, and it is manufactured in the liver. Hereditary factors also affect your cholesterol level. Because of these factors outside your control, you cannot assume you have a low blood cholesterol level just because you eat well.

High blood cholesterol levels are very common in the United States. About 71 million people, or a third of the population, have high levels of low-density lipoprotein (LDL), the *bad* type of cholesterol.[1] This is due in part to a generally poor diet and lack of exercise. Cholesterol affects cardiovascular health because it is deposited in the arteries along with other substances as plaque **(Figure 5-1).** A buildup of **plaque** leads to the condition called **atherosclerosis,** a narrowing and "hardening" of the arteries. Atherosclerosis in coronary arteries can cause a heart attack and in arteries in the brain can cause a stroke.

FIGURE 5-1

High blood cholesterol levels contribute to buildup of plaque inside arteries.

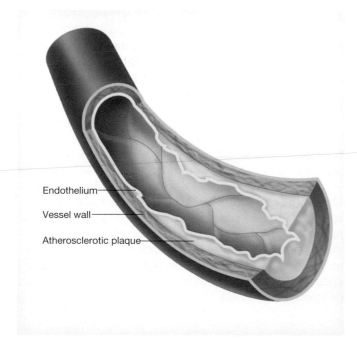

Endothelium
Vessel wall
Atherosclerotic plaque

Because high blood cholesterol levels double a person's risk for cardiovascular disease, adults need regular testing. Increasingly, pediatricians are testing children as well. Only a blood test can determine your cholesterol level.

If you are found to have high blood levels of LDL, you can take several steps to control this risk factor:

- Avoid high-cholesterol foods, such as animal fats.

- Maintain a healthy weight (cholesterol levels rise in overweight people).

- Get more exercise (cholesterol levels generally rise with inactivity). Make it your goal to get 30-60 minutes of exercise on most or all days of the week.

- Talk with your health care provider about whether a cholesterol-lowering medication is appropriate for you. If you do take a medication, do so consistently. For a variety of reasons, less than half of people prescribed these medications are still taking them a year later even though they still need them – perhaps because they feel fine. Remember that usually you can't feel the results of plaque building up in your arteries and threatening your health.

[1]*Centers for Disease Control and Prevention, cdc.gov/dhdsp/ data_statistics/fact_sheets/fs_cholesterol.htm Accessed January 2016.*

Exercise

It has become a cliché but is nonetheless true: Most children and adults do not get enough exercise. Almost 40% of the population reports no leisure-time physical activity at all, with many more not engaging in any activity regularly. Television, computer games and the Internet have contributed to children becoming more sedentary than decades ago. Adults often say they are too busy with work and family responsibilities to engage in activities that provide exercise.

Exercise is good not only for the muscles but for the heart, lungs and blood vessels. Like diet, exercise helps both adults and children be healthier now while building a foundation for future cardiovascular health and a longer, healthier, happier life. **Box 5-2** provides the federal recommendations for physical activity for different groups of people. Both children and adults get more exercise if it is fun. Almost all age-appropriate sports and energetic activities that children enjoy are good forms of cardiovascular exercise. Adults can choose from a full range of exercise programs developed for use at home or at a fitness center. Even brisk walking counts.

Consume a healthy eating pattern that accounts for all foods and beverages within an appropriate calorie level.

A healthy eating pattern includes:

- A variety of vegetables from all of the subgroups — dark green, red and orange, legumes (beans and peas), starchy and other

- Fruits, especially whole fruits

- Grains, at least half of which are whole grains

- Fat-free or low-fat dairy, including milk, yogurt, cheese and/or fortified soy beverages

- A variety of protein foods, including seafood, lean meats and poultry, eggs, legumes (beans and peas), and nuts, seeds and soy products

- Oils

A healthy eating pattern limits:

- Saturated fats and trans fats, added sugars and sodium

Key recommendations that are quantitative are provided for several components of the diet that should be limited. These components are of particular public health concern in the United States, and the specified limits can help individuals achieve healthy eating patterns within calorie limits:

- Consume less than 10% of calories per day from added sugars[1]

- Consume less than 10% of calories per day from saturated fats[2]

- Consume less than 2,300 milligrams (mg) per day of sodium[3]

- If alcohol is consumed, it should be consumed in moderation – up to one drink per day for women and up to two drinks per day for men – and only by adults of legal drinking age.[4]

Notes

[1]*The recommendation to limit intake of calories from added sugars to less than 10% per day is a target based on food pattern modeling and national data on intakes of calories from added sugars that demonstrate the public health need to limit calories from added sugars to meet food group and nutrient needs within calorie limits. The limit on calories from added sugars is not a Tolerable Upper Intake Level (UL) set by the Institute of Medicine (IOM). For most calorie levels, there are not enough calories available after meeting food group needs to consume 10% of calories from added sugars and 10% of calories from saturated fats and still stay within calorie limits.*

[2]*The recommendation to limit intake of calories from saturated fats to less than 10% per day is a target based on evidence that replacing saturated fats with unsaturated fats is associated with reduced risk of cardiovascular disease. The limit on calories from saturated fats is not a UL set by the IOM. For most calorie levels, there are not enough calories available after meeting food group needs to consume 10% of calories from added sugars and 10% of calories from saturated fats and still stay within calorie limits.*

[3]*The recommendation to limit intake of sodium to less than 2,300 mg per day is the UL for individuals ages 14 years and older set by the IOM. The recommendations for children younger than 14 years of age are the IOM age- and sex-appropriate ULs.*

[4]*It is not recommended that individuals begin drinking or drink more for any reason. The amount of alcohol and calories in beverages varies and should be accounted for within the limits of healthy eating patterns. Alcohol should be consumed only by adults of legal drinking age. There are many circumstances in which individuals should not drink, such as during pregnancy.*

Source: U.S. Departments of Health and Human Services (HHS) and of Agriculture (USDA), health. gov/dietaryguidelines/2015/guidelines/chapter-1/key-recommendations/ Accessed January 2016.

Adults who are presently out of shape, especially those older than 50 who have become sedentary, should talk to their health care provider before beginning an exercise program. Often it is best to begin slowly and gradually increase your workouts to a comfortable yet effective level.

As with other lifestyle changes, it is important to have a realistic attitude when beginning an exercise or fitness program. People often join a fitness club or purchase exercise equipment for home use, begin strenuously, and soon quit. A long-term commitment

is needed, developing a plan that realistically fits your lifestyle and personal interests.

Make physical activity a routine part of the day, not a special requirement at certain times. Everyone needs to think of physical activity as being as "normal" in their life as eating or sleeping, not something special to be done just when you feel like it or only to meet a specific weight goal. It is important to help children to develop this attitude, too.

BOX 5-2: PHYSICAL ACTIVITY GUIDELINES FOR AMERICANS

Key Guidelines for Children and Adolescents

- Children and adolescents should do 60 minutes (1 hour) or more of physical activity daily.

  - **Aerobic:** Most of the 60 or more minutes a day should be either moderate- or vigorous-intensity aerobic physical activity, and should include vigorous-intensity physical activity at least 3 days a week.

  - **Muscle-strengthening:** As part of their 60 or more minutes of daily physical activity, children and adolescents should include muscle-strengthening physical activity on at least 3 days of the week.

  - **Bone-strengthening:** As part of their 60 or more minutes of daily physical activity, children and adolescents should include bone-strengthening physical activity at least 3 days of the week.

- It is important to encourage young people to participate in physical activities that are appropriate for their age, that are enjoyable, and that offer variety.

Key Guidelines for Adults

- All adults should avoid inactivity. Some physical activity is better than none, and adults who participate in any amount of physical activity gain some health benefits.

- For substantial health benefits, adults should do at least 150 minutes (2 hours and 30 minutes) a week of moderate-intensity, or 75 minutes (1 hour and 15 minutes) a week of vigorous-intensity aerobic physical activity, or an equivalent combination of moderate- and vigorous-intensity aerobic activity. Aerobic activity should be performed in episodes of at least 10 minutes, and preferably, should be spread throughout the week.

- For additional and more extensive health benefits, adults should increase their aerobic physical activity to 300 minutes (5 hours) a week of moderate intensity, or 150 minutes a week of vigorous intensity aerobic physical activity, or an equivalent combination of moderate- and vigorous-intensity activity. Additional health benefits are gained by engaging in physical activity beyond this amount.

- Adults should also do muscle-strengthening activities that are moderate or high intensity and involve all major muscle groups on 2 or more days a week, as these activities provide additional health benefits.

Key Guidelines for Older Adults

The Key Guidelines for Adults also apply to older adults. In addition, the following Guidelines are just for older adults:

- When older adults cannot do 150 minutes of moderate-intensity aerobic activity a week because of chronic conditions, they should be as physically active as their abilities and conditions allow.

- Older adults should do exercises that maintain or improve balance if they are at risk of falling.

- Older adults should determine their level of effort for physical activity relative to their level of fitness.

- Older adults with chronic conditions should understand whether and how their conditions affect their ability to do regular physical activity safely.

Key Guidelines for Safe Physical Activity

To do physical activity safely and reduce the risk of injuries and other adverse events, people should:

- Understand the risks yet be confident that physical activity is safe for almost everyone.

- Choose to do types of physical activity that are appropriate for their current fitness level and health goals, because some activities are safer than others.

- Increase physical activity gradually over time whenever more activity is necessary to meet guidelines or health goals. Inactive people should "start low and go slow" by gradually increasing how often and how long activities are done.

- Protect themselves by using appropriate gear and sports equipment, looking for safe environments, following rules and policies, and making sensible choices about when, where, and how to be active.

- Be under the care of a health-care provider if they have chronic conditions or symptoms. People with chronic conditions and symptoms should consult their health-care provider about the types and amounts of activity appropriate for them.

5 • Cardiovascular Emergencies and Cardiopulmonary Resuscitation

BOX 5-2: PHYSICAL ACTIVITY GUIDELINES FOR AMERICANS (CONTINUED)

Key Guidelines for Women During Pregnancy and the Postpartum Period

- Healthy women who are not already highly active or doing vigorous-intensity activity should get at least 150 minutes of moderate-intensity aerobic activity a week during pregnancy and the postpartum period. Preferably, this activity should be spread throughout the week.

- Pregnant women who habitually engage in vigorous-intensity aerobic activity or who are highly active can continue physical activity during pregnancy and the postpartum period, provided that they remain healthy and discuss with their health-care provider how and when activity should be adjusted over time.

Key Guidelines for Adults with Disabilities

- Adults with disabilities, who are able to, should get at least 150 minutes a week of moderate-intensity, or 75 minutes a week of vigorous-intensity aerobic activity, or an equivalent combination of moderate- and vigorous-intensity aerobic activity. Aerobic activity should be performed in episodes of at least 10 minutes, and preferably, should be spread throughout the week.

- Adults with disabilities, who are able to, should also do muscle-strengthening activities of moderate or high intensity that involve all major muscle groups on 2 or more days a week, as these activities provide additional health benefits.

- When adults with disabilities are not able to meet the Guidelines, they should engage in regular physical activity according to their abilities and should avoid inactivity.

- Adults with disabilities should consult their health-care provider about the amounts and types of physical activity that are appropriate for their abilities.

Key Messages for People with Chronic Medical Conditions

- Adults with chronic conditions obtain important health benefits from regular physical activity.

- When adults with chronic conditions do activity according to their abilities, physical activity is safe.

- Adults with chronic conditions should be under the care of a health-care provider. People with chronic conditions and symptoms should consult their health-care provider about the types and amounts of activity appropriate for them.

Source: U.S. Department of Health and Human Services, health.gov/paguidelines/guidelines/summary.aspx Accessed January 2016.

WEIGHT CONTROL

Two-thirds of adults in the United States are overweight or obese by current standards. Overweight and obesity contribute to many other diseases in addition to cardiovascular disease. The National Institutes of Health reports[1]:

- More than 2 in 3 adults are considered to be overweight or obese.

- More than 1 in 3 adults are considered to be obese.

- More than 1 in 20 adults are considered to have extreme obesity.

- About one-third of children and adolescents ages 6-19 are considered to be overweight or obese.

- More than 1 in 6 children and adolescents ages 6-19 are considered to be obese.

[1]*National Institutes of Health, niddk.nih.gov/health-information/ health-statistics/Pages/overweight-obesity-statistics.aspx Accessed January 2016.*

Overweight and obesity are categorized in relation to a person's **body mass index (BMI),** a measure of weight in relation to a person's height. The higher the BMI number, the greater the percentage of fat in a person's body. Overweight is defined as a BMI of 25 to 30, and obesity is a BMI of 30 or higher. The chart in **Figure 5-2** provides an approximate BMI for adults based on height and weight.

The habits that lead to overweight start early in life. Prevention is a better approach than having to lose weight later on and keep it off. The earlier recommendations for diet and exercise, while promoting good health generally, are also the keys to preventing a weight problem from developing.

The cornerstones of all effective weight-loss programs combine a healthy diet with adequate physical activity, as detailed in the previous section. Many different programs have been developed, including a large number of programs that involve fad diets or dietary supplements that promise to burn off the fat. Research shows, however, that controlling caloric intake and getting exercise are the only factors that result in successfully losing weight and keeping it off. Like other major lifestyle changes, such as quitting smoking, weight control requires commitment, a realistic attitude and plan, and time and effort. An excellent starting point is talking with your health care provider to learn what kind of program will work best for you.

HIGH BLOOD PRESSURE

As noted earlier, about 70 million people in the United States have high blood pressure – and in many this condition is not controlled. Hypertension is often called the *silent killer* because in most people it causes no symptoms and the person can be completely unaware of having it. Yet hypertension is linked to high death rates caused by heart attack, stroke or other diseases.

Although in some cases hypertension is caused by an underlying condition that may be treated, in the great majority of cases it exists without a specific known cause that can be addressed. Hypertension is diagnosed by regular blood pressure tests. The current standards classify different levels of hypertension according to seriousness. Normal blood pressure is defined as a systolic pressure less than 120. Prehypertension is a systolic blood pressure of 120 to 139. Hypertension is 140 or above. By these standards, even those in the prehypertension category are at some risk and should take steps to control their blood pressure. Because blood pressure generally rises with age, it is now estimated that by age 55, adults have more than a 50% chance of being hypertensive – a percentage that rises more than 70% by age 75.[1]

[1]*Centers for Disease Control and Prevention, cdc.gov/ bloodpressure/facts.htm Accessed January 2016.*

Recommendations for controlling blood pressure involve both lifestyle changes and medications. For those with prehypertension, lifestyle changes alone are generally sufficient:

- Maintain a normal weight.

- Get more physical activity.

- Reduce salt intake.

Many individuals with hypertension will also need medication to lower their blood pressure. The risks of hypertension are among the reasons that everyone should have periodic physical examinations by a health care provider, who will give appropriate recommendations for controlling high blood pressure.

FIGURE 5-2 BODY MASS INDEX

	NORMAL						OVERWEIGHT					OBESE									
BMI	19	20	21	22	23	24	25	26	27	28	29	30	31	32	33	34	35	36	37	38	39
Height (inches)											BODY WEIGHT (pounds)										
58	91	96	100	105	110	115	119	124	129	134	138	143	148	153	158	162	167	172	177	181	186
59	94	99	104	109	114	119	124	128	133	138	143	148	153	158	163	168	173	178	183	188	193
60	97	102	107	112	118	123	128	133	138	143	148	153	158	163	168	174	179	184	189	194	199
61	100	106	111	116	122	127	132	137	143	148	153	158	164	169	174	180	185	190	195	201	205
62	104	109	115	120	126	131	136	142	147	153	158	164	169	175	180	186	191	196	202	207	213
63	107	113	118	124	130	135	141	146	152	158	163	169	175	180	186	191	197	203	208	214	220
64	110	116	122	128	134	140	145	151	157	163	169	174	180	186	192	197	204	209	215	221	227
65	114	120	126	132	138	144	150	156	162	168	174	180	186	192	198	204	210	216	222	228	234
66	118	124	130	136	142	148	155	161	167	173	179	186	192	198	204	210	216	223	229	235	241
67	121	127	134	140	146	153	159	166	172	178	185	191	198	204	211	217	223	230	236	242	249
68	125	131	138	144	151	158	164	171	177	184	190	197	203	210	216	223	230	236	243	249	256
69	128	135	142	149	155	162	169	176	182	189	196	203	209	216	223	230	236	243	250	257	283
70	132	139	146	153	160	167	174	181	188	195	202	209	216	222	229	236	243	250	257	264	271
71	136	143	150	157	165	172	179	186	193	200	208	215	222	229	236	243	250	257	265	272	279
72	140	147	154	162	169	177	184	191	199	206	213	221	228	235	242	250	258	265	272	279	287
73	144	151	159	166	174	182	189	197	204	212	219	227	235	242	250	257	265	272	280	288	295
74	148	155	163	171	179	186	194	202	210	218	225	233	241	249	256	264	272	280	287	295	303
75	152	160	168	176	184	192	200	208	216	224	232	240	248	256	264	272	279	287	295	303	311
76	156	164	172	180	189	197	205	213	221	230	238	246	254	263	271	279	287	295	304	312	320

Source: National Institutes of Health, nhlbi.nih.gov/health/educational/lose_wt/BMI/bmi_tbl.htm Accessed January 2016.

Stress

Stress is an emotional or mental state that is generally considered a risk factor for cardiovascular disease. Long-term, frequent stress is thought to have various negative effects on a person's physical health, although it is difficult for research studies to study the exact effects of stress because of issues of quantifying and measuring stress and separating this factor from other risk factors. Nonetheless, there is some evidence that excessive stress lowers the body's immune functions and has other negative effects, and that stress reduction in some cases has a positive benefit. Interestingly, some of the other healthy lifestyle decisions described previously, such as exercise and a good diet, also help one to control or reduce stress. Those who frequently feel stressed, however, would benefit from talking to their health care provider about programs for stress reduction.

Respiratory Emergencies

Any illness or injury that causes a victim to stop breathing, or to breathe so ineffectively that the body is not receiving enough oxygen, is a respiratory emergency. The two primary types of breathing emergencies are respiratory arrest and respiratory distress.

All body tissues need a continual supply of oxygen to function and to maintain life. As described in **Chapter 3,** the respiratory system, working primarily with the cardiovascular system, provides this needed oxygen. In the lungs, oxygen moves out of the air into the blood, which is then circulated throughout the body. Carbon dioxide, a waste product of cellular metabolism, is also picked up from the tissues by the blood and eliminated in the lungs. The functioning of the respiratory and cardiovascular systems also depends on the muscles of breathing and on the nervous system's control of breathing and the heartbeat. A problem in any of these areas can result in a respiratory emergency. For example:

- A physical obstruction in the airway, such as food blocking the pharynx, or immersion in water, can make it impossible for air to reach the lungs.

- An injury to the chest can penetrate the lungs and hinder the movement of air into and out of the lungs with breathing.

- Breathing in carbon monoxide from a faulty furnace or smoke from a fire can reduce the availability of oxygen in the lungs and cause less oxygen to be present in the blood for body tissues.

- A heart problem can result in insufficient blood being circulated in the body, reducing the amount of oxygen available for tissues.

- An electric shock can disrupt the nervous system's control of either breathing or the heartbeat, thereby disrupting the flow of oxygen to the body.

- A drug overdose or poisoning can depress nervous system control of breathing such that insufficient oxygen reaches body tissues.

These are just a few of the many ways in which respiratory emergencies may occur. Regardless of the cause, body cells begin to die soon after losing their oxygen supply. Brain cells are very susceptible to low levels of oxygen and begin to die as soon as 4 minutes after oxygen is cut off. Within 6 minutes brain damage is likely **(Figure 5-3).** Death is likely soon after.

FIGURE 5-3

Without oxygen, vital organs soon begin to die.

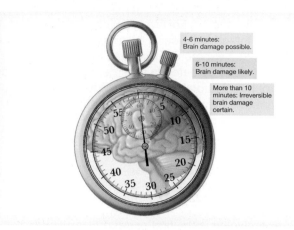

4-6 minutes: Brain damage possible.

6-10 minutes: Brain damage likely.

More than 10 minutes: Irreversible brain damage certain.

RESPIRATORY ARREST AND RESPIRATORY DISTRESS

Respiratory arrest means that breathing has completely stopped. Again, this condition may result from many different causes. You do not need to know the exact cause, however, because the BLS steps for respiratory arrest are the same in all cases.

With **respiratory distress,** on the other hand, the victim is still breathing, but the breathing is difficult and may become so ineffective that the victim's blood-oxygen content drops to a life-threatening level. Respiratory distress may occur with different illnesses and injuries. Someone with asthma, for example, may experience great difficulty breathing when tissues of the airway swell and make it difficult to move air into and out of the lungs. A severe allergic reaction may cause a similar problem.

The first aid for victims of respiratory distress is somewhat different because the victim is still breathing. In this case, care focuses on easing the breathing crisis and addresses the cause of the problem, if possible. Conditions causing respiratory distress are described in **Chapter 16.** Note, however, that respiratory distress can progress to respiratory arrest, in which case the victim needs CPR as described in this chapter.

PREVENTION OF RESPIRATORY ARREST

Respiratory arrest can be prevented by preventing its common causes, including drowning and sudden infant death syndrome (SIDS), as well as all general injury prevention measures. The prevention of choking, a common cause of respiratory arrest, is described in **Chapter 7.** Because breathing stops when the heart stops, preventing cardiac arrest also prevents respiratory arrest.

Preventing Drowning

Every year about 3,900 people in the United States die from drowning. About one in five of these are children under age 14. For every child who dies from drowning, another five receive emergency department care for nonfatal submersion injuries. More than 50% of drowning victims treated in emergency departments require hospitalization or transfer for further care. These nonfatal drowning injuries often cause severe brain damage caused by lack of oxygen during submersion or related factors, which may result in long-term disabilities.[1]

[1]Centers for Disease Control and Prevention,cdc.gov/ HomeandRecreationalSafety/Water-Safety/waterinjuries- factsheet.html Accessed January 2016.

Although drowning is the first or second leading cause of injury-related death for children ages 1-14 years old[2], most parents say they do not worry about their child drowning. This overconfidence and lack of concern is likely a significant factor in the poor supervision of children around water. Among children, the huge majority of drownings occur with an adult "supervising" but distracted by other factors.

The prevention of drowning is based on understanding the primary risk factors:

- Most infant victims drown in bathtubs, buckets or toilets. An infant should never be left unsupervised near water, even to a depth of an inch or two, for even a moment.

- Most victims 1-4 years old drown in residential swimming pools with one or both parents at home at the time – with the child usually out of sight for less than 5 minutes. Never leave a young child alone in or near the water, even if the child has had beginning swimming lessons or promises to stay out of the water in your absence. All children should be supervised by an adult who maintains continuous visual contact and does not engage in distracting activities such as talking on the telephone or reading. Pools should have protective barriers with effective locks. Parents should never trust floating toys, rafts or inner tubes to keep their children afloat.

- Up to half of drowning deaths in the age group with the most drownings, adolescents and adults, are associated with alcohol use during water recreational activities. Alcohol influences balance, coordination and judgment, which are key factors in situations that lead to drowning. Prevention is simple: Do not drink and go into or near the water. Swim with a buddy, never dive into shallow or unknown water and wear a life jacket during water sports.

- About 70% of the more than 500 annual boating deaths result from drowning, according to the Centers for Disease Control and Prevention. More than 90% of these drowning victims were not wearing a personal flotation device (PFD), and about 40% of cases involved alcohol. Following safe boating guidelines would have prevented most of these drowning deaths.[3]

[2]National Safety Council. (2015). Injury Facts®, 2015 Edition. Itasca, IL: Author.

[3]Centers for Disease Control and Prevention, cdc.gov/features/ boatingsafety Accessed December 2015.

PREVENTING SUID AND SIDS[4]

About 3,500 infants die each year of sudden unexpected infant death (SUID). This is the term for an infant death that cannot be explained, usually while the infant is sleeping, occurring most commonly between 2 and 4 months of age. Researchers cannot know how many of these deaths may occur from suffocation in soft bedding or another person rolling on top of or against a sleeping infant. Sudden infant death syndrome (SIDS) is the term for the sudden death of an infant of unexplained causes after a thorough Investigation including an autopsy. Of the 3,500 SUID deaths, about 1,500 occur from SIDS, which is the most common cause of infant death from 1 to 12 months of age.

[4]Centers for Disease Control and Prevention: cdc.gov/sids/ aboutsuidandsids.htm Accessed December 2015.

To reduce the risk of SIDS and suffocation:

- Always place infants on their backs to sleep. This step alone can lower the risk of SIDS by more than 50%.

- Use a firm, flat crib mattress that meets safety standards.

- Remove pillows, comforters, toys and other soft objects from the crib.

- Do not cover the infant's head during sleep.

- If a blanket must be used, use a thin blanket, tuck it under the edges of the mattress, and keep it at chest level and below to reduce the likelihood of the infant pulling it over his or her face.

- Avoid smoking. When a woman smokes during pregnancy, the infant is three times more likely to have SIDS, and an infant exposed to passive smoke has a much higher than normal risk.

- Avoid overheating during sleep; dress the infant in light sleep clothing and keep the room at a temperature that is comfortable for an adult.

- Do not have the infant sleep in a bed shared with siblings or parents. Experts recommend having the infant's crib beside the bed when parents wish to be close and to facilitate breastfeeding.

- Give an infant aged 1-12 months a clean, dry pacifier at bedtime.

Cardiac Chain of Survival

Any victim whose breathing or heart stops needs CPR. Cardiac arrest and respiratory arrest victims both need CPR. **Cardiac arrest** refers to a sudden stop in the beating of the heart. **Respiratory arrest** refers to a cessation of breathing, in which case cardiac arrest will also soon occur.

The **Cardiac Chain of Survival (Figure 5-4) emphasizes** the urgent need for quick, effective actions to save the lives of cardiac arrest victims. This chain has five crucial links:

1. **Recognition and activation of the emergency response system.** *Recognize that a victim whose heart has stopped needs help immediately!* It is also important that you recognize the signs and symptoms of a potential life-threatening condition, such as a heart attack or a stroke in a responsive person (see **Chapter 16**). Do not wait until a person becomes unresponsive to start the chain of events needed to keep him or her alive. Call 9-1-1 and get help on the way. The victim needs early access to advanced medical care.

2. **Immediate high-quality CPR.** For an unresponsive victim who is not breathing normally, start CPR immediately. This helps keep the brain and other vital organs supplied with oxygen until the AED arrives.

3. **Rapid defibrillation**. An AED, now present in many public and work places, can help get the heart beating normally again after a cardiac arrest. Send someone right away to get the AED.

4. **Basic and advanced emergency medical services.** The sooner the victim is treated by emergency care professionals, the better the chance for survival. You can help make sure the victim reaches this link in the chain by acting immediately with the earlier links.

5. **Advanced life support and post-arrest care.** Following early care, the victim needs continued advanced medical care by a team of medical professionals, typically within a hospital or other advanced medical center.

FIGURE 5-4

Cardiac Chain of Survival.

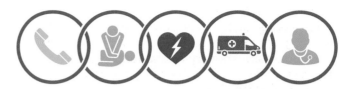

IF SOMEONE'S HEART STOPS, QUICK ACTION IS NEEDED!

Call First/Call Fast

In any situation in which you recognize that a victim of injury or illness is unresponsive, if someone else is present at the scene, have that person call for help immediately. Shout for anyone who may hear you, and have them get help or call 9-1-1 and go for an AED.

An unresponsive victim who is not breathing normally should generally be assumed to need an AED and EMS as soon as possible because of the likelihood of cardiac arrest. If you are alone and you have a cell phone or other mobile device, contact EMS immediately so that an AED and other emergency equipment and personnel can be on their way as soon as possible. At the same time, you can begin your simultaneous assessment for breathing and a pulse – in order to provide CPR right away.

When alone with an unresponsive victim likely to be in cardiac arrest, and you do not have a mobile device with which to call EMS, the priority is still to get EMS and an AED as soon as possible, even if you must leave the victim to call for help and get a nearby AED ("call first"). These victims are more likely to require defibrillation, and calling EMS *immediately* starts the process of getting an AED to the victim sooner.

With an unresponsive child or infant victim who was not seen to collapse suddenly, however, an airway obstruction is more likely than cardiac arrest, so provide about 5 cycles of CPR (about 2 minutes) before leaving the victim, if alone without a mobile device, to call EMS ("call fast").

For unresponsive victims whose circumstances suggest a likely asphyxial arrest, such as a drowning victim or a victim with an airway obstruction, call fast. Give about 5 cycles of CPR (about 2 minutes) before stopping to call EMS.

5 • Cardiovascular Emergencies and Cardiopulmonary Resuscitation

1. Select the best answer. CPR stands for –

    a. cardiac position for recovery.

    b. cardiopulmonary resuscitation.

    c. chest pump rescue.

    d. None of the above

2. Put a check mark next to risk factors for cardiovascular disease.

    ☐ Smoking

    ☐ Regular aspirin use

    ☐ High blood pressure

    ☐ Growing older

    ☐ High cholesterol levels

    ☐ Inactivity

    ☐ Family history of heart disease

    ☐ Working full-time

3. Fill in the correct answer. The first crucial link in the Cardiac Chain of Survival is

    _____ .

4. If alone without a cell phone, go to call for help (before starting CPR) for which of these victims? (Check all that apply.)

    ☐ Unresponsive adult not breathing normally

    ☐ Unresponsive infant not breathing normally

    ☐ Unresponsive child not breathing normally

CPR

CPR is used for all unresponsive victims who are not breathing normally. Remember that airway and respiratory problems can cause breathing to stop, followed by cardiac arrest. Cardiac arrest is also commonly caused by:

-   Heart attack or other heart disease

-   Drowning

-   Suffocation

-   Stroke

-   Allergic reaction

-   Diabetic emergency

-   Prolonged seizures

-   Drug overdose

-   Electric shock

-   Certain Injuries

You do not need to know the cause of cardiac or respiratory arrest, however, before starting CPR. The technique for CPR is the same regardless of cause.

CPR helps keep the victim alive by circulating some oxygenated blood to vital organs. Compressions on the **sternum** (breastbone) increase pressure inside the chest, resulting in movement of some oxygen-carrying blood to the brain and other tissues. Rescue breaths move oxygen into the lungs, where it is picked up by the blood. The circulation of blood resulting from CPR is not nearly as strong as the circulation from a heartbeat, but it can help keep brain and other tissues alive until a normal heart rhythm is restored. Often an electric shock from an AED (see **Chapter 6**) or other medical procedures called **advanced cardiac life support (ACLS)** are needed to restore a heartbeat – and CPR can keep the victim viable until then. In some instances, the heart may start again spontaneously with CPR.

CPR has been demonstrated to save lives in many circumstances. With the most common cause of cardiac arrest, a heart attack, CPR and defibrillation within 3-5 minutes after the victim collapses can save more than 50% of victims. Given that sudden out-of-hospital cardiac arrest occurs in about 900 people with heart disease every day, CPR and use of an AED could save many thousands of lives every year (American Heart Association, *2015 Heart Disease and Stroke Statistics Update*[1]). Remember that CPR is only one step in the cardiac chain of survival; however, in most cases of cardiac arrest, CPR only helps keep the victim alive until an AED and/or EMS professionals arrive at the scene.

[1]*American Heart Association, circ.ahajournals.org/content/131/4/ e29.extract Accessed January 2016.*

CHEST COMPRESSIONS IN CPR

The general technique of CPR involves alternating chest compressions and rescue breaths. After determining the victim is unresponsive and not breathing normally, start CPR with chest compressions followed by rescue breaths. For a victim of any age, these are the general steps of CPR:

1. Bare the chest and find the correct hand position on the lower half of the breastbone in the middle of the chest in adults and children **(Figure 5-5).** In infants, the position is just below the nipple line. For adults, place the heel of 1 hand in the correct position; then put the second hand on top of the first and interlock fingers. For children, depending on their size and your strength, use both hands or the heel of 1 hand. For infants, use 2 fingers.

2. Compress the chest hard and fast at a rate of 100-120 compressions per minute. Compressions in an adult should be at least 2 inches deep but not more than 2.4 inches. In an infant or child, compressions should be at least ⅓ the depth of the chest (about 1½ inches in an infant or about 2 inches in a child). Between compressions let the chest return to its normal height by taking your weight off your hands (do not lean on the chest), but do not remove your hands (or fingers for infants) from the chest.

3. Alternate 30 chest compressions and 2 rescue breaths for all victims. For all victims, give each breath over 1 second.

FIGURE 5-5

Proper placement for compressions.

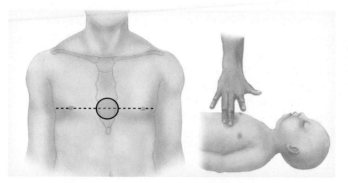

RESCUE BREATHS IN CPR

Giving rescue breaths is the technique of blowing air into a nonbreathing victim's lungs to oxygenate the blood. Rescue breaths are given along with chest compressions, which help circulate the oxygenated blood to vital organs, keeping the victim alive until the victim is resuscitated or EMS personnel arrive to give advanced care.

Rescue breaths are given with the first aider's own air unless special equipment is available. The air around us contains about 21% oxygen, and the breath we exhale contains about 16% oxygen – still enough oxygen to increase the oxygen level in the victim's blood to maintain life. When a first aider blows air into the victim's mouth or nose, this air moves into the lungs in a manner similar to natural breathing. The chest rises as the lungs expand, and oxygen moves into the blood in the small vessels within the lungs. After each breath, the chest is allowed to fall and the air is "exhaled" out, then the next breath is given.

Rescue breaths are given along with chest compressions to any victim who is not breathing normally. An unresponsive victim who is occasionally gasping is not breathing and needs CPR. Also have someone call 9-1-1 immediately. If an AED is available, send someone to get it (see **Chapter 6**).

TECHNIQUES FOR GIVING RESCUE BREATHS

After beginning CPR with 30 chest compressions, open the victim's airway to give 2 rescue breaths. This is done by tilting the head back and lifting the chin as shown in **Figure 5-6.** This is called the head tilt–chin lift. This position moves the tongue away from the opening into the throat to allow air to pass through the airway. Then you can give the rescue breaths.

FIGURE 5-6

Head tilt–chin lift.

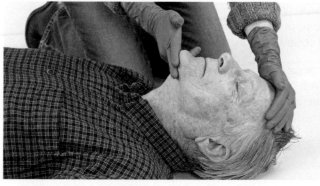

Use a barrier device, if you have one, to protect against disease transmission, but do not delay giving rescue breaths to get one. Even without a barrier device the risk of contracting an infectious disease from rescue breathing is very low.

The basic technique is to blow air slowly into the victim while watching the chest rise to make sure your air is going into the lungs. Do not try to rush the air in or blow too forcefully. Do not take a big breath in order to exhale more air into the victim; just take a normal breath. Give each breath over about 1 second. If the breath does not go in – if you feel resistance or do not see the victim's chest rise – then try again to open the airway. If your breath still does not go in, then the victim has an airway obstruction and needs care for choking (see **Chapter 7**). If your initial breath does go in, give a second breath over 1 second and then resume chest compressions.

Remember these key points:

- Do not blow harder than is needed to make the victim's chest rise.

- After each breath, remember to let the air escape and the chest fall.

- Blowing in too forcefully or for too long is ineffective and may put air in the stomach, which may cause vomiting.

- Avoid excessive ventilation (too many breaths or too large a volume) during CPR.

Mouth to Barrier

Barrier devices are always recommended for giving rescue breaths and should be kept in the first aid kit **(Figure 5-7)**. The two most common types of barrier devices are pocket masks and face shields. Both types of devices offer protection from the victim's saliva and other fluids, as well as from the victim's exhaled air when equipped with a one-way valve. With either device, keep the victim's head positioned to maintain an open airway as you deliver rescue breaths through the device.

A pocket mask is positioned on the victim's face over both the mouth and nose. A one-way valve in the mouthpiece lets your air flow into the victim but directs the victim's exhaled air out another way so that it does not reach you directly during rescue breathing. With a face mask, as with any barrier device, make sure it is well sealed to the victim's face, and watch the victim's chest rise to confirm that your air is going into the victim.

A face shield is also positioned over the victim's mouth as a protective barrier. The victim's nose is pinched closed when giving a rescue breath to prevent the air from coming out the nose instead of entering the lungs.

FIGURE 5-7

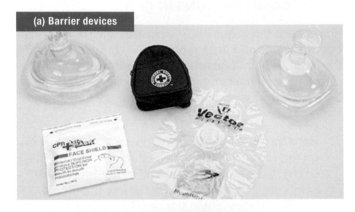
(a) Barrier devices

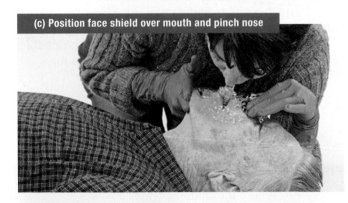
(b) Position pocket mask over mouth and nose

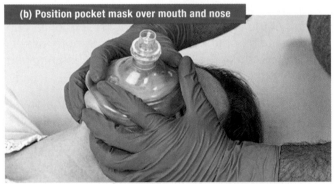
(c) Position face shield over mouth and pinch nose

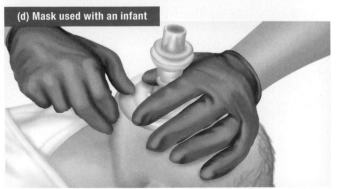
(d) Mask used with an infant

Mouth-to-Mouth

If you do not have a barrier device, pinch the victim's nose shut and seal your mouth over the victim's mouth. Blow into the victim's mouth, watching the chest rise to confirm that the air is going in.

Mouth-to-Nose

If the victim's mouth cannot be opened or is injured, or if you cannot get a good seal with your mouth over the victim's mouth, you can give rescue breaths through the nose. Hold the victim's mouth closed, seal your mouth over the nose to blow in, and then allow the mouth to open to let the air escape.

Mouth-to-Stoma

Because of past illness or injury, some people breathe through a hole in their lower neck called a **stoma (Figure 5-8).** In the initial assessment, check this hole to see if the victim is breathing normally. To give rescue breaths through a stoma, cup your hand over the victim's nose and mouth to prevent your air from leaving by the nose and mouth instead of going to the lungs. Then seal your mouth over the stoma, and give rescue breaths as usual. Or you can use a round pediatric face mask if you have one.

FIGURE 5-8

Victim with a stoma.

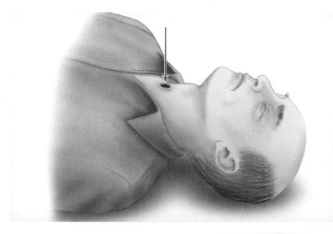

Mouth-to-Nose-and-Mouth

Because of their smaller size, infants and very small children are generally given rescue breaths through both their mouth and nose. Seal your mouth over both the nose and mouth and give gentle breaths as usual, watching to see the chest rise with each breath.

RESCUE BREATHS FOR INFANTS

Rescue breathing for infants is similar to that for adults and children, with these differences:

- Gently tilt the head back to open the airway and check breathing – do not overextend the neck.

- If no barrier device is available, cover both mouth and nose with your mouth to give breaths. (Use the mouth or nose only if you cannot cover both.)

SPECIAL CIRCUMSTANCES FOR RESCUE BREATHS

In some circumstances you may have to adjust how you give rescue breaths, including a victim vomiting, a victim wearing dentures, and a victim with facial injuries.

Vomiting

In some cases, the air provided with rescue breaths may move into the stomach rather than the lungs. If the airway is not sufficiently open, if rescue breaths are given too quickly, or if you continue to blow in air even after the lungs have expanded and the chest has risen, air may be forced into the stomach. In this situation, not only is the victim possibly not receiving enough air in the lungs to oxygenate the blood, but the air in the stomach makes vomiting more likely. Vomiting presents two problems. First, if an unresponsive victim vomits during BLS care, you have to roll the victim onto his or her side to drain the victim's mouth, and then wipe the mouth clean before continuing. The time required to do this takes time away from the chest compressions of CPR, which are essential for moving oxygenated blood to vital organs. Second, when the victim vomits there is a risk of aspiration, which is the movement of vomit or other fluids or solids into the lungs, which can cause a serious infection and other problems. For these reasons, when giving rescue breaths be sure to:

- Open the airway first.

- Watch the chest rise as you give breaths.

- Blow slowly and steadily rather than too quickly.

- Stop each breath when the chest rises rather than continuing to blow.

- Let the chest fall between breaths.

Dentures

A victim's dentures are usually left in place during rescue breathing. If they are loose and make it difficult to give breaths or may fall back in the mouth and block the airway, remove dentures before giving rescue breaths.

Facial Injuries

If the victim's mouth cannot be opened or is injured, or if you cannot get a good seal with your mouth over the victim's mouth, you can give rescue breathing through the nose. Hold the victim's mouth closed, seal your mouth over the nose to blow in, and then allow the mouth to open to let the air escape.

Note: A victim with injuries may have blood in the mouth, which needs to be drained before giving rescue breathing. If suction equipment is available and you are trained in its use, you may suction either blood or vomit from the victim's mouth (see **Appendix A**).

 LEARNING CHECKPOINT 3

1. Select the best answer. Rescue breaths are needed to –

   a. get oxygen into the victim's blood.

   b. circulate the blood to vital organs.

   c. open the victim's airway.

   d. All of the above

Circle **True** or **False** for the following statement:

2. Blow as hard as you can into the victim's mouth during rescue breathing.

   True   False

3. What is the best way to confirm that your breaths are going into the victim's lungs? Select the best answer.

   a. Listen at the victim's mouth for escaping air.

   b. Place one hand on the victim's abdomen to feel movement.

   c. Watch the victim's chest rise and fall.

   d. None of the above

4. Fill in the correct answer:
   When giving rescue breaths, give each breath over _____ second(s).

TECHNIQUE OF CPR FOR ADULTS AND CHILDREN

See the Skill: "CPR for Adults, Children, and Infants" (1 Rescuer) for the steps for combining chest compressions with rescue breaths in CPR for adults and children.

COMPRESSION-ONLY CPR

An unresponsive victim who is not breathing normally needs both rescue breaths and chest compressions to move oxygenated blood to vital organs. However, if for any reason you cannot or will not give rescue breaths, you should still give the victim chest compressions. This gives the victim a better chance for survival than doing nothing.

STEP 1

Activate the emergency response system. Determine that the unresponsive victim is not breathing normally.

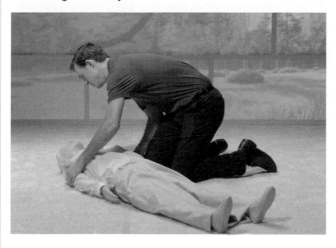

STEP 2

Expose the chest. Put your hand on the lower half of the breastbone in the middle of the chest for chest compressions. For an adult, put your second hand on top of the first and interlock the fingers. For a child, use 1 or both hands. For an infant, put your 2 middle fingers of 1 hand just below the nipple line.

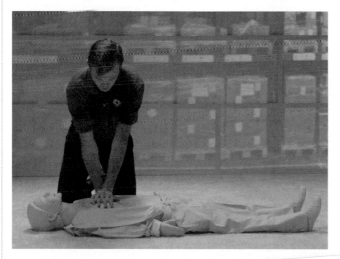

STEP 3

Give 30 chest compressions hard and fast at least 2 inches deep in an adult (but not more than 2.4 inches) and at least ⅓ the depth of the chest in an infant (about 1½ inches) or child (about 2 inches) at a rate of 100-120 per minute. Count aloud for a steady fast rate: "One, two, three..." Then give 2 breaths.

STEP 4

Open the airway and give 2 rescue breaths, each lasting 1 second, to cause a visible chest rise. (If the first breath does not go in, reposition the victim's head and try again; if the second breath still does not go in, give choking care (see **Chapter 7**).

STEP 5

Continue cycles of 30 compressions and 2 breaths.

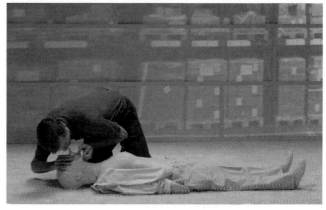

STEP 6

Continue CPR until:

- The victim wakes up and is breathing normally.

- An AED is brought to the scene and Is ready to use.

- Personnel with more training arrive and take over.

- If the victim starts breathing normally but is unresponsive, put the victim in the recovery position and monitor breathing.

STEP 7

When an AED arrives and is ready to be used, start the AED sequence for a victim who is not breathing normally.

5 • Cardiovascular Emergencies and Cardiopulmonary Resuscitation

Chest Compressions

- Be careful with your hand position for chest compressions. Keep fingers off the chest (except the 2 fingers for an infant).

- Do not give compressions over the bottom tip of the breastbone.

- When compressing, keep your elbows straight and keep your hands in contact with the chest at all times.

- Remember to compress the chest hard and fast, but let the chest recoil completely between compressions. Do not lean on the chest.

- Minimize the amount of time used giving rescue breaths between sets of compressions.

- Performing chest compressions only is called Hands-Only (compression-only) CPR. It can be used by any bystander to treat adult victims of out-of-hospital, cardiac arrest.

BOX 5-3: PROBLEMS WITH CPR TECHNIQUE

It is well known that CPR saves lives and that CPR training is needed to effectively use this procedure. CPR is taught in the classroom using manikins, of course, and thus the skill is typically learned in ideal circumstances rather than real-life situations, which may be very different. It is often difficult to evaluate the effectiveness of CPR given in the field because of the many variables that determine victim outcome.

Studies have shown two key problems in the chest compression technique of many rescuers. Often compressions are not delivered steadily and constantly at all times during the resuscitation efforts. Equally important, compressions are often too shallow, resulting in ineffective blood flow.

Studies have also shown that only high-quality CPR improves the victim's chances of survival. The quality depends mostly on giving chest compressions at the correct rate and depth.

This research clearly indicates the importance of performing CPR as learned – especially the depth and rate of chest compressions. Understanding the importance of these factors should help first aiders remember to focus on their technique in order to provide the quality CPR the victim needs to survive.

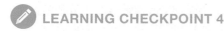 **LEARNING CHECKPOINT 4**

1. When is it appropriate to start CPR? Select the best answer.

   a. As soon as you determine the victim is unresponsive.

   b. As soon as you determine the victim is not breathing normally.

   c. As soon as you determine the victim is both unresponsive and not breathing normally.

   d. Only when you have called 9-1-1 and the dispatcher tells you to start CPR.

2. Describe how to find the site for chest compressions in an adult or child victim.

   _____

   _____

   _____

3. Fill in the correct answers: Chest compressions in an adult should be at least _____ inches deep but not more than _____ inches deep. In an infant or child, compress to a depth of at least _____ of the chest depth.

4. What is the correct ratio of chest compressions to breaths in single-rescuer CPR? Select the best answer.

   a. 15 to 1

   b. 15 to 2

   c. 30 to 1

   d. 30 to 2

5. If you are performing CPR on an adult victim when an AED is brought to the scene and is ready to use, what action should you take? Select the best answer.

   a. Use the AED as soon as it is ready.

   b. Continue CPR for at least 15 cycles before using the AED.

   c. Use the AED only if you can feel the victim's heart quivering in his or her chest.

   d. Use the AED only if the victim showed signs and symptoms of having a heart attack; otherwise, do not use it but continue CPR.

 CONCLUDING THOUGHTS

Remember to check for normal breathing in any unresponsive victim. If an unresponsive victim is gasping or is not breathing normally, give CPR beginning with chest compressions. Remember also that, as important as CPR is for sustaining life, in many cases of cardiac arrest the victim also needs defibrillation to restore a normal heartbeat. The use of an AED, the final step for lay rescuers in basic life support, is described in **Chapter 6.**

 ADDITIONAL ACTIVITIES AND RESOURCES

Much research has been conducted in the last decade into the effectiveness of CPR and the problems of poor CPR technique. You might research such studies on the Internet and report your findings to the class. This helps emphasize the crucial importance of using good technique when providing CPR.

 REVIEW QUESTIONS

Select the best answers.

1. Preventable risk factors for cardiovascular disease include –

   a. smoking.

   b. high cholesterol levels.

   c. inactivity.

   d. All of the above

2. For the purposes of CPR, when does an infant become a child?

   a. At 6 months

   b. At 1 year

   c. At 15 pounds

   d. At 25 pounds

3. Call 9-1-1 first before beginning CPR for –

   a. an unresponsive adult who is not breathing normally.

   b. an unresponsive child or infant who is not breathing normally.

   c. a responsive adult.

   d. a responsive child or infant.

4. The correct hand position for chest compressions in adults is –

   a. on the top of the breastbone below the neck.

   b. on the lower end of the breastbone just above the abdomen.

   c. on the lower half of the breastbone in the middle of the chest.

   d. three finger-widths above where the ribs join.

5. How long should it take to deliver one rescue breath?

   a. ½ second

   b. 1 second

   c. 1½ seconds

   d. 2 seconds

6. Why should a barrier device be used with rescue breaths?

   a. To help get more air into the victim

   b. To prevent vomiting

   c. To protect against infectious disease

   d. To prevent air from entering the esophagus

7. Vomiting during rescue breaths may result from –

   a. blowing in too forcefully.

   b. blowing in for too long.

   c. blowing in too fast.

   d. All of the above

8. The correct ratio of chest compressions to breaths in single-rescuer CPR is –

   a. 5 to 2.

   b. 10 to 2.

   c. 15 to 2.

   d. 30 to 2.

9. If a victim begins breathing normally after you have given CPR but remains unresponsive, what do you do?

   a. Put the victim in the recovery position.

   b. Continue chest compressions and rescue breaths.

   c. Continue giving only chest compressions.

   d. Give rescue breaths only.

10. When should you send someone to bring an AED to the scene when you encounter an unresponsive adult?

   a. As soon as you see the victim is unresponsive

   b. As soon as the 9-1-1 dispatcher tells you to

   c. After 1 minute of CPR

   d. It depends on the cause of the victim's condition

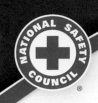

CHAPTER 6

Automated External Defibrillators (AEDs)

LESSON OBJECTIVES

- Explain how AEDs work to correct an abnormal heart rhythm.

- Describe when an AED should be used and the basic steps for use.

- Demonstrate how to use an AED with an adult, child or infant victim.

- List special considerations to be aware of when using an AED with certain types of victims or situations.

You are called to the scene where a man is lying unresponsive on the floor. Someone has already called 9-1-1. You know where an AED is located in the building, and you send someone for it as you check the victim for normal breathing. The victim is not breathing, and you begin CPR starting with chest compressions. About 1 minute later, the other person returns with an AED and first aid kit. What series of actions should you now take?

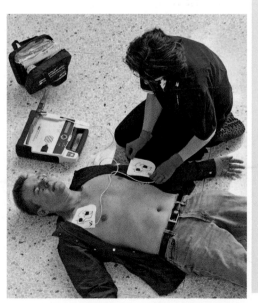

Not every victim who receives BLS needs an AED, but many do. In many cases of cardiac arrest, the victim's heart has an abnormal rhythm that does not circulate the blood, and this rhythm can often be corrected with the AED. Remember the Cardiac Chain of Survival: AED should be used with any unresponsive victim who is not breathing or only gasping. The early use of an AED for a heart attack victim doubles the chances for survival, and the American Heart Association estimates that the widespread availability and use of AEDs could save the lives of many thousands of people every year in the United States.[1]

[1]*American Heart Association. http://cpr.heart.org/idc/groups/ heart-public/@wcm/@ecc/documents/downloadable/ ucm_456455.pdf Accessed January 2016*

Public Access to AEDs

To give a victim of cardiac arrest the best chance for resuscitation, CPR and **defibrillation** must begin as soon as possible. Ideally, an AED should reach the victim within minutes. All ambulances and many other emergency responders, such as police officers, carry AEDs and reach the scene quickly after 9-1-1 is called, but the availability of AEDs in public places where people may experience heart attacks helps ensure that a unit is present when needed by a trained first aider or first responder. Public access to defibrillation (PAD) programs has worked to make AEDs available in workplaces, public gathering places and other facilities for use by trained rescuers and first aiders. Signs indicating where AEDs are located are becoming increasingly more visible in public places **(Figure 6-1)**. Many states have laws requiring AEDs to be present in various public places.

In many areas, a health care provider oversees the placement and use of the AED as well as AED training. For professional rescuers, this is called medical direction. Your course instructor will inform you how to meet any legal requirements in your area for using an AED. The Food and Drug Administration approves nonprescription AEDs for home use, and AED units that do not require specific training are present in homes and other settings. These devices have been demonstrated to be safe for use by lay people who follow the instructions printed on the device and the device's voice prompts during use. AED training will always offer benefits, but AEDs are generally simple and safe to use.

FIGURE 6-1

AEDs are increasingly common in public places.

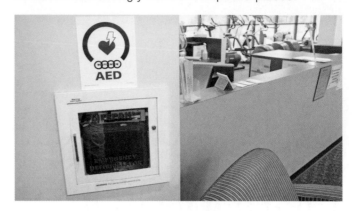

The Heart's Electrical System

The heart pumps blood to the lungs to pick up oxygen, and then pumps oxygenated blood to all parts of the body. The heart consists of 4 chambers: the left atrium, the right atrium and the left and right ventricles. The ventricles, which are the lower chambers of the heart, do most of the pumping. The heart's electrical system keeps the 4 chambers of the heart synchronized and working together. The sinoatrial (sinus) and atrioventricular (AV) nodes help organize and control the rhythmic electrical impulses that keep the heart beating properly **(Figure 6-2)**.

With a heart attack or other heart problems, this rhythmic electrical control may be disrupted, causing an abnormal heart rhythm such as ventricular fibrillation.

VENTRICULAR FIBRILLATION

Ventricular fibrillation (V-fib) is an abnormal heart rhythm that commonly occurs with heart attacks and stops circulation of the blood. Although we say a victim in V-fib is in cardiac arrest, the heart is not actually completely still but is beating abnormally. **Fibrillation** means the ventricles of the heart are quivering instead of beating rhythmically. Blood is not filling the ventricles and is not being pumped out to the lungs or body as usual.

Heart attack is the most common cause of cardiac arrest, and V-fib is a common arrhythmia that may result from heart attack, electrocution, hypothermia,

FIGURE 6-2

The heart's electrical system.

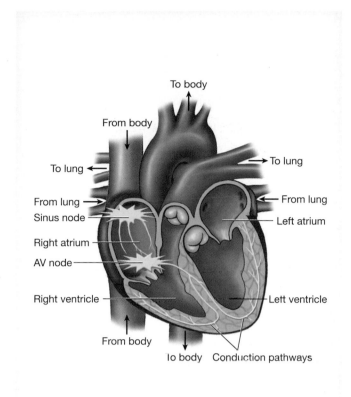

FIGURE 6-3

An AED gives a shock to the heart.

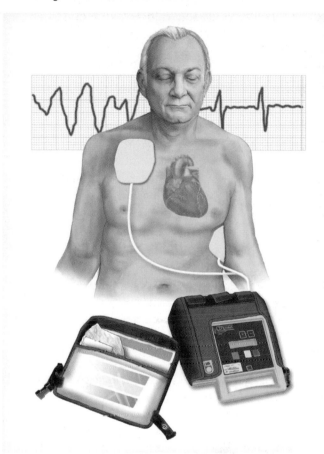

trauma and other causes. Studies show that in approximately half the cases of cardiac arrest, the victim's heart is in fibrillation, and therefore, would benefit from a shock delivered by the AED.

How AEDs Work

The AED automatically checks the victim's heart rhythm and advises whether the victim needs a shock. The pads placed on the victim's chest are connected by cables to the main unit, which contains wires through which an electrical current passes.

The pads monitor the heart's electrical activity, and the unit determines whether an abnormal rhythm is present for which a shock is needed. If the victim's heart is in V-fib, the machine will advise giving an electric shock to return the heart to a normal rhythm. This is called defibrillation, or stopping the fibrillation of the heart **(Figure 6-3).**

The AED's **electrodes**, or pads, are placed on the victim's chest (or, with some AED models, on the front and back of the chest of a small child). When the unit delivers a shock, electricity travels through the cables to the pads, then through the body to the heart, and "jolts" the heart's electrical system in an attempt to restore a normal heartbeat. Because electrical current passes through the pads, it is important to position them correctly on the body and to avoid water, metal and any other substance that conducts electricity.

AEDs are simple to use, but they must be used right away. With every minute that goes by before defibrillation begins, the victim's chances for survival drop by about 10%.

THE AED UNIT

AEDs are complex inside despite their ease of use. They contain a battery and are portable.

Some models have a screen that tells you what to do; all models give directions in a clear voice. AED models vary somewhat in other features, but all work in the same basic way **(Figure 6-4).**

FIGURE 6-4

A variety of AEDs.

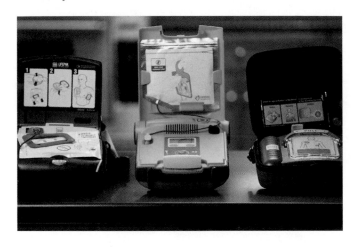

 LEARNING CHECKPOINT 1

Circle **True** or **False** for each of the following statements:

1. An AED works by giving a shock to a fibrillating heart to restore it to a normal rhythm. **True** **False**

2. It is very risky to use an AED because the unit cannot tell whether the victim's heart is beating normally or not. **True** **False**

3. About what proportion of cardiac arrest victims are in fibrillation and require a shock?

_____

Using an AED

In any situation in which a victim suddenly collapses or is found unresponsive, be thinking about the possibility of cardiac arrest even as you approach. If someone else is present and you know an AED is available nearby, send that person to call 9-1-1 and get the AED. It is better to have it right away and not use it than to need it and have to wait for it.

DETERMINE THE NEED FOR AED

As always, with any unresponsive victim, send someone to call 9-1-1 and to get an AED. If the victim is not breathing normally, you will need to use the AED.

START CPR

Remember BLS and the Cardiac Chain of Survival. Give CPR until the AED arrives at the scene and is ready to use. If you arrive at the victim with an AED, check the victim for normal breathing and then use the AED immediately on a victim before starting CPR. If another rescuer is present, one should begin CPR while the other sets up the device. Continue CPR until the unit is ready to analyze the victim's heart rhythm, and then stop and follow the unit's instructions.

ATTACH AED PADS TO VICTIM

Be sure the victim is not in water or in contact with metal. Water and metal conduct electricity that may pose a risk to you or others. Place the AED near the victim's shoulder next to the rescuer who will operate it. Turn it on, and attach the pads (electrodes) to the victim's chest. Most AED units have a diagram on the pads or the unit itself to remind you where to position the pads **(Figure 6-5).** Typically, the first pad is placed on the right side below the collar bone and to the right of the breastbone. The second pad is placed below and to the left of the left nipple and above the lower rib margin. On an infant or small child, the AED unit may indicate to position the pads on the front and back of the chest instead. If you have only adult pads, use them on the infant or child because this is their only hope; position the pads on the front and back of the chest if they would be too close together on the anterior chest and possibly cause an electrical arc between them.

Attach the AED pads to the victim only if the victim is unresponsive and not breathing. Expose the victim's chest, and dry the skin with a towel or dry clothing (heart attack victims are often sweating). If the victim has heavy chest hair, quickly shave the pad areas. If a razor is not available, use scissors or trauma shears (which should be kept with the AED) to trim the hair and allow skin contact with the pads. Remove the backing from the pads and apply the pads firmly on the victim's chest. If required with your AED model, plug the pad cables into the main unit.

FIGURE 6-5

AED pads usually include diagrams showing correct pad placement.

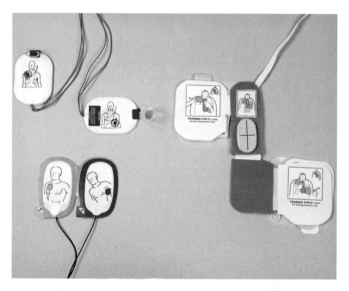

ANALYZE AND SHOCK

With the pads in place and the AED unit on, most AED models then automatically analyze the victim's heart rhythm. Do not move or touch the victim while it is analyzing. After it analyzes the heart rhythm, the unit will advise you whether to give a shock or to resume CPR. If a shock is advised, be sure no one is touching the victim. Look up and down the victim and say, "Everybody clear!" Once everyone is clear, administer the shock (when advised) or stay clear as the AED automatically gives the shock. After the shock, immediately resume CPR, beginning

with chest compressions, until the AED prompts to analyze the victim's heart rhythm again, usually after about 2 minutes. Then, the AED will advise another shock if needed or prompt you to continue CPR (with the pads left in place).

Note that different AEDs may use slightly different prompts. Follow the unit's voice and visual prompts through this process. Some units are programmed to administer the shock automatically rather than prompt the user to push the shock button; in this case, always follow the unit's prompts.

If the victim recovers (moves and is breathing normally), put an unresponsive breathing victim in the recovery position (who has not experienced trauma, especially a neck, back, hip or pelvic injury) and continue to monitor his or her breathing. Keep the AED pads in place as some victims may return to V-fib and require defibrillation again.

The AED may also say no shock is indicated. This means the victim's heart will not benefit from defibrillation. If this is so, immediately continue CPR (see Skill: "Using an AED").

STEP 1

Position the victim away from water and metal. Place the unit by the victim's shoulder and turn it on.

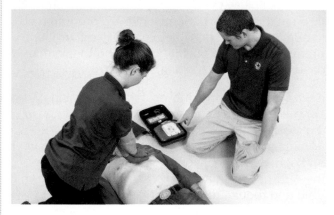

STEP 2

Expose the victim's chest, and quickly dry or shave the pad placement area if necessary.

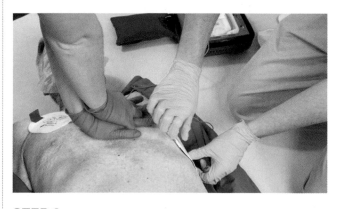

STEP 3

Apply the pads to the victim's chest as shown on the pads. If needed, plug the cables into the unit. Use adult pads for a victim 8 or older. For an infant or child younger than 8, use pediatric pads if available, applied as directed by the unit; if pediatric pads are unavailable, use adult pads.

STEP 4

Stay clear during rhythm analysis.

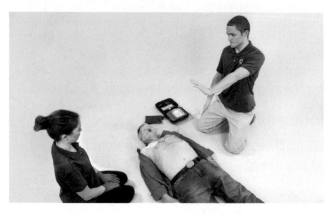

STEP 5

Follow prompts from the AED unit to do 1 of 3 things: (1) Press the shock button, (2) stay clear while the AED automatically delivers a shock or (3) do not shock but immediately give CPR with the pads remaining in place, starting with chest compressions.

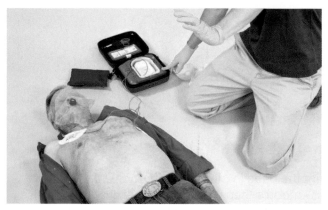

STEP 6

Follow the AED's prompts to analyze the rhythm again after 5 cycles of CPR (about 2 minutes).

STEP 7

Continue Steps 5 and 6 until the victim wakes up or more advanced help arrives and takes over.

STEP 8

If the victim begins breathing normally but is unresponsive, put the victim (if no trauma to the neck, back, hip or pelvis) in the recovery position (with pads remaining in place) and continue to monitor breathing and pulse.

- Move the victim away from metal or standing water before using the AED.

- Remove any medication pads with a gloved hand, and dry the victim's chest well before attaching the electrodes.

- Avoid any flammable materials, including oxygen flowing through a mask. Do not use alcohol to wipe the victim's skin.

- Do not use the AED when in motion in a vehicle or boat.

- Do not use a cell phone or 2-way radio within 6 feet of the AED.

- Remember not to touch the victim while the AED is analyzing the rhythm or administering a shock.

LEARNING CHECKPOINT 2

1. Which statement is true about the pads (electrodes) of an AED? Select the best answer.

   a. The AED has 2 pads that must be correctly positioned.

   b. The AED has 4 pads that must be correctly positioned.

   c. The AED has 2 pads, but only one needs to be put on the victim's chest (the other is a spare).

   d. The pads are used only if a heart rhythm is not detected when the machine is placed in the center of the victim's chest.

2. If the AED unit advises you to give a shock, what do you do next? Select the best answer.

   a. Continue CPR while asking someone else to push the shock button.

   b. Place a wet towel over the victim's chest and push the shock button.

   c. Make sure everyone is clear of the victim and then push the shock button.

   d. Wait about 1 minute for the unit to confirm analysis of a shockable rhythm.

3. What do you do immediately after the AED administers a shock?

Special Considerations

Some situations involve special considerations in the use of the AED.

AED USE IN CHILDREN

AEDs are designed and recommended to be used for both children and infants. Follow the adult guidelines for children older than 8.

Although sudden cardiac arrest in younger children is more rare, it can occur from causes such as:

- Sudden infant death syndrome

- Poisoning

- Drowning

- A heart problem

Most AED units can be used with children and infants, using different pads specially designed for children and infants **(Figure 6-6).** It is important to use only approved pediatric AED electrode pads when available, which are smaller than those for adults and produce lower-energy shocks on a child younger than 8. Usually, the pads have a distinctive appearance to prevent confusing adult and pediatric pads, such as pink connectors and teddy-bear emblems. If pediatric pads are not available, however, using adult pads is better than not using the AED at all. Pediatric pads should not be used for an adult, however, because the lower energy is insufficient to affect the heart rhythm.

Be sure to follow the device's instructions for pad placement on a small child. For example, the pediatric pads shown on the right in **Figure 6-6** should be placed on the front and back of the child's chest. Testing has demonstrated that with small children, it can be difficult to position both of the pads on the front of the chest, and studies have shown that placement on the front and back also delivers an effective shock.

FIGURE 6-6

The pads on the left are adult pads, while the pads on the right are for pediatric use.

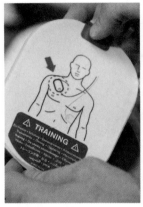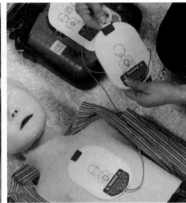

INTERNAL PACEMAKER OR DEFIBRILLATOR

When you expose the victim's chest to apply the AED pads, you may see a bulge or lump beneath the victim's skin from an implanted **pacemaker** or defibrillator, often on the upper left side of the chest **(Figure 6-7)**. Do not place a pad directly over this area, but instead, place it at least 1 or more inches away. If the victim's chest or body is jerking, there may be an implanted defibrillator that is giving shocks; wait until jerking has ended before applying the pads. Even if you suspect that an implanted defibrillator has activated, still apply the external AED after jerking has ended; if the internal defibrillator has malfunctioned, a shock from the external AED may be needed.

FIGURE 6-7

Vary AED pad placement if the victim has an implanted device.

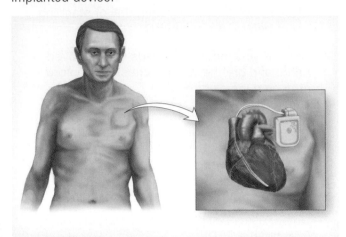

HYPOTHERMIA VICTIMS

Detecting breathing in a victim of hypothermia (low body temperature) can be difficult. Handle a hypothermic victim very carefully because jarring may cause cardiac arrest.

MEDICATION PATCH ON CHEST

If the victim has a medication patch or paste on the chest, remove it with a gloved hand and wipe the chest before applying the AED pads **(Figure 6-8)**.

FIGURE 6-8

Remove medication patches prior to AED use.

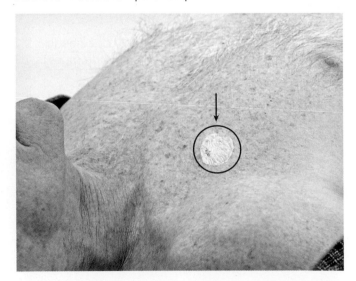

Potential AED Problems

An AED must be maintained regularly and the battery kept charged. With regular maintenance, an AED should not have any problems during use.

The AED may also prompt you to avoid problems. If you get a low-battery prompt, change the battery before continuing. Another prompt may advise you to avoid moving the victim if the AED detects motion.

AED Maintenance

AEDs require regular maintenance. Check the manufacturer's manual for periodic scheduled maintenance and testing of the unit.

A daily inspection of the unit helps ensure that the AED is always ready for use and all needed supplies are present. Professional rescuers usually inspect the unit at the beginning of their shift. Most facilities with an AED use a daily checklist form **(Figure 6-9).** A checklist should always be adapted for the specific AED model, including the manufacturer's daily maintenance guidelines. In addition, many units come with a simulator device used to check that the AED is correctly analyzing rhythms and delivering shocks; this may be part of the daily inspection routine.

FIGURE 6-9

Example of an AED inspection checklist.

AED INSPECTION CHECKLIST

Date: _____ Location: _____ AED Model: _____

Inspected by: _____ Signed: _____

Criteria	ok/no	Corrective action/remarks
AED unit		
Verify correctly placed	____	_____
Clean, clear of objects	____	_____
No cracks or damage to case	____	_____
Cables/connectors present and not expired	____	_____
Fully charged battery in place	____	_____
Charged spare battery present	____	_____
Check status/service light indicator	____	_____
Check absence of service alarm	____	_____
Power on, self-test	____	_____
Supplies		
Two sealed sets of electrode pads	____	_____
Verify expiration date on pad packages	____	_____
Razor	____	_____
Medical examination gloves	____	_____
Hand towels	____	_____
Scissors or trauma shears	____	_____
Pocket mask or face shield	____	_____

🖉 **LEARNING CHECKPOINT 3**

1. Name at least 1 situation in which a young child may experience sudden cardiac arrest and could benefit from the use of a pediatric AED.

   _____

   _____

   _____

2. Describe where to put the AED pads if you see that a victim has an implanted pacemaker or defibrillator.

   _____

   _____

   _____

3. What should you do with the AED pads if the victim has a medication patch on his or her chest?

   _____

   _____

   _____

TABLE 6-1

Summary of Basic Life Support

Step	Infant (younger than 1 year)	Child (1 – puberty, except 1-8 for AED)	Adult
1. Check for responsiveness and normal breathing.	Stimulate to check response. Observe whether breathing normally.	Tap shoulder and shout "Are you OK?" while checking for normal breathing (only gasps are not normal).	
2. If unresponsive, have someone call for help.	Send someone to call 9-1-1 and get an AED. If alone, give 2 minutes of care before calling 9-1-1 (and getting AED).	Send someone to call 9-1-1, and get an AED. If alone, unless the child has a known heart problem, give 2 minutes of care before calling 9-1-1 (and getting AED).	Send someone to call 9-1-1, and get an AED. If alone, call 9-1-1 and get an AED immediately (give 2 minutes of care first for a drowning victim).
3. If unresponsive and not breathing normally, give CPR, starting with chest compressions.	For compressions, use 2 fingers just below the nipple line. Compress chest to at least ⅓ the depth of chest (about 1½ inches).	For compressions, use 1 or 2 hands in the center of the chest between nipples. Compress chest to at least ⅓ the depth of chest (about 2 inches).	For compressions, use both hands, 1 on top of other, in the center of the chest between nipples. Compress chest at least 2 inches but not more than 2.4 inches.
3a. Chest compressions in CPR.	Chest compressions at a rate of 100-120 per minute		
3b. Ratio of compressions and breaths	Cycles of 30 compressions and 2 breaths		
4. Give 2 breaths.	Use barrier device or cover mouth, nose or stoma. Each breath lasts 1 second.		
4a. If breaths do not go in, reposition head and try again.	Each breath lasts 1 second.		
4b. If breaths still do not go in, continue with chest compressions.	Continue with chest compressions. Check the mouth for an object each time breaths are given, and remove it if seen.		
5. Use AED as soon as available.	Use pediatric electrode pads if available. If not available, use adult pads.		Use adult AED electrode pads.
6. If victim recovers normal breathing, put in recovery position.	Hold infant and monitor breathing.	Lay on side in recovery position and monitor breathing.	

CONCLUDING THOUGHTS

Remember that an AED is needed for most victims who are in cardiac arrest – CPR alone is often not enough. Always call or send someone for an AED for a victim who is unresponsive and not breathing normally.

 CRITICAL THINKING CHALLENGE QUESTIONS

👥 SCENARIO 1

A coworker who had been feeling ill suddenly clutches at his chest and then collapses. You check and find he is not breathing. A coworker calls 9-1-1 and runs to get a nearby AED while you start CPR. When the coworker returns with the AED, what should you do first?

_____

_____

_____

_____

👥 SCENARIO 2

An AED unit is present in your office suite, just down the hall from your office. One evening, you are driving home from your 6-year-old son's soccer game when you remember you need to get something from your office. Your son goes in with you. He has been alone in your office for only a couple minutes, but when you walk back in, you find him unresponsive on the floor. You find he is not breathing normally.

a. What is your first action?

_____

_____

_____

👥 SCENARIO 2 continued

b. After 30 chest compressions, you open his airway and give him 2 breaths. The breaths go in, and you watch his chest rise and fall. How long should you continue CPR?

_____

_____

_____

c. After 2 minutes, he is still motionless and not breathing, and you call 9-1-1 as you run for the AED. You apply the pediatric pads to his chest and let the unit analyze his rhythm. It advises giving a shock, and you push the shock button. Now what should you do?

_____

_____

_____

_____

_____

✏️ ADDITIONAL ACTIVITIES AND RESOURCES

1. Identify places where an AED is located on your campus or in the community, and estimate the time it would take to retrieve the nearest AED to your classroom.

2. Because AEDs continue to evolve rapidly, with newer units including more advanced features, you should understand what features and capabilities you may encounter in new models. If your instructor asks, you may research certain new AED models and share the information you find with the class. All major manufacturers maintain easily found websites with information about their current models, and several commercial sites provide information about a range of different units.

6 • Automated External Defibrillators (AEDs)

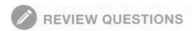

Select the best answers.

1. What is occurring during ventricular fibrillation?
   a. The ventricles of the heart have stopped moving.
   b. The ventricles of the heart are contracting too slowly.
   c. The ventricles of the heart are quivering rather than pumping.
   d. The ventricles of the heart are contracting with opposing rhythms.

2. An AED administers a shock to the victim –
   a. whenever you turn it on.
   b. automatically, about 15 seconds after the unit is turned on.
   c. when you push the shock button after being prompted to do so.
   d. about 3 seconds after the pads are applied to the victim.

3. What should you do before using an AED?
   a. Ensure that the victim is not breathing.
   b. Administer CPR until the AED is ready to use.
   c. Place it next to the victim and turn it on.
   d. All of the above

4. The AED pads should be positioned where on the victim?
   a. Where the diagram on the unit indicates placement
   b. Below the nipples on both sides of the chest
   c. In both armpits
   d. One on the chest and the other on the abdomen

5. While the AED is analyzing the victim's heart rhythm –
   a. continue CPR.
   b. do not touch the victim.
   c. push the shock button.
   d. push down on the pads to hold them in place.

6. If the AED indicates no shock is needed, you should then –
   a. wait 20 seconds and try again.
   b. give CPR, starting with chest compressions.
   c. give a lower-power shock.
   d. take the pads off and reposition them.

7. An AED may be used with a child 1-8 years old, ideally with –
   a. special pediatric pads.
   b. the voltage knob turned to a lower setting.
   c. the pads on the legs to lower the voltage through the heart.
   d. petroleum jelly between the skin and the pads.

8. When using an AED with a victim of hypothermia –
   a. briskly rub the victim's chest to warm up the skin below the pads.
   b. handle the victim very carefully.
   c. put oil on the pads to provide better conductivity.
   d. wait until you have fully warmed the body before applying the pads.

CHAPTER 7

Airway Obstructions

LESSON OBJECTIVES

- List ways to prevent choking.

- Demonstrate choking care for a responsive adult, child and infant.

- Demonstrate choking care for an unresponsive adult, child and infant.

You are having a cup of tea in the lunch room when you see a woman at the next table suddenly bring her hands up to her throat. She looks frantic and her mouth is open, but she is not speaking. The others at her table are looking at her, but no one has moved to help – they do not seem to know what to do. You approach the woman, who you think may be choking. What should you say and do?

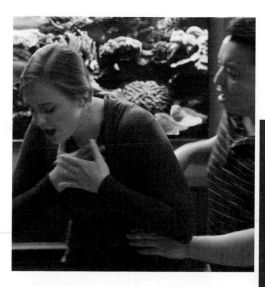

As described in **Chapter 5,** the inability to breathe is a life-threatening emergency, and body cells not receiving oxygen begin to die within minutes. The inability to breathe because of an airway obstruction is commonly called choking. Choking is a common cause of respiratory arrest (the stopping of breathing). Because time is so critical in these emergencies, it is important to be prepared to give immediate care to responsive and unresponsive choking victims.

Choking Emergencies

With airway obstructions, the victim cannot breathe because the airway is blocked by a foreign object, an anatomical structure such as the tongue, or fluid or vomit. These emergencies require immediate care to clear the obstruction and enable the victim to breathe **(Figure 7-1).**

FIGURE 7-1

(a) Food lodged in the airway, obstructing breathing.

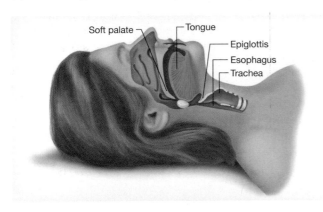

(b) The tongue blocking the airway in an unresponsive victim.

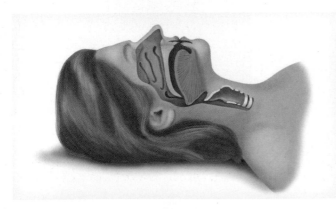

Preventing Choking

Choking is common in both adults and children. About 4,500 people die from choking each year in the United States. Although people often think of choking as a problem primarily for infants and young children, the age group that experiences choking most frequently is adults 65 and older, who are more than twice as likely to die from choking as younger adults. Virtually all cases of choking could have been prevented.[1]

In adults, choking often results from trying to swallow large pieces of food that have not been chewed sufficiently, either from eating too quickly or from eating while engaged in other activities. Choking is more common in people under the influence of alcohol or drugs. Choking is also more likely in those wearing dentures, apparently because of a diminished sensation for how well food has been chewed before attempting to swallow.

Choking is a serious threat to infants and children up to 3-4 years of age and a significant cause of death. An infant or young child may put any small object in his or her mouth, and nonfood items account for most choking deaths in young children. Coins, balloons, small balls and toy parts are the most common causes of choking in young children. In older children, the most common items choked on are food, candy and gum. Follow these guidelines to prevent choking in infants and children:

- Do not leave any small objects within reach of an infant (such as buttons, beads, coins, etc.). Ensure that small parts cannot break off toys or other items around the infant or young child.

- Feed infants only soft foods that do not require chewing.

- Have children sit in a highchair or at a table to eat. Never let a child move around while eating.

- Teach children not to eat too fast or to talk or laugh while eating.

- Cut up foods a child could choke on, such as hot dogs, into small pieces.

- Do not give children younger than 3 foods such as:

  - Peanuts
  - Popcorn
  - Grapes
  - Gum
  - Chunks of raw vegetables (such as baby carrots) or fruits
  - Marshmallows

- Supervise young children while they eat, and be prepared to care for a child who chokes.

[1]*National Safety Council. (2015). Injury Facts®, 2015 Edition. Itasca, IL: Author.*

 LEARNING CHECKPOINT 1

1. List at least 4 situations in which choking is a risk for an adult.

_____

_____

_____

_____

2. Put a check mark next to food items that should not be given to a child younger than 3.

   ☐ Popcorn

   ☐ Jell-O

   ☐ Marshmallows

   ☐ Spaghetti

   ☐ Grapes

   ☐ Corn kernels

   ☐ Soft bread slices

   ☐ Gum

Airway Obstruction

A victim is choking when the airway is obstructed either partially or fully. A victim can choke on:

- Food or other foreign bodies in the mouth

- The tongue (in an unresponsive victim lying on his or her back)

- Teeth or other body tissues resulting from injury

- Vomit

A complete **airway obstruction** means the victim is getting no air at all and consequently no oxygen is entering the blood. This victim will soon become unresponsive, and not long after breathing stops, the heart will stop too. Choking care is urgently needed.

A partial obstruction means something is partially blocking the airway, but the victim is still getting some air into the lungs around the obstructing object. The victim may be getting enough air to cough out

the obstructing object – or breathing may be very difficult, and the victim might not be able to cough strongly enough to expel the object.

ASSESSING CHOKING

Most cases of choking in adults occur while eating. Most cases of choking in infants and children occur while eating or playing. Therefore, someone is often present and recognizes the choking event while the victim is still responsive. With a partial obstruction, the victim is usually coughing forcefully in an attempt to expel the object. The victim is getting some air and may be making wheezing or high-pitched sounds with breaths, along with coughing. Do not interrupt the person's coughing or attempts to expel the object, and do not pound the person on the back in an effort to help.

With a complete obstruction, however, the victim is getting very little air or none at all. The person may look frantic and be clutching at the throat **(Figure 7-2).** You may notice a pale or bluish coloring (cyanosis) around the mouth and nail beds. A victim who is coughing very weakly and silently, or not coughing at all, is unlikely to expel the obstructing object. The victim cannot speak. Simply ask the victim if he or she is choking. If the victim cannot answer but indicates that he or she is choking, ask for permission to help, and begin choking care for a responsive victim.

FIGURE 7-2

The universal sign of a responsive victim who is choking.

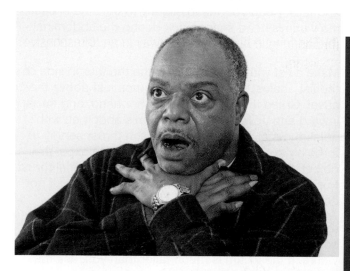

An unresponsive victim who may be choking receives the same initial assessment as any unresponsive victim as described in **Chapter 4.** If the victim is not breathing normally, start CPR with 30 chest compressions. If your first breath does not go into the victim after opening the airway, try again to open the airway and attempt a second breath. If it still does not go in, then assume the victim has an obstructed airway.

CHOKING CARE FOR ADULTS AND CHILDREN

Choking care depends on whether the victim is responsive or unresponsive:

- For a **responsive choking victim who is coughing,** encourage the victim to continue coughing to clear the object. Stay with the victim, and call 9-1-1 if the object is not immediately expelled.

- For a **responsive choking victim who cannot speak or cough forcefully,** give abdominal thrusts as described in the Skill: "Choking Care for Responsive Adult or Child."

- For **an unresponsive choking victim who is not breathing normally and who may be choking,** immediately have someone call 9-1-1 and begin CPR.

With a responsive victim, after quickly asking for consent, telling the victim what you intend to do, and having someone call 9-1-1, stand behind the victim and reach around to the abdomen. Place 1 leg forward between the victim's legs bracing yourself in case the victim becomes unresponsive and falls. Keep your head slightly to the side in case the victim's head snaps back during the abdominal thrusts.

Make a fist with 1 hand, and place the thumb side of the fist against the victim's abdomen just above the navel. Grasp the fist with your other hand, and thrust inward and upward into the victim's abdomen with quick thrusts. The pressure of each thrust serves to force air from the lungs up the trachea to expel the object. Pause only briefly after each abdominal thrust to see if the victim is able to breathe or cough; if not, continue with additional thrusts.

If you are giving abdominal thrusts to a child or someone much shorter than you, kneel behind the victim. If the victim is much taller than you, ask the victim to kneel or sit, because it is important that your thrusts go upward as well as inward, which is impossible if you have to reach up to the victim's abdomen.

Note that because abdominal thrusts may sometimes cause internal injury, a victim who is given abdominal thrusts is recommended to be examined by a health care provider.

When a complete airway obstruction is not cleared, the victim will become unresponsive within minutes. You may have found the victim in an unresponsive condition, or the victim may become unresponsive while you are giving abdominal thrusts if the object is not expelled. In the latter case, quickly and carefully lower the victim, and lay him or her on his or her back on the floor. Make sure 9-1-1 has been called. Begin the CPR sequence as usual, with 30 chest compressions delivered hard and fast. Then, when you open the victim's mouth to give a rescue breath, look first for an object in the mouth. If you see an object in the victim's mouth, remove it. If the object is expelled, give 2 rescue breaths as usual and continue CPR unless the victim recovers and is breathing normally.

If the obstruction remains, the chest compressions of CPR may expel the foreign object. Each time you open the victim's mouth to give breaths, check first to see if an object is visible; if so, remove it.

CARE FOR CHOKING INFANTS

If a responsive choking infant can cry or cough, watch carefully to see if the object comes out. If the infant is responsive but cannot cry or cough, have someone call 9-1-1, and assume the airway is obstructed. Give alternating back blows (slaps) and chest thrusts in an attempt to expel the object. Support the infant in 1 hand against your thigh as you sit or stand, keeping the infant's head lower than the body. To prevent spinal injury, be sure to support the infant's head and neck during these maneuvers. The detailed steps for back blows (slaps) and chest thrusts are described in the Skill: "Choking Care for Responsive Infant."

If an infant to whom you were giving responsive choking care then becomes unresponsive, be sure 9-1-1 has been called, and start CPR with chest compressions. If you are alone with the infant, give 2 minutes of CPR before stopping to call 9-1-1 yourself. As with an adult or child, the chest compressions may cause the object to be expelled. Check for an object in the mouth each time you open the airway before you give a breath, and remove any object you see. Never do a finger sweep of the mouth if you do not see an object, because this could force an object deeper into the throat.

STEP 1

Stand behind an adult victim with 1 leg forward between the victim's legs. Keep your head slightly to 1 side. For a child, move down to the child's level or kneel behind the child. Reach around the abdomen.

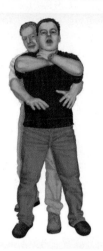

STEP 2

Locate the person's navel with a finger from 1 hand. Make a fist with the other hand and place the thumb side of the fist against the person's abdomen just above the navel.

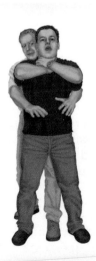

STEP 3

Grasp your fist with your other hand and thrust inward and upward into the victim's abdomen with quick thrusts. Continue abdominal thrusts until the victim expels the object or becomes unresponsive.

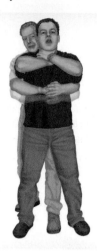

STEP 4

For a responsive pregnant victim, or any victim you cannot get your arms around or cannot effectively give abdominal thrusts to, give chest thrusts in the middle of the breastbone from behind the victim. Avoid squeezing the ribs with your arms.

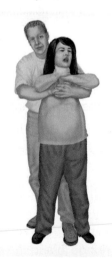

When you encounter an unresponsive infant, have someone call 9-1-1 immediately. Check quickly for normal breathing. If the infant is not breathing normally, begin CPR with chest compressions. If you are alone with the infant, give CPR for 2 minutes before calling 9-1-1 yourself. If your first breath does not go in after opening the airway and the infant's chest does not rise, try again after repositioning the infant's head to open the airway. If the second breath does not go in, assume that the infant has an airway obstruction and continue CPR, checking the mouth for an object each time you open it to give a rescue breath.

⚙ SKILL: CHOKING CARE FOR UNRESPONSIVE ADULT, CHILD OR INFANT

STEP 1
If the victim is unresponsive and not breathing normally, start CPR with 30 chest compressions at least 2 inches deep in an adult (but not more than 2.4 inches), and at least ⅓ the depth of the chest in a child (about 2 inches) or infant (about 1½ inches) at a rate of 100-120 per minute. Count aloud for a steady fast rate: "1, 2, 3 ... ."

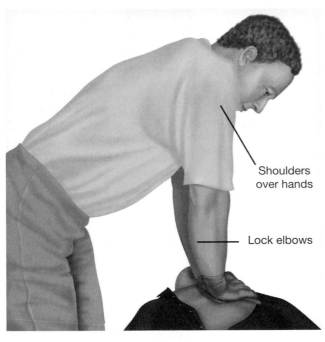

Shoulders over hands

Lock elbows

STEP 2
Open the airway with the head tilt–chin lift.

STEP 3
Give 2 rescue breaths, each lasting 1 second. If the first breath does not go in and the chest does not rise, position the victim's head again to open the airway, and try again.

STEP 4
If breaths still do not go in, continue CPR with chest compressions, in a ratio of 30 compressions and 2 breaths.

STEP 5
Look inside the mouth before giving breaths after each cycle of compressions, and remove any object you see. Then, give 2 breaths.

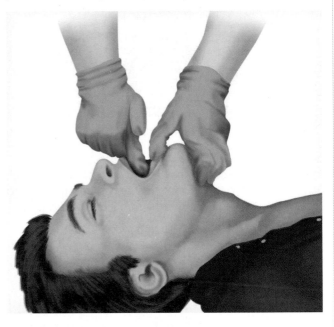

STEP 6
Continue CPR until:

• The victim recovers and is breathing normally.

• Professional help arrives and takes over.

STEP 1

Support the infant face down by holding the head in 1 hand, with the torso on your forearm against your thigh. Give up to 5 back blows (slaps) between the shoulder blades with the heel of your hand.

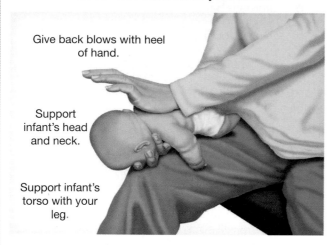

Give back blows with heel of hand.

Support infant's head and neck.

Support infant's torso with your leg.

STEP 2

Check for an expelled object. If not present, continue with next step.

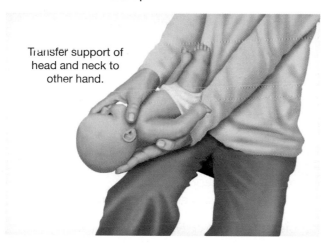

Transfer support of head and neck to other hand.

STEP 3

With your other hand on the back of the infant's head, roll the infant face up, supporting the back of the infant's head with your hand.

STEP 4

Give up to 5 chest thrusts with 2 fingers on sternum just below the nipple line, about 1 per second. Each thrust should be 1½ inches deep. Check mouth for expelled object.

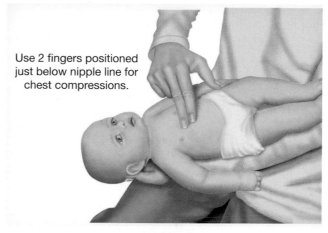

Use 2 fingers positioned just below nipple line for chest compressions.

STEP 5

Continue cycles of 5 back blows (slaps), 5 chest thrusts and checking the mouth. If alone, call 9-1-1 after 2 minutes. Continue until the object is expelled or the infant becomes unresponsive. If the infant becomes unresponsive, give CPR. Look inside the mouth before giving breaths and after each cycle of compressions, removing any object you see.

SELF-TREATING CHOKING

If you are choking when alone, give yourself abdominal thrusts to try to expel the object. You may try using your hands or leaning over and pushing your abdomen against the back of a chair or other firm object **(Figure 7-3)**.

FIGURE 7-3

Abdominal self-thrusts.

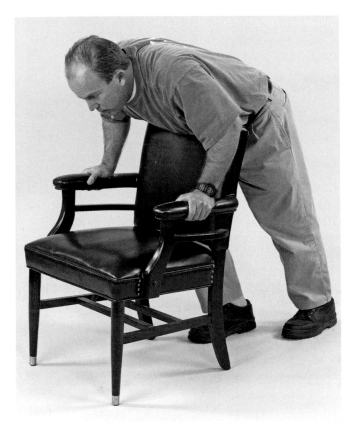

1. Select the best answer. For a responsive adult victim who is choking and cannot cough, you should –

   a. start CPR immediately.

   b. alternate back blows and chest thrusts.

   c. give abdominal thrusts.

   d. wait until the victim becomes unresponsive.

Circle **True** or **False** for each of the following statements:

2. A choking victim who is coughing forcefully is still able to breathe and may be able to cough out the foreign body.

   True   False

3. A choking victim who is unable to breathe will soon become unresponsive.

   True   False

4. Select the best answer. For a responsive choking infant –

   a. support the head as you position the infant.

   b. alternate back blows (slaps) and chest thrusts.

   c. check the infant's mouth for an expelled object.

   d. All of the above

5. Explain why CPR is given to a choking victim who becomes unresponsive.

   _____

   _____

   _____

   _____

   _____

⏱ **CONCLUDING THOUGHTS**

You have now learned the basic life support skills of CPR, AED use, and care for choking victims. **Chapter 8** continues with another important Skill: "Controlling Bleeding." Severe bleeding is another life-threatening condition.

SCENARIO 1

A friend is visiting you in your home. You have had a nice meal and are enjoying the cookies the friend brought, when the telephone rings with an important call you have to take. When you return to the kitchen 5 minutes later, you find your friend collapsed in her chair, unresponsive.

a.   Describe what to do first.

_____

_____

_____

b.   You do not see normal breathing, so you position her on her back on the floor and begin CPR with chest compressions. After 30 chest compressions, what is your next step?

_____

_____

_____

c.   You try to give the first rescue breath, but air does not go in, and her chest does not rise. Now what do you do?

_____

_____

_____

d.   After repositioning her head to open the airway and trying to give a second breath, air still does not go in. Now what do you do?

_____

_____

_____

e.   After the second cycle of 30 chest compressions, you open her airway to give a rescue breath, and when you look inside, you see a chunk of food. What do you do?

_____

_____

f.   You remove the food but she is still not breathing. You give 2 rescue breaths, and this time, they go in and you see her chest rise. Now what should you do?

_____

_____

_____

The section on choking prevention in this textbook chapter is necessarily short and only an overview. If you live in a home where small children or elderly people are present, you should learn more detailed guidelines for prevention. Conduct an Internet search using the key phrase, "choking prevention," and report your findings to the class.

 REVIEW QUESTIONS

Select the best answers.

1. What increases the risk of choking in an adult?

    a. Taking high blood pressure medication

    b. Overcooking foods

    c. Having gum disease

    d. Drinking alcohol with meals

2. A victim with a complete airway obstruction –

    a. cannot speak or cough forcefully.

    b. cannot speak but can cough forcefully.

    c. can speak and cough weakly.

    d. can speak but only in short sentences.

3. To give abdominal thrusts to a responsive choking adult, what hand position is used?

    a. Both hands together on the bottom edge of the breastbone

    b. Both hands together just above the navel

    c. 1 hand at the navel and 1 hand at the "V" where the lower ribs meet

    d. 1 hand on the bottom rib at each side

4. What is important when giving choking first aid to a responsive infant?

    a. Alternate series of back blows (slaps) and chest thrusts

    b. Keep the infant's head raised above the body.

    c. Give CPR in the usual way.

    d. Perform a more gentle version of the adult-responsive choking technique.

CHAPTER 8

Controlling Bleeding

LESSON OBJECTIVES

- Explain the effects of blood loss and the body's mechanisms to control bleeding.

- Describe the different types of external bleeding.

- Demonstrate the steps for controlling external bleeding.

- Demonstrate the steps for applying a pressure bandage.

- List the steps for caring for a bruise.

- List the signs and symptoms of internal bleeding and describe the first aid to give.

You receive a call that a worker in the shipping department is injured. You grab the first aid kit and arrive at the scene within a minute. The injured woman is holding a bloody rag wrapped around her hand. She says she was using a box cutter, which slipped and made a gash in her hand. She unwraps the rag to show you, and you see a deep laceration that is still bleeding. What are the important steps you should take?

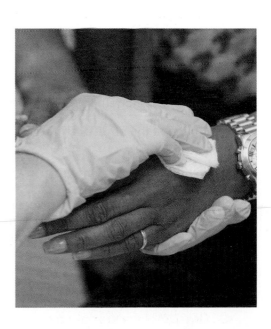

Blood carries oxygen from the lungs to all parts of the body. Many kinds of injuries damage blood vessels and cause external or internal bleeding. Bleeding may be minor or life threatening. Severe loss of blood can threaten the ability of the cardiovascular system to get the needed oxygen to vital organs. Severe bleeding, therefore, can be as great a threat to life as respiratory or cardiac arrest. This is why the victim is examined for severe bleeding in the initial assessment. Fortunately, most external bleeding is not that severe and can be controlled with first aid techniques.

Effects of Blood Loss

As you learned in **Chapter 3,** the cardiovascular system has several important functions. Of all these, none is more important than transporting oxygen to the body. Without oxygen, vital tissues begin to die within minutes. Although the other functions of blood are also essential for life, the lack of oxygenation resulting from severe blood loss is the most serious first aid issue.

Fortunately, the body can compensate for a small blood loss without ill effects **(Figure 8-1).** This is why it is possible for a healthy person to donate blood periodically without problems. A larger blood loss, however, can have serious effects, potentially leading to death. **Table 8-1** shows the amount of blood loss that causes shock and the amount of blood loss that becomes lethal if not immediately corrected. Note that in infants and children, severe bleeding becomes critical more quickly than in adults because the same amount of blood lost represents a higher percentage of the body's blood volume.

When a blood vessel is damaged and blood escapes, the body attempts to control the bleeding through three processes:

- **Vascular spasm** is a mechanism in which the damaged blood vessel constricts to slow the bleeding and to allow clotting to occur. With an injured small vessel, this constriction may be sufficient to stop the bleeding, but with a larger vessel bleeding usually still occurs.

- **Platelets** in the blood then stick to each other and to the walls of the injured vessel to form a **platelet plug,** which may reduce or stop minor bleeding.

- **Clotting** (coagulation) is the process in which **fibrin** produced from blood proteins clumps together with platelets and other blood cells in a fibrin web to seal the leak in the vessel **(Figure 8-2).**

These three mechanisms working together may be able to stop or reduce bleeding after an injury. In a more serious injury, however, these mechanisms may not be sufficient to stop the bleeding, or bleeding may continue long enough that the victim shows the effects of reduced blood volume. Controlling bleeding is therefore an important first aid action.

Bleeding occurs when blood from injured vessels escapes the body through a wound (external bleeding) or gathers in a body space or cavity (internal bleeding). Although many of the signs and symptoms of each are different, as is the first aid given, both external and internal bleeding can be life threatening when severe and uncontrolled.

FIGURE 8-1

Effects of blood loss.

Class 1	**Class 2**	**Class 3**	**Class 4**
Blood loss up to 15% of body blood volume	Blood loss of 15-30% of body blood volume	Blood loss of 30-40% of body blood volume	Blood loss of >40% of body blood volume

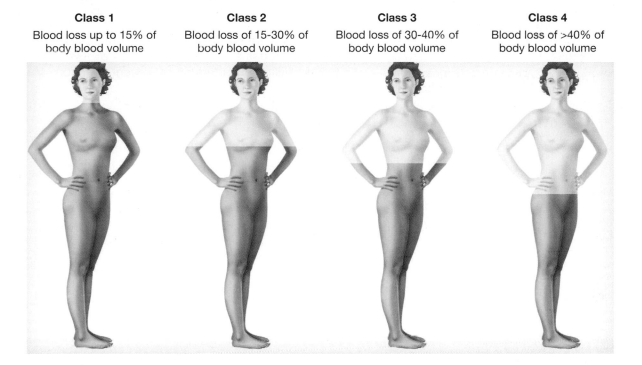

Blood loss after an injury may occur quickly with severe bleeding, but usually the body passes through a series of stages as blood volume drops:

With a loss of up to 15% of blood volume, the body can compensate for the loss of volume by constricting (shrinking) blood vessels to maintain blood pressure and can continue to transport oxygen to organs. The victim remains alert, and blood pressure and pulse are close to normal.

With a loss of 15%-30% of blood volume, constricting blood vessels maintain blood flow to vital organs, such as the brain and heart, while reducing blood flow to other body areas. The skin looks pale or ashen, cool and dry. Heart and respiratory rates increase in an attempt to compensate. The victim may feel restless and confused.

With a loss of 30%-40% of blood volume, the body can no longer compensate. Blood pressure falls, and the victim experiences **shock,** a serious condition in which vital organs are not receiving enough oxygenated blood. The victim is confused or anxious. Without medical treatment soon, vital organs will fail and the victim will die.

With a loss of more than 40% of blood volume, blood pressure falls further and vital organs begin to fail. The victim becomes lethargic, stuporous and eventually unresponsive. Death occurs when the brain and other vital organs fail from lack of oxygen.

FIGURE 8-2

View of blood clot showing blood cells in a web of fibrin.

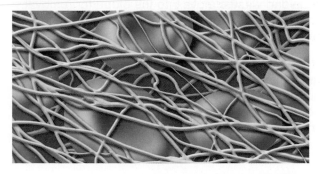

TABLE 8-1

Lethal Blood Loss

Hemorrhage	Percentage of Total Blood Volume Lost	Effects
Class I	Less than 15%	Generally well tolerated
Class II	15%-30%	Shock occurs, victim needs rapid transport
Class III	30%-40%	Severe shock occurs, victim needs immediate transfusion
Class IV	More than 40%	Rapidly fatal

Note: A 15% volume loss in a 150-lb. person is about 750 mL. A 30% loss is about 1.5 liters and a 40% loss is about 2 liters.

External Bleeding

External bleeding typically occurs when skin and other underlying tissues are damaged by trauma, and blood from cut or torn blood vessels flows out through the wound. The rate at which bleeding occurs depends on the size and type of the vessel(s) damaged. Larger blood vessels are *usually* deeper in the body and more protected, and therefore most superficial wounds damage only smaller blood vessels **(Figure 8-3).** This is not true in all body areas, however, and a wound where a major vessel is close to the skin surface may result in very heavy bleeding, such as at the wrist or neck.

TYPES OF EXTERNAL BLEEDING

There are three types of blood vessels: **arteries,** which carry blood from the heart to body tissues; **veins,** which carry blood back to the heart from body tissues; and **capillaries,** which are tiny vessels between the arteries and veins where oxygen and nutrients in the blood pass into tissues and carbon dioxide and wastes move into the blood for removal. Therefore, there are three types of external bleeding **(Figure 8-4):**

• **Bleeding from injured arteries** is more likely with deep injuries and is generally more serious. The blood is bright red and may spurt from the wound; blood loss can be very rapid. This bleeding needs to be controlled immediately.

• **Bleeding from injured veins** is generally slower and steady but can still be serious. The blood is darker red and flows steadily rather than spurting. This bleeding is usually easier to control.

• **Bleeding from capillaries** oozes from shallow cuts or scrapes and often stops soon by itself. The wound still needs attention to prevent infection.

FIGURE 8-3

Arteries of the leg. Note that the larger arteries are deeper within the leg, and the arteries nearer the skin surface are generally much smaller and will bleed less.

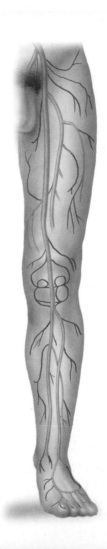

FIGURE 8-4

Arterial, venous and capillary bleeding.

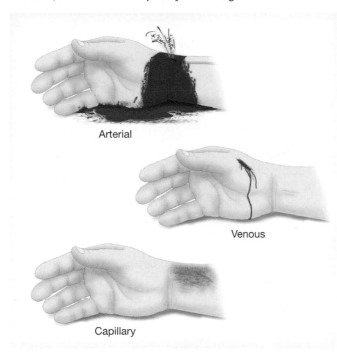

Arterial

Venous

Capillary

CONTROLLING EXTERNAL BLEEDING

For minor bleeding that stops by itself, clean and dress the wound as described in **Chapter 10**. The bleeding should stop by itself or with light pressure on the dressing, such as the pressure provided by an adhesive bandage around a cut finger.

For more serious bleeding, first aid is needed immediately to stop the bleeding.

Applying direct pressure on the wound is sufficient to stop the bleeding in most cases (see Skill: "Controlling Bleeding"). Direct pressure on the wound controls bleeding by squeezing shut the bleeding vessel at the point where it is damaged. Press directly on the wound with a sterile dressing and your gloved hand. If gloves are not available, you can improvise with any impermeable substance as a barrier to prevent contact between the victim's blood and your skin. This pressure stops the blood from flowing out. When the blood stops flowing, the natural body processes involved in clotting have a chance to function more effectively because platelets and fibrin are not "washed out" of the damaged area by the flow of blood. This is why sometimes pressure is needed only for a short time; the body's natural processes control the bleeding once they have the opportunity to work. With more severe vessel damage, however, pressure may have to be maintained for some time before clotting is successful. Releasing the pressure on the wound too soon would allow the normal blood pressure to break through the "dam" made of platelets, fibrin and other cells. This is also the reason why you should add more dressings on top of blood-soaked bandages when bleeding continues, rather than removing the first dressings – because removing them would release pressure and remove blood that is clotting.

Direct pressure should not be put on certain wounds, such as skull fractures or objects impaled in the wound, because the pressure may cause additional damage. In such cases, pressure is applied around the wound or object, as described in **Chapter 10**.

Call 9-1-1 for any severe bleeding or bleeding that does not stop quickly. The victim should seek medical attention for any significant wound (see **Chapter 10**). Do not remove the dressing or bandage; the wound will be cleaned later by medical personnel.

HEMOSTATIC DRESSINGS

Hemostatic dressings are a relatively new, special kind of dressing available over the counter in most locations. Hemostatic dressings may be present in a first aid kit you are using for a bleeding victim, and they can be a valuable when direct pressure alone is not sufficient to stop bleeding. Hemostatic dressings promote rapid blood clotting to help control bleeding. Most are designed to absorb water from the blood, which acts to concentrate the clotting factors in blood at the wound site. Some hemostatic dressings are also impregnated with substances that promote fibrin formation.

If you have a hemostatic dressing and are unable to control bleeding with direct pressure alone, consider using the hemostatic dressing as described in the Skill: "Controlling Bleeding." Save the packaging of the dressing and give it to responding EMS personnel.

STEP 1

Put on gloves.
Improvise a barrier if no barrier is available.

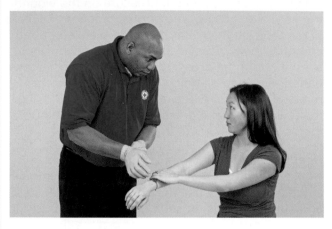

STEP 2

Place a sterile dressing or clean cloth on the wound.

STEP 3

Apply firm direct pressure with your hand for about 5 minutes.

- Do not put pressure on an object in a wound.

- Do not put pressure on the scalp if the skull may be injured.

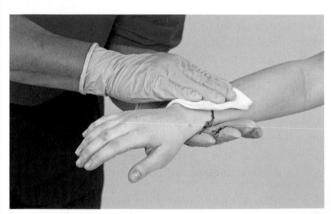

STEP 4

Reevaluate the bleeding.

a. If direct pressure does not control the bleeding and you have a hemostatic dressing, remove dressings already used and apply the hemostatic dressing directly on the wound using direct pressure.

b. If a hemostatic dressing is not available, continue to apply direct pressure. If blood soaks through the first dressing, place additional dressings on top of the blood-soaked dressing and keep applying pressure.

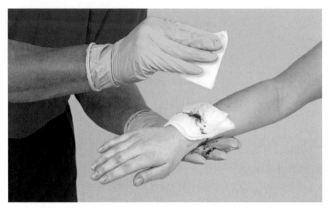

STEP 5

If needed, apply a pressure bandage to keep pressure on the wound, wrapping from the end of the extremity toward the center of the body. *The pressure is sufficient if the bandage is snug but you can slip a finger under it. Use a tourniquet when direct pressure and a pressure bandage do not control severe bleeding from a limb.*

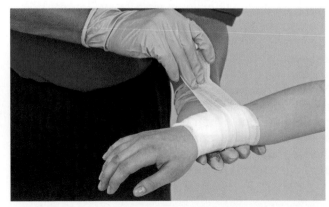

STEP 6

If appropriate, treat the victim for shock (see **Chapter 9**), and call 9-1-1.

SKILL: APPLYING A PRESSURE BANDAGE

STEP 1

Place a sterile dressing or clean cloth on wound. Start wrapping an elastic or self-adhering roller bandage below the wound dressing, wrapping from the end of the extremity toward the center of the body.

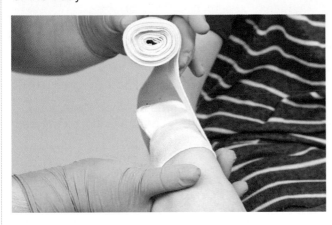

STEP 2

Make several circular turns, then overlap turns by about ½ of previous turn.

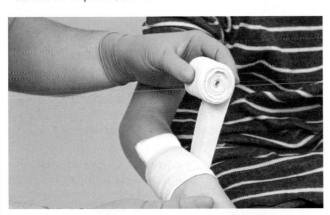

STEP 3

Work up the limb to cover the dressing completely. The pressure is sufficient if the bandage is snug but a finger can be slipped under it.

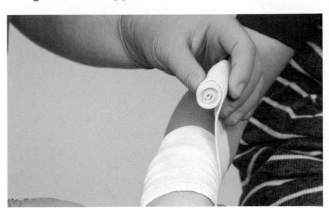

STEP 4

Fix or tie the end of the bandage in place.

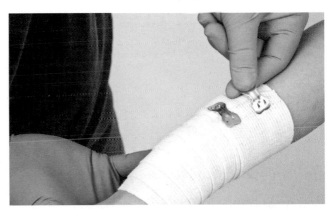

PRESSURE BANDAGES

To control severe bleeding as quickly as possible, apply direct pressure with your gloved hand on a sterile dressing (or clean cloth) placed on the wound. If needed, you may apply a **pressure bandage** over a wound in an extremity to maintain this pressure so you can give other first aid as needed. Wrap a bandage around the limb to completely cover the wound and to maintain sufficient pressure to keep bleeding from starting again (see Skill: "Applying a Pressure Bandage").

Whenever you apply a bandage around an extremity, be sure that it is not so tight that it cuts off circulation to the limb. As a general rule, the pressure is sufficient if the bandage is snug but a finger can be slipped under it. Periodically check the victim's fingers or toes for signs of good circulation: normal skin color, warmth, and sensation (not a tingling or numbness). If you find signs that circulation is reduced, loosen the bandage and apply it less tightly. Note that injuries often cause swelling that may increase after you apply the bandage, making the bandage tighter and possibly cutting off circulation. Therefore continue to check for signs of circulation until the victim receives medical attention. **Chapter 10** describes bandaging more fully.

Tourniquets

With severe bleeding from an extremity that cannot otherwise be controlled, a tourniquet may be effective. A tourniquet may also be appropriate if a pressure bandage does not control serious bleeding and you are unable to maintain manual pressure, such as when:

- There are multiple victims to care for.

- The victim has multiple injuries requiring care.

- The environment is unsafe and you need to evacuate the victim.

- You are unable to access the wound.

Use a commercial tourniquet if available, following the manufacturer's steps for its correct use. Only apply a tourniquet if you are trained in their use.

FIGURE 8-5

Commercial tourniquet.

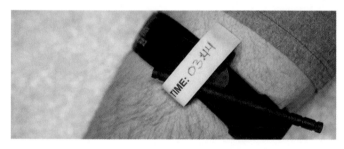

Using an Improvised Tourniquet

Following are steps for using an improvised tourniquet:

1. To make a tourniquet, use a non-stretchy material, such as terry cloth or a triangular bandage), folded lengthwise to be 1-2 inches wide.

2. Tie the tourniquet around the injured arm or leg, several inches above the injury. If the injury is below the elbow or knee, you may need to tie the tourniquet above the joint. Use a common square knot (like tying your shoes without the bow).

3. Above the first knot in the tourniquet, position a stick or other long object as a windlass that can be twisted to tighten the tourniquet, and tie a second square knot. Use any long object that is strong enough to hold the tourniquet and can be secured in place (a pencil, stick, spoon, pipe, etc.).

4. Twist the windlass to increase the pressure until the bleeding stops.

FIGURE 8-6

Improvised tourniquet.

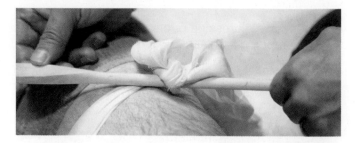

5. Secure the windlass in place by tying one or both ends to the victim's arm or leg.

6. If possible, mark the time the tourniquet was placed by putting a "T" on the victim's forehead with the time/day.

PREVENTING BLOODBORNE INFECTION

When giving first aid to control bleeding, remember to follow standard precautions to prevent disease transmission. If you do not have medical exam gloves with you, put your hand in a plastic bag or use a barrier, such as plastic wrap, between your hand and the wound. If nothing is available to use as a barrier, you can use the victim's own hand to apply pressure on the wound.

After providing care for bleeding, remember also not to touch your face or other parts of your body until you have thoroughly washed your hands. Because objects or surfaces contaminated with blood can remain infectious for some time afterward, be sure to dispose of soiled supplies properly and disinfect all contaminated items. **Chapter 2** describes guidelines for preventing bloodborne disease transmission.

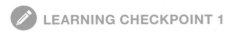

LEARNING CHECKPOINT 1

Circle **True** or **False** for each of the following statements:

1. Arterial bleeding is the most serious because blood loss can be very rapid.   True   False

2. The first thing to do with any bleeding wound is wash it and apply antibiotic ointment.   True   False

3. Describe the skin characteristics of a victim who has been bleeding severely.

_____

_____

_____

_____

_____

4. If you do not have medical exam gloves with you, what other materials or objects can be used as a barrier between your hand and the wound when applying direct pressure?

_____

_____

_____

_____

_____

_____

Internal Bleeding

Internal bleeding is any bleeding within the body in which the blood does not escape from an open wound. Internal bleeding is typically caused by a blunt impact on the body. The body may be impacted by a large force, such as being struck by a car, or a smaller force that leaves only a bruise. A serious injury can cause organs deep within the body to bleed severely. This bleeding, although unseen, can be life threatening. A closed wound resulting from a minor injury may involve only minor local bleeding in the skin and other superficial tissue, appearing as a bruise (also called a contusion). Internal bleeding may also occur in the absence of trauma, such as with a bleeding ulcer.

Because you cannot see internal bleeding, it is important to consider the mechanism of injury when you assess the victim. With any injury involving a fall or a moving vehicle, even a bicycle, consider the possibility of internal bleeding. The victim may complain of pain. With internal bleeding the victim may experience shock – which may cause cool, clammy skin that is pale or bluish or ashen – thirst, and possible confusion or light-headedness. In some cases, the victim may vomit or cough up blood, or blood may be present in urine or stool (bloody or black). With bleeding into the abdominal cavity, the victim's abdomen may be tender, swollen, bruised or hard.

Minor bleeding just below the skin surface can be reduced to some extent with a cold pack or ice and wrapping an injured extremity (see First Aid: "Simple Bruises"). Deeper internal bleeding cannot be controlled by first aid. Call 9-1-1 immediately if you suspect internal bleeding, and treat for shock (see **Chapter 9**). Be prepared to give basic life support if the victim's condition worsens (see First Aid: "Internal Bleeding").

First Aid: Simple Bruises

Signs, Symptoms and Care

WHEN YOU SEE

- Bruising
- Signs of pain

DO THIS FIRST

1. Check for signs and symptoms of a fracture or sprain (see **Chapter 14**) and give appropriate first aid.

2. Place a plastic bag or damp cloth with an ice-water mix on the injured area to reduce swelling and lessen pain; put a wet barrier, such as a cloth, between the plastic bag and the skin. A cold pack also can be used. Apply the cold for 20 minutes (or 10 minutes if it produces discomfort), then remove it for 30 minutes. Repeat the process for 24-48 hours or until the victim receives medical help.

3. With an arm or leg, wrap the area with an elastic roller bandage. Keep the part raised to help reduce swelling.

ADDITIONAL CARE

- Seek medical attention if you suspect a more serious injury such as a fracture or sprain.

First Aid: Internal Bleeding

Signs, Symptoms and Care

WHEN YOU SEE

- Abdomen is tender, swollen, bruised or hard

- Blood vomited or coughed up, or present in urine or stool (bloody, black or tarry)

- Cool, clammy skin; may be pale, bluish or ashen in color

- Thirst

- Possible confusion or lightheadedness

DO THIS FIRST

1. Have the victim lie on his or her back (if no suspected trauma, especially a neck, back, hip or pelvic injury).

2. Call 9-1-1.

3. Be alert for vomiting. Put a victim who vomits or becomes unresponsive in the recovery position (if no trauma).

4. Keep the victim from becoming chilled or overheated.

5. If the victim becomes unresponsive, monitor breathing and be ready to give basic life support (BLS) if needed.

ADDITIONAL CARE

- Calm and reassure the victim.

- Treat for shock (see **Chapter 9**).

ALERT

- Do not give the victim anything to drink even if he or she is thirsty.

LEARNING CHECKPOINT 2

Circle **True** or **False** for the following statement:

1. Internal bleeding is seldom life-threatening because there is no loss of blood from the body.　　True　　False

2. Put a check mark next to the signs and symptoms of internal bleeding.

    ☐　Cool, clammy skin

    ☐　Vomiting or coughing up blood

    ☐　Tender, swollen or hard abdomen

    ☐　Confusion or light-headedness

    ☐　Blood in urine or stool

    ☐　Bruise

3. Select the best answer. First aid for serious internal bleeding includes –

    a.　calling 9-1-1.

    b.　positioning the victim lying down.

    c.　keeping the victim from becoming chilled or overheated.

    d.　All of the above

 CONCLUDING THOUGHTS

Many people are frightened of or upset by bleeding. Fortunately, in most cases, the body's own mechanisms make it easy to control external bleeding with direct pressure. Because serious bleeding can be life threatening, however, always call 9-1-1. In **Chapter 9,** you will learn more about caring for a victim who is in shock as a result of serious bleeding.

 CRITICAL THINKING CHALLENGE QUESTIONS

SCENARIO 1

A coworker who was repairing a piece of equipment suddenly yells and grabs at his arm. You see blood flowing from between his fingers. You check him and see the blood is spurting from a severed artery.

a. What do you do to try to stop the bleeding?

_____

_____

b. Even with your pressure on the wound, the bleeding continues through the dressing. What do you do next?

_____

_____

_____

SCENARIO 2

You are riding the bus home from work in the evening. As the bus stops where you will get off, an inebriated passenger in front of you staggers and trips on the last step and lands on the sidewalk. Not seeing what happened, the bus driver pulls away. The man rolls over and you see that his shirt over his shoulder is rapidly becoming soaked with blood – he apparently landed on a piece of broken glass. You have neither a cell phone nor first aid kit with you. What do you do?

_____

_____

SCENARIO 3

You respond to a scene where a construction worker is lying unresponsive on his back. Another worker tells you that a few minutes ago the victim was struck in the abdomen by a concrete block that tumbled from on top of a wall. This other person unbuttoned the man's shirt to see if he was bleeding, and although his skin is abraded and bruised, there is no active external bleeding.

a. What are the first actions you should take?

_____

_____

b. You carefully check his abdomen. It is hard and swollen, and his skin is cool and moist. Now what should you do?

_____

_____

REVIEW QUESTIONS

Select the best answers.

1. The body attempts to slow or stop bleeding from a damaged blood vessel by –

   a. skeletal muscle contraction.

   b. blood clotting.

   c. producing more red blood cells.

   d. stopping the heartbeat.

2. Which type of bleeding is usually most serious?

   a. Arterial bleeding

   b. Venous bleeding

   c. Capillary bleeding

   d. All bleeding is equally serious.

3. To prevent bloodborne disease transmission, apply pressure on a bleeding wound with –

   a. your gloved hand.

   b. any impermeable substance.

   c. the victim's hand.

   d. Any of the above

4. What do you do if blood soaks through the pressure bandage?

   a. Ignore the blood but maintain the pressure.

   b. Put a new bandage on top of the first and maintain pressure.

   c. Call 9-1-1 and ask for instructions.

   d. Apply a tourniquet on top of the bandage.

5. A pressure bandage is applied –

   a. around the extremity from the joint above the wound to the joint below the wound, to apply equal pressure to the whole area.

   b. above the wound to cut off the blood flow.

   c. on the wound to control bleeding.

   d. both above and below the wound to control blood flow and bleeding.

6. Which is a sign or symptom that a pressure bandage is too tight on the arm?

   a. Red color under the fingernails

   b. Hot fingers

   c. Cold fingers

   d. Extreme thirst

7. Internal bleeding into the abdomen may result in the abdomen feeling –

   a. hard.

   b. hot.

   c. pulsing.

   d. soft and squishy.

8. Severe internal bleeding may cause –

   a. the victim to feel thirsty.

   b. the victim's skin to be cool and clammy.

   c. the victim to be confused.

   d. All of the above

CHAPTER 9

Shock

LESSON OBJECTIVES

- Explain what happens inside the body with severe blood loss.

- List common causes of shock.

- Describe first aid for a victim in shock.

- Describe ways to prevent exposure to known allergens.

- Describe the first aid for anaphylaxis.

- Demonstrate how to use an emergency epinephrine auto-injector (if trainers are available).

Seated at a nearby table at a local Mexican restaurant are a woman, her two daughters, and her daughter's friend. They are sharing a variety of dishes and having a good time – until the friend abruptly puts down her fork and leans back in her seat, looking ill. You notice her face seems puffy around the mouth, and she is obviously having trouble breathing. The mother and two daughters are asking her if she is OK but don't seem to know what to do. With your first aid training, you recognize the situation as a possible food allergy. What should you do?

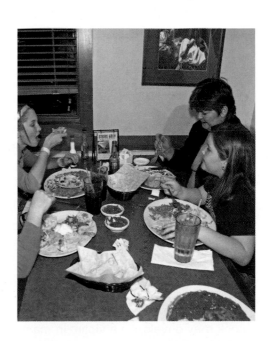

Shock is a dangerous condition in which not enough oxygen-rich blood reaches vital organs in the body. The brain, heart and other organs need a continuous supply of oxygen. Anything that happens to or in the body that significantly reduces blood flow can cause shock. Severe bleeding is a common cause of shock in first aid situations.

Shock is a life-threatening emergency. It may develop quickly or gradually. Always call 9-1-1 for a victim in shock.

Shock

For enough blood to reach the body's vital organs and keep them well oxygenated, three general conditions must be met:

1. The heart must be efficiently pumping blood.

2. Blood volume in the body must be sufficient to fill blood vessels so the pumping action circulates blood to vital organs.

3. Blood vessels throughout the body must be intact and functioning normally. A loss of blood through injured blood vessels may reduce the blood volume to the point where not enough blood is circulated to vital organs. Certain conditions may also dilate blood vessels to the extent that there is not enough blood volume to fill blood vessels.

Normally the body easily meets these conditions. The heart rate varies as needed to pump more or less blood throughout the body. The body controls blood volume by moving fluid into or out of the blood as needed. Blood vessels constrict or dilate in different conditions to ensure that enough blood is circulated to vital organs at all times. In a healthy person these mechanisms work automatically to provide the constant supply of oxygen that the brain, heart and other vital organs need.

In cases of injury or illness, however, one or more of these necessary conditions may be disrupted. Disruption of the heart, the blood volume or the blood vessels may reduce the blood flow to vital organs, causing shock **(Figure 9-1)**.

TYPES AND CAUSES OF SHOCK

Shock may develop in a victim in many different situations. Following are descriptions of the primary types of shock. You do not need to know which exact type a victim has, as long as you recognize the

FIGURE 9-1

Shock may result from disruption of the heart, blood volume or blood vessels.

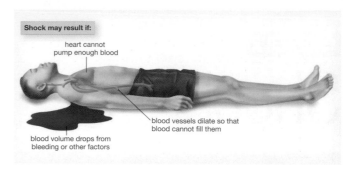

problem and give appropriate first aid. **Box 9-1** lists the specific types of injuries and conditions that may lead to shock.

- **Hypovolemic shock** occurs when blood volume drops. Severe bleeding, either external or internal, is a common cause of shock when not enough blood is left circulating in the body to bring required oxygen to vital organs (this is called hemorrhagic shock). Other conditions may also lower blood volume. Severe burns result in a loss of fluid from the blood. Severe vomiting or diarrhea, or other causes of dehydration, may also result in the body moving fluid from the blood to meet other body needs, causing shock. Infants and young children are especially vulnerable to hypovolemic shock caused by persistent vomiting or diarrhea.

- **Cardiogenic shock** occurs when any condition causes the heart function to be reduced to the point that blood is not circulating sufficiently. Heart attack is a common cause. An abnormal heartbeat, such as ventricular fibrillation, is another cause of inadequate circulation. As described in the chapters on basic life support, CPR and an AED are used to restore a normal heartbeat and keep blood moving to vital organs, thereby helping to prevent the occurrence of shock.

- **Neurogenic shock** occurs when a problem related to the nervous system's control of blood vessels allows vessels to dilate excessively. If blood vessels throughout the body expand too much, the volume of blood is not sufficient to fill blood vessels, and not enough blood can be pumped to vital organs. Certain spinal cord injuries may cause neurogenic shock. A similar condition may result from extreme fear or similar emotions that cause fainting when blood vessels temporarily dilate because of the nervous system reaction.

- **Anaphylactic shock** is an extreme allergic reaction, typically to an insect sting, a particular food, medication, or some other substance. Anaphylaxis produces shock because part of the allergic reaction causes the dilation of blood vessels and the movement of fluid out of the blood through capillary walls. Because anaphylaxis causes other signs and symptoms and requires different first aid treatment, it is discussed separately later in this chapter.

BOX 9-1: INJURIES AND CONDITIONS THAT MAY CAUSE SHOCK

- Severe bleeding
- Severe burns
- Heart failure
- Heart attack
- Head or spinal injuries
- Severe allergic reactions
- Dehydration (common with heat stroke or severe vomiting or diarrhea)
- Electrocution
- Extreme emotional reactions (temporary, less dangerous form of shock)

FIRST AID FOR SHOCK

A victim in shock has various signs and symptoms depending on the cause and severity. Note, however, that the victim's signs and symptoms are not always correlated with the severity of the shock; therefore all cases of shock should be treated as severe. A victim with any serious injury should be assumed to be at risk of shock, even if you do not see all the signs and symptoms. Remember that internal bleeding can be life threatening even though you cannot see it or know for certain whether it is occurring.

Shock generally occurs in stages that may progress either gradually or so quickly that the victim is in full shock very soon after the injury. In the first stage, compensatory shock, early signs include feelings of anxiety, restlessness or fear, along with increased breathing and heart rates. In the second stage, decompensatory shock, mental status continues to deteriorate, leading to confusion, disorientation or sleepiness. Breathing becomes rapid and shallow, and the heartbeat becomes rapid (but the pulse weak because of decreased blood volume). The skin becomes pale or ashen and cool as blood is shunted from the extremities to vital organs. Nausea and thirst occur as blood is shunted from the digestive system. As oxygen levels drop in body tissues, the lips and

nail beds may look bluish. The victim ultimately becomes unresponsive. Without medical treatment, the third stage, irreversible shock, leads to respiratory and cardiac arrest. Once it develops, shock cannot be reversed without professional medical care, so it is important to recognize situations in which shock is likely or is beginning to occur and to give care to minimize it.

Not all victims experience all symptoms of shock or have them in the same order. But a victim who has several of these signs and symptoms after a serious injury is probably beginning to experience shock. It is crucial to call 9-1-1 immediately because, once it begins, shock will continue to develop unless medical treatment begins. EMS professionals often refer to the "golden hour" – the period of time from when a shock-producing traumatic injury occurs until the victim is receiving emergency medical treatment in a hospital. A victim reaching medical care later has a much lower chance of survival. Calling 9-1-1 immediately is necessary to start the emergency response process so the victim can receive help before shock leads to death.

After EMS is called, first aid for shock is directed at helping minimize or delay the onset; first aid at the scene cannot reverse shock. If the victim is bleeding, it is essential to control the bleeding immediately to prevent further blood loss. Then, position the victim lying on his or her back with legs raised such that the feet are 6-12 inches above the ground, unless the victim may have a spinal injury or head injury or may have had a stroke. This is often called the *shock position*. Put a victim who is having breathing difficulty into the position of easiest breathing, typically a reclining position partly sitting up. Ensure that the airway is open. Help the victim to maintain normal body temperature, if necessary, by covering him or her with a blanket or coat, but avoid overheating. Outdoors in cold weather, put a blanket or coat under the victim unless the victim may have a spinal injury (see First Aid: "Shock").

Blood loss in infants or children may quickly lead to shock. Young children and infants are also more susceptible to shock caused by dehydration resulting from repeated vomiting or diarrhea. Call 9-1-1 for any infant or child with persistent vomiting or diarrhea; do not wait for the signs of shock to develop.

Early shock may be less obvious in children because a child's body is generally more efficient at compensating initially for the blood volume decrease. By the time the classic signs of shock occur, the child's blood volume is usually already very low. As shock progresses, the child's condition declines very rapidly. An infant or child in shock may become limp and unresponsive, with eyes partially open or closed and the skin pale, bluish or ashen. Call 9-1-1 immediately. Treatment is the same as for adults, but because the child's decline is rapid, you should be prepared to give basic life support as needed.

First Aid: Shock

Signs, Symptoms and Care

WHEN YOU SEE

- Anxiety, confusion, agitation or restlessness

- Dizziness, light-headedness

- Cool, clammy or sweating skin; pale, bluish or ashen in color

- Rapid, shallow breathing

- Thirst

- Nausea or vomiting

- Changing responsiveness

DO THIS FIRST

1. Check for responsiveness, normal breathing and severe bleeding.

2. Call 9-1-1 and care first for life-threatening conditions, such as severe bleeding.

3. Be ready to give CPR if needed.

4. a. If there is no evidence of trauma, position a responsive victim on his or her back using a blanket or coat as a pad. If the movement or position does not cause the victim pain, raise the legs such that the feet are 6-12 inches above the ground.

   b. Put a breathing, unresponsive victim (if no suspected trauma, especially a neck, back, hip or pelvic injury) in the recovery position.

5. Loosen any tight clothing.

6. Be alert for the possibility of vomiting; if vomiting occurs, turn the victim's head to drain the mouth.

7. Try to maintain the victim's normal body temperature. If necessary, maintain the victim's body heat with a blanket or coat over the victim.

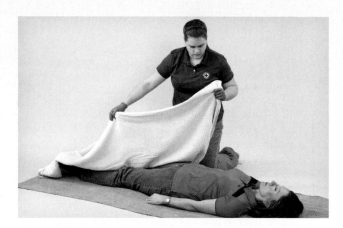

ADDITIONAL CARE

- Stay with the victim and offer reassurance and comfort.

- Keep bystanders from crowding around the victim.

ALERT

- Do not let a shock victim eat, drink or smoke.

- Note that sweating in a shock victim is not necessarily a sign of being too warm. If in doubt, it is better to maintain a shock victim's body temperature by keeping the victim warm.

LEARNING CHECKPOINT 1

Circle **True** or **False** for each of the following statements:

1. Because a shock victim is thirsty and may be dehydrated, offer clear fluids to drink.

   True   False

2. A spinal injury can cause shock.

   True   False

3. Which of these actions should you take *first* for a victim in shock because of external bleeding? Select the best answer.

   a. Stop the bleeding.

   b. Raise the legs.

   c. Loosen tight clothing.

   d. Cover the victim with a blanket.

4. A shock victim is likely to have which signs and symptoms? Select the best answer.

   a. Vomiting; diarrhea; red, blotchy face

   b. Nausea, thirst or clammy skin

   c. Incontinence, hives or swollen legs

   d. Headache, painful abdomen or coughing

5. What is the most important action to take for *all* shock victims?

   _____

   _____

   _____

Anaphylaxis

As described earlier, **anaphylaxis,** also called anaphylactic shock, involves a severe allergic reaction that can be fatal if not treated. In addition to the circulatory problems of shock, the victim's airway may swell, making breathing difficult or impossible. The breathing problem is usually the immediate life-threatening emergency. Always call 9-1-1 for an anaphylaxis emergency.

CAUSES OF ANAPHYLAXIS

The immune system has several mechanisms that protect the body from foreign substances that enter the body. When the individual is allergic to the substance (called an **allergen**), such as pollen that is inhaled or a food that is ingested, the normal action of the immune system results in a physiological response that includes various signs and symptoms, depending on the type and strength of the allergy. Typical mild allergic reactions include nasal congestion, watery eyes, or itching, blotchy skin.

Anaphylaxis, or anaphylactic shock, is a more extreme allergic reaction in some people that causes severe signs and symptoms that can rapidly become life threatening. The most common causes of anaphylaxis are[1]:

- Certain drugs (such as penicillins and sulfa)

- Certain foods (such as peanuts, shellfish and eggs)

- Insect stings and bites (such as bees or wasps)

The signs and symptoms of anaphylactic shock may begin within minutes, even seconds, of the victim's contact with the allergen. As a general rule, the more quickly the reaction occurs, the more serious it is likely to be. Anaphylaxis is frightening and demands immediate action because you cannot know if the reaction will continue to worsen and become fatal without medical care. Even if the victim has had what feels like a similar reaction in the past, he or she cannot know that it will not be worse this time.

[1]*National Institute of Allergy and Infectious Diseases. niaid.nih.gov/topics/anaphylaxis/Pages/default.aspx Accessed January 2016.*

PREVENTION OF ANAPHYLAXIS

Prevention of anaphylaxis resulting from an allergic reaction depends on avoiding the specific allergen.

Allergies to food, medications and insect stings are the most common cause of anaphylaxis. Unfortunately, most reactions occur in people without a history of reaction because allergic reactions develop from repeated exposures to the particular allergen, making prevention difficult. Health care professionals are trained to watch for the early effects of an anaphylactic reaction, however, and to provide early treatment. Following are preventive actions for people with known medication allergies:

• Maintain a complete history of medication reactions and share this with health care providers.

• Wear a medical alert ID in case you cannot communicate about an allergy in an emergency.

• For people allergic to nonprescription medications, read product labels carefully; many products include a number of unexpected ingredients.

Food allergies affect an estimated 5% percent of children younger than 5 and 4% of children ages 5-17 years old and adults.[1] Peanut and nut allergies are the most common; other common foods causing allergies include milk, eggs, wheat, soy, fish and shellfish. Approximately 9,500 children younger than 18 are hospitalized each year due to a food allergy.[2] Preventing reactions depends on avoiding foods known to cause a reaction, which can be more difficult than it may seem:

• Check food product labels for alternate names of foods.

• In restaurants and other settings where exact ingredients cannot be known, do not trust what wait staff or other people may say. Avoid foods that may contain hidden ingredients, such as sauces that may have been prepared using equipment contaminated by an allergenic food.

• Educate a child's caretakers, teachers and friends' parents about an allergy and its dangers to prevent the child from eating something shared by another child.

About 3% of adults and 1% of children have an allergic reaction to the venom of stinging insects, including honeybees, hornets, wasps, yellow jackets and fire ants. As many as 90-100 deaths every year in the United States are attributed to anaphylactic reactions to such stings.[3] Again, prevention is based on avoiding stinging insects whenever possible. When outdoors, these actions help you to avoid attracting or provoking stinging insects:

• Stay away from insect nesting areas. Check around the home for insect nests to destroy.

• Do not wear bright colors or sweet-smelling perfumes or colognes.

• Wear clothing that covers arms and legs; wear shoes to prevent stings caused by stepping on insects.

• Do not swat at or try to wave insects away.

• When getting into a car, if the windows were left open, check for insects that may have flown in.

• Be cautious when near areas where insects gather, such as around flowering plants and garbage cans.

• If stung, do not pull out the stinger with your fingers because the attached venom sac may eject more venom when squeezed; instead, scrape it off with something similar in size and rigidity to a credit card **(Figure 9-2)**. **Chapter 19** provides additional information about bites and stings.

Immunotherapy, often called *allergy shots*, is also available to lessen a person's reaction to insect venoms. Injections, usually given over three years, gradually desensitize the body, eventually preventing allergic reactions in most people undergoing therapy. People with severe insect allergies should see their health care provider for information about immunotherapy.

As described in the following section, emergency medication is also available for people at risk for severe allergic reactions. Although this medication cannot prevent the exposure to the allergen, it can stop the progress of an allergic reaction and prevent the victim from experiencing anaphylaxis.

[1]*National Institute of Allergy and Infectious Diseases niaid.nih. gov/topics/allergicDiseases/Pages/default.aspx Accessed January 2016.*

[2]*Centers for Disease Control and Prevention cdc.gov/nchs/data/ databriefs/db10.htm Accessed January 2016.*

[3]*Centers for Disease Control and Prevention. cdc.gov/niosh/ topics/insects/default.html Accessed January 2016.*

FIGURE 9-2

Use a rigid piece of plastic to scrape away a stinger.

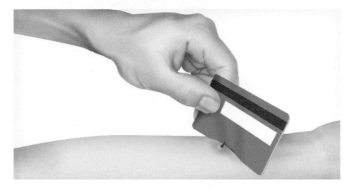

FIRST AID FOR ANAPHYLAXIS

If the victim knows he or she has the allergy and knows about the exposure, the victim may be able to tell you about the allergy when the reaction begins. Following the guidelines for the SAMPLE history in **Chapter 4,** ask all victims about allergies and the things they ate or drank most recently. For example, a victim who is severely allergic to bee stings, and who has just been stung, may say he or she needs medication immediately to prevent anaphylaxis. Or, someone who is allergic to nuts may feel the start of the reaction and wonder if there were nuts in something he or she just ate. In many cases, however, the person may not know about the allergy and may not have had an allergic reaction before. Therefore you cannot depend on having this information but should suspect an allergic reaction based on the situation and the victim's signs and symptoms

The early signs and symptoms of anaphylaxis include skin flushing, itching or burning and rash; sneezing and watery eyes and nose; coughing or a feeling of a tickle or lump in the throat that does not go away; and gastrointestinal upset. As symptoms worsen, the victim becomes anxious and may have the feeling that the throat is closing and the chest is becoming tight. Other signs include fast breathing, coughing, wheezing or hoarseness and altered mental status. The victim may have severe headache, a feeling of weakness or fainting and pale or ashen skin or cyanosis (bluish color of lips and nail beds), along with other shock signs and symptoms.

First aid begins with making sure 9-1-1 is called; medical care is urgently needed because first aid usually cannot stop or reverse anaphylactic shock. Help the victim into a position for easiest breathing and offer reassurance. Be prepared to give basic life support, if needed. If the victim becomes unresponsive, put him or her in the recovery position and continue to monitor breathing.

Some people who know they have a severe allergy carry an emergency epinephrine auto-injector, such as an EpiPen, EpiPen Jr. (for children), or Twinject **(Figure 9-3).** This medication usually will stop the anaphylactic reaction temporarily. Ask a victim about this and help him or her to open and use the auto-injector as needed. If the victim cannot use his or her prescribed EpiPen auto-injector, you may administer it yourself if permitted by state law. The EpiPen is removed from its case and the safety release cap removed. The tip is then jabbed into the outer part of the thigh muscle and held there for 10 seconds while the medication is injected. The effects of the emergency epinephrine will last 15-20 minutes, during which time you should stay with the victim until EMS professionals arrive and take over care. You may observe the victim experiencing the side effects of epinephrine: fast heartbeat, breathing difficulty, nausea and vomiting, dizziness or nervousness, and headache (see First Aid: "Use of an Emergency Epinephrine Auto-Injector").

FIGURE 9-3

Emergency epinephrine auto-injectors.

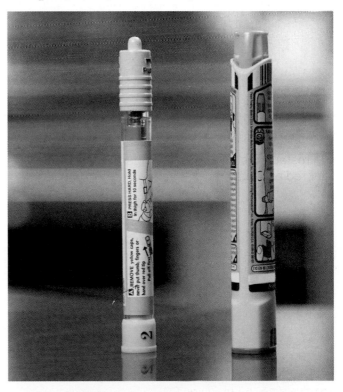

First Aid: Use of an Emergency Epinephrine Auto-Injector

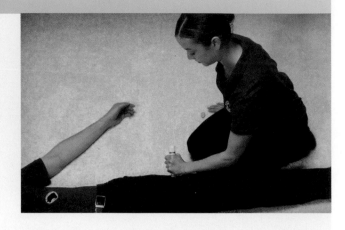

Signs, Symptoms and Care

WHEN YOU SEE

- Difficulty breathing, wheezing

- Complaints of tightness in throat or chest

- Swelling of the face and neck or puffy eyes

- Anxiety or agitation

- Nausea or vomiting

- Changing levels of responsiveness

DO THIS FIRST

1. Call 9-1-1.

2. Help a responsive victim use his or her emergency epinephrine auto-injector. If the victim cannot use his or her prescribed auto-injector, you may administer it yourself if permitted by state law.

3. Take the EpiPen out of its case and remove the cap or protective cover.

4. To administer the medication, press the auto-injector firmly against the outer thigh and hold it there while the medication is injected (follow the product instructions for how long). You should feel a "click" when the injection starts.

a. The medication should provide relief for 15-20 minutes.

b. If symptoms continue after the first dose of epinephrine has been given, and if EMS personnel are not expected to arrive within 5-10 minutes, administer a second dose of epinephrine, using a second auto-injector.

5. Monitor the victim's breathing and be ready to give CPR if needed.

6. Help a responsive victim sit up in a position of easiest breathing. Put an unresponsive victim who is breathing in the recovery position.

ADDITIONAL CARE

Stay with the victim and offer reassurance and comfort.

LEARNING CHECKPOINT 2

Circle **True** or **False** for each of the following statements:

1. Ask a victim having an anaphylactic reaction about any allergies and medication for allergies.　　True　False

2. A bee sting can cause a severe allergic reaction.　　True　False

3. Select the best answer. The major risk for a victim in anaphylaxis is –

   a. swelling around the eyes.

   b. heart attack.

   c. internal bleeding.

   d. breathing problems.

4. How should a victim in anaphylaxis be positioned if he or she is having trouble breathing?

_____

_____

 CONCLUDING THOUGHTS

Most commonly, shock is caused by heavy blood loss, so the most important thing to do for a victim who is bleeding is to control the bleeding as quickly as possible. Call 9-1-1 because shock is a serious threat to life. In most cases the first aid for a victim in shock is primarily supportive, but a victim with severe allergies may carry an emergency medication auto-injector that can be used to treat anaphylactic shock caused by an allergic reaction.

 CRITICAL THINKING CHALLENGE QUESTIONS

SCENARIO 1

The rear bumper of a truck backing up to the loading dock strikes a man's leg above the knee, knocking him down. The man is yelling with pain, and his leg looks twisted and distorted above the knee. By the time you reach him he has become quiet and seems confused about what happened. He is sweating but his skin is cool and clammy. What should you do?

_____

_____

_____

SCENARIO 2

You are finishing lunch in a restaurant with a coworker when she says she doesn't feel well. She is wheezing and short of breath and holding her throat. Her eyes look puffy. You ask her if she has any allergies and she says she is allergic to peanuts, but she didn't think there were any nuts in the sauce on her food. Her wheezing becomes worse and she is very agitated. What do you do?

_____

_____

_____

SCENARIO 3

While working outdoors, your coworker is stung by a bee. He says he is allergic to bees. Almost immediately he starts having difficulty breathing. What is the first thing you should ask him?

_____

_____

_____

ADDITIONAL ACTIVITIES AND RESOURCES

1. If you or a family member has a severe allergy, tell the class how you take precautions – such as asking the waiter questions in restaurants, etc. Share your personal precautions with others who may need a better understanding of preventive actions.

2. Research stories in Internet news sites about people with food or other allergies. Unfortunately, the stories that reach the media usually have negative outcomes, such as a story about a teenage girl who died from anaphylaxis after kissing her boyfriend who had just eaten a peanut butter sandwich. The point is to become more aware of how serious a severe reaction can be.

 REVIEW QUESTIONS

Select the best answers.

1. Which is fundamental to the definition of shock?
   a. Not enough oxygen reaching vital organs
   b. Too much waste building up in the urine
   c. The heartbeat stopping
   d. An abdominal injury

2. When should you call 9-1-1?
   a. Call only if the shock victim becomes unresponsive.
   b. Call only for blood loss of more than 30% of blood volume.
   c. Call for all victims in shock.
   d. Call for all victims who had any bleeding.

3. Which is a possible cause of shock?
   a. Bleeding
   b. Spinal cord injury
   c. Severe burn
   d. All of the above

4. Which is a part of first aid for shock?
   a. Giving the victim water to drink to replace lost fluids
   b. Raising the victim's legs
   c. Keeping the victim moving to prevent his or her becoming unresponsive
   d. Applying ice to the injury

5. Signs and symptoms of shock include –
   a. confusion.
   b. rapid, shallow breathing.
   c. pale, bluish, or ashen skin.
   d. All of the above

6. Shock in a child is similar to shock in an adult except –
   a. a child's condition may decline more rapidly.
   b. early shock is more dramatically obvious in a child.
   c. a greater blood loss is required in a child to produce shock.
   d. a child's skin does not become pale with shock.

7. Anaphylaxis is commonly caused by a severe allergic reaction to –
   a. campfire smoke.
   b. insect stings.
   c. poison ivy.
   d. other people.

8. How soon may a severe allergic reaction occur following exposure?
   a. Within seconds or minutes
   b. Within about 30 minutes
   c. Within 1 to 2 hours
   d. Within 6 to 12 hours

9. If a person who has just been stung by a bee says he is allergic to bee stings, you should –
   a. call 9-1-1 immediately.
   b. wait for the development of signs and symptoms, then call 9-1-1.
   c. send someone to the nearest drugstore to buy an EpiPen.
   d. use the shock position and see if that reverses the problem.

10. First aid for a victim experiencing anaphylaxis includes –
    a. cooling the victim's body with ice packs.
    b. giving the victim an aspirin as quickly as possible.
    c. positioning the victim for easiest breathing.
    d. using pressure points on arms and legs.

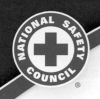

CHAPTER 10

Wounds and Soft Tissue Injuries

LESSON OBJECTIVES

- Describe how to clean a wound.

- Describe the signs and symptoms of an infected wound and what to do about it.

- List standard guidelines for using dressings and bandages.

- Explain how to determine when a wound needs medical attention.

- Describe first aid for punctures, wounds with impaled objects, avulsions and amputations, injuries of the genitals, scalp and specific facial areas.

Your coworker has cut his arm while trying to repair some office equipment. It is not bleeding heavily, but the wound seems dirty. You get the first aid kit and put on gloves, then take him to a nearby sink. How should you wash the wound? What other first aid should you give?

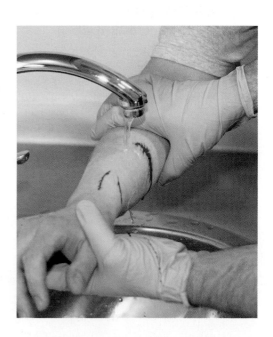

A wound is an injury to the skin, and sometimes, other deeper soft tissues. In an **open wound,** the skin is torn or cut open, often leading to bleeding. Different types of wounds require specific types of first aid, but all wounds have a risk for becoming infected by pathogens that may enter the body through the break in the skin. In addition to controlling bleeding (see **Chapter 8**), first aiders should also know how to care for different kinds of wounds and how to apply dressings and bandages.

Wound care involves cleaning and dressing a wound to prevent infection and protecting the wound so healing can occur. Remember: *Do not waste time cleaning a wound that is severely bleeding. Controlling bleeding is always the priority.* Health care personnel will clean the wound as needed.

This chapter describes first aid for open wounds. Care of internal bleeding caused by **closed injuries** is described in **Chapter 8.** The care of musculoskeletal injuries, another type of closed injury, is described in **Chapter 14.**

Types of Open Wounds

Different mechanisms of injury cause different types of damage to soft tissues. The main types of open wounds discussed in this chapter are abrasions, lacerations, punctures, avulsions and amputations. The type and amount of bleeding caused by an injury depend on the type of wound, its location and its depth. Different types of wounds also have different implications for first aid.

• **Abrasions** occur when the top layers of skin are scraped off **(Figure 10-1).** Skinned elbows or knees, for example, are common in children. Abrasions are often painful but are not serious injuries because underlying tissues are not usually injured. Bleeding is usually limited to capillary bleeding that typically stops soon by itself. Foreign material may be present in the wound, which can cause infection.

FIGURE 10-1

Abrasion.

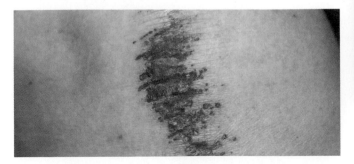

• **Lacerations,** or cuts, frequently penetrate the skin and may also damage underlying tissue **(Figure 10-2).** Lacerations are either smooth cuts with straight edges (called incisions), such as those caused by knives or other sharp objects, or jagged cuts with rough edges. Depending on the depth and location of the cut, lacerations may cause heavier bleeding. A laceration through a major artery may cause life-threatening bleeding.

FIGURE 10-2

Laceration.

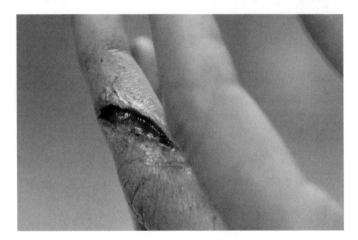

• **Punctures** occur when sharp objects penetrate the skin and possibly deeper tissues **(Figure 10-3).** The wound may penetrate through the body part, as with a gunshot wound, causing both entrance and exit wounds. Puncture wounds are more likely to trap foreign material in the body, increasing the risk for infection.

FIGURE 10-3

Puncture.

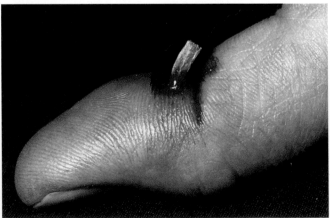

- An **avulsion** is an area of skin or other soft tissue torn partially from the body, like a flap **(Figure 10-4)**. Any area of skin, or a whole soft tissue structure like the ear, may be avulsed.

FIGURE 10-4

Avulsion.

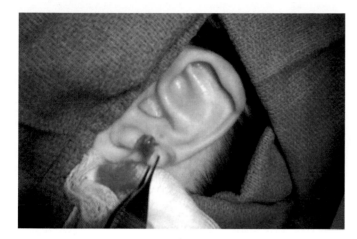

- An **amputation** is the complete cutting or tearing off of all or part of an extremity: a finger or toe, hand or foot, arm or leg. This wound is often called a traumatic amputation to distinguish it from an amputation performed surgically. Depending on the nature of the wound and the time that passes before the victim reaches the hospital, the amputated part may be reattached.

- **Burns** are damage caused to skin and other tissue by heat, chemicals or electricity. Because of the significant differences among first aid approaches for burns, burn care is covered in detail in **Chapter 11.**

First aid care for open wounds varies depending on their location on the body. Wounds to certain body areas require special first aid measures as described later in this chapter.

Cleaning Wounds

When a wound is bleeding heavily, the first aid priority is to control the bleeding (see **Chapter 8**). Do not delay or interrupt efforts to stop bleeding in order to clean the wound. Health care professionals who treat the victim later will clean the wound. Even after you have stopped the bleeding with direct pressure or other means, do not remove the dressing from the wound in order to clean it. Removing the dressing may disturb clotted blood and start the wound bleeding again.

Unless the wound is very large, deep or bleeding seriously, or the victim has other injuries needing attention, the first step in minor wound care is to clean the wound to help prevent infection. Wash your hands first and wear gloves if available. You may need to expose the wound first by removing clothing, taking care to avoid contact with the wound. Then, gently wash a shallow wound or abrasion with large amounts of warm or room-temperature water with or without soap to remove dirt. Irrigate a deeper wound under large amounts of running water to remove foreign matter **(Figure 10-5).** Do not merely soak the wound in water. Instead, actively run water over it. Washing out a wound under running water is called **irrigation.** Then, carefully pat the wound dry. Apply antibiotic ointment only to an abrasion or superficial wound and only if the victim is not allergic to the antibiotic. Apply a sterile dressing and bandage to protect and keep the dressing in place (see First Aid: "Wound Care").

FIGURE 10-5

Irrigate a shallow wound with running water to help clean it.

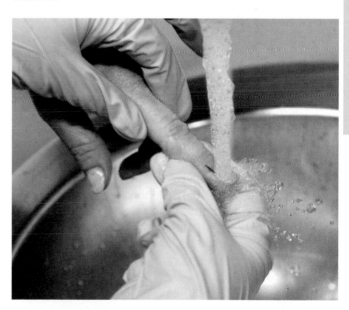

First Aid: Wound Care

Signs, Symptoms and Care

WHEN YOU SEE

- A shallow, open wound

DO THIS FIRST

1. Wash your hands and put on gloves if available.

2. Gently wash shallow wounds and abrasions with large amounts of warm or room temperature water with or without soap to remove dirt.

3. Irrigate a deeper wound that is not severely bleeding under large amounts of running water to remove foreign matter.

4. Do not use alcohol, hydrogen peroxide or iodine on the wound.

5. Pat the area dry.

6. Apply antibiotic ointment only to an abrasion or superficial wound, and only if the victim is not allergic to the antibiotic.

7. Cover the wound with a sterile dressing and bandage (or adhesive bandage with nonstick pad).

ADDITIONAL CARE

- Change the dressing daily or if it becomes wet. (If a dressing sticks to the wound, soak it in water first.)

- Seek medical attention for the following:

  - If the person's tetanus vaccination is out of date

  - The wound may be infected

  - A deep or puncture wound

  - An impaled object

  - A wound that may require stitches (cuts on the face or hands when the edges do not close together, gaping wounds and cuts longer than 1 inch)

ALERT

- Do not try to clean a major wound after controlling bleeding – it may start bleeding again. Health care personnel will clean the wound as needed.

- Do not put antibiotic ointment on a puncture wound or deep wound; use only on abrasions and shallow wounds.

- Do not use alcohol, hydrogen peroxide or iodine on the wound. Such substances may not kill pathogens or may damage healthy body tissue along with pathogens.

- Avoid breathing or blowing on the wound, since this may transmit pathogens.

- Do not attempt to remove clothing stuck to a wound; cut around the clothing and leave it in place for health care providers to manage.

- Do not scrub a wound, as this can cause further tissue damage.

Wound Infection

Infection is an invasion of the body by a pathogen that may potentially cause disease. Because a wound lacks the protection offered by intact skin and allows pathogens into body tissues and/or the blood, infection may occur with any open wound. Some pathogens cause local tissue damage, while others spread throughout the body and may become life threatening. The bloodborne diseases described in **Chapter 2** may be transmitted from one person to another through an open wound, but many other pathogens are also present in the environment. Pathogens may be transmitted into a wound by the object that caused the wound, by any substance that comes into contact with the wound or even by pathogens in the air. Because infection is an ever-present threat, wound care includes steps to prevent infection.

Although infection is a risk with all open wounds, some types of wounds are at greater risk, including wounds resulting from bites (even human bites); puncture wounds; wounds contaminated with dirt or other substances; and wounds with jagged, uneven edges that are not easily cleaned.

As noted earlier, to help healing and prevent infection, **antibiotic** ointment may be used on abrasions or shallow wounds in a person who is not allergic to the antibiotic, after the wound is cleaned. Antibiotic ointment should not be used on other types of open wounds because the ointment may seal the wound and block the drainage that is part of the normal healing process. If you see signs of infection occurring in a wound, do not just apply an antibiotic ointment and hope it will kill the pathogen. See a health care provider before the infection becomes worse **(Box 10-1).**

Any wound can become infected **(Figure 10-6),** in which case medical attention is needed. The signs and symptoms of an infection are:

• Wound area is red, swollen and warm.

• Pain

• Pus

• Fever

• Red streaks or trails on the skin near the wound are a sign the infection is spreading – see a health care provider immediately.

FIGURE 10-6

An infected wound.

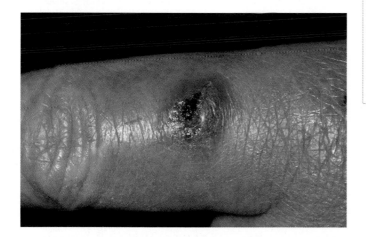

BOX 10-1: TETANUS

Tetanus, also called lockjaw because a stiff neck and jaw is an early symptom, is an infection caused by common bacteria. Tetanus bacteria are found in soil, on skin surfaces and elsewhere in the environment, including the home and other indoor locations. The bacteria enter the body through a wound, multiply and produce a powerful toxin that acts on the nervous system, causing death in up to 15% of cases.

The number of cases of tetanus in the United States has fallen dramatically since immunization became common in the late 1940s. In the most recent year reported, only 19 cases were reported, leading to 2 deaths.[1] Tetanus immunization is included in routine childhood vaccinations, but adults need a tetanus booster at least every 10 years. A tetanus booster may be recommended before 10 years in a victim with a significant wound. Tetanus infection is more common following puncture wounds or deep lacerations, but can also occur with abrasions or any break in the skin, including burns, dental infections and animal bites. It is important, therefore, for adults to maintain their immunization status with periodic boosters. In addition, medical attention should be sought for any deep or puncture wound. A tetanus shot must be given soon after receiving a wound to be effective.

[1]*Centers for Disease Control and Prevention cdc.gov/ vaccines/pubs/surv-manual/chpt16-tetanus.html Accessed January 2016.*

Dressing and Bandaging Wounds

DRESSINGS

Dressings are placed on wounds to help stop bleeding, prevent infection and protect the wound while it is healing.

Types of Dressings

First aid kits should include sealed sterile dressings in many sizes **(Figure 10-7).** Common types of dressings include:

- Gauze squares of various sizes

- Roller gauze

- Nonstick pad dressings

- Hemostatic dressings to help control bleeding (see **Chapter 9**)

- Adhesive strips, such as Band-Aids, and other dressings combined with a bandage

- Bulky dressings, also called **trauma dressings** (for large wounds or to stabilize an object impaled in a wound)

- **Occlusive dressings** (which create an airtight seal over certain types of wounds)

In some situations, it may be necessary to improvise a dressing. If a sterile dressing is not available, use a clean cloth as a dressing; non-fluffy cloth works best because it is less likely to stick to the wound. Look for a clean towel, handkerchief or other material. Avoid using cotton balls or cotton cloth if possible because cotton fibers tend to stick to wounds. To improvise bulky dressings, use sanitary pads if available, which, although not sterile, are generally individually wrapped and very clean. Bulky dressings can also be made of towels, baby diapers or many layers of gauze. A ring dressing can be used around an area on which direct pressure should not be used **(Box 10-2).**

FIGURE 10-7

A variety of dressings.

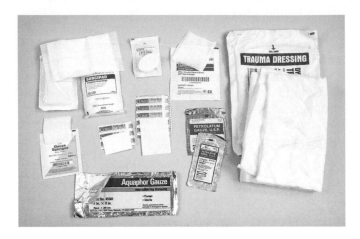

Guidelines for Using Dressings

After washing and drying the wound, apply the dressing this way:

1. Wash hands and wear gloves.

2. Choose a dressing larger than the wound. Do not touch the part of the dressing that will contact the wound.

3. Carefully lay the dressing on the wound (do not slide it on from the side). Cover the entire wound **(Figure 10-8).**

4. If blood seeps through, do not remove the dressing; instead, add more dressings on top of it. (See **Chapter 9** for use of hemostatic dressings if bleeding continues.)

5. Apply a bandage to hold the dressing in place.

When a dressing is later removed – to clean the wound or change a soiled dressing, for example – do not tug on a dressing that sticks to the wound. Soak it in warm water to release the dressing.

FIGURE 10-8

Cover the wound with a sterile dressing and apply a bandage.

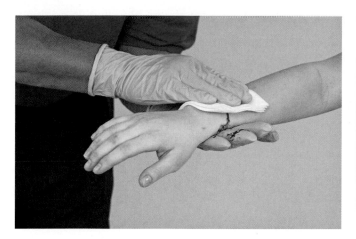

FIGURE 10-9

Types of bandages.

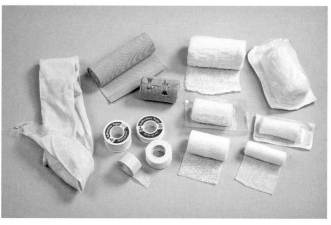

BANDAGES

Bandages are used for covering a dressing, keeping the dressing on a wound and maintaining pressure to control bleeding. Because only dressings touch the wound itself, bandages need to be clean but not necessarily sterile. As described in **Chapter 14,** bandages are also used to support or immobilize an injury to bones, joints or muscles, and to reduce swelling.

Types of Bandages

Different types of bandages are available for different uses **(Figure 10-9).** The following are common types of bandages:

- Adhesive compresses or strips for small wounds that combine a dressing with an adhesive bandage, such as Band-Aids

- Adhesive tape rolls (cloth, plastic or paper)

- Tubular bandages for fingers or toes

- Elastic bandages

- Self-adhering bandages

- Gauze roller bandages

- Triangular bandages (or folded square cloths)

- Any cloth or other material improvised to meet the purposes of bandaging

Guidelines for Bandaging

Follow these guidelines for bandaging:

1. To put pressure on a wound to stop bleeding or to prevent the swelling of an injury, apply the bandage firmly, but not so tightly that it cuts off circulation. The pressure is sufficient if the bandage is snug but you can slip a finger under it. Never put a circular bandage around the neck. With a bandage around a limb, check the fingers or toes for color, warmth and sensation (normal touch, not tingling) to make sure circulation is not cut off. If there are signs of reduced circulation, unwrap the bandage and reapply it less tightly.

2. Do not cover fingers or toes unless they are injured. Keep them exposed so they can be checked for adequate circulation.

3. Because swelling continues after many injuries, keep checking the tightness of the bandage. Swelling may make a loose bandage tight enough to cut off circulation.

4. With a bandaged wound, be sure the bandage is secure enough that the dressing will not move and expose the wound to possible contamination.

5. With elastic and roller bandages, anchor the first end and tie, tape, pin or clip the ending section in place. Loose ends could get caught on something and pull the bandage loose or disrupt the wound.

6. Use an elastic bandage to make a pressure bandage around a limb to control bleeding and protect the wound (see **Chapter 8**).

7. An elastic bandage is used to support a joint and prevent swelling. At the wrist or ankle, a figure-8 wrap is used (see **Chapter 14**).

8. Wrap a bandage from the bottom of the limb upward toward the heart to avoid cutting off circulation.

9. Avoid bending a joint once it has been bandaged because movement may loosen the dressing or cut off circulation.

When to Seek Medical Attention for a Wound

Remember: Call 9-1-1 for severe bleeding. In addition, the victim should see a health care provider as soon as possible in the following cases:

- Bleeding that is not easily controlled

- Any deep or large wound (e.g., wounds into muscle or bone)

- Significant wounds on the face

- Signs and symptoms that the wound is infected

BOX 10-2: RING PAD

Direct pressure should not be used over the entire surface of certain types of wounds. For example, pressure should not be put on a skull fracture (see **Chapter 12**), a fractured bone protruding from a wound (see **Chapter 14**) or an object impaled in a wound. Cover the open wound with a sterile dressing as usual, but do not apply direct pressure on the wound. In these cases, bleeding is controlled around the object or fracture. A dressing made into a pad in a ring shape is appropriate for controlling bleeding and dressing such wounds.

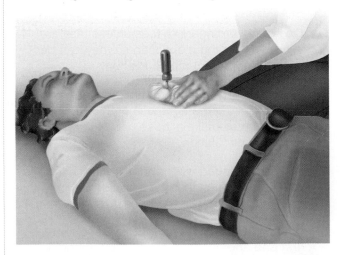

Make a ring pad from a long strip of gauze or other material. First, make a circular wrap the right size to surround the area. With the remainder of the strip or an additional strip, wrap around the circular wrap to give the ring more bulk. Then, position the ring around the wound and apply indirect pressure as needed.

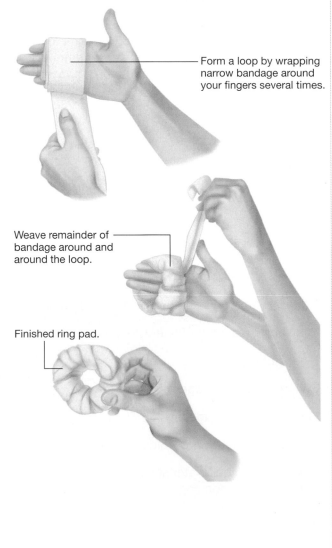

Form a loop by wrapping narrow bandage around your fingers several times.

Weave remainder of bandage around and around the loop.

Finished ring pad.

- Any bite from an animal or human

- Foreign object or material embedded in the wound

- Puncture wounds

- The victim is unsure about tetanus vaccination

- Any wound you are unsure about

- Wounds that may require stitches **(Figure 10-10)**

- Cuts on the face or hands when the edges do not close together

- Gaping wounds

- Cuts longer than 1 inch

FIGURE 10-10

A large, open wound may require stitches.

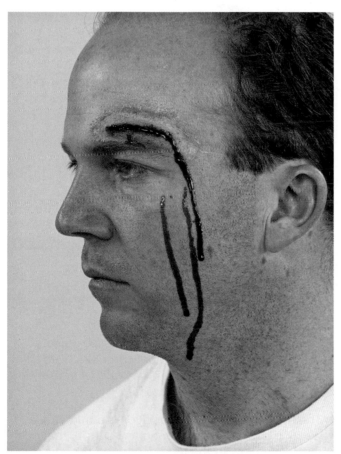

✎ **LEARNING CHECKPOINT 1**

1. Check off the actions that are included in wound care:

   ☐ Irrigate minor wounds with running water.

   ☐ Pour rubbing alcohol on any wound.

   ☐ Wash major wounds to help stop the bleeding.

   ☐ Cover any wound with a sterile dressing and bandage.

   ☐ Let a scab form before washing a minor wound.

   ☐ See a health care provider for a deep wound or puncture wound.

   ☐ Blow on a minor wound to cool the area and relieve pain.

2. If you are changing a wound dressing a day after the injury and the dressing sticks to the wound, what should you do?

   _____

   _____

   _____

Circle **True** or **False** for each of the following statements:

3. Puncture wounds have little risk for infection.　　True　False

4. You don't need to bother putting on gloves to dress a minor wound if you know the victim well.　　True　False

5. For what type(s) of wound(s) is an antibiotic ointment appropriate?

   _____

   _____

6. Check off which signs and symptoms may indicate a wound is infected:

   ☐ Headache

   ☐ Warmth in the area

   ☐ Cool, clammy skin

   ☐ A scab forms that looks dark brown

   ☐ Red, swollen area

   ☐ Nausea and vomiting

   ☐ Fever

   ☐ Pus drains from the wound

7. Which of these victims need to seek medical attention? (Check all that apply.)

   ☐ José has a deep laceration from a piece of equipment, but you managed to stop the bleeding in 15 minutes.

   ☐ Rebecca had lunch in a nearby park and was bitten by a squirrel she was feeding, but the bleeding was minor and stopped almost immediately.

   ☐ Carl scraped his knee when he fell off his bicycle on the way to work, but the abrasion washed out clean and you have applied an antibiotic ointment.

   ☐ Kim got a bad gash on her cheek when a bottle broke in the supply room, but she had already stopped the bleeding by the time you saw her.

Circle **True** or **False** for the following statement:

8. To control bleeding, make a pressure bandage as tight as you can get it. | True | False |

9. You have put a pressure bandage around a victim's arm to control bleeding from a laceration. A few minutes later, she says her fingers are tingling. You feel her hand, and her fingers are cold. What should you do?

   _____

   _____

   _____

   _____

10. Select the best answer. When applying a bandage over a dressing, the bandage should –

    a. hold down only the corners of the dressing so the wound can breathe.

    b. be soaked first in cold water.

    c. cover the entire dressing.

    d. be loose enough so it can be slid to one side to change the dressing.

Special Wounds

In addition to the general guidelines for all wounds, certain types of wounds require special first aid considerations. These include puncture wounds, impaled objects, amputations and injuries to the genitals, head or face.

INJURY PREVENTION

Wounds may occur anywhere in the body as a result of any kind of trauma. Prevention focuses on injury prevention in general, as described throughout this text. Following are guidelines for preventing certain special kinds of wounds:

- Many traumatic amputations result from industrial emergencies and the use of power tools in the home. Always follow OSHA guidelines in the work setting to prevent injury, and when using power tools at home, follow the specific guidelines provided by the tool's manufacturer. Never disassemble safeguards built into tools or equipment.

- Wearing the appropriate helmet at work or during sports and recreational activities can prevent skull injuries and injuries to the face and ears.

- Eye injuries frequently result from small objects or particles being unexpectedly propelled into the eye. Eye shields should be worn whenever one is working with power equipment.

- The American Dental Association recommends wearing a mouthguard during any activity that can result in a blow to the face or mouth. Ask your dentist about having a custom mouthguard made to provide a safe, comfortable fit.

- To avoid breaking a tooth, do not chew ice, hard candy or popcorn kernels.

- To prevent injuries to the genitals, males engaging in contact sports should wear an athletic cup; females should wear a pelvic shield or groin pad or protector.

- To prevent stretching and potentially tearing ligaments and other supportive breast tissues, women should wear a sports bra during exercise or sport activities.

PUNCTURE WOUNDS

Puncture wounds may involve deeper injuries you cannot see. If the puncturing object may have penetrated the body, check also for an exit wound. In general, puncture wounds carry a greater risk of infection than other types of wounds because often they bleed less, and therefore, germs may not be flushed out. In addition to routine wound care, follow these steps:

1. Irrigate the wound with large amounts of warm or room-temperature water with or without soap to remove foreign matter.

2. Gently press on wound edges to promote bleeding.

3. Dry the area. Do not put any medication inside or over the puncture wound.

4. Cover the wound with a sterile dressing and bandage.

5. Seek medical attention.

IMPALED OBJECTS

Removing an object from a wound could cause more injury and bleeding, because oftentimes, the object is sealing the wound or damaged blood vessels. Leave it in place and dress the wound around it **(Figure 10-11)**. Use bulky dressings (trauma dressings) to stabilize the object and keep it from moving. If there is blood or sweat on the skin, adhesive tape may not stick well enough to hold bulky dressings in place; use a roller bandage or strips of cloth to tie the bandage in place around the impaled object. Follow these guidelines:

1. Control bleeding by applying direct pressure around the edges of the object.

2. Dress the wound around or over the object.

3. Stabilize the object in place with large dressings or folded cloths.

4. Support the object while bandaging the dressings in place.

5. Keep the victim still and seek medical attention.

An impaled object in the eye or the cheek is a unique circumstance requiring special care, as described in the later sections on eye and cheek injuries.

FIGURE 10-11

Leave an impaled object in place and use bulky dressings to keep it from moving.

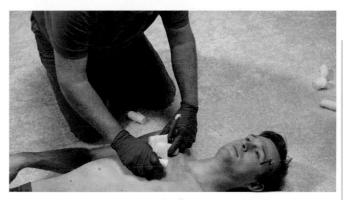

AVULSIONS AND AMPUTATIONS

An avulsion is a piece of skin or other soft tissue torn partially from the body, like a flap. Try to move the skin or tissue back into its normal position unless the wound is contaminated, and then control bleeding and provide wound care.

If the avulsed tissue is completely separated from the body, care for it the same as you would for an amputated part.

In an amputation, a part has been severed from the body. Control the bleeding and care for the victim and the wound first, then recover and care for the amputated part. Bleeding can usually be controlled with the same measures as for other wounds, using bulky dressings. Follow these steps to care for the severed body part, which surgeons may be able to re-attach to the victim:

1. Wrap the severed part in a dry, sterile dressing or clean cloth. Do not wash it.

2. Place the part in a plastic bag or container and seal it.

3. Place the sealed bag in another bag or container with ice. Do not let the part touch water or ice directly, and do not surround it with ice **(Figure 10-12)**.

4. Make sure the severed part is given to emergency personnel or taken with the victim to the emergency department.

FIGURE 10-12

Keep amputated part cold but not directly touching ice.

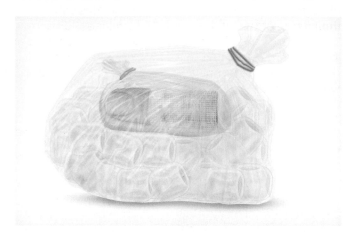

FIGURE 10-13

Apply a triangular bandage like a diaper to secure dressings in the genital area.

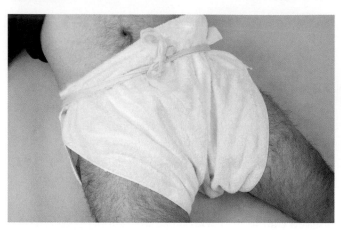

GENITAL INJURIES

Injuries to the genitals are rare because of their protected location. Injuries may occur from blunt trauma, an impact that creates a wound or sexual abuse. Provide privacy for a victim when giving first aid for a wound in the genital area. Follow these guidelines:

- Use direct pressure with a sterile dressing or sanitary pad to control external bleeding. Then, use a large triangular bandage applied like a diaper to secure the dressings in place **(Figure 10-13).**

- For injured testicles, provide support with a towel wrapped between the legs like a diaper. For a closed injury caused by blunt trauma, a cold pack may help reduce pain.

- For vaginal bleeding, have the woman press a sanitary pad or clean folded towel to the area to control the bleeding.

- Call 9-1-1 for severe or continuing bleeding, significant pain or swelling or the possibility of sexual abuse.

- In the case of rape or sexual abuse, preserve evidence for law enforcement personnel by following the guidelines in **Chapter 21.**

HEAD AND FACE WOUNDS

Wounds to the head or face may require special first aid. The following sections provide guidelines for these special injuries. Skull injuries, such as fractures, are described in **Chapter 12.**

With any significant injury to the head, the victim may also have a neck or spinal injury. If you suspect a spinal injury, be careful not to move the victim's head while giving first aid for head and face wounds.

SCALP WOUND WITHOUT SUSPECTED SKULL FRACTURE

If signs and symptoms of a skull fracture are not present, and the wound is restricted to the scalp, apply a dressing and use direct pressure as usual to control bleeding. Then apply a roller bandage, or a triangular bandage folded into a cravat, around the head to secure the dressing. *Never wrap a bandage around the neck because of the risk of impeding breathing if the injury causes swelling* (see First Aid: "Scalp Wound Without Suspected Skull Fracture").

First Aid: Scalp Wound Without Suspected Skull Fracture

Signs, Symptoms and Care

WHEN YOU SEE

- Bleeding from the head

- No sign of skull fracture

DO THIS FIRST

1. Replace any skin flaps and cover the wound with a sterile dressing.

2. Use direct pressure to control bleeding.

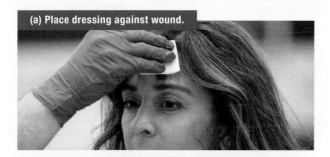

(a) Place dressing against wound.

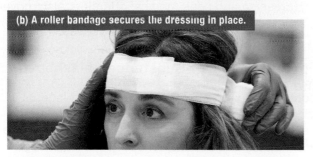

(b) A roller bandage secures the dressing in place.

3. Put a roller or triangle bandage around the victim's head to secure the dressing.

ADDITIONAL CARE

- Position the victim with head and shoulders slightly raised to help control bleeding.

- Seek medical attention if the victim later experiences nausea and vomiting, persistent headache, drowsiness or disorientation, stumbling or lack of coordination or problems with speech or vision. (See discussion of concussion in **Chapter 12**.)

EYE INJURIES

Eye injuries are serious because vision may be affected. Eye injuries include blows to the eye, impaled objects in the eye, dirt or small particles in the eye, and chemicals or other substances splashed into the eye. When caring for any eye injury, avoid putting pressure directly on the eyeball because this tissue is easily injured.

With most eye injuries, movement of the eye will continue to worsen the injury. Bandaging or otherwise covering an injured eye discourages the victim from moving it. Because the eyes move together, the unaffected eye must also be covered; otherwise, the victim, when using the unaffected eye, will also be moving the injured eye. Having both eyes covered or bandaged is often frightening, especially to an injured victim. Explain what you are doing and why before covering the good eye. To minimize anxiety, keep talking to the victim or have another person offer reassurance with conversation and touch.

For a Blow to the Eye:

1. If the eye is bleeding or leaking fluid, call 9-1-1 or get the victim to the emergency department immediately.

2. Put a cold pack over the eye, with a barrier such as cloth between the cold pack and the eye, for up to 15 minutes to ease pain and reduce swelling, but do not put pressure on the eye. If the victim is wearing a contact lens, do not try to remove it **(Figure 10-14)**.

3. Have victim lie still. Cover the uninjured eye.

4. Seek medical attention if pain persists or vision is affected in any way.

For a Large Object Embedded in the Eye:

1. Do not remove the object. Stabilize it in place with dressings or bulky cloth. Be careful not to put any pressure on the eye from the object. With a large impaled object or one that may move, use a paper cup or something similar to stabilize the object and keep it from moving in the eye **(Figure 10-15).**

2. Cover both eyes, because movement of the uninjured one causes movement of the injured one.

3. Call 9-1-1 or get the victim to the emergency department immediately.

FIGURE 10-14

For a blow to the eye, hold a cold pack on the eye.

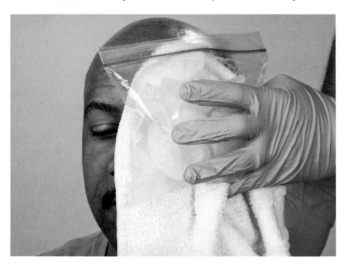

FIGURE 10-15

Stabilize an object impaled in the eyeball.

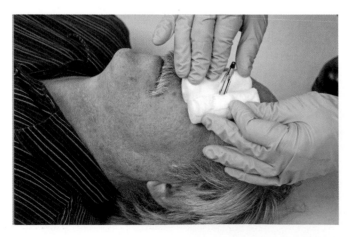

For Dirt or a Small Particle in the Eye:

If the victim complains of something small caught in the eye, do not let the victim rub the eye with his or her hands, which could cause scratching of the eye or other soft tissue. The body's natural way to remove small particles from the eye is to wash it out with tears and blinking. Wait a minute to see if the victim's tears flush out the object. If not, try these methods:

1. Gently pull the upper eyelid out and down over the lower eyelid. This allows the lower lashes to catch a particle caught under the upper eyelid.

2. If the particle remains, gently flush the eye with water from a medicine dropper or water glass. Have the victim tilt the head so that the affected eye is lower than the other; this prevents water from flowing into the unaffected eye. Flush from the corner nearer the nose. Ask the victim to hold the eyelids open with his or her fingers if needed, and to look in all directions and blink during the flushing.

3. If the particle remains and is visible, carefully try to brush it out gently with a wet, sterile dressing. Lift the upper eyelid and swab its underside if you see the particle **(Figure 10-16).**

4. If the particle remains or the victim has any vision problems or pain, cover the eye with a sterile dressing and seek medical attention. Also, cover the uninjured eye to prevent movement of the injured one.

For a Chemical or Substance Splashed in the Eye:

1. Continuously flush the victim's eye with large amounts of clean, running water for at least 15 minutes or until EMS arrives. If tap water is not available, use normal saline or a commercial eye irrigation solution.

2. Have a victim wearing contact lenses remove them.

3. Tilt the victim's head so the water does not run into the unaffected eye.

4. For a responsive victim, call the Poison Control Center (800 222-1222) immediately and follow its instructions. For an unresponsive victim or if the Poison Control Center is not available, call 9-1-1 or seek help from a medical provider.

FIGURE 10-16

Carefully remove a particle from the eyelid.

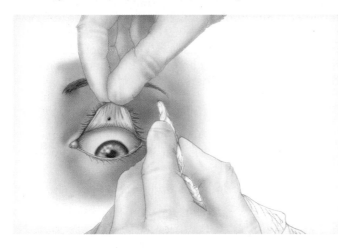

EAR INJURIES

With bleeding from the external ear, control the bleeding with direct pressure and dress the wound.

Remember that bleeding or clear fluid (cerebrospinal fluid) from within the ear can be a sign of a serious head injury. Do not use direct pressure to try to stop fluid from coming out of the ear. Give care as described in **Chapter 12.**

If the victim complains of a foreign object in the ear, do not try to remove it with any tool or object. Never insert tweezers, a pin or cotton swab into the ear in an attempt to remove an object. The object may be pushed further into the ear, or the tool may damage the eardrum or other tissues. Leave the object in place and seek medical attention. Only if the foreign object is clearly visible and easily grasped with your fingers is it safe to remove an object, but do not remove an impaled object. Occasionally, an insect may crawl into the ear when a person is sleeping. If you see or know that an insect is in the ear, gently pour lukewarm water into the ear to try to float it out. If it does not come out, seek medical attention.

For bleeding from within the ear, follow the guidelines in First Aid: "Ear Injuries."

First Aid: Ear Injuries

Signs, Symptoms and Care

WHEN YOU SEE

- Bleeding or fluid from inside the ear

- Signs of pain

- Possible deafness

DO THIS FIRST

1. Clear fluid or watery blood from the ear could mean a skull fracture. Call 9-1-1.

2. Help victim to sit up, tilting the affected ear lower to let blood or other fluid drain.

3. Cover the ear with a loose, sterile dressing, but do not apply pressure.

4. Seek medical attention immediately if 9-1-1 was not called.

ADDITIONAL CARE

- Keep the ear covered to reduce the risk of infection.

ALERT

- Do not plug the ear closed to try to stop bleeding.

NOSE INJURIES

Injury to the nose can cause heavy bleeding. Nosebleeds can also be caused by pressure changes or a child picking at the nose. Nosebleeds can usually be controlled, usually within a few minutes, by positioning the victim leaning slightly forward and pinching the nostrils closed until bleeding stops. For an unresponsive victim or a victim who cannot sit leaning forward, position the victim on one side with the head turned to allow drainage from the nose and mouth while you pinch the nostrils closed. Do not try to pack the nostrils with a dressing in an effort to control the bleeding.

Bleeding that runs from the back of the nose down the throat is more serious and needs immediate medical attention. Do not tilt the victim's head backward, but keep the victim positioned to allow blood to drain out of the mouth so that the airway is not threatened (see First Aid: "Nose Bleed").

Small children often put small objects in their noses. If a foreign object is clearly visible and easily grasped with tweezers, you may safely remove it, but do not remove an impaled object. Do not push tweezers or your finger into the nostril to try to remove an object because of the risk of pushing it in deeper. Do not have a child try to blow an object out, because it may be sucked in deeper instead.

First Aid: Nose Bleed

Signs, Symptoms and Care

WHEN YOU SEE

- Blood coming from either or both nostrils

- Blood possibly running from back of nose down into the mouth or throat

DO THIS FIRST

1. Have the victim sit and tilt head slightly forward with mouth open. Carefully remove any object you see protruding from the nose, but do not probe inside the nose.

2. Have the victim pinch the nostrils together, just below the bridge of the nose, for 10 minutes. Ask victim to breathe through the mouth and not speak, swallow, cough or sniff.

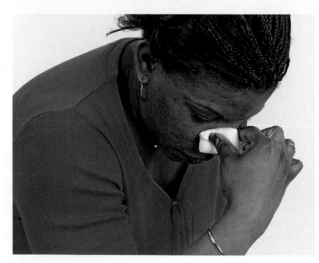

3. If victim is gasping or choking on blood in the throat, call 9-1-1.

4. Place a cold compress on the bridge of the nose.

5. After 10 minutes, release the pressure slowly. Pinch the nostrils again for another 10 minutes if bleeding continues.

ADDITIONAL CARE

- Place a cold compress on the bridge of the nose.

- Seek medical attention if:

  - Bleeding continues after 2 attempts to control it.

  - You suspect the nose is broken.

  - There is a foreign object in the nose.

  - The victim has high blood pressure.

- Have the person rest for a few hours and avoid rubbing or blowing the nose.

ALERT

- Do not tilt the victim's head backward.

- Do not have the victim lie down.

CHEEK INJURIES

A wound on the outside of the cheek is cared for by following the general guidelines for wounds. If an object is impaled in a wound in the cheek, check inside the mouth to see if the object has penetrated through. If you can see both sides of the object and can remove it safely, do so. *This is the one exception to the rule about not removing an impaled object from a wound.* The object may pose a risk to the airway if it protrudes into the mouth or later falls into the mouth. Gently pull the object out, in the direction from which it penetrated the cheek, taking care with a sharp object not to cut the cheek further. Then, place a dressing inside the mouth between the cheek wound and the teeth; watch that this dressing does not come out of position and block the airway. Apply another dressing to the outside of the wound, applying pressure as needed to control bleeding. For an unresponsive victim, roll the victim's body as a unit to position the head so that blood and other fluid will run out of the mouth (as described in **Chapter 12**).

TEETH AND MOUTH INJURIES

Injuries to the mouth may cause bleeding anywhere in the mouth and may knock out a tooth. Bleeding is controlled with direct pressure on a dressing over the wound. A tooth that has been knocked out can usually be replanted if the tooth is properly cared for. The priority of first aid for the mouth is always to ensure that the airway is open, and that blood can drain from the mouth until bleeding is controlled.

A tooth that has been knocked out requires care if it is to be successfully replanted because delicate tissues attached to the tooth may quickly die. Do not try to put the tooth back in the socket. The tooth should not be allowed to dry out; immerse it in milk or water.

If a tooth is knocked loose enough that there is a risk it may fall out, make a pad from rolled gauze and have the victim bite down on it to keep the tooth in place until the victim reaches the dentist. If a tooth is broken, rinse the victim's mouth with saline or tap water, and then apply a cold pack to reduce swelling and pain; see a dentist as soon as possible.

For a Knocked-Out Tooth:

1. Have the victim sit with head tilted forward to let blood drain out.

2. Rinse the wound with saline solution or tap water.

3. Control the bleeding by having the victim bite down for 20-30 minutes on a gauze pad or cotton ball placed over the tooth socket **(Figure 10-17)**.

4. Save the tooth. Pick it up by the crown and place it in a solution, such as Hank's Balanced Salt Solution – a specialized tooth-preserving solution, or whole milk. Do not clean or scrub the tooth.

5. Have the victim see a dentist immediately.

For Other Bleeding in the Mouth:

1. Have the victim sit with head tilted forward to let blood drain out.

2. **For a wound penetrating the lip:** Put a rolled dressing between the lip and the gum. Hold a second dressing against the outside lip.

3. **For a bleeding tongue:** Put a dressing on the wound and apply pressure.

4. Do not repeatedly rinse the mouth (this may prevent clotting).

5. Do not let victim swallow blood, which may cause vomiting.

6. When the bleeding stops, tell the victim not to drink anything warm for several hours.

7. Seek medical attention if bleeding is severe or does not stop.

FIGURE 10-17

Stop bleeding with dressing over tooth socket.

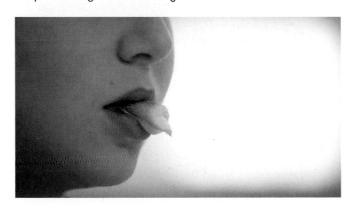

BLISTERS

Blisters usually occur because of friction on the skin, as when a shoe rubs the back of the ankle or heel. They can be painful and may become infected after breaking. Burns may cause a different kind of blister (see **Chapter 11**).

Blisters can usually be prevented by protecting the feet with socks or with tape where socks rub. A small blister can be protected with an adhesive bandage. Try to prevent it from breaking open, which can lead to infection. For a larger blister, cut a hole in several layers of gauze or moleskin, and position this dressing over the blister with the blister itself protected within the hole (see First Aid: "Blisters").

If a blister breaks, wash the area and care for it as you would care for a wound (see **Chapter 10**).

First Aid: Blisters

Signs, Symptoms and Care

WHEN YOU SEE

- A raised, fluid-filled blister, often surrounded by red skin

DO THIS FIRST

1. Wash the blister and surrounding area with soap and water. Rinse and gently pat dry.

2. Cover the blister with an adhesive bandage big enough that the gauze pad covers the entire blister. Bandages with an adhesive strip on all 4 sides are best because they keep the area cleaner if the blister breaks. For a larger blister, use a donut-shaped dressing to surround the blister and prevent pressure on it.

ADDITIONAL CARE

- Prevent continued friction in the area.

ALERT

- Never deliberately break a blister. This could lead to infection.

SPLINTERS

You can remove a splinter in the skin by coaxing it out with a sterile needle and then grasping the end with tweezers or your fingers. Cleanse the area with soap and water.

CRUSH INJURIES

A crush injury is caused when strong pressure is exerted against the body. Depending on the force involved, a crushing injury can result in muscle, bone, nerve and tissue damage; shock; and internal and/or external bleeding.

Provide care for the injuries you find and call 9-1-1.

 LEARNING CHECKPOINT 2

1. Name one circumstance in which you might want to promote bleeding.

_____

_____

_____

Circle **True** or **False** for each of the following statements:

2. The first thing to do when you see an impaled object in a wound is to pull it out so you can put direct pressure on the wound to stop the bleeding.   True   False

3. An amputated part should be kept cold but not put in direct contact with ice.   True   False

4. With an eye injury, why would you cover the *uninjured* eye, too?

_____

_____

_____

5. Describe 3 ways you can try to remove a small particle from the eye.

_____

_____

_____

_____

Circle **True** or **False** for the following statement:

6. For bleeding from within the ear, roll a piece of gauze into a plug and try to seal the ear with it.　　True　False

7. Fill in the correct answer. A nose bleed victim should first try to stop the bleeding by pinching the nostrils closed for ____ minutes. During this time, list 2 or 3 things the victim should *not* do.

_____

_____

Circle **True** or **False** for the following statements:

8. A knocked-out tooth can be reimplanted if it is carefully preserved and the victim reaches a dentist soon.　　True　False

9. Repeatedly rinsing the mouth with cool water is the best way to stop bleeding in the mouth.　　True　False

 CONCLUDING THOUGHTS

Wounds are among the most common injuries requiring first aid. In most cases, the care is simple and straightforward: Clean the wound, apply a dressing and cover and secure the dressing with an appropriate bandage. Particular kinds of wounds and injuries in certain areas of the body require additional specific care. Following these guidelines will, in most cases, prevent infection of the wound and lead to effective healing.

 CRITICAL THINKING CHALLENGE QUESTIONS

📷 SCENARIO 1

A coworker's young son, playing outside, falls and gets a nasty scrape on his palm. The bleeding soon stops by itself, but the wound is full of dirt. Describe the steps to take with this wound.

_____

_____

_____

📷 SCENARIO 2

You are using an ice pick to chip away ice around a frozen door when you slip and the tip of the ice pick penetrates your palm. The wound does not seem too deep and it is not bleeding. How do you care for this wound?

_____

_____

_____

📷 SCENARIO 3

A carpenter at your worksite is using a nail gun to install new siding. As he is putting the tool down, it fires and a nail is shot into the calf muscle of his leg. You cut open his pants leg and see the head of the nail sticking out about an inch, with bleeding around the nail. How do you care for this wound?

_____

_____

_____

 ADDITIONAL ACTIVITIES AND QUESTIONS

If you play organized sports, what kinds of special equipment do you use to prevent injuries of the mouth, eyes and head? Tell others in your class about these safety items. If you are employed in a job involving physical labor or risks, tell others about the safety equipment you use.

✏ REVIEW QUESTIONS

Select the best answers.

1. What is the first priority for a severely bleeding wound?

   a. Seeking medical attention

   b. Controlling the bleeding

   c. Preventing infection

   d. Irrigating the wound

2. Infection is more likely in which kind of wound?

   a. Puncture

   b. Laceration

   c. Abrasion

   d. Avulsion

3. What is the best way to clean a wound?

   a. Soak in alcohol.

   b. Apply iodine.

   c. Irrigate with water.

   d. Apply a cool, moist compress.

4. Antibiotic ointment may be used on what kinds of wounds?

   a. Abrasions

   b. Punctures

   c. Deep burns

   d. Open abdominal wounds

5. A pressure bandage to control bleeding –

   a. should be applied directly over the wound.

   b. should be as tight as you can get it to stop the bleeding.

   c. should be applied above the wound like a tourniquet.

   d. All of the above

6. Signs of good circulation in a limb below a pressure bandage include –

   a. cool skin.

   b. normal skin color.

   c. tingling sensations.

   d. ability to move fingers or toes.

7. What wounds should be seen by a health care provider?

   a. Wounds through the skin into muscle tissue

   b. Human bite wounds

   c. Wounds that may require stitches

   d. All of the above

8. How would you best care for a traumatically amputated finger?

   a. Wash it under running water and put it in a glass or jar of ice water.

   b. Wrap it in a dressing, place it inside a plastic bag and put the bag on ice.

   c. Keep it dry and at body temperature (held against victim's body).

   d. Put it in a plastic bag, and place the bag in the freezer until help arrives.

9. For a nonbleeding but painful blow to the eye –

   a. flush constantly with warm, running water for up to 30 minutes.

   b. have victim sit in a dark room with both eyes covered for 30 minutes.

   c. put a cold pack over the eye for up to 15 minutes.

   d. give the victim aspirin or ibuprofen.

10. Care for a nose bleed includes –

   a. having the victim "blow" the nose into a handkerchief to clear out blood.

   b. pinching the nostrils closed for up to 10 minutes.

   c. packing the nose with sterile gauze.

   d. having the victim tilt head back while sucking on ice chips.

CHAPTER 11

Burns

LESSON OBJECTIVES

- Explain common causes of fires and burns and how to prevent them.

- Describe what happens in the body with a burn.

- List differences among first-, second- and third-degree burns.

- Describe first aid for first-, second- and third-degree heat burns.

- Describe first aid for smoke inhalation.

- Describe first aid for chemical burns.

- Describe first aid for electrical burns and shocks.

While visiting your aunt at her home, you join her in the kitchen as she cooks pasta for dinner. On the stove's front burner is a large pot of boiling water. She is telling you about something that happened earlier that day and is not paying close attention to her cooking. Before you can react to stop her, you see her reach across the boiling water for the kettle on the back burner. She yelps as the steam burns her forearm, and jerks her arm back. What should you do immediately? Then, what additional care should you give for this burn?

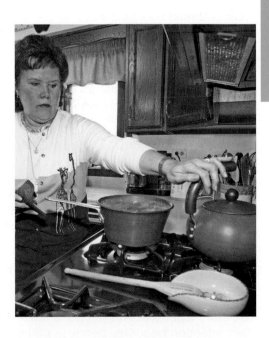

Fires and burns are a major cause of death and injury. There are about 2,400 deaths a year in the United States caused by fires and burns, and about 393,000 burn injuries leading to emergency department visits.[1] Fires and burns may occur in almost any setting, but the great majority occur in the home, and experts believe that most fires and burns can be prevented. Even with preventive steps, however, it is essential to know what to do when fire occurs and how to treat burn victims.

Burns of the skin or deeper tissues may be caused by the sun, heat, chemicals or electricity. Mild heat burns and sunburn may need only simple first aid, but severe burns can be a medical emergency.

[1]*National Safety Council [NSC]. (2015). Injury Facts®, 2015 Edition. Itasca, IL: Author.*

What Happens with a Burn?

A burn is an injury to the skin and potentially deeper structures caused by heat, electricity or chemicals. Burns can cause severe adverse effects in the body because the skin has several important functions:

- *Protection.* The skin protects the body against the entry of **pathogens** that can cause infection, as well as other harmful substances. Specialized cells also have an immune function.

- *Fluid retention.* The skin prevents the loss of fluids and other important substances, such as electrolytes.

- *Temperature regulation.* The skin has a major role in controlling the body's temperature, preventing heat loss in cold environments and promoting heat loss in hot environments.

- *Sensation.* The skin contains sensory and other nerves and blood vessels.

Although a minor burn like a sunburn may damage only the **epidermis,** the outer layer of skin, more severe burns damage the **dermis,** or middle layer, which contains nerves and blood vessels, or the deepest layer of **subcutaneous** tissue, through which larger blood vessels and nerves pass **(Figure 11-1).**

Burns that extend into the dermis expose tissues to the outside environment and carry a high risk of infection from pathogens present almost everywhere. The more extensive and deeper a burn, the more likely infection becomes because pathogens may enter more easily, and medical treatment becomes more difficult.

Burns extending into the dermis or deeper also cause fluid loss. Injured capillaries in the dermis leak fluid; this is the cause of watery blisters in second-degree burns. Deeper burns cause fluid loss from larger blood vessels. Significant fluid loss from severe burns can cause shock, a further threat to the burn victim that can be life threatening (see **Chapter 9**).

To function well, the human body must maintain a fairly consistent internal temperature. Because the skin helps regulate this function, a severe burn can cause a loss of body heat, further stressing vital organs. Therefore, a victim with extensive severe burns should not be cooled with water over much of the body because of the increased risk of **hypothermia,** which would further threaten the victim's condition.

Because the skin is rich in sensory nerves, burns can be very painful due to damage to these nerves. With burns entirely through the skin, however, the victim may not feel pain because the nerve endings are completely destroyed. In such cases, there are often less severely burned areas around the pain-free areas that do cause significant pain. Pain is, therefore, present in most burns, but is not an indication of the burn's severity.

Finally, burns may damage body tissues other than just the skin. A full-thickness burn that penetrates all the way through the skin may damage muscle and fat tissue beneath as well as underlying organs, resulting in additional trauma to the body and increasing the urgency for medical treatment. Victims with burns caused by fires may also have respiratory damage caused by inhaling smoke, fumes or hot air. Respiratory tract tissues may swell, causing breathing difficulty.

FIGURE 11-1

Layers of the skin.

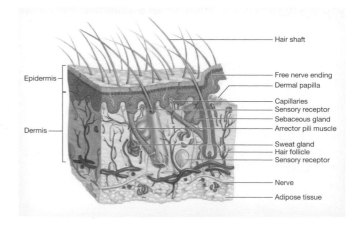

Prevention of Fires and Burns

COMMON CAUSES OF FIRES RESULTING IN BURNS

The huge majority of all deaths by fire and burns occur in the home. Following are some sobering facts and statistics about fires in the home:[1]

- In 2014, United States fire departments responded to an estimated 1,298,000 fires.

- On average, a fire department responded to a fire every 24 seconds.

- Fire claimed 3,275 lives.

- Cooking is the leading cause of home fires and home fire injuries.

- Smoking has been the leading cause of home fire deaths for decades.

- Almost all United States homes have at least one smoke alarm, but three out of five home fire deaths resulted from fires in homes without working smoke alarms.

- Children younger than 5 and older adults face the highest risk of home fire death, but young adults face a higher risk of home fire injury.

The following are the most common causes of fires leading to injury or death:

- Smoking

- Heating

- Cooking

- Playing with fire

- Electrical wiring

- Open flames

- Appliances or other equipment

[1]National Fire Protection Association. nfpa.org/research/reports-and-statistics/fires-in-the-us Accessed January 2016.

PREVENTING BURNS

Preventing burns involves both preventing fires and preventing burns from hot water and other sources of heat, such as stoves.

PREVENTING FIRES

Follow these guidelines to prevent a fire in the home and other settings **(Figure 11-2)**:

- Make your home and workplace safe:

  - Make sure enough smoke detectors are installed and change batteries twice a year when you change your clocks for daylight saving time.

  - Do not allow smoking, or ensure that it is done safely and materials are safely extinguished. Never allow smoking in bed.

  - Keep curtains and other flammable objects away from fireplaces and stoves; use fireplace screens.

  - Have chimneys regularly inspected and cleaned to prevent chimney fires.

  - Never store gasoline or other highly flammable liquids indoors.

- Prevent fires in the kitchen:

  - Keep a fire extinguisher in the kitchen and know how to use it.

  - Tie back long hair or loose clothing when cooking or working around flames.

  - If food catches on fire in a microwave or toaster oven, leave the food there and turn off the appliance; keep other objects away until the flames go out.

- Prevent fires caused by electricity:

  - Keep power cords safely out of the way and away from children.

  - Check appliance cords for damaged areas or fraying.

  - Do not overload electrical outlets or use multiple extension cords.

  - Unplug appliances and extension cords when not in use.

- Keep children from playing with fire:

  - Store matches, lighters, candles and other ignition sources away from children.

  - Teach young children that matches, candles and lighters are only for adult use, and model safe behavior when using them yourself.

- Accept that "child-resistant" lighters are not childproof, but can be used even by toddlers to start fires.

- Understand that children who know that fire is "bad" are likely to play with matches or lighters in their bedrooms or elsewhere where they think they will not be caught.

- Any child may play with fire because of peer pressure or simple curiosity. Teach all children the dangers of fire, and keep matches and ignition sources away from them. Remember that almost 50,000 structure fires every year are set by children.[1]

- Protect children from burns caused by fire:

  - Purchase only flame-resistant pajamas and bedding.

  - Plan escape routes and teach children where to go if a fire breaks out.

  - Teach children to "stop, drop and roll" if their clothing catches on fire.

[1]National Fire Protection Association, nfpa.org/safety-information/for-consumers/arson-and-youth-fire-setting/young-firesetters Accessed January 2016.

FIGURE 11-2

Inspect all rooms for fire hazards, and keep children away from flames and sources of heat.

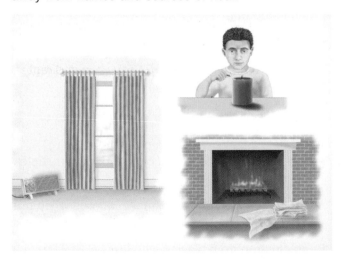

IF A FIRE OCCURS

Because a fire may occur even when you try to prevent it, know what to do if one should break out:

- Evacuate everyone first. Do not delay evacuation while you call 9-1-1 or use a fire extinguisher. Follow the rehearsed evacuation route.

- Do not use an elevator.

- Feel doors before opening them, and do not open a door that is hot.

- If the air is smoky, stay near the floor where there is more oxygen.

- Do not throw water on an electrical or grease (cooking) fire.

- If you cannot escape a building on fire, stuff clothing or rags in door cracks and vents; call 9-1-1 and give the dispatcher your exact location.

PREVENTING HEAT BURNS

After house fires, the most common cause of serious burns to children and the elderly is scalding from hot gases and liquids. Follow these guidelines to prevent burns from *anything* that may be hot:

- Do not use steam vaporizers; if you do, keep them away from areas children can reach.

- Keep hot irons, curling irons, toasters and similar appliances away from children. Never leave a child alone in a room with a hot object.

- Do not use space heaters on the floor or anywhere children can reach them. Install heat guards around radiators and heaters. Move a child's bed away from radiators or other heat sources.

- Keep children away from barbecue grills, which stay hot for a long time after use.

- Keep children away from campfires, which contain hot or burning coals many hours after the fire was "put out." Never leave children unsupervised near a fire or use flammable liquids to start a campfire. Keep tents and other gear well away.

- Never let children use fireworks.

- In the bathroom:

  - Prevent scalding burns by turning down the temperature of the water heater to 120°F or lower. If you cannot do this (as in an apartment building with shared hot water), purchase an anti-scald device from a children's store or hardware store.

- Check the temperature of bath water with your wrist. Stir the water with your hand to prevent hot spots.

- Supervise children in the bathtub.

- In the kitchen:

  - When cooking, use the back burners on the stove and keep pot handles turned toward the back of the stove.

  - Do not store food near the stove because children may attempt to reach it on their own.

  - Do not hold an infant when cooking or drinking a hot liquid.

  - Do not open the oven door with a child nearby.

  - Check the temperature of microwaved baby food or a baby bottle before feeding it to an infant.

  - Do not let young children use a microwave oven by themselves.

  - Keep high chairs away from the stove and counters where hot foods or electrical cords may be present.

PREVENTING HEAT BURNS IN THE ELDERLY

The elderly are less likely to hear, see or feel fire and burn threats, and are less able to escape a fire. In addition to the guidelines described previously, take these preventive actions in a home with an elderly family member:

- Ensure that all exits are kept clear.

- Keep eyeglasses, a telephone and needed walking aids next to the bed.

- Wear short sleeves or tight garments when cooking, and use oven mitts for protection.

- Avoid cooking when sleepy or when taking medications that cause drowsiness.

- Do not let anyone smoke near a device that supplies oxygen.

- Use a timer to remind you to turn off electric heating pads and blankets.

- Be aware of the special risks of hot objects, such as cooking materials and utensils.

- Understand the limitations imposed by any physical impairments or cognitive deficits.

- Contact an organization, such as the American Burn Association (ameriburn.org), for additional safety tips on preventing burns among the elderly.

PREVENTING SUNBURN

Sunburns cause pain and damage the skin. Because repeated sunburns can cause skin cancer later in life, steps should always be taken to prevent sunburns.

- Keep infants younger than 12 months out of direct sunlight as much as possible. Sun-blocking clothing and shade are recommended for infants younger than 6 months, although sunscreen can safely be used on small areas of skin. Protect an infant's eyes from sunlight, as well.

- For everyday outdoors activities, the American Cancer Society recommends applying sunscreen or sunblock with a **sun protection factor (SPF)** of at least 15 on all exposed areas of skin 20 minutes before sun exposure, and at least every 2 hours while in the sun **(Figure 11-3).** Use a higher SPF for prolonged sun exposure.

- Wear a wide-brimmed hat and protective clothing, and keep infants and young children covered with light clothing, hats and sunglasses.

- Limit sun exposure between 10 a.m. and 4 p.m.

- Be aware that reflective surfaces, such as water and snow, increase the risk of burning.

- Use sunscreen even on cloudy, hazy or foggy days, because sunburn may still occur.

- Use a lip balm with at least 15 SPF when in direct sun for an extended time.

FIGURE 11-3

Protect against sunburn with frequent use of sunscreen.

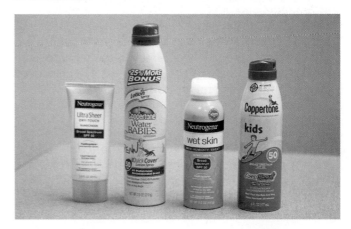

Heat Burns

Heat burns may be caused by flames or contact with steam or any hot object. The severity of a burn depends on the amount of damage to the skin and other tissues under the skin.

PUT OUT THE FIRE!

If the victim's clothing is on fire, use a blanket or water to put out any flames, or have the victim roll on the ground. Even when the fire is out, the skin will keep burning if it is still hot, so cool the burn area with water immediately, except with very severe burns. Also, remove the victim's clothing and jewelry, if it is possible to do so without further injuring the victim, because they may still be hot and continue to burn the victim.

ASSESSING A BURN

Assess burns to determine the appropriate first aid to give and decide whether to call 9-1-1 or transport the victim to medical care. Assessment involves consideration of several factors:

• What type of burn(s) does the victim have (first-, second- or third-degree)?

• How extensive is the burn (how much body area)?

• What specific body areas are burned?

• Are special circumstances present (the victim's age and health status)?

Because these variables can be complex, there is no one simple rule for determining when to call 9-1-1 or seek medical care. Whenever any burn may be serious, call 9-1-1 and let medical professionals guide your decision.

CLASSIFICATION OF BURNS

Burns are classified according to their depth into or through the skin:

• **First-degree burns** (also called **superficial burns**) damage only the skin's outer layer, the epidermis, like a typical sunburn. The skin is red, typically dry, and painful. These minor burns usually heal well by themselves but may require medical attention if they cover an extensive area.

• **Second-degree burns** (also called **partial-thickness burns**) damage the skin's deeper layer, the dermis. The skin is red, may look mottled and is very painful. Blisters are often present and may be weeping clear fluid. Scarring may be present after healing. Depending on size and other factors, second-degree burns may require medical attention.

• **Third-degree burns** (also called **full-thickness burns**) damage the skin all the way through the subcutaneous layer and may burn muscle or other tissues. The skin is charred or blackened or may look white and leathery. Pain is not present where the skin has burned through but is likely in adjacent areas. These burns are medical emergencies. Often a victim with serious burns has a mix of different burn classifications. One area may have a third-degree burn, for example, while nearby areas have first- or second-degree burns. Follow the first aid guidelines for the most severely burned area first.

ASSESSING BURN SIZE AND SEVERITY

In addition to burn depth, the size of the burned area is an important part of the assessment. This is usually calculated as a percentage of body surface area. A common method used by medical professionals to estimate the body surface area of a burn is the **rule of nines.** In this system, the adult body is divided into a number of areas with percentages based on increments of 9%. As shown in **Figure 11-4,** the percentages are different for a small child.

• Each arm is 9% (front or back alone is 4.5%).

• Each leg is 18% (front or back alone is 9%).

• The front of the torso is 18% (9% for abdomen and 9% for chest).

• The back of the torso is 18% (9% for lower back and buttocks, 9% for upper back).

• The head is 9% (face or back of head alone is 4.5%).

• The genital region is 1%.

FIGURE 11-4

The rule of nines for calculating body surface area burned. These numbers represent one-half (front or back) of the body.

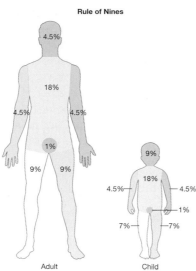

Rule of Nines

Adult

Child

In some cases, the percentage of body surface area burned influences the decision to call EMS and determines some aspects of advanced medical care. Any third-degree burn larger than a 50-cent piece or second-degree burn over more than 10% of the body in an adult (5% in a child or older adult) is an emergency. Seek medical attention also for a first-degree burn over more than 50% of the body.

Also important is the location of the burn on the body. Second- or third-degree burns on the face, genitals, hands or feet are considered emergencies and require immediate medical care. Circumferential burns that wrap around an extremity or a finger or toe should also receive immediate medical attention. Burns around the nose and mouth may affect breathing and are medical emergencies.

Finally, consider the victim's age and health. A burn in a child younger than 5 or an adult older than 55 is more serious than in a younger adult. Many **chronic** health disorders also make burns more serious. When in doubt about whether a victim needs immediate emergency treatment, call 9-1-1 **(Box 11-1).**

BOX 11-1: WHEN TO CALL 9-1-1 FOR A BURN

- The victim has a third-degree burn.

- The victim has a second-degree burn that is large (over 10% of body area in adult, or 5% of body area in a child, older adult or someone with chronic illness) or that affects the head, genitals, hands or feet.

- The victim is having trouble breathing.

- The victim may have inhaled smoke or fumes.

LEARNING CHECKPOINT 1

1. List at least 3 of the most common activities during which fires occur.

_____

_____

_____

2. Describe at least 3 things you can do to help prevent fires from occurring in the kitchen.

_____

_____

_____

Circle **True** or **False** for the following statement:

3. If a fire breaks out in a building where you and others are present, the first thing you should do is call 9-1-1.   True   False

4. Name 4 factors that affect how serious a burn may be.

_____

_____

_____

_____

First Aid for Heat Burns

First aid for heat burns is based on 4 general principles of burn care:

1. Stop the burning and cool the area.

2. Protect the burned area from additional trauma and pathogens.

3. Provide supportive care.

4. Ensure medical attention.

The specific first aid varies somewhat depending on the severity of the burn.

CARE FOR FIRST-DEGREE BURNS

First-degree burns include most cases of sunburn and minor burns caused by heat or scalding. The skin is pink or red and remains unbroken, but some swelling may occur. Although first-degree burns may seem minor, they still cause pain and damage the skin. The first goal, as with all burns, is to stop the burning by removing the heat source and cooling the area with running cool or cold, potable water, such as tap water; do not use ice, which can cause further damage. Be sure to use running water so that the water stays cold – a wet cloth put on a burn, for example, might absorb the burn's heat and no longer be cold. Because swelling may occur, jewelry and constrictive clothing should be removed from the area. Thereafter, protect the burned skin from contact with objects that may rub or put pressure on it. Do not apply ointment or other oily or greasy substances on the burn, although **aloe vera** gel may later provide some comfort (see First Aid: "First-Degree Burns").

First Aid: First-Degree Burns

Signs, Symptoms and Care

WHEN YOU SEE

- Skin is red, dry and painful

- May be some swelling

- Skin not broken

DO THIS FIRST

1. Stop the burning by removing the heat source.

2. Immediately cool the burn with running cool or cold, potable water, such as tap water, for at least 10 minutes. (Do not put ice on a burn, which could cause tissue injury.)

3. Remove clothing and jewelry or any other constricting item before the area swells.

4. Protect the burn from friction or pressure.

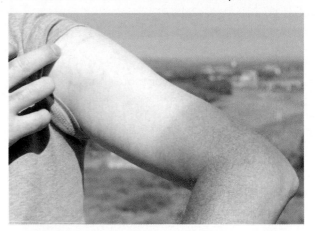

ADDITIONAL CARE

- Aloe vera gel can be used on the skin for comfort.

ALERT

- Do not put butter on a burn. Natural remedies, such as honey or potato peel dressings, should not be applied to a burn.

- Do not use ice on a burn because even though it may relieve pain, the cold may cause additional damage to the skin. Ice-cold water should not be used.

CARE FOR SECOND-DEGREE BURNS

A second-degree burn is deeper than a first-degree burn, involving the dermis and causing more damage to capillaries and nerve endings. The skin is red and swollen, often blotchy in appearance, and has blisters that may leak a clear fluid. If blisters break, pathogens may enter the skin and cause infection; first aid, therefore, includes protecting the skin. Pain is more severe than with a first-degree burn.

A small, second-degree burn (smaller than your palm) may be treated at home, but a larger burn requires immediate medical attention. If larger than 10% of the body surface area (or 5% in a child, older adult or person with chronic illness), the burn should be treated as an emergency and 9-1-1 called. Stop the burning immediately and cool the area with running cool or cold potable water, such as tap water. Remove jewelry and constricting clothing from the area. While waiting for medical care, keep the burn covered with a dry, loose, nonstick dressing. As with all burns, do not apply ointment or other substances to the burn (see First Aid: "Second-Degree Burns").

First Aid: Second-Degree Burns

Signs, Symptoms and Care

WHEN YOU SEE

- Skin is swollen and red, may be blotchy or streaked

- Blisters that may be weeping clear fluid

- Signs of significant pain

DO THIS FIRST

1. Stop the burning by removing the heat source.

2. Immediately cool the burn with running, cool or cold, potable water, such as tap water, for at least 10 minutes. (Do not put ice on a burn, which could cause tissue injury.)

3. Remove constricting items, such as clothing and jewelry.

4. For large second-degree burns, call 9-1-1.

5. Protect the burn area from friction or pressure. Put a sterile, dry dressing over the burn to protect the area, but keep it loose and do not tape it to the skin.

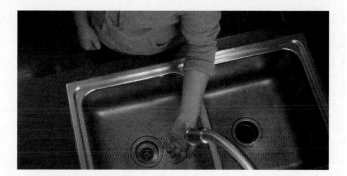

6. Keep burn blisters intact. This reduces pain and improves healing by preventing infection. Natural remedies, such as honey or potato peel dressings, should not be applied to a burn.

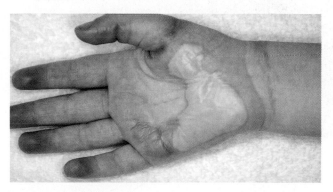

ADDITIONAL CARE

- For burns on the face, genitals, hands or feet, seek medical attention.

ALERT

- Do not break skin blisters; this could cause an infection.

- Be gentle when covering the area.

CARE FOR THIRD-DEGREE BURNS

Third-degree burns are usually emergencies, and when large, may be life threatening. Third-degree burns penetrate all the way through the skin and may damage underlying tissues. Infection is likely. It is important to act immediately to stop the burning and cool the burn, although a very large burn area (over 20% of body surface area) should not be immersed in water because of the risk of causing hypothermia. The victim may rapidly develop the signs of shock, a life-threatening condition requiring treatment in addition to the burn first aid. Call 9-1-1.

Stop the burning immediately and cool the area with running cool or cold, potable water, such as tap water. Remove jewelry and constricting clothing from the area. Cover the burn with a dry, loose, nonstick dressing. As with all burns, do not apply ointment or other substances to the burn. While waiting for emergency personnel, treat the victim for shock by having the victim lie down, elevating the legs and maintaining normal body temperature. Monitor the victim's breathing and give basic life support (BLS), if needed (see First Aid: "Third-Degree Burns").

First Aid: Third-Degree Burns

Signs, Symptoms and Care

WHEN YOU SEE

- Skin damage, charred skin or white, leathery skin

- May have signs and symptoms of shock (clammy, pale or ashen skin; nausea and vomiting; fast breathing)

DO THIS FIRST

1. Stop the burning by removing the heat source.

2. Immediately cool the burn with running cool or cold, potable water, such as tap water, for at least 10 minutes. (Do not put ice on a burn, which could cause tissue injury.) With a large burn, monitor the victim for hypothermia.

3. Remove clothing and jewelry before the area swells.

4. Call 9-1-1.

5. Prevent shock: Have the victim lie down, elevate the legs if trauma is not suspected and maintain normal body temperature.

6. Carefully cover the burn with a nonstick dressing; keep it loose and do not tape it to the skin. Do not apply a cream or ointment.

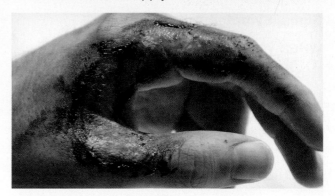

ADDITIONAL CARE

- Watch the victim's breathing and be ready to give basic life support BLS, if needed.

ALERT

- Do not attempt to cool the burn with cold water if it is larger than 20% of the body (e.g., one whole leg or torso from neck to waist), or 10% for child, because of the risk of hypothermia and shock.

- Do not touch the burn or put anything on it.

- Do not give the victim anything to drink.

- Do not try to remove any clothing stuck to the burn area.

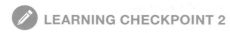 **LEARNING CHECKPOINT 2**

Circle **True** or **False** for the following statement:

1. For a victim with a second-degree burn, you should break skin blisters and cover the area with a burn ointment to promote faster healing.

    True   False

2. Fill in the correct answer: For a victim with a third-degree burn, you should cool only a _____ area with water because of the risk of shock or hypothermia.

3. As you are leaving work, you see a man working on his car in the parking lot. He suddenly screams and backs away, his clothing on fire. What do you do? List in correct order the first four actions you should take.

    _____

    _____

    _____

Smoke Inhalation

Any victim who was in the vicinity of a fire could have airway or lung injuries from inhaling smoke or other fumes resulting from fires. Even hot air can cause such injuries. This can be a medical emergency. The lining of the airway may swell and make breathing difficult. The small sacs in the lungs where oxygen enters the lungs, the alveoli, may be damaged and affect the ability of the body to receive enough oxygen through normal breathing. A victim of smoke inhalation may also have carbon monoxide poisoning (see **Chapter 17**).

The signs and symptoms of smoke inhalation include coughing, wheezing or hoarseness; burns or blackening around the mouth or nose; coughing up a sooty substance; and difficulty breathing. Note that symptoms from smoke inhalation may not become obvious for up to 48 hours after exposure.

CARE FOR SMOKE INHALATION

First, get the victim to fresh air or fresh air to the victim. A victim who can safely be moved should be assisted outdoors or to an area of fresh air. If the victim cannot be moved, ventilate the area by any means available to remove smoke and fumes. Call 9-1-1 immediately, even if the victim is not experiencing signs and symptoms, because injury may have occurred even though the effects are not yet showing. While waiting for medical care, help the victim into a position for easiest breathing (often semi-reclining) and keep him or her calm. If the victim becomes unresponsive, position him or her in the recovery position and monitor breathing. Be prepared to give basic life support if needed (see First Aid: "Smoke Inhalation").

First Aid: Smoke Inhalation

Signs, Symptoms and Care

WHEN YOU SEE

- Smoke visible in area

- Coughing, wheezing or hoarse voice

- Possible burned area on face or chest

- Difficulty breathing

DO THIS FIRST

1. Get the victim to fresh air or fresh air to the victim.

2. Call 9-1-1.

3. Help the victim into a position for easiest breathing.

ADDITIONAL CARE

- Put an unresponsive victim in the recovery position.

- Be ready to give BLS if needed.

11 • Burns

Chemical Burns

Many strong chemicals found in workplaces and the home can burn skin on contact. Sometimes the burn develops slowly and in some cases the victim may not be aware of the burn for up to 24 hours. Acids and alkalis, liquids and solids can all cause serious chemical burns **(Figure 11-5)**.

FIGURE 11-5

A chemical burn.

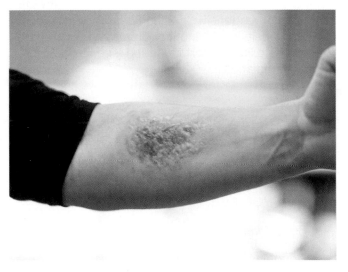

PREVENTING CHEMICAL BURNS

- Read directions before using any household products. Heed warnings on products, and keep all products in their original containers. Do not mix different products.

- Protect hands with heavy rubber gloves, and cover other exposed areas of the body.

- Ensure adequate ventilation when using products with dangerous fumes.

CARE FOR CHEMICAL BURNS

In most cases you can see the substance on the victim's skin, and the victim feels a burning or stinging sensation. Because the chemical reaction can continue as long as the substance is on the skin, you must remove it immediately. In a work setting, check safety data sheets (SDS – formerly called material safety data sheets, or MSDS) for the care of a burn caused by the specific chemical. For a dry chemical, brush it off with a gloved hand, cloth, piece of cardboard or paper, spare article of clothing or any other item available. Be careful not to get the chemical on your own skin or to spread it to other areas of the victim's skin. Wear gloves if available. Then, flush the area with large amounts of running water as soon as possible. Flush until EMS personnel arrive to give definitive care or until a toxic-specific solution is available. Remove any clothing and jewelry from the burned area. For a liquid spilled on the victim's skin, start flushing with water immediately.

Call 9-1-1 for any chemical burn, and keep flushing the burned area with water until medical care arrives (see First Aid: "Chemical Burns"). Remember that a chemical may give off fumes, even if you cannot smell them; therefore the victim should be moved (if safe) to fresh air. Even a dry chemical may give off fumes once it is in contact with water. Note: Do not try to neutralize an acid by applying an alkaline substance, or vice versa, because of the risk of further damage caused by the chemical reaction.

First Aid: Chemical Burns

Signs, Symptoms and Care

WHEN YOU SEE

- A chemical on the victim's skin or clothing

- Complaints of pain or a burning sensation

- A spilled substance on or around an unresponsive victim

- A smell of fumes in the air

DO THIS FIRST

1. Send someone to check the SDS for the chemical involved.

2. Move the victim away from fumes or ventilate the area.

3. With a gloved hand or piece of cloth, brush off any dry chemical, but do not contaminate skin that has not been in contact with the chemical.

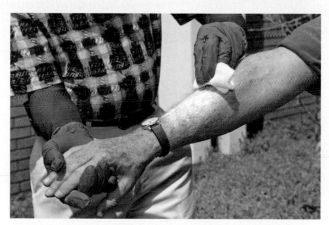

4. Remove clothing and jewelry from the burn area while flushing with water.

5. Flush the entire area as quickly as possible with large amounts of running water. Flush until EMS personnel arrive to give definitive care or until a toxic-specific solution is available.

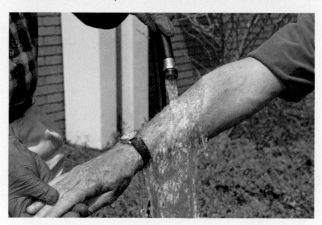

6. Call 9-1-1 for any chemical burn.

ALERT
Chemical in the Eyes

- For a chemical splashed into the eye, continuously flush the victim's eye with large amounts of clean running water for at least 15 minutes or until EMS arrives. If tap water is not available, use normal saline or a commercial eye irrigation solution.

- Have the victim remove contact lenses.

- Tilt the victim's head so the water runs away from the face and not into the unaffected eye.

- For a responsive victim, call the Poison Control Center (800-222-1222) immediately and follow its instructions. For an unresponsive victim or if the Poison Control Center is not available, call 9-1-1 or seek help from a medical provider.

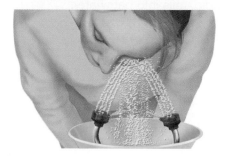

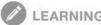

1. A coworker has splashed an unknown liquid in her eye and is holding her hand over the eye. What should you do first? Select the best answer.

   a. Have her keep holding the eye closed so her tears will wash out the chemical.

   b. Call 9-1-1 and wait for health care personnel to take care of her eye.

   c. Immediately flush the eye with large amounts of running water.

   d. Mix baking soda with water and pour it into her eye.

2. Describe the first action to take if a victim has a dry chemical on the skin.

   _____

   _____

   _____

   _____

Circle **True** or **False** for the following statement:

3. If a person who was in a smoky area near a fire does not have any signs and symptoms within an hour, that person does not need medical care.   True   False

Electrical Burns and Shocks

An electrical burn or shock occurs whenever any part of the body comes in contact with electricity. Typical electrical injuries occur from faulty appliances or power cords, or when an appliance comes into contact with water. Water easily conducts electricity to anyone who touches the water. Many deaths caused by electricity occur when an appliance, such as a hair dryer or radio, falls into bathwater.

PREVENTING ELECTRICAL SHOCKS AND BURNS

Electricity may cause life-threatening shocks as well as electrical burns. Follow these guidelines to stay safe **(Figure 11-6)**:

• Use outlet caps to block unused electrical outlets.

• Do not use a night-light that looks like a toy in a young child's bedroom; it can cause an electrical burn if the child tries to play with it.

• Never use electrical appliances near water or when your hands are wet.

• Inspect electric cords for broken or frayed insulation.

• Be careful not to touch the wire prongs when inserting or removing electrical plugs from a receptacle. Pull the plug itself out, not the cord.

• Install a **ground fault circuit interrupter (GFCI)** in outlets in bathrooms and kitchens; this device automatically turns off electricity when appliances become wet.

• Outdoors, keep everyone away from downed power lines, and do not let children play near electrical poles or fly kites near electrical wires.

FIGURE 11-6

Overloaded outlets or extension cords pose a risk of fire or electrical shocks.

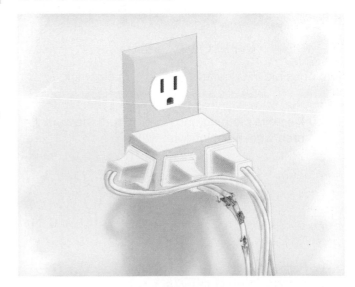

PREVENTING LIGHTNING STRIKES

Each year, an estimated 700 people in the United States are struck by lightning, causing significant injuries and about 50 deaths.[1] If you are caught outdoors in a thunderstorm, follow these guidelines:

- Know that the lightning is a risk even if the storm seems far off. Seek shelter if you hear thunder within 30 seconds of seeing a lightning strike. Lightning has been known to "jump" miles away from a storm cloud.

- Get out of water immediately, or off a boat.

- Try not to be the tallest object around. Crouch near the ground or get beneath a group of trees – but not a tall, isolated tree. Avoid high ground and open spaces.

- Stay away from metal fences and power lines. Do not take shelter near metal objects.

- A closed motor vehicle is safer than being caught in the open. Keep the doors and windows completely shut.

- If you are caught in the open, crouch or squat down (but do not lie down) with your feet together. A group of people should stay about 15 feet away from each other.

- Indoors, stay away from doors and windows, and do not use electrical appliances or devices. Also keep away from telephone lines and plumbing fixtures.

[1]*National Weather Service, lightningsafety.noaa.gov/fatalities. shtml Accessed January 2016.*

INJURIES FROM ELECTRICITY

Two possible injuries may occur from electricity:

- External burns caused by the heat of electricity

- Electrical injuries caused by electricity flowing through the body

High-voltage electricity flowing through the body can cause significant injuries to many different tissues. Heart damage may cause heart rhythm irregularities that threaten the victim's circulation or cause the heart to stop **(Box 11-2).**

As with all types of burns, the urgent first step is to stop the burning. If the victim is still in contact with a source of electricity, ensure that the power is disconnected or turned off immediately. Do not touch a victim still in contact with electricity because of the risk of receiving a shock or burn yourself.

BOX 11-2: HIGH-VOLTAGE SHOCKS

HIGH POWER LINES

If a power line is down, do not approach a victim in contact with the line. Call 9-1-1 immediately. Do not try to move the wire away using any object. Wait for emergency workers to arrive, and keep others away from the scene.

LIGHTNING STRIKES

Lightning strikes often cause serious injury. In addition to burns, the electrical shock may affect the heart and brain and cause temporary blindness or deafness, unresponsiveness or seizures, bleeding, bone fractures or cardiac arrest. Call 9-1-1 immediately and give basic life support, treating the most serious injuries first.

External burns resulting from heat or flames caused by electricity are cared for in the same manner as heat burns. Electrical injuries may cause only minor external burns where the electricity entered and left the body; these are called **entrance** and **exit wounds (Figure 11-7).**

Internal damage caused by an electric shock is seldom as obvious as an external burn. Signs and symptoms may include seizures or changing levels of responsiveness. Call 9-1-1 and monitor the victim's breathing while waiting for medical assistance. Be prepared to give basic life support if needed (see First Aid: "Electrical Burns").

FIGURE 11-7

An electrical burn.

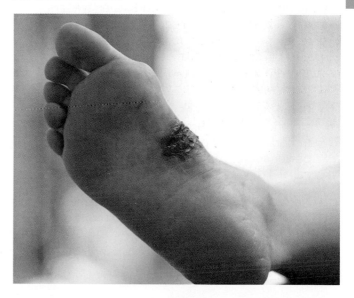

First Aid: Electrical Burns

Signs, Symptoms and Care

WHEN YOU SEE

- A source of electricity near the victim: bare wires, power cords, an electrical device

- Burned area of skin or possibly both entrance and exit wounds

- Changing levels of responsiveness

DO THIS FIRST

1. Do not touch the victim until you know the area is safe. Unplug or turn off the power.

2. Call 9-1-1.

3. For an unresponsive victim, give BLS.

4. Care for the burn (stop the burning, cool the area, remove clothing and jewelry and cover the burn with a sterile dressing).

5. Treat for shock by having the victim lie down, elevating the legs, and maintaining normal body temperature.

ADDITIONAL CARE

- Keep an unresponsive breathing victim in the recovery position (if no suspected trauma, especially a neck, back, hip or pelvic injury) and monitor breathing until help arrives. Be ready to give CPR if needed.

ALERT
Electrical Shock

- Do not touch a victim you think is receiving an electrical shock! First make sure the power is turned off or the person is well away from the power source. Turn off the circuit breaker and call 9-1-1.

- Note that electrical burns can cause massive internal injuries even when the external burn may look minor.

 LEARNING CHECKPOINT 4

Circle **True** or **False** for the following statement:

1. The first thing to do for an unresponsive victim in contact with an electrical wire is pour water over the area of contact.   True   False

2. What is the safest way to stop the electricity when someone is shocked by an electrical appliance? How should you *not* try to stop it?

_____

_____

_____

3. Select the best answer. Driving home from work, you are stopped behind a car that has struck a telephone pole. You get out to help the driver and see a power line dangling from the pole, in contact with the roof of the car. Your first action should be to –

   a. use your cell phone to call 9-1-1.

   b. look for a stick or piece of wood to push the wire away from the car.

   c. try to pull the victim out the car window.

   d. give any needed first aid by leaning in the car window.

 CONCLUDING THOUGHTS

First aid for burns may seem complex because of the variations in care depending on the type of burn, its size and location on the body, and its depth. Most important, remember the general first aid principles for all burns:

- Act fast to stop the burning.

- Cool the area.

- Seek help.

- Protect the victim.

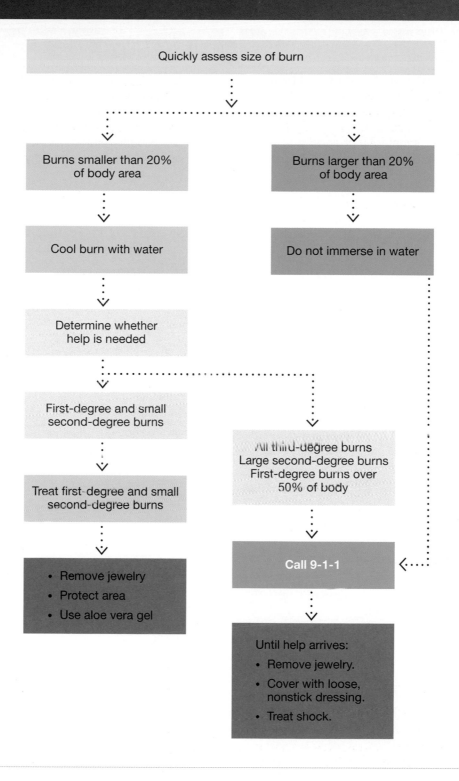

Quickly assess size of burn

Burns smaller than 20% of body area

Burns larger than 20% of body area

Cool burn with water

Do not immerse in water

Determine whether help is needed

First-degree and small second-degree burns

All third-degree burns
Large second-degree burns
First-degree burns over 50% of body

Treat first-degree and small second-degree burns

Call 9-1-1

- Remove jewelry
- Protect area
- Use aloe vera gel

Until help arrives:

- Remove jewelry.
- Cover with loose, nonstick dressing.
- Treat shock.

11 • Burns

SCENARIO 1

A welder just completed welding a broken piece of wrought iron fence. Before anyone can stop her, the daughter of an employee, playing in the area, runs by, trips and falls against the hot iron. The skin on her palm is instantly charred black. Describe the immediate actions you should take.

_____

_____

_____

_____

SCENARIO 3

A coworker ignores a "Wet Floor" sign and while walking fast down a wet hallway slips and falls. Without thinking, he rubs his bruised face. Immediately his eye hurts with a burning sensation, and you see his hand is wet from the liquid that was on the floor. How should you care for him?

_____

_____

_____

_____

SCENARIO 2

In the employee break room, someone emptied an ashtray into a trashcan, which then caught on fire and ignited the window curtains nearby. After evacuating everyone, you put out the fire with a fire extinguisher. Your throat feels a little raw, but otherwise you feel fine. The next morning, however, you are hoarse and coughing. Is this just "normal," or do you need medical attention?

_____

_____

_____

_____

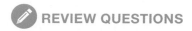

Select the best answers.

1. Most fires occur –
   a. in the home.
   b. in the workplace.
   c. in schools.
   d. in public gathering places.

2. A first-degree burn is characterized by –
   a. the presence of white, fluid-filled blisters.
   b. pink or red skin.
   c. white, leathery areas of skin.
   d. bleeding.

3. Factors that influence the severity of a burn include –
   a. the depth of the burn.
   b. the percentage of body area burned.
   c. the location of the burn.
   d. All of the above

4. Which of the following is true about burns?
   a. The deeper the burn, the more painful it is.
   b. Third-degree burns are more painful than others.
   c. The level of pain is not an indicator of burn severity.
   d. Blisters are more painful than charred or red skin.

5. Which of the following is the best substance to put on a burn immediately after it has occurred?
   a. Antibiotic ointment
   b. Aloe vera
   c. Butter
   d. Cold running water

6. The purpose of putting a dressing over a second- or third-degree burn is to –
   a. protect the area.
   b. absorb the fluid from blisters.
   c. keep the area moist for 24 hours.
   d. prevent swelling.

7. Using icy water to cool a burn that covers 25% of the body may result in –
   a. hypothermia and shock.
   b. shock and cardiac arrest.
   c. hypothermia and severe bleeding.
   d. electrolyte imbalances and infection.

8. A ring should be removed from a burned finger because –
   a. gold and silver are toxic metals on exposed skin.
   b. swelling may cut off circulation.
   c. the ring is a likely source of infection.
   d. the ring makes it difficult to cool the burn.

9. First aid for a dry chemical burn includes –
   a. neutralizing an acid with an alkaline substance.
   b. neutralizing an alkaline burn with an acidic substance.
   c. brushing off the chemical and then flushing the skin with water.
   d. tightly taping a dressing over the burn.

10. Call 9-1-1 for –
    a. a second-degree burn larger than 10% of body surface area in an adult victim.
    b. a second-degree burn larger than 5% of body surface area in an elderly victim.
    c. a third-degree burn.
    d. All of the above

11 • Burns

CHAPTER 12

Head and Spinal Injuries

LESSON OBJECTIVES

- List the signs and symptoms of head and spinal injuries.

- Perform a physical examination of a victim with head or spinal injury.

- Describe the first aid for a victim with a possible brain injury.

- Explain why a victim with a possible spinal injury should not be moved unnecessarily.

- Perform manual spinal motion restriction.

- With other rescuers, perform a log roll of a victim with a spinal injury.

You have stopped by a neighborhood school on your way home to see a friend who helps coach the girls' gymnastic team. While talking in a corner of the gym, you are horrified to see a young girl on the uneven bars attempt a release move and miss the bar. You run to her and find that she is unresponsive. What should you do?

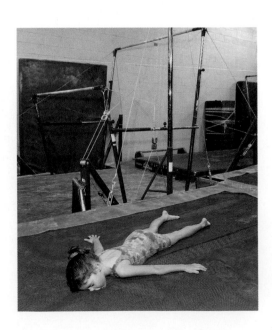

Head and spinal injuries may be life threatening or may cause permanent damage to the brain or spinal cord, producing nervous system deficits, such as paralysis. Any trauma to the head, neck or back may result in a serious injury. Injuries that cause unresponsiveness or loss of sensation in a body part are especially likely to be serious, but even injuries without immediate, obvious signs and symptoms may create a potentially life-threatening problem.

Because of the forces involved, any injury to the head may also injure the spine. Whenever you find a serious head injury, suspect a neck or back injury.

This chapter considers head and spinal injuries that involve deeper injuries to the skull or spine, including bone and nerves. **Chapter 10** describes the first aid for more superficial wounds to the head and face.

Preventing Head and Spinal Injuries

Motor vehicle crashes are the leading cause of head and spinal injuries in people younger than 65, with about 200,000 people dying each year from brain injuries and another 500,000 hospitalized for treatment.[1] Falls are the leading cause of these injuries in people older than 65. Violence, sports and recreation activities are additional leading causes of spinal cord injuries. About 12,000 people in the United States suffer a spinal injury each year, and an estimated 259,000 Americans live with a disability resulting from a spinal cord injury.[2]

[1]*Physicians Desk Reference, pdrhealth.com/diseases/brain-and-spinal-cord-injury Accessed January 2016.*

[2]*BrainandSpinalCord.org, brainandspinalcord.org/spinal-cord-injury/statistics.htm Accessed January 2016.*

Many head and spinal injuries can be prevented by following accepted guidelines for safety in vehicles, during recreation and at work.

- Always wear safety belts and shoulder restraints in vehicles.

- Use approved car seats for infants and small children, and make sure they are installed correctly (incorrect installation is a frequent cause of injury).

- Wear appropriate helmets, headgear or hard hats for bicycling, skating, skateboarding, other sports and work activities.

- At work, follow appropriate OSHA guidelines for equipment and safety practices.

- Avoid risky activities, including driving, when you are under the influence of drugs, alcohol or medications that produce drowsiness.

- Ensure that children's playground surfaces are made of a shock-absorbing material.

- Store firearms in a locked cabinet with ammunition in a separate secure location.

- Do not dive into murky or shallow water (less than 9 feet deep).

- To prevent falls, keep yourself and your house safe for children and older adults:

  - To reach high shelves, use a step stool with a grab bar.

  - Make sure all stairways have handrails.

  - Use safety gates at the top and bottom of stairs when young children are present.

  - Remove tripping hazards, such as small area rugs and loose electrical cords.

  - Use nonslip mats in the tub and shower.

  - Install grab bars by the toilet and in the tub or shower.

- Exercise regularly to improve strength, balance and coordination.

- See an eye doctor regularly for vision checks.

- Because falls often result from dizziness caused by medications, have your health care provider review your medications.

Assessing Head and Spinal Injuries

Assessing a victim with a potential head and spinal injury begins with considering the cause of the injury and the forces involved. An understanding of the general signs and symptoms of head and spinal injuries helps you to focus the physical examination.

It is essential to recognize the possibility of a head or spinal injury immediately because the possibility of a spinal injury determines how and when a victim is positioned and moved.

CAUSES OF HEAD AND SPINAL INJURIES

Any trauma to the head may cause a head or spinal injury. In addition, spinal injuries may be caused by forces to the back, chest or even the pelvis or legs by indirect force. Common causes of head and spinal injuries include the following:

- Motor vehicle crashes (including whiplash injuries without direct impact to the head)

- Falls from a height of more than a few feet

- Diving emergencies involving impact to the head (even blows that do not cause bruises or wounds)

- Skiing emergencies and other sports injuries

- Any forceful blow to the head, neck or back

Suspect a spinal injury in an injured victim who has these risk factors:

- Victim is 65 or older

- Child older than 2 with trauma to head or neck

- Motor vehicle or bicycle crash involving driver, passenger or pedestrian

- Falls from more than the person's standing height

- Victim feels tingling in hands or feet, pain in back or neck, muscle weakness or lack of feeling in torso or arms

- Victim is intoxicated or not alert

- Any painful injury, particularly to the head, neck or back

In addition, if you encounter an unresponsive victim with an unknown mechanism of injury, suspect a spinal injury when wounds or other injuries in the body suggest large forces were involved. If so, observe the victim carefully and thoroughly for the signs and symptoms of a head or spinal injury even as you are carrying out the initial assessment.

GENERAL SIGNS AND SYMPTOMS OF HEAD AND SPINAL INJURIES

Head and spinal injuries are closely related because a traumatic injury to one may injure the other as well. For example, a blow to the head that fractures the skull may also put enough force on vertebrae in the neck that a spinal injury occurs. Although a head injury may occur in a victim without a spinal injury, and a spinal injury may occur in a victim without a head injury, the assessment of a victim with such injuries should look for both head and spinal injuries.

The general signs and symptoms of head and spinal injuries may overlap in victims with an injury of the head, neck or back. Suspect a head or spinal injury in a victim if any of these signs and symptoms is present:

- Lump or deformity in the head, neck or back

- Changing levels of responsiveness, drowsiness, confusion, dizziness (see AVPU scale in **Chapter 4**)

- Unequal pupils

- Headache

- Clear or bloody fluid from the nose or ears

- Stiff neck

- Inability to move any body part

- Tingling, numbness or lack of feeling in feet or hands

Noting any of these signs and symptoms in the initial assessment or physical examination of a victim should lead to a more specific assessment for a head or spinal injury. These specific injuries are described in following sections in this chapter.

PHYSICAL EXAMINATION OF HEAD AND SPINAL INJURIES

Chapter 4, "Assessing the Victim," describes general procedures for assessing all victims, including a physical examination of a victim not being treated for a life-threatening injury. In the initial assessment of an unresponsive victim, consider whether the victim may have a spinal injury based on the risk factors listed above and these factors:

- The cause of the victim's injuries (e.g., blow to the head, a fall, strong forces)

- Observations of bystanders at the scene who saw the injury occur

- Immediately apparent injuries and wounds (e.g., a serious head wound, or the neck twisted at an unusual angle) – but do not take the time to do a physical examination if the victim is not breathing

- Any observed sign of a head or spinal injury

During the initial assessment of the victim, you may have to position the victim to open the airway, to check breathing, to give CPR, to control bleeding or to allow blood, vomit or other fluid to drain from the mouth. If you suspect that the victim may have a spinal injury, take great care when moving or repositioning the victim, as described later in this chapter. Unless it is necessary, do not move the victim.

If the victim is unresponsive and the initial assessment does not reveal a life-threatening condition for which you must care, do not perform a full physical examination but observe the victim for other injuries. If an unresponsive victim may have a spinal injury, do not move the victim unless it is necessary. Check only for serious injuries, such as bleeding that must be controlled. Otherwise, maintain the victim's head position to restrict movement and wait for EMS professionals.

If the victim is responsive and you suspect the possibility of a spinal injury, carefully assess for the signs and symptoms of spinal injury during the physical examination. Ask the victim to stay in position and not move more than you ask during the examination, to prevent further damage to the spine.

Perform the physical examination as described in **Chapter 4,** paying particular attention to signs and symptoms of a head or spinal injury. Gently feel the skull for bumps or depressions. Check the ears and nose for blood or a clear fluid. Check the pupils of both eyes, which should be of equal size and should respond to light when you cover and uncover the eyes with your hand. Check the neck for deformity or swelling, bleeding or pain. When checking the torso, observe for impaired breathing and loss of bladder or bowel control (a sign of nerve damage). When assessing the extremities, check for sensation and the ability to move the hand or foot, comparing strength from one side of the body to the other.

If you suspect a head or spinal injury, call 9-1-1 and keep the victim still until EMS professionals arrive. Note that it can be very difficult for first aiders without advanced training to recognize a spinal injury with certainty. **Do not depend on any specific assessment of a victim to decide whether the victim may have a spinal injury. Do not assume a victim without specific symptoms does not have a possible spinal injury.** Consider the forces involved in the injury, and when in doubt, keep the victim's head immobile while waiting for help to arrive. With a responsive victim, encourage the victim not to move, and with an unresponsive victim, hold the head in place to restrict movement.

In addition, the results of the examination are not always clear-cut. For example, even though the spinal cord may be intact, an injury may put pressure on the cord that results in limited sensation, pain, or partial inability to move. If the victim can move a hand or foot only weakly, for example, assume a spinal injury has occurred.

Follow this assessment approach for all suspected cases of head or spinal injuries (see Skill: "Assessing Head and Spinal Injuries").

STEP 1
Check the victim's head.

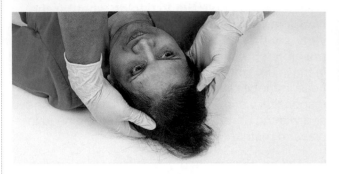

STEP 2
Check neck for deformity, swelling and pain.

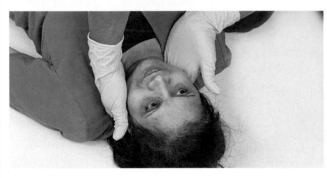

STEP 3
Touch toes of both feet and ask victim if the sensation feels normal.

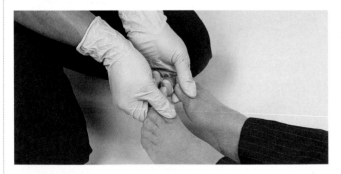

STEP 4
Ask victim to point toes.

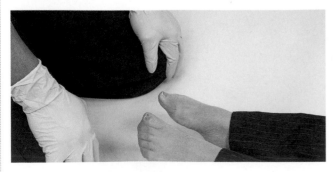

STEP 5
Ask victim to push against your hands with the feet.

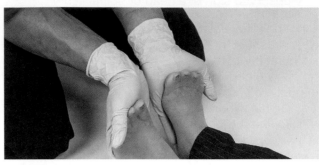

STEP 6
Touch fingers of both hands and ask victim if the sensation feels normal.

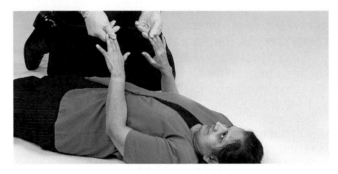

STEP 7
Ask victim to make a fist and curl (flex) it in.

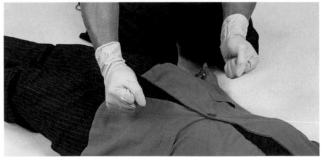

STEP 8
Ask victim to squeeze your hands.

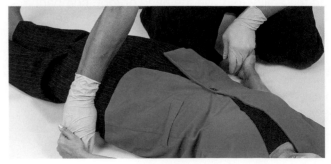

Skull Fracture

If the victim had a blow to the head, consider the possibility of a skull fracture or a brain injury. The skull is generally strong and is fractured only with severe trauma. When you find bleeding from the scalp, check carefully for a possible skull fracture before applying direct pressure to the wound. If the skull is fractured, direct pressure on the wound could push bone fragments into the brain, causing serious injury.

Feel the scalp gently for signs of a skull fracture: a depressed or spongy area or the presence of bone fragments. Blood or a clear fluid leaking from the nose or ears may also be a sign of a skull injury. In such a case, to control bleeding, apply pressure around the wound rather than directly on it. Note that a skull fracture may occur even without an open wound.

A skull fracture is life threatening. Call 9-1-1 immediately. Note that a skull fracture often also causes injuries to the brain (see First Aid: "Skull Fracture").

First Aid: Skull Fracture

Signs, Symptoms and Care

WHEN YOU SEE

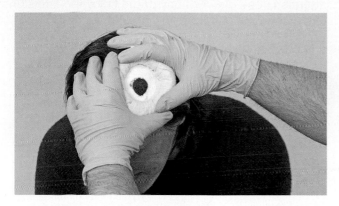

- A deformed area of the skull

- A depressed area in the bone felt during the physical examination

- Blood or fluid coming from the ears or nose

- Eyelids swollen shut or becoming discolored (bruising)

- Bruising behind the ears

- Unequal pupils

- Impaled object in the skull

DO THIS FIRST

1. Call 9-1-1 and stay with the victim.

2. Put a breathing unresponsive victim in the recovery position unless you suspect a neck, back, hip or pelvic injury. Monitor breathing and be ready to give CPR if needed.

3. *Do not* clean the wound, press on it or remove an impaled object.

4. Cover the wound with a sterile dressing.

5. If there is significant bleeding, apply pressure only around the edges of the wound, not on the wound itself. You may use a ring dressing to apply pressure around the wound (see **Chapter 10**). Do not apply pressure if you feel bone fragments move.

6. Do not move the victim unnecessarily because there may also be a spinal injury.

ADDITIONAL CARE

- Do not raise the victim's legs.

Brain Injuries

Brain injuries may occur with a blow to the head with or without an open wound. A brain injury is likely with a skull fracture. Injury results when the traumatic force is transmitted to brain tissue, causing bleeding or swelling of the brain and concussion. Brain injuries may cause a range of signs or symptoms, including headache, altered mental status, confusion or unresponsiveness; weakness, numbness, loss of sensation or **paralysis** of body areas; nausea and vomiting; seizures; and unequal pupils **(Figure 12-1).** If breathing is impaired, the victim may need basic life support.

FIGURE 12-1

The signs of a brain injury.

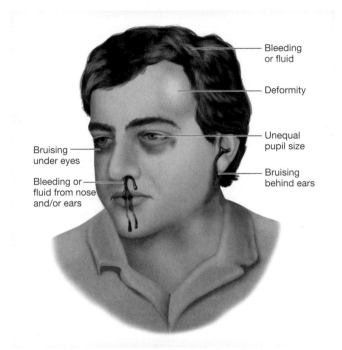

Bleeding or fluid

Deformity

Unequal pupil size

Bruising under eyes

Bleeding or fluid from nose and/or ears

Bruising behind ears

Call 9-1-1 for any victim with a suspected brain injury. Even if the signs and symptoms seem mild at first, swelling and/or bleeding in the brain may continue, and the victim's condition may rapidly deteriorate and become life threatening. Stay with the victim and be prepared to give basic life support if needed. With any force strong enough to injure the brain, suspect a possible spinal injury as well and support the victim's head to restrict movement while waiting for help to arrive. Because vomiting commonly occurs with brain injuries, be prepared to move the victim into the recovery position to allow fluid to drain from the mouth. Enlist the help of bystanders to keep the victim's head in line with the body whenever you move the victim (see First Aid: "Brain Injuries").

In some cases after a blow to the head, the victim does not immediately have the signs and symptoms of brain injury and does not seek medical care. Signs and symptoms may appear within the next 48 hours that indicate a more serious injury. Seek medical attention immediately if any of the following late signs and symptoms occurs following a head injury:

• Nausea and vomiting

• Severe or persistent headache

• Changing levels of responsiveness

• Lack of coordination, movement problems

• Problems with vision or speech

• Seizures

First Aid: Brain Injuries

Signs, Symptoms and Care

WHEN YOU SEE

- A head wound suggesting a blow to the head occurred
- Changing levels of responsiveness, drowsiness
- Confusion, disorientation or memory loss about the injury
- Headache
- Dizziness
- Seizures
- Nausea or vomiting
- Breathing problems or irregularities
- Unequal pupils

DO THIS FIRST

For a responsive victim:

1. Have the victim lie down.

2. Keep the victim still and protect him or her from becoming chilled or overheated.

3. Call 9-1-1 and monitor the victim's condition until help arrives.

4. Support the head and neck, even in a responsive victim, if you suspect a spinal injury.

For an unresponsive victim:

1. Call 9-1-1.

2. Monitor the victim's breathing without moving the victim unless necessary.

3. Suspect a spinal injury and restrict movement of the head and neck.

4. Control serious bleeding and cover any wounds with a dressing.

ALERT

- Do not let the victim eat or drink anything.

CONCUSSION

A **concussion** is a type of brain injury that can result from a blow to the head, or as a result of sudden, violent movement of the head, such as in whiplash. Concussion often involves a temporary impairment of brain function but usually not permanent damage. Usually there is no head wound, and the victim may not have many of the signs and symptoms of a more serious brain injury. Most concussions do not involve a loss of consciousness, or the victim may have been "knocked out" by a blow to the head but regained consciousness quickly. A concussion typically causes these signs and symptoms:

- Temporary confusion or feeling stunned or dazed
- Memory loss about the traumatic event
- Brief loss of responsiveness
- Mildly or moderately altered mental status
- Nausea

- Dizziness
- Visual disturbances, sensitivity to light and noise
- Unusual behavior
- Headache or head pressure

Concussion cannot easily be determined, so it is best to take a cautious approach after any blow to the head. Although the victim may seem to recover quickly and to experience no signs or symptoms, it is generally difficult to determine the seriousness of the injury. More serious signs and symptoms may occur over time. Therefore it is important to seek medical care for all suspected brain injuries. If a concussion is suspected, call 9-1-1 and keep the victim still and give supportive care while waiting for help to arrive. In no situation should a victim with a suspected head injury, no matter how mild, continue an activity, such as a sport, in which a second injury may occur (see **Box 12-1**).

BOX 12-1: SECOND IMPACT SYNDROME

The American College of Sports Medicine estimates that 1.6-3 million concussions occur each year, with only about 15% diagnosed.[1] Such brain injuries are more likely to occur in contact sports, such as football. In the last two decades, sports physicians have become increasingly aware of the fact that a second head impact after even a mild concussion can cause severe brain swelling that may lead to death. Both high school and college football players have died of brain swelling after a second impact. In some cases the first injury was so mild that the player did not tell the coach at all before returning to play. Even mild injuries can have this cumulative fatal effect. Because an athlete with only a mild concussion may not tell anyone, statistics are lacking for how often "second impact syndrome" occurs.

The problem occurs in part because it is difficult to diagnose a concussion quickly and to know whether it is safe for the player to get back into the game. Pressure from coaches and other players to stay in the game may contribute to an athlete's not admitting to a mild injury.

There is hope, however, that the situation may improve with increased awareness of second impact syndrome among athletes, athletic trainers and coaches. In addition, new methods have been devised for testing whether a player has sustained a concussion. The goal is to prevent a player with a concussion from returning to play and risking another injury.

[1]*American College of Sports Medicine, acsm.org/public-information/articles/2012/01/13/sport-related-concussions Accessed January 2016.*

LEARNING CHECKPOINT 1

1. List two or three signs of a possible skull fracture. What is one thing you should *not* do to stop bleeding from the head if you suspect a skull fracture?

_____

_____

_____

_____

Circle **True** or **False** or the following statement:

2. You can easily distinguish a mild concussion from a serious brain injury by the signs and symptoms.   True   False

3. Check off the possible signs and symptoms of a brain injury:

   ☐ Headache

   ☐ Rapid blinking

   ☐ Memory loss

   ☐ Fingernail beds look blue

   ☐ Dizziness or confusion

   ☐ Nausea and vomiting

4. Select the best answer. The one sure way to know whether the victim has a spinal injury is –

   a. pain in the neck.

   b. headache.

   c. unresponsiveness.

   d. None of the above

5. How long after a blow to the head might signs and symptoms of a more serious injury appear?

_____

_____

_____

_____

Spinal Injuries

A fracture of the neck or back is a spinal injury. These injuries are always serious because of possible damage to the **spinal cord** – the bundle of nerves that runs down from the base of the skull and through the neck to branch off to all parts of the body. As **Figure 12-2** shows, these nerves pass through openings in the **vertebrae,** the bones of the neck and back. Even a small displacement or fracture of these bones can damage the soft tissue of the spinal cord or the nerves that lead from the cord to the body. Spinal injuries are serious because the spinal cord, unlike bones and some soft tissues, cannot grow back to heal the injury. Although medical care can improve the condition of a victim with partially damaged nerves, if the spinal cord is severed by the injury, the victim will have usually permanent paralysis and loss of function.

FIGURE 12-2

The spinal cord passes through openings in the vertebrae. Nerve branches exit the spinal cord to reach all body areas.

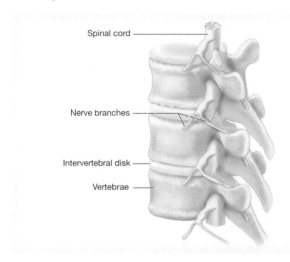

The effects of nerve damage caused by a spinal injury depend on the nature and location of the injury. In general, body functions controlled by nerves exiting the spinal cord below the level of injury may be affected. An injury to the lower spine may result in paralysis of the legs, for example, while an injury to the spinal cord at a higher level may paralyze the arms as well as the legs. If the nerves controlling the muscles involved in breathing are damaged, the victim may have a life-threatening breathing problem. Any spinal cord damage can cause permanent paralysis.

Although an injury to the spine may cause immediate nerve damage with immediate signs and symptoms,

in some cases nerve damage may not yet have occurred. For example, a fractured vertebra in the neck could put the nerves of the spinal cord at risk for damage if the neck vertebrae were to move. The victim may not have signs and symptoms of a spinal injury, but if the neck were moved carelessly, fractured bone could damage nerve tissue and cause permanent paralysis or a life-threatening condition. Similarly, when signs and symptoms of spinal nerve damage are present, movement of the head or neck could make the injury worse. Therefore it is critical to restrict head and neck movement in all victims suspected of having a spinal injury.

The primary care for a suspected spinal cord injury is to prevent movement of the spine by restricting movement of the head, neck and body. Unless you must move the victim, support the victim's head in the position in which you find the victim **(Figure 12-3).** Although it is generally better for the head to be in line with the body, *do not move the victim's head to put it in line with the body*. Damage to the spinal cord and nerves could be worsened by any unnecessary movement of the head. If the victim's head is already in line with the body when you reach the scene, support it in that position; this can be done with the victim lying down or sitting up. This technique is called **spinal motion restriction,** which simply means to restrict movement of the head and neck by supporting them manually in line with the body (see Skill: "Spinal Motion Restriction"). A responsive victim is likely to be in this position, and you should encourage the victim not to move while you provide support. If the victim is unresponsive and must be moved in order to give CPR, keep the head in line with the body while you move the victim with assistance from others.

If a victim with a suspected spinal cord injury is wearing a helmet, the helmet should remain in place unless the victim is experiencing respiratory difficulty and the helmet prevents giving care to the victim.

While supporting the victim's head manually until help arrives, continue to maintain the victim's open airway if needed, and monitor the victim's breathing (see First Aid: "Spinal Injuries").

FIGURE 12-3

Support the head in the position in which you find the victim.

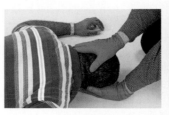
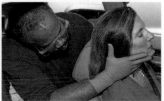

STEP 1
Ask a responsive victim what happened. If he or she has any of the risk factors, explain the need to hold the head still to restrict spinal movement and spinal cord injury. With an unresponsive victim, check for risk factors for suspected spinal injury.

STEP 2
Hold the victim's head and neck with both hands in the position found to restrict movement.

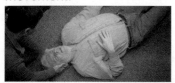

STEP 3
Monitor the victim's breathing and be ready to provide basic life support.

STEP 4
Have someone call 9-1-1.

STEP 5
Reassure a conscious victim and tell him or her not to move.

STEP 6
Continue to stabilize the head and spine, and monitor the victim's breathing until help arrives.

First Aid: Spinal Injuries

Signs, Symptoms and Care

WHEN YOU SEE

For a responsive victim:

- Inability to move any body part

- Tingling or a lack of sensation in hands or feet

- Deformed neck or back

- Breathing problems

- Headache

For an unresponsive victim:

- Deformed neck or back

- Signs of blow to head or back

- Nature of the emergency suggests possible spinal injury

Suspect a spinal injury in an injured victim who has these risk factors:

- 65 or older

- Child older than 2 with trauma of head or neck

- Motor vehicle or bicycle crash involving driver, passenger or pedestrian

- Fall from more than the person's standing height

- Victim feels tingling in hands or feet, pain in back or neck, muscle weakness or lack of feeling in torso or arms

- Victim is intoxicated or not alert

- Any painful injury, particularly to the head, neck or back

DO THIS FIRST

1. Ask a responsive victim what happened. If they have any of the risk factors, explain the need to hold the head still to restrict spinal movement. With an unresponsive victim, check for risk factors for suspected spinal injury.

2. Hold the victim's head and neck with both hands in the position found to restrict movement of the neck and spine.

3. Monitor the victim's breathing and be ready to give CPR if needed.

4. Have someone call 9-1-1.

ADDITIONAL CARE

- Reassure a responsive victim and tell him or her not to move.

- Continue to stabilize the head and spine, and monitor the victim's breathing until help arrives.

POSITIONING THE VICTIM

Generally you support the victim's head and neck in the position found. Move the victim only if absolutely necessary. If the victim is lying on his or her back and vomits, you must roll the victim onto his or her side to let the mouth drain and allow breathing. If the victim is lying on his or her side or face-down and requires CPR, you must move the victim onto his or her back.

The help of two or three others is necessary to keep the back and neck aligned during the move.

The technique called a log roll is used by multiple rescuers to turn the victim while keeping the head supported in line with the body (see Skill: "Rolling a Victim with Spinal Injury [Log Roll]"). Continue to monitor the victim's breathing until help arrives.

If you are alone and the victim vomits, move him or her into the recovery position, supporting the head and neck at all times.

☻ SKILL: ROLLING A VICTIM WITH SPINAL INJURY (LOG ROLL)

STEP 1

Hold the victim's head with hands on both sides over ears.

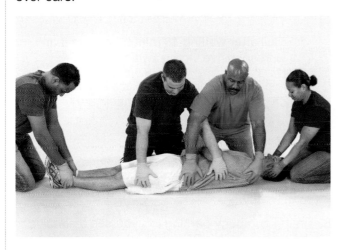

STEP 2

The first aider at the victim's head directs others to roll the body as a unit.

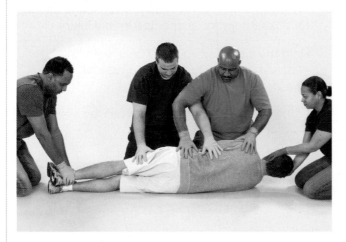

STEP 3

Continue to support head in new position on side.

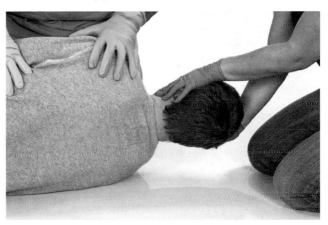

INJURIES TO LOWER BACK

Spinal injuries include lower back injuries that may not damage the spinal cord or be as serious as other spinal injuries. Such injuries generally occur as a result of a stressful activity rather than a traumatic injury, such as a fall or blow to the head or neck. For example, the victim may have been lifting or moving a heavy object or working in an unusual position. A strained muscle or ligament may result, or a disk (soft tissue between vertebrae) may be damaged. Such injuries may not be emergencies, although often they require medical attention.

Signs and symptoms of a less serious lower back injury may include sharp pain in the lower back, stiffness and reduced movement in the back, and possible sharp pain in one leg. If any of the signs and symptoms of a spinal injury are present, call 9-1-1 and keep the victim from moving. Otherwise, the victim should see a health care provider.

 LEARNING CHECKPOINT 2

Circle **True** or **False** or the following statement:

1. Suspect a spinal injury in any victim with a serious head injury. **True   False**

2. Select the best answer. For an unresponsive victim you suspect may have a spinal injury –

    a. immediately place the victim on his or her back in case you have to give CPR.

    b. monitor the victim's breathing in the position in which you found the victim.

    c. turn the head to one side in case the victim vomits.

    d. move all body parts to see if anything feels broken.

3. A spinal injury should be suspected in which of these situations? (Check all that apply.)

    ☐ The victim fell from a roof 20 feet high.

    ☐ A victim with diabetes passes out at lunch.

    ☐ The victim was in a car that hit a telephone pole.

    ☐ A piece of heavy equipment fell from a shelf onto the victim's head.

    ☐ You find a victim slumped over in a desk chair.

4. Which of these are signs and symptoms of a spinal injury? (Check all that apply.)

    ☐ Victim cannot stop coughing

    ☐ Victim's hands are tingling

    ☐ Victim has a breathing problem

    ☐ Victim's face is bright red

    ☐ Unresponsive victim has a fever

    ☐ Victim's neck seems oddly turned

5. When do you call 9-1-1 for a victim with a potential spinal injury? Select the best answer.

    a. Call for all victims with potential spinal injury.

    b. Call only if the victim is unresponsive.

    c. Call for a responsive victim only if feeling is lost on one side of the victim's body.

    d. Call after waiting 10 minutes to see if an unresponsive victim awakes.

6. In what position do you stabilize the head of a victim with a suspected spinal injury?

    _____

7. Fill in the correct answer: Roll a victim with a suspected spinal injury onto his or her side only if the victim _____.

8. In the company parking lot, you see a car skid on an icy patch and smash into another car. The driver is still behind the wheel and looks dazed. Her forehead is bleeding. You ask her how she feels, and she does not answer but just stares ahead. What should you do?

    _____

    _____

    _____

    _____

CONCLUDING THOUGHTS

Because of the risk of brain damage or paralysis, head and spinal injuries can be frightening experiences. Most important, remember that you do not have to assess the injury with certainty before acting. Any time you suspect a victim has a head or spinal injury, call 9-1-1 and keep the victim still until help arrives.

 CRITICAL THINKING CHALLENGE QUESTIONS

SCENARIO 1

A coworker slips on ice in the parking lot, smashing his head against the side of a car. You rush over and ask him how he feels, and he says he's dizzy. He seems disoriented and is staggering, and then he suddenly vomits. What should you do?

_____

_____

_____

_____

SCENARIO 2

While skiing, you come across another skier who has fallen at the edge of the trail, apparently after having hit a tree. He is lying in the snow on his back, unresponsive. Several people have gathered around. His skis have been removed. From the bruise on his forehead, you think that he hit his head against the tree. You check and find that he is breathing. Suddenly he vomits. Describe what you should do (and how to do it safely).

_____

_____

_____

_____

 ADDITIONAL ACTIVITIES AND RESOURCES

1. Organizations such as the National Spinal Cord Injury Association (spinalcord.org) provide information about the long-term needs and care of victims of spinal cord injuries, as well as information about ongoing research for new treatments and hopes for the future.

2. If you work in lifeguarding or are training for a career as an athletic trainer, conduct Internet research on spinal injuries related to diving or contact sports; focus on both prevention strategies and immediate treatment in out-of-hospital settings.

 REVIEW QUESTIONS

Select the best answers.

1. Assessing a victim with a potential head or spinal injury includes –

    a. considering the risk factors in an injured victim.

    b. asking the victim to turn his or her head to the side.

    c. assessing how the victim holds his or her head when sitting.

    d. comparing skin color in different parts of the body.

2. Which of the following is *not* a sign or symptom of possible head or spinal injury?

    a. Unequal pupils

    b. Sudden red rash around neck

    c. Tingling in hands

    d. Headache

3. What is the best way to stop bleeding from the scalp at the site of a skull fracture?

    a. Apply direct pressure on the wound.

    b. Apply indirect pressure on the pulse point in the neck.

    c. Apply pressure only around the edges of the wound.

    d. Tightly bandage the wound but do not apply pressure at all.

4. What is the one sure way for a first aider to know whether a head injury victim has a serious brain injury?

   a. The victim feels temporarily confused.

   b. The victim is acting unusually.

   c. The victim was briefly unconscious.

   d. There is no certain way.

5. A spinal cord injury can cause –

   a. paralysis.

   b. a breathing problem.

   c. numbness in the feet.

   d. All of the above

6. You find an unresponsive victim at the base of a ladder with his head turned to one side. He is breathing normally. You should –

   a. support the head in the position found.

   b. gently move the head in line with the body.

   c. roll the victim onto his side.

   d. try to move his body in line with his head.

7. In your physical examination of a victim with a suspected spinal injury, the victim squeezes your hand only very softly with her left hand. To further assess this victim you can –

   a. squeeze her hand hard and ask what she feels.

   b. ask her to squeeze with both hands at the same time and compare them.

   c. ask her to snap her fingers with her left hand.

   d. have her clasp her hands together and pull with each, to see which arm pulls the other.

8. When might you have to move a victim with a suspected spinal injury?

   a. To position the victim for CPR

   b. To drain vomit from the victim's mouth

   c. To escape an encroaching fire

   d. All of the above

9. When should you call 9-1-1 for a suspected spinal injury?

   a. Call only if the victim is unresponsive.

   b. Call only if the victim is unresponsive, or if a responsive victim is experiencing a severe headache.

   c. Call for any suspected spinal injury.

   d. Call if no one else is present to help you transport the victim to the emergency department.

CHAPTER 13

Chest, Abdominal and Pelvic Injuries

LESSON OBJECTIVES

- Explain why chest injuries may be life threatening and list the general signs and symptoms of chest injuries.

- Describe the specific first aid steps for broken ribs, flail chest, an impaled object in the chest and a sucking chest wound.

- Describe the signs and symptoms of a closed abdominal injury and the first aid to give.

- Explain how to care for an open abdominal wound.

- Describe the signs and symptoms of a pelvic fracture and the first aid to give.

The car in front of you suddenly swerves to the right and runs into the back of a parked car. Fortunately, it was not moving very fast at the time. You pull over and get out to see if you can help. The driver is slumped forward against the steering wheel, apparently not wearing a safety belt and shoulder harness. As you approach, at first he seems unresponsive, but then he leans back and opens the car door. He gets out, holding his chest on one side, and staggers a few feet before you reach him. He does not seem to be bleeding but is obviously in pain. What do you do?

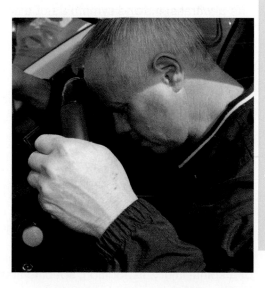

Injuries to the chest, abdomen, or pelvis can result from either blunt or penetrating forces. Blunt trauma typically occurs from motor vehicle crashes, falls, industrial emergencies, fights and similar events. Open injuries can result from any object that breaks the skin, including gunshots and stab wounds. Both closed and open injuries to the chest, abdomen, and pelvis can be life threatening when bleeding is severe or internal organs are injured. Shock often occurs. Always call 9-1-1 for these injuries.

Chest Injuries

The chest contains many important structures that may be damaged from a chest injury, including the heart, lungs and large blood vessels. Trauma may injure the chest wall – including the ribs and soft tissues – or structures within the chest, or both. Serious chest injuries include broken ribs, objects impaled in the chest, and sucking chest wounds in which air passes in and out of the chest cavity. These wounds can be life threatening if breathing is affected. Chest injuries may result from such things as:

• Striking the steering wheel in a motor vehicle crash

• A blow to the chest

• A fall from a height

• Sports injuries

• Physical assault

• A penetrating injury or impaled object

The general signs and symptoms of a serious chest injury include:

• Breathing problems

• Severe pain

• Bruising or swelling

• Deformity of the chest

• Coughing blood

Because the condition of a victim with a chest injury may be life threatening and may worsen over time, it is essential to continue checking the victim's breathing and provide basic life support as needed. The forces involved may also suggest the possibility of a spinal injury. In addition, specific first aid is given for the particular injury.

CLOSED CHEST INJURIES

Common chest injuries involving the lungs include pneumothorax and hemothorax, which may occur with either open or closed injuries. In a pneumothorax, air escapes from an injured lung into the thoracic cavity – the space inside the chest around the lungs – causing collapse of some or all of the lung and resulting in respiratory distress. In a hemothorax, blood from an injury accumulates in the thoracic cavity, compressing the lung and causing respiratory distress and possibly shock.

The fact that the skin is not broken in a closed chest injury does not mean that there is no serious underlying damage. Because organ damage or internal bleeding could be serious, call 9-1-1 and monitor the victim's breathing while waiting for help to arrive. In an unresponsive victim, maintain an open airway and keep checking breathing. Let a responsive victim find the position that is most comfortable and allows for easiest breathing.

BROKEN RIBS

Rib fractures typically result from blunt trauma to the chest. Rib fractures are more common in the lower ribs and along the side. Rib fractures usually cause severe pain, discoloration and swelling at the site of the fracture. The pain is often sharper upon breathing in, and the victim may be breathing shallowly. Another sign of a rib fracture is the victim holding or supporting the area. Many rib fractures involve only the fracture, but with severe trauma there also may be injuries to the lungs or other underlying organs **(Figure 13-1)**. Because of the possibility of serious injury and the risk that the injury may become worse with movement, always call 9-1-1 when you suspect a rib fracture.

The first aid for rib fractures is primarily supportive. Let a responsive victim assume a comfortable position. The victim may sit or stand and often leans toward the side of the injury with an arm compressed against the rib. Use a pillow or blanket to help immobilize the area and reduce pain. Do not tightly wrap a bandage or padding around the chest, because this could restrict breathing (see First Aid: "Broken Ribs").

FIGURE 13-1

The rib cage protects underlying organs in the chest.

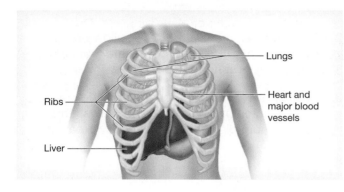

Lungs

Ribs

Heart and major blood vessels

Liver

First Aid: Broken Ribs

Signs, Symptoms and Care

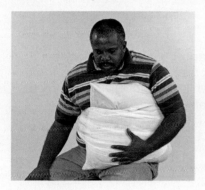

WHEN YOU SEE

- Signs of pain with deep breathing or movement
- Victim holding ribs
- Shallow breathing

DO THIS FIRST

1. Help the victim to sit or stand in the position of easiest breathing.

2. Support the ribs with a pillow or soft padding loosely bandaged over the area and under the arm.

3. Call 9-1-1.

ADDITIONAL CARE

- Monitor the victim's breathing while waiting for help

- If helpful, immobilize the arm with a sling and binder (see **Chapter 15**) to prevent movement and ease pain

FLAIL CHEST

A **flail chest** may result from fracture of two or more ribs in two or more places **(Figure 13-2)**. Flail chest usually results from a severe blow to the chest. The injury actually separates a segment of the chest wall from the remainder of the chest.

With breathing, the flail segment moves in the opposite direction from the rest of the chest wall in what is called **paradoxical movement**. This part of the chest wall moves outward during exhalation because of the increased pressure within the chest. During inhalation the segment moves inward. The larger the flail segment, the greater the threat to the victim's respiratory function.

First aid for flail chest includes monitoring the victim's breathing and supporting the affected chest area with a bulky dressing, towel, or pillow secured with tape or bandages (see First Aid: "Flail Chest").

FIGURE 13-2

In flail chest, a section of the chest wall moves in and out opposite to the normal motion of breathing.

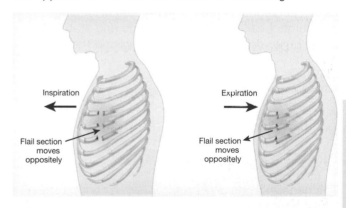

Inspiration

Expiration

Flail section moves oppositely

Flail section moves oppositely

First Aid: Flail Chest

Signs, Symptoms and Care

WHEN YOU SEE

- Victim holding ribs
- Shallow breathing
- Paradoxical movement of chest segment
- Severe pain
- Swelling or chest deformity

DO THIS FIRST

1. Help the victim sit in a comfortable position for easiest breathing.

2. Splint the flail area with a small pillow or thick padding loosely bandaged in place (but not completely around the chest).

3. Position the victim lying on the injured side to give more support to the area, unless this causes more discomfort or difficulty breathing.

4. Call 9-1-1.

ADDITIONAL CARE

- If padding is not available to splint the flail area, support it with pressure from your hand.

- Monitor the victim until help arrives.

IMPALED OBJECT

Removing an impaled object from the chest could cause additional bleeding, injury and breathing problems. Leave the object in place and stabilize it using bulky dressings bandaged around the object, as described in **Chapter 8**. Call 9-1-1 and treat the victim for shock (see **Chapter 9**). Monitor the victim's breathing while waiting for help to arrive (see First Aid: "Impaled Object").

First Aid: Impaled Object

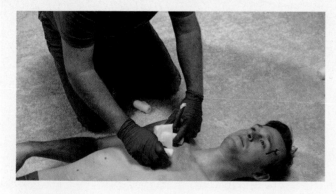

Signs, Symptoms and Care

WHEN YOU SEE

- An object impaled in a chest wound

DO THIS FIRST

1. Keep victim still in the position found.

2. Stabilize the impaled object with bulky dressings.

3. Call 9-1-1.

ALERT

- Do not give the victim anything to eat or drink.

- If you note air moving in or out of a penetrating chest wound, do not block the airflow with a dressing.

ADDITIONAL CARE

- Reassure the victim.

- Monitor the victim's breathing until help arrives.

SUCKING CHEST WOUND

A **sucking chest wound** is an open wound in the chest caused by a penetrating injury that lets air move in and out of the chest during breathing. When the chest expands during inhalation, the pressure inside the chest decreases, and air is sucked in through the wound. When the chest contracts during exhalation, air is forced out through the wound. You may hear a gurgling or sucking sound and may see air bubbles in the blood around the wound.

A sucking chest wound **(Figure 13-3)** can be life threatening because breathing can be affected. When providing first aid for any chest wound when you see air moving in and out of the chest wound, do not block the airflow with a dressing or bandage.

FIGURE 13-3

A sucking chest wound.

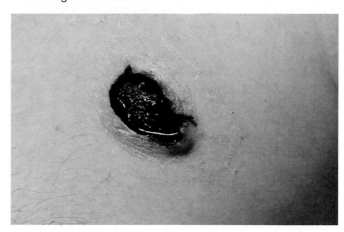

First Aid: Sucking Chest Wound

Signs, Symptoms and Care

WHEN YOU SEE

- Air moving in or out of a penetrating chest wound
- Sucking sounds on inhalation

DO THIS FIRST

1. Put a sterile dressing around the wound but do not block airflow into or out of the wound.

2. Position victim lying down inclined toward the injured side, unless this causes more discomfort or difficulty breathing.

3. Call 9-1-1.

ADDITIONAL CARE

- Monitor the victim's breathing until help arrives.
- Treat the victim for shock.

🖉 **LEARNING CHECKPOINT 1**

Circle **True** or **False** for the following statement:

1. Broken ribs are treated by taping the entire rib cage tightly. **True False**

2. Select the best answer. Immobilize the arm of a victim with a rib fracture to –

   a. prevent movement.

   b. ease pain.

   c. help immobilize that side of the chest.

   d. All of the above

3. What should you do with a screwdriver you see embedded in the chest of an unresponsive friend after an explosion in his garage?

   _____

4. A gunshot victim has a small, bleeding hole in the right side of his chest. You open his shirt to treat the bleeding and see air bubbles forming in the hole as air escapes. How do you dress this wound?

   _____

Abdominal Injuries

Abdominal injuries include closed and open wounds that result from a blow to the abdomen or a fall. Because large blood vessels are present within the abdomen along with many organs, injury may cause internal and/or external bleeding. The abdominal cavity is not protected from injury as the chest is by the ribs. The posterior abdomen is afforded some protection by the spine and lower part of the rib cage, but the anterior abdomen is relatively unprotected **(Figure 13-4)**. Internal organs may be damaged, and organs may protrude from an open wound.

The external appearance of an injured abdomen can sometimes be deceptive, even when serious or life-threatening injuries to organs are present. Often the only indication of abdominal injury is a small bruise or wound. Because of the potential for serious injury, all abdominal wounds should be regarded as potentially life threatening and treated accordingly.

FIGURE 13-4

Abdominal organs have little protection from injury.

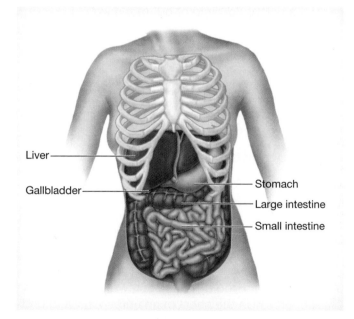

Liver

Gallbladder

Stomach

Large intestine

Small intestine

CLOSED ABDOMINAL INJURY

A closed abdominal injury can threaten life because internal organs may have ruptured and there may be serious internal bleeding. Blunt abdominal trauma commonly occurs in motor vehicle crashes but may also result from sports injuries, falls, physical assault or industrial emergencies.

The signs and symptoms of abdominal trauma can vary. Often, the only symptom is pain. The physical examination may reveal bruising or an obvious abdominal wound. If bleeding is severe, shock may also be present and the abdomen may appear very firm, almost rigid. Abdominal muscles may also contract to minimize movement or agitation of the affected site, a condition called guarding.

First aid for a victim with an abdominal injury includes monitoring the victim's breathing and giving supportive care as well as first aid for an open wound. Do not move the victim, who should try to avoid coughing or straining. Keep the victim warm. Do not give the victim anything to eat or drink because emergency surgery may be needed (see First Aid: "Closed Abdominal Injury").

First Aid: Closed Abdominal Injury

Signs, Symptoms and Care

WHEN YOU SEE

- Signs of severe pain, tenderness in area or victim protecting the abdomen

- Bruising

- Swollen or rigid abdomen

- Rapid, shallow breathing

- Nausea or vomiting

DO THIS FIRST

1. Carefully position the victim on his or her back and loosen any tight clothing. Bending the knees may relax the abdominal muscles, reducing the pain.

2. Call 9-1-1.

3. Treat the victim for shock, monitor the victim's breathing and be ready to give CPR if needed.

ALERT

- If you suspect a spinal injury, do not move the victim from the position found.

- Do not let the victim eat or drink.

ADDITIONAL CARE

- Continue to monitor the victim's breathing until help arrives.

OPEN ABDOMINAL WOUND

An open abdominal injury usually injures internal organs such as the intestines, liver, kidneys or stomach. A large wound in the abdominal wall may allow abdominal organs to protrude through the wound **(Figure 13-5);** this is called **evisceration**.

This is a serious emergency because organs can be further damaged by drying out, bleeding from associated blood vessels or infection.

First aid includes positioning the victim as you would for a closed abdominal injury and providing wound care and treatment for shock. If abdominal organs are protruding through an open wound, do not touch them or try to push them back into the abdomen. Do not pack the wound with dressings. Instead, cover the wound with a moist, sterile dressing or a dry, nonadherent dressing, and cover with an occlusive dressing or plastic wrap loosely taped in place to keep the organs from drying out (see First Aid: "Open Abdominal Wound").

FIGURE 13-5

Open abdominal wound.

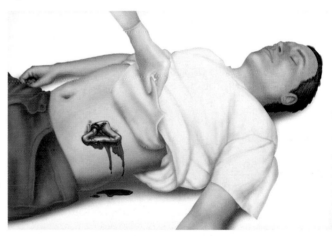

First Aid: Open Abdominal Wound

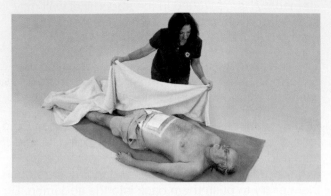

Signs, Symptoms and Care

WHEN YOU SEE

- Open abdominal wound
- Bleeding
- Severe pain
- Organs possibly protruding from wound
- Signs of shock

DO THIS FIRST

1. Lay the victim on his or her back and loosen any tight clothing.

2. Cover the wound with a moist, sterile dressing or a dry, nonadherent dressing.

3. Cover the dressing with a large, occlusive dressing or plastic wrap, taped loosely in place. Then cover the area with a blanket or towel to help maintain warmth.

4. Call 9-1-1.

5. Treat the victim for shock. Monitor the victim's breathing and be ready to give CPR if needed.

ALERT

- If you suspect a spinal injury, do not move the victim from the position found.
- Do not push protruding organs back inside the abdomen, but keep them from drying out with an occlusive dressing or plastic covering.
- Do not apply direct pressure on the wound.

ADDITIONAL CARE

- Monitor the victim until help arrives

✏ LEARNING CHECKPOINT 2

1. You find an unresponsive victim who has suffered a sports injury on the ground. Which of the following are signs and symptoms he may have a closed abdominal injury? (Check all that apply.)

   ☐ Bruises below the rib cage

   ☐ Blotchy skin around the eyes

   ☐ Abrasions on the chest

   ☐ Swollen abdomen

   ☐ Skin feels hot all over

   ☐ Tight skin around the neck

2. Describe the best position for a victim with either an open or closed abdominal wound.

Circle **True** or **False** for the following statement:

3. To treat a victim for shock, help maintain normal body temperature.   True   False

4. If the victim has an organ protruding from an open abdominal wound, what should you do? Select the best answer.

   a. Push the organ back into the abdomen.

   b. Spray clean water over the organ to keep it moist.

   c. Leave the wound exposed to the air.

   d. Cover the wound with a nonadherent dressing and plastic wrap.

5. In what circumstances do you call 9-1-1 for a victim with an open or closed abdominal wound?

Pelvic Injuries

The most common pelvic injury is fracture of the pelvis. Such fractures in healthy adults are usually caused only by large forces, which are likely to cause other injuries as well. Pelvic fractures are more common in the elderly and may be caused by lesser forces, such as falls. Pelvic fractures are generally very serious. A broken pelvis may cause severe internal bleeding and organ damage. A broken pelvis can be life threatening. With severe bleeding, the victim may be in shock.

A victim with a pelvic fracture cannot move and often has severe pain. In the physical examination you may note instability in the pelvic area. The victim may be bleeding from the genitalia or rectum or leaking urine.

Because of the large forces that typically cause the injury, consider that the victim also may have a spinal injury, and support the head and neck accordingly. The care for a suspected pelvic fracture is primarily supportive. Do not move the victim or let the victim move. Take steps to minimize shock, including maintaining the victim's body temperature, but do not elevate the legs (see First Aid: "Pelvic Injuries").

 LEARNING CHECKPOINT 3

1. Fill in the correct answer: First aid for a pelvic fracture prevents _____ of the area.

Circle **True** or **False** for each of the following statements:

2. Internal bleeding can be severe with a broken pelvis. True False

3. For a victim with a broken pelvis, raise the victim's feet and legs to treat for shock. True False

 CONCLUDING THOUGHTS

Victims with serious injuries to the chest, abdomen or pelvis usually have experienced significant trauma, and often there are injuries to internal organs you cannot observe. The victim may have other wounds or injuries as well, complicating the situation. Most important, ensure that 9-1-1 is called immediately to get help on the way. Then care for any life-threatening conditions first and provide specific first aid for the injuries.

First Aid: Pelvic Injuries

Signs, Symptoms and Care

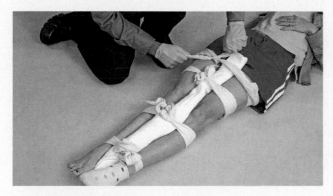

WHEN YOU SEE

- Signs of pain and tenderness around the hips

- Inability to walk or stand

- Signs and symptoms of shock

DO THIS FIRST

1. Support the victim in the position found.

2. Call 9-1-1.

3. If help may be delayed, immobilize the victim's legs by padding between the legs and then bandaging them together, unless this causes more pain.

4. Treat the victim for shock. Monitor the victim's breathing and be ready to give CPR if needed.

ADDITIONAL CARE

- Monitor the victim until help arrives.

- Care for any open wounds, such as wounds to the genitals.

SCENARIO 1

A heavy metal piece breaks loose from machinery in motion and strikes a co-worker in the side, knocking him to the floor. He is sitting up, clutching his side and wincing in pain with each breath taken. You find heavy bruising beginning a few inches below his armpit but no bleeding or open wounds. He is responsive but says it hurts to breathe or move. What do you do?

_____

_____

_____

SCENARIO 2

An electrician working on wiring behind the ceiling falls off a ladder onto a computer monitor on a desk. The glass of the monitor breaks and slices through the skin over her abdomen. She is still responsive but disoriented and confused. The gash in her abdomen is not bleeding heavily, but a purplish-white organ is pushing through the wound. How do you care for this victim?

_____

_____

_____

SCENARIO 3

An elderly customer loses his grip on his cane and falls, twisting sideways as he hits the floor. He is responsive but pale, unable to stand or move his legs, and says his left hip hurts badly. What first aid should you give?

_____

_____

_____

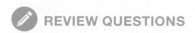

Select the best answers.

1. Chest injuries may be life threatening because –

   a. breathing may be affected.

   b. rib fractures usually involve nerve damage.

   c. chest abrasions can bleed heavily.

   d. All of the above

2. First aid for a rib fracture includes –

   a. tightly bandaging around the chest to prevent movement.

   b. using a pillow or blanket to help support the area.

   c. taping the arm against the side down to the waist.

   d. applying rigid splints on both sides of the thorax.

3. When should an impaled object be removed from the chest wall?

   a. Always

   b. Only when there is no heavy bleeding around it

   c. Only when air bubbles from the lungs are escaping around it

   d. Never

4. The dressing and bandaging of a sucking chest wound should –

   a. allow air to escape but prevent air from being sucked in.

   b. allow air to be sucked in but prevent air from escaping.

   c. allow air to flow in and out of the wound.

   d. prevent air from flowing in or out of the wound.

5. Which of the following is a sign of a closed abdominal injury with severe internal bleeding?

   a. Breathing is slow and very deep.

   b. The area of skin below the umbilicus looks red.

   c. The abdomen feels hard.

   d. The victim always has a fever.

6. The position that is usually most comfortable for a victim with an abdominal injury is –

   a. curled up on side in fetal position.

   b. lying on back.

   c. standing.

   d. lying face down.

7. Internal organs protruding from an abdominal wound should be protected by –

   a. covering them with the victim's shirt.

   b. covering them with a sterile, moist dressing.

   c. pushing them back into the body.

   d. placing the victim's hand over them.

8. What should you do if you suspect the victim has a pelvic fracture?

   a. See if the victim can stand up.

   b. Carefully roll the victim into a face-down position.

   c. Elevate the legs to prevent shock.

   d. Keep the victim still and call 9-1-1.

CHAPTER 14

Bone, Joint and Muscle Injuries

LESSON OBJECTIVES

- Describe ways to prevent common sports and recreation injuries.

- Explain what to look for when assessing musculoskeletal injuries.

- Demonstrate how to use RICE to care for a musculoskeletal injury.

- Describe the first aid for fractures, dislocations and sprains.

- Explain the differences among strains, contusions and cramps and describe the first aid for each.

On a Saturday morning you are jogging on a trail at a local park when you see a woman jogging some distance in front of you suddenly tumble to the ground. When you reach her, she is holding her ankle, which she says really hurts. She says she came down on the side of her foot and felt her ankle twist. She thinks it is sprained, but she doesn't know what to do. How can you help?

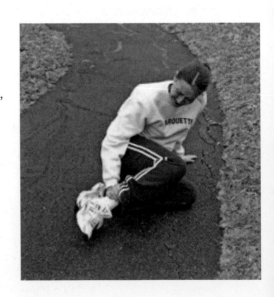

Injuries of the bones, joints and muscles are among the most common injuries in the home, at work, and in sports and recreation **(Table 14-1).** Injuries may result from a blow, the impact of a body part against an object or surface (as in a fall), or other forces acting on the body's bones, joints or muscles. Most sports injuries are musculoskeletal injuries. Although this chapter focuses on first aid for more serious injuries, the most common musculoskeletal injuries are less serious, such as muscle strains resulting from overexertion, and they are seldom an emergency.

This chapter covers musculoskeletal injuries to the extremities. Injuries to the skull or spine are discussed in **Chapter 12,** and injuries to the rib cage and pelvis are discussed in **Chapter 13.**

CLASSIFICATION OF MUSCULOSKELETAL INJURIES

Musculoskeletal injuries are generally classified as injuries of bones **(fractures), joints** (dislocations and sprains) or muscles (strains, contusions, cramps). A **dislocation** is movement of a bone out of its usual position in a joint. A **sprain** is a tearing of **ligaments** in a joint. A **strain** is the tearing of a muscle or tendon, and a **contusion** is a bruised muscle. It is not necessary to know the exact nature of the injury, however, to provide effective first aid. Remember always to assess the victim's breathing first and look for any threats to life before looking for musculoskeletal injuries.

PREVENTION OF SPORTS AND RECREATION INJURIES

Injuries from almost all sports and recreational activities are very common. Death from such injuries, although rare, is usually caused by head injuries in victims not wearing helmets, but emergency department visits are very common. In addition to causing pain and temporary disability, sports injuries may cause long-term or even permanent disability.

Following are some key statistics about sport injuries[1]:

- More than 3.5 million children ages 14 and younger get hurt annually playing sports or participating in recreational activities.

- More than 775,000 children, ages 14 and younger, are treated in hospital emergency rooms for sports-related injuries each year. Most of the injuries occurred as a result of falls, being struck by an object, collisions and overexertion during unorganized or informal sports activities.

TABLE 14-1

Unintentional injuries at work by industry, United States, 2013

Industry division	Hours worked[a] (millions)	2013 Deaths[a]	Medically consulted injuries[c]
All industries	268,127	3,738	4,800,00
Agriculture[b]	4,238	459	120,000
Mining[b]	2,508	153	30,000
Construction	16,972	770	320,000
Manufacturing	30,211	272	600,000
Wholesale trade	7,484	169	120,000
Retail trade	27,936	134	530,000
Transportation and warehousing	10,477	625	250,000
Utilities	1,802	22	20,000
Information	5,489	33	40,000
Financial activities	18,889	49	120,000
Professional and business services	31,046	349	250,000
Educational and health services	39,936	102	880,000
Leisure and hospitality	21,514	104	410,000
Other services[b]	12,429	132	160,000
Government	37,095	365	960,000

Source: National Safety Council, Injury Facts 2015. Deaths are preliminary data from the Bureau of Labor Statistics (BLS) Census of Fatal Occupational Injuries. All other figures are National Safety Council estimates based on data from BLS.

[a]Deaths include persons of all ages. Workers and death rates include persons 16 or older. The rate is calculated as: (number of fatal work injuries x 200,000,000/total hours worked). The base for 100,000 full-time equivalent workers is 200,000,000 hours. Prior to 2008, rates were based on estimated employment – not hours worked.

[b]Agriculture includes forestry, fishing, and hunting. Mining includes oil and gas extraction. "Other services" excludes public administration.

[c]See Technical Appendix for the definition of medically consulted injury.

- Playground, sports, and bicycle-related injuries occur most often among children between ages 5 and 14 years old.

- The highest rates of injury occur in sports that involve contact and collisions.

- More severe injuries occur during individual sports and recreational activities.

- Most organized sports-related injuries (62%) occur during practice.

- Numbers of children ages 5-14 treated in hospital emergency rooms for selected activities and sports:

  - Basketball   170,000
  - Baseball and softball   110,000
  - Bicycling   200,000
  - Football   215,000
  - Ice hockey   20,000
  - In-line and roller skating   47,000
  - Skateboarding   66,000
  - Sledding or toboggan   16,000
  - Snow skiing or snowboarding   25,000
  - Soccer   88,000
  - Trampolines   65,000

¹Stanford Children's Health, stanfordchildrens.org/en/ topic/ default?id=sports-injury-statistics-90-P02787 Accessed January 2016.

Preventing sports and recreational injuries begins with the correct use of sports equipment, such as helmets and other protective gear, and following established safety guidelines for the particular sport. No sport can be made 100% safe, however, and specific sports have certain risks for injury – a factor that should be considered by those involved and the parents of young athletes. Sports medicine is increasingly investigating the long-term effects of some types of sports injuries, such as the potential for disabling conditions, such as arthritis or pain from hairline fractures that appear years or decades after the injury.

To reduce the risk of injury, before beginning a strenuous new activity, check with a health care provider. To prevent common sprains and strains in sports and recreational activities, the following are recommended:

- Maintain a healthy, well-balanced diet to keep muscles strong.

- Maintain a healthy weight.

- Practice safety measures to help prevent falls. For example, keep stairways, walkways, yards, and driveways free of clutter, and salt or sand icy patches in the winter.

- Wear shoes that fit properly. Replace athletic shoes as soon as the tread wears out or the heel wears down on one side.

- Do stretching exercises daily.

- Drink enough water to stay hydrated and prevent heat exhaustion and heat stroke.

- Be in proper physical condition to play a sport.

- Warm up and stretch before participating in any sports or exercise. Use a cool-down routine afterwards.

- Schedule regular days off.

- Wear protective equipment when playing.

- Avoid exercising or playing sports when tired or in pain.

- Run on even surfaces.

Assessing Musculoskeletal Injuries

Remember to first perform the initial assessment of any victim and to care for any life-threatening conditions before performing a physical examination. Musculoskeletal injuries are usually not life threatening, except in cases of severe bleeding, but they may nonetheless be serious and result in pain and disability.

When assessing the injury, consider the type and size of the forces involved. Ask a responsive victim what happened and what he or she felt when the injury occurred. **Figure 14-2** describes common mechanisms of injury.

FIGURE 14-2

Common mechanisms of injury.

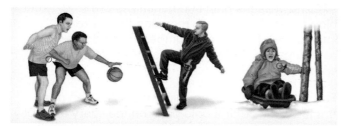

Direct forces, such as a blow to a bone, joint or muscle, often injure that impacted area of the body; the larger the force, the more likely it is a serious injury, such as a fracture.

An **indirect force** may also be transferred up or down an extremity, as when falling on one leg. Similarly falling on an outstretched arm may cause dislocation of shoulder bones.

Twisting forces occur when the body moves in one direction but a force keeps some part of an extremity from moving with the rest of the body. Twisting forces may cause fractures or dislocations of bones at joints.

If large forces were involved in the injury, consider the potential for a spinal injury, and assess the victim accordingly (see **Chapter 12**). Particularly, if the victim is unresponsive, do not move him or her unnecessarily to assess a musculoskeletal injury.

When you perform a physical examination on an injured extremity, remember to look for the following signs and symptoms **(Figure 14-3).** Compare an injured arm or leg to the opposite one.

- Pain when an area is touched
- Bleeding or other wounds
- Swelling
- An area that is deformed
- Skin discoloration
- Abnormal sensation (numbness, tingling)
- Inability to move the area
- Difference in temperature
- Guarding: Because of pain, victim holds the area to prevent movement

In addition, with a fracture, you may hear the broken bone ends grating together, or the victim may feel them grinding together. This is called **crepitus.**

FIGURE 14-3

Signs of a musculoskeletal injury.

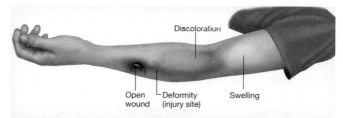

Carefully remove the victim's clothing as needed to examine an injured area and check for an open wound that may require care. Pain occurs with most musculoskeletal injuries and may be more severe with serious injuries, although less painful injuries should not be assumed to be minor. When checking for the ability to move the extremities, do not ask the victim to move an injured area that causes pain. A lack of sensation in the injured area or below it (for example, the finger or toes) may be a symptom of a serious injury involving nerve damage. Swelling occurs in most musculoskeletal injuries because of bleeding in injured tissues, but the amount of swelling is not a good indication of the severity of the injury. An obvious deformity or difference between the injured extremity and its uninjured opposite is usually a sign of a fracture or dislocation, both of which are serious injuries. Skin discoloration may include the black and blue color of bruising or a pale or light blue skin color (ashen in dark-skinned individuals) that, along with cool skin, may indicate a lack of blood flow below the injured area, a sign of a serious injury.

General First Aid for All Musculoskeletal Injuries

Later sections in this chapter describe the specific care for fractures, dislocations, sprains, strains and other injuries. The general first aid for all musculoskeletal injuries is similar, however, based on the same principles of care. You do not have to know the specific type of injury before caring for the victim. The general first aid for most bone, joint and muscle injuries involves four steps that are summarized in the acronym **RICE (Box 14-1):**

R = Rest

I = Ice

C = Compression

E = Elevation

BOX 14-1: "RICE" AND OTHER ACRONYMS

RICE is a widely used acronym to help first aiders remember the treatment for most musculoskeletal injuries, but other acronyms also have been devised for the care of these injuries.

One that is becoming more commonly used now is PRICE, in which the P stands for "protection." This is intended to remind the first aider to protect the injured area by immobilizing it either with a splint (when appropriate) or by protecting the area from movement until the victim is seen by emergency personnel. (Some would argue that this protection is already implied by the R in RICE – resting the injured area.)

Other old standards are PIE (pressure, ice, elevation) and PIES (pressure, ice, elevation, splinting). The P for pressure is equivalent to the C for compression – both referring to wrapping the injury. Proponents of these acronyms suggest the R in RICE for rest is not necessary because the pain and discomfort of the injury will force the victim to rest the area anyway. Still other acronyms that have been used as memory aids include ICE, ICES and PRICES. Occasionally the same acronym has been defined in different ways, such as having I stand for ice in one definition but immobilization in another, and C for cold in one definition but compression in another.

What matters, of course, is remembering the first aid steps behind the acronym.

REST

Any movement of a musculoskeletal injury can cause further injury, pain and swelling. With a fracture or dislocation, for example, any movement of the extremity could cause movement of the bone, further injuring soft tissues, such as blood vessels and nerves, around the bone. In addition, movement generally increases blood flow, which may increase internal bleeding and swelling. For serious injuries, call 9-1-1 and have the victim rest until help arrives. Usually the victim can assume whatever position is the least painful. For less serious injuries, when the victim will be transported to a health care provider or home, minimize movement of the injured extremity as much as possible. For a fracture or dislocation, if medical care may be delayed or the victim must be moved, use a **splint** to immobilize the injured area, as described in **Chapter 15.**

Rest is also important for healing. The victim should follow the health care provider's advice to continue to rest the injured area after treatment.

ICE

Cold applied to a musculoskeletal injury reduces swelling, lessens pain and minimizes bruising. Broken blood vessels constrict, reducing the bleeding into tissues. Nerves are numbed by cold, thereby reducing pain. Cold also helps relieve muscle spasms.

For any musculoskeletal injury other than an open fracture, put ice or a cold pack on the injury as soon as possible. A plastic bag with an ice-water mix is preferred; a commercial cold pack or a cloth pad soaked in cold water can be used. A cold pack that undergoes a phase change (melts) is preferred to refreezable gel packs. The ice or cold pack should be wrapped in a damp cloth, or a damp cloth barrier placed between it and the skin, to prevent injury caused by cold in direct contact with the skin.

Cold works best if applied to the injury as soon as possible, preferably within 10 minutes. Apply the cold for 20 minutes (or 10 minutes if it produces discomfort), then remove it for 30 minutes. Repeat the process for 24-48 hours or until the victim receives medical help. For any injury for which the victim sees a health care provider, follow the provider's instructions for the use of cold (and later heat) after the injury and during the healing period **(Box 14-2).**

BOX 14-2: COLD FIRST, HEAT LATER

People sometimes become confused about applying cold to an injury because they know heat is also used to treat musculoskeletal injuries. It is true that heat is beneficial for healing – just not soon after the injury.

Heat is beneficial for the healing of sprains and strains in part because it causes blood vessels to dilate, or enlarge, which allows more blood to reach the injured area. This increased circulation helps speed up the body's healing processes.

But heat should not be used for about 3 days, or until the initial swelling of the injury is diminished. Heat applied too early would have the opposite of the desired effect of cold: Heat would encourage more internal bleeding because of the increased circulation, would increase swelling, and would make nerve endings more sensitive to pain. Follow your health care provider's guidelines and wait at least 72 hours after the injury, or until the swelling goes down, before soaking the injured area in warm water or applying a heat pad.

COMPRESSION

Compression provides comfort and support and may prevent swelling. Compression of an injured extremity is done with an elastic bandage. Wrap the bandage over the injured area, starting at least 2 inches below the injury and using overlapping turns for at least 2 inches above the injury. The bandage should be firm but not so tight that it cuts off circulation. Compare the fingers or toes on the injured side to those on the other extremity to ensure that circulation is not impeded by the bandage. If the fingers or toes look pale and feel cold compared with the other side, or feel numb or tingling, loosen the bandage (see Skill: "Applying a Spiral Bandage," Skill: "Applying a Figure-8 Bandage to the Wrist" and "Skill: Applying a Figure-8 Bandage to the Ankle").

A compression bandage can also be applied around a cold pack. Remove the bandage just long enough to remove the cold pack after 20 minutes (or 10 minutes if it produces discomfort), and then rewrap it until it is time to apply cold again. Because in some cases swelling may increase after bandaging and cause the bandage to become tighter, it is necessary to continue checking the fingers or toes for circulation.

A compression bandage can be used for 24-48 hours as long as it is not too tight and the person can assess the injury to ensure that the bandage is not too tight.

ELEVATION

Elevating an injured arm or leg uses gravity to help slow the blood flow to the injury, thereby helping to minimize swelling and internal bleeding. First, apply cold and a compression bandage, and then elevate the injured area above the level of the heart if possible **(Figure 14-4).** Do not try to elevate an extremity with a suspected fracture or dislocation – or move it at all – without first splinting it as described in **Chapter 15.** In all cases, elevate the injured extremity only if moving the limb does not cause pain (see Skill: "RICE for Wrist Injury").

FIGURE 14-4

Remember the acronym RICE for treatment of musculoskeletal injuries.

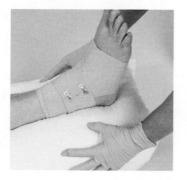

SKILL: APPLYING A SPIRAL BANDAGE

STEP 1

Anchor the starting end of the elastic bandage below the injured area, farther from the trunk.

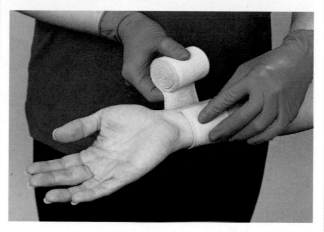

STEP 2

Wrap the bandage in spirals up the limb toward the center of the body.

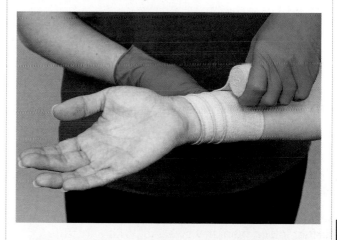

STEP 3

Secure the end of the bandage with clips or tape.

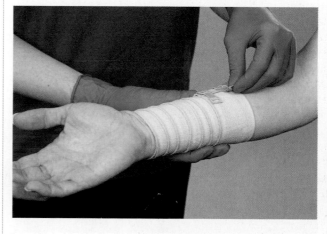

⊙ SKILL: APPLYING A FIGURE-8 BANDAGE TO THE WRIST

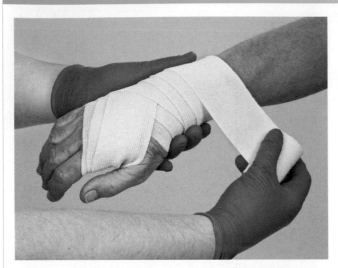

STEP 1
Anchor the starting end of the roller bandage.

STEP 2
Turn the bandage diagonally across the wrist and back around the hand (forming a figure 8).

STEP 3
Continue overlapping the figure-8 turns by about ¾ of the previous turn.

STEP 4
Secure the end of the bandage with clips or tape.

⊙ SKILL: APPLYING A FIGURE-8 BANDAGE TO THE ANKLE

STEP 1
Anchor the starting end of the bandage.

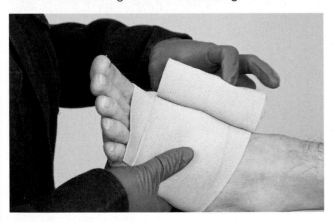

STEP 2
Turn the bandage diagonally across the top of foot and around the ankle, and bring the bandage around in a figure 8.

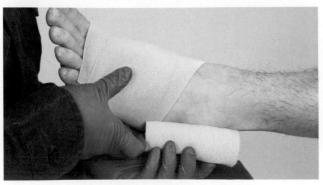

STEP 3
Continue overlapping the figure-8 turns by about ¾ of the previous turn.

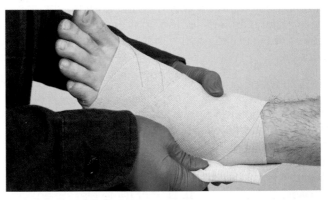

STEP 4
Secure the end of the bandage with clips or tape.

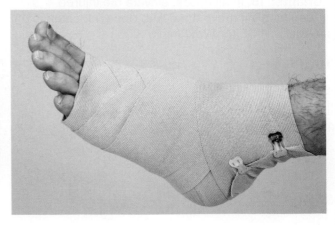

STEP 1

Rest the injured wrist.

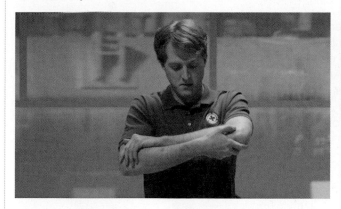

STEP 2

Put ice or a cold pack on the injured area.

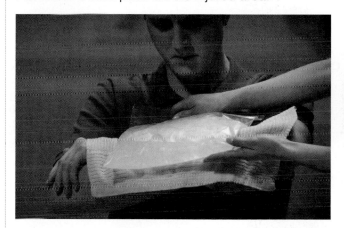

STEP 3

Compress the injured area with an elastic bandage.

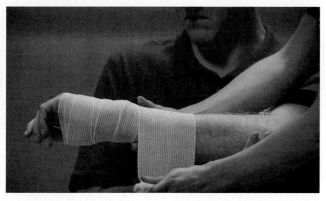

STEP 4

Elevate the injured area. Use a sling to hold the wrist in place.

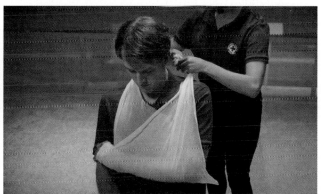

LEARNING CHECKPOINT 1

1. Select the best answer. Use RICE for –

   a. most musculoskeletal injuries.

   b. fractures only.

   c. muscle injuries only.

   d. muscle and joint injuries only.

Circle **True** or **False** for the following statement:

2. Putting a bag with an ice-water mixture or a commercial cold pack directly on the skin is the best way to relieve pain and reduce swelling.   True   False

3. What is important about how you apply a compression bandage? Select the best answer.

   a. Using an elastic bandage

   b. Putting the cold pack under the bandage if needed

   c. Checking that circulation is not cut off

   d. All of the above

4. Describe the steps you would follow to use RICE for an injured ankle.

   _____

   _____

Fractures

A fracture is a broken bone. The bone may be completely broken with the pieces separated or still together, or it may only be cracked.

With a closed fracture, the skin is not broken. Internal bleeding may occur. With an open fracture, there is an open wound at the fracture site, and the bone end may protrude through the wound **(Figure 14-5).** An open fracture can be more serious because there is a greater chance of infection and more serious bleeding. **Figure 14-6** describes common types of fractures.

FIGURE 14-5

Closed and open fractures.

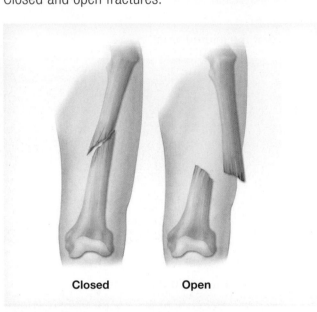

| Closed | Open |

FIGURE 14-6

Common types of fractures.

Transverse	Greenstick	Comminuted fracture	Hairline fracture	Impacted
The fracture line crosses the bone at a right angle.	An incomplete fracture and bending of bone that is more likely in children whose bones are soft.	The bone is broken into more than two fragments.	The bone fragments do not separate.	One fragment is driven into the bone of the other fragment.

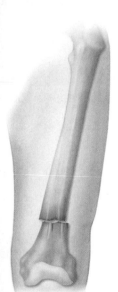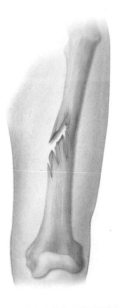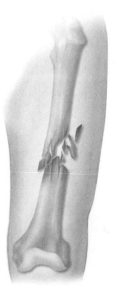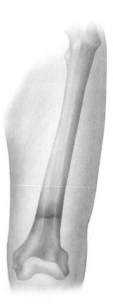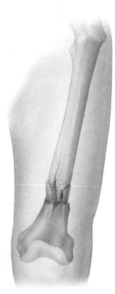

First Aid: Fractures

Signs, Symptoms and Care

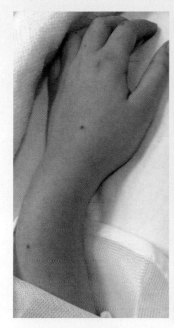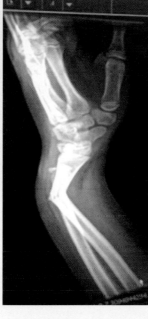

WHEN YOU SEE

- A deformed body part (compare to other side of body)

- Signs of pain

- Swelling or discoloration of skin

- Inability to use the body part

- Bone exposed in a wound

- Victim heard or felt a bone snap

- Possible signs and symptoms of shock

DO THIS FIRST

1. Immobilize the area. For an extremity, also immobilize the joints above and below the fracture.

2. Call 9-1-1 for a large bone fracture. A victim with a fracture in the hand or foot may be transported to the emergency department.

3. For an open fracture, cover the wound with a dressing and apply gentle pressure around the fracture area only if needed to control bleeding.

4. Apply RICE.

5. If help may be delayed or if the victim is to be transported, use a splint to keep the area immobilized (see **Chapter 15**). Elevate a splinted arm.

ADDITIONAL CARE

- Treat the victim for shock.

- Monitor the victim's breathing.

- Remove clothing and jewelry if they may cut off circulation as swelling occurs.

ALERT

- Do not try to align the ends of a broken bone.

- Do not put pressure on bone ends when controlling bleeding.

- Do not give the victim anything to eat or drink.

Although most fractures are not life threatening, external or internal bleeding can be severe with fractures of large bones, such as the femur (thigh bone). Nerves and organs nearby may also be injured. A fracture can also result in extended or permanent disability. Fractures are more likely in elderly adults whose bones are often weaker due to osteoporosis, a gradual thinning of bone with aging. In more severe cases of osteoporosis, a bone may fracture with relatively little force.

A fracture causes pain, swelling, bruising, deformity and an inability to use the affected body part. You may hear, or the victim may feel, the broken bone ends grating together. With severe bleeding, the victim may also experience shock. With a fracture of a long bone like the femur, muscle spasms in the area may occur, possibly further damaging blood vessels or nerves. Check the victim first for any life-threatening conditions, and then care for the fracture. Assess the victim's fingers or toes below the injury to determine if circulation has been disrupted; if so, call 9-1-1 immediately. Also call 9-1-1 for fractures of large bones or bones of the spine, head or trunk. The first aid for fractures includes resting and immobilizing the area, the use of ice or a cold pack, the use of a compression bandage (except for open fractures), and, when practical, elevating a splinted arm (never elevate a leg with a leg fracture). The victim needs to see a health care provider as soon as possible (see First Aid: "Fractures"). The splinting of specific injuries is described in **Chapter 15.**

Joint Injuries

In joints, bones are held in place by ligaments and other structures that allow for movement. Every joint allows a certain range of motion. Forcing a body part beyond the normal range of a joint, or in a direction in which the joint normally cannot move, causes a joint injury.

Injuries to joints include dislocations and sprains. In a dislocation, one or more bones have been moved out of their normal position in a joint; this usually involves the tearing of ligaments and other joint structures. In a sprain, the bones remain in place in the joint, but ligaments and other structures are injured. Both kinds of joint injuries often look similar to a fracture and may be just as serious. When in doubt about the seriousness of any injury, assume the worst: Treat the injury as severe and call 9-1-1.

DISLOCATIONS

In a dislocation, one or more of the bones at the joint are displaced from their normal position when the ligaments that normally hold the bone in place are torn **(Figure 14-7)**. Dislocations typically result from strong forces and are sometimes accompanied by bone fractures or other serious injuries.

FIGURE 14-7

In a dislocation, the bones at the joint are not in normal position.

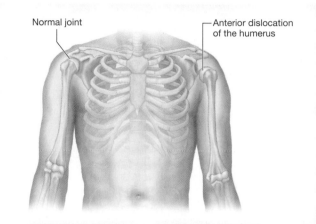

Normal joint — Anterior dislocation of the humerus

Pain, swelling, and bruising usually occur. The victim is unable to use the joint because of both pain and structural damage in the joint. Because major blood vessels and nerves are located near joints in many parts of the body, a significant displacement of the bones can damage nearby nerves and cause serious bleeding. If the dislocation is severe, the joint or limb will look deformed. Dislocations can be serious because of the potential for nerve and blood vessel injury, which may be indicated by a loss of sensation or cool, pale skin in the extremity below the injury.

It is not always possible to tell a dislocation from a closed fracture, but the first aid is very similar for both. With severe bleeding, the victim may experience shock. Check the victim first for any life-threatening conditions, and then care for the dislocation. Assess the victim's fingers or toes below the injury to determine if circulation has been disrupted; if so, call 9-1-1 immediately. Except for a dislocation in the hand or foot, which can be immobilized so that the victim can be transported to a hospital, call 9-1-1 for a suspected dislocation. First aid includes resting and immobilizing the area, using ice or a cold pack, using a compression bandage and, when practical, elevating a splinted hand or foot (see First Aid: "Dislocations"). The splinting of specific injuries is described in **Chapter 15.**

First Aid: Dislocations

Signs, Symptoms and Care

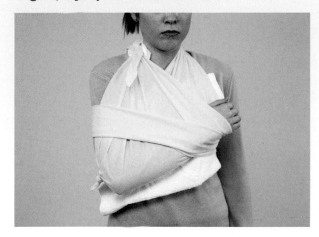

WHEN YOU SEE

- The joint is deformed (compare to other side of body)
- Signs of pain
- Swelling
- Inability to use the body part

DO THIS FIRST

1. Immobilize the area in the position in which you find it.

2. Call 9-1-1. A victim with a dislocated bone in the hand or foot may instead be transported to an emergency department.

3. Apply RICE, but do not use a compression bandage or elevate the injured area if moving the joint causes pain.

4. If help may be delayed or if the victim is to be transported, use a splint to keep the area immobilized in the position in which you find it (see **Chapter 15**).

ADDITIONAL CARE

- Treat the victim for shock.
- Monitor the victim's breathing.
- Remove clothing and jewelry if they may cut off circulation as swelling occurs.

ALERT

- Do not try to put the displaced bone back in place.
- Do not let the victim eat or drink.

BOX 14-3: WHEN TO SEE A HEALTH CARE PROVIDER FOR A MUSCULOSKELETAL INJURY

Because you cannot always judge the type or severity of an injury by the signs and symptoms, you may be unsure about whether you need medical attention. You should see a health care provider if any of the following is true:

- You have the signs and symptoms of a fracture or dislocation.
- The injury causes severe pain.
- You cannot put any weight on an injured leg or walk more than a few steps without significant pain, or the leg buckles when you try to walk.
- An injured joint or the area around it is very tender to touch or feels numb.

- The injured area looks different from the same area on the other extremity (other than swelling).
- The injured joint cannot move.
- Redness or red streaks spread out from the injured area.
- An area that has been injured several times before is reinjured.
- You are unsure how serious an injury is or what treatment to give.

SPRAINS

A sprain is a joint injury involving the stretching or tearing of ligaments. Sprains typically occur when the joint is overextended or forced beyond the range of normal movement, as when the ankle is twisted by a sideways force on the foot. Sprains can range from mild to severe. The ankles, knees, wrists and fingers are the body parts most often sprained.

Sprains cause swelling, pain, bruising and an inability to use the joint because of the pain. The swelling may be considerable and often occurs rapidly. It can be difficult to tell a severe sprain from a fracture, but the first aid is similar for both. Check the victim first for any life-threatening conditions, and then care for the sprain. Assess the victim's fingers or toes below the injury to determine if circulation has been disrupted; if so, call 9-1-1. Use RICE, immobilize the joint with a splint if the victim is to be moved and seek medical attention (see First Aid: "Sprains"). The splinting of specific sprains is described in **Chapter 15**.

First Aid: Sprains

Signs, Symptoms and Care

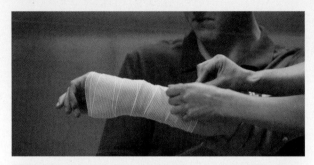

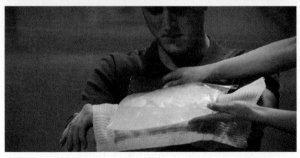

WHEN YOU SEE

- Signs of pain

- Swollen joint

- Bruising of joint area

- Inability to use joint

DO THIS FIRST

1. Immobilize the area in the position in which you find it.

2. Apply RICE.

3. Use a soft splint (bandage, pillow or blanket) to immobilize and support the joint.

4. Seek medical attention.

ADDITIONAL CARE

- Remove clothing or jewelry if they may cut off circulation as swelling occurs.

BOX 14-4: REMOVING A RING

When an injury to the hand or fingers causes swelling, the victim's watch or rings can cut off circulation. Try to remove a watch and rings before swelling occurs. Removal of a ring is easier if you first soak the finger in cold water or wrap it in a cold pack, and then put oil or butter on the finger.

 LEARNING CHECKPOINT 2

Circle **True** or **False** for the following statement:

1. Call 9-1-1 for a fracture of a large bone, such as the thigh bone.   True   False

2. When you are immobilizing a fracture injury, what body area should be immobilized? Select the best answer.

    a. The immediate fracture area

    b. The fracture area and the joint above it

    c. The fracture area and the joints both above and below it

    d. The entire victim

Circle **True** or **False** for the following statement:

3. For a fracture, you may also need to treat the victim for shock. True False

4. The signs and symptoms of a bone or joint injury include which of the following? (Check all that apply.)

   ☐ Deformed area

   ☐ Pain

   ☐ Small or unequal pupils

   ☐ Inability to use body part

   ☐ Skin is hot and red

   ☐ Fever

   ☐ Swelling

   ☐ Spasms and jerking of nearby muscles

Circle **True** or **False** for the following statement:

5. A victim with a sprained ankle should "walk it off." True False

Muscle Injuries

Common muscle injuries include strains, contusions and cramps. These injuries are usually less serious than fractures and joint injuries. Muscle injuries are often easy to identify because, unlike sprains and dislocations, they do not usually involve the joint. Muscle injuries are typically caused by overexertion, careless or sudden uncoordinated movements or poor body mechanics, such as lifting a weight with back bent or twisted. Repetitive forces, as frequently occur in some sports, may also inflame or injure tendons. Repeated injury can lead to chronic problems.

STRAINS

A strain is a tearing of a muscle or a tendon, which connects the muscle to bone. Usually the tear is partial, but in extreme cases the muscle or tendon may tear completely. A strain occurs when the muscle is stretched too far by overexerting the body area. The victim experiences pain, swelling and sometimes an inability to use the muscle. Back strains are common occupational injuries, and strains

First Aid: Strains

Signs, Symptoms and Care

WHEN YOU SEE

- Signs of dull or sharp pain when muscle is used

- Stiffness in the area of the injury

- Weakness or inability to use the muscle normally

DO THIS FIRST

1. Apply RICE.

2. Keep the cold pack on the area for 20 minutes (or 10 minutes if it produces discomfort), then remove it for at least 30 minutes; reapply for 20 (or 10) minutes, then remove again for 30 minutes.

ADDITIONAL CARE

- Seek medical attention if pain is severe or persistent, or if there is a significant or prolonged (3 days or more) impairment of function.

First Aid: Contusion

Signs, Symptoms and Care

WHEN YOU SEE

- Signs of pain

- Swollen, tender area

- Skin discoloration (black and blue)

DO THIS FIRST

1. First treat any injury that caused the bruising.

2. Apply RICE. Do not massage the muscle.

3. Keep the cold pack on the area for 20 minutes (or 10 minutes if it produces discomfort), then remove it for 30 minutes. Repeat the process for 24-48 hours as needed.

ADDITIONAL CARE

- Seek medical attention if pain is severe or impaired function persists.

in extremities are common in sports. In most cases, strains can be prevented by avoiding overexertion, using good body mechanics and following accepted guidelines for sports safety.

Use RICE to treat strains (see First Aid: "Strains"). Follow-up light exercise may help with healing and later muscle strengthening. With a very serious muscle or tendon tear, surgical repair may be required.

CONTUSIONS

A contusion is a bruised muscle that may result from a blow. The blow causes blood vessels within the muscle to rupture, leaking blood into the muscle tissue. This injury often occurs when the muscle is compressed between the object causing the blow and an underlying bone. Contusions cause pain, swelling and discoloration **(Figure 14-8)** and are treated with RICE (see First Aid: "Contusion"). The discoloration may persist up to a month.

FIGURE 14-8

Contusion.

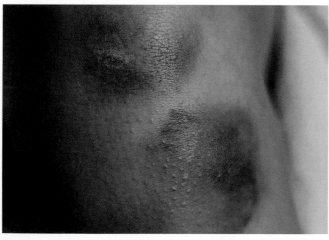

MUSCLE CRAMPS

A muscle **cramp** is a tightening of a muscle that usually results from prolonged use but may occur with no apparent cause. Cramps are most common in the thigh and calf muscles, but they may also occur in abdominal or back muscles, in any muscle that is overused or with dehydration. These cramps are different from heat cramps, which result from fluid loss in hot environments (see **Chapter 20**). A cramp may last only a few seconds or up to 15 minutes. You may see the muscle bunching up or twitching under the skin. Cramps are treated with gentle stretching, a cold pack and massage after the cramping stops (see First Aid: "Muscle Cramp"). Cramps may be prevented with flexibility exercises and stretching before engaging in physical activity.

First Aid: Muscle Cramp

Signs, Symptoms and Care

WHEN YOU SEE

• Signs of muscle pain and tightness

DO THIS FIRST

1. Have the victim stop the activity.

2. Gently stretch out the muscle, if possible.

3. Gently massage the muscle after active cramping stops, if this provides relief.

4. Place a cold pack on the area for 20 minutes (or 10 minutes if it produces discomfort), then remove it for 30 minutes.

ADDITIONAL CARE

• Give the victim a carbohydrate-electrolyte drink, such as a sports drink, to promote rehydration. (Other beverages, such as 2% milk and coconut water, are also effective.) If a carbohydrate-electrolyte drink is not available, give the victim water.

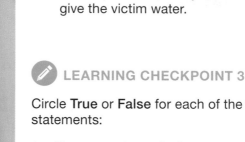 LEARNING CHECKPOINT 3

Circle **True** or **False** for each of the following statements:

1. For a muscle strain, keep an ice pack on the injury for at least 2 hours.   True   False

2. Vigorous massage is the best treatment for a muscle contusion.   True   False

3. You can distinguish a contusion from a fracture because only a contusion causes an area of skin discoloration.   True   False

4. Name three things you can do to ease a muscle cramp.

_____

_____

_____

CONCLUDING THOUGHTS

Millions of people every year go to the emergency department with musculoskeletal injuries. Countless others sustain less serious injuries that do not require a health care provider's attention. Most people will experience at least one sprain or strain in their lifetime and will also care for another person with such an injury. Fortunately, most of these injuries are not life threatening or very severe, and the victim recovers well. Giving the appropriate first aid, however, is important for making a good recovery without future disability. Remember that you do not have to know the exact nature of the injury before helping: use RICE (Rest, Ice, Compression, Elevation) for most injuries, and call 9-1-1 or seek medical attention for more serious injuries.

CRITICAL THINKING CHALLENGE QUESTIONS

SCENARIO 1

An employee riding his bicycle to work hits a pothole as he enters the parking lot, loses control and swerves into the path of a moving pickup truck. The truck's bumper strikes his leg below the knee. By the time you reach the scene, the victim has been helped into a position lying down. He is responsive but in significant pain. You carefully cut open his pants leg and see an open wound that is bleeding, in which you can see the end of a broken bone. Describe what care to give.

_____

_____

_____

_____

SCENARIO 2

A worker has been carrying heavy equipment and supplies all morning to a construction site, and he now stumbles and falls. He says the muscle in his leg is "all cramped up" and really hurts when he walks on that leg. You see no sign of a fracture or other serious injury. What should you do?

_____

_____

_____

_____

SCENARIO 3

While using a long pole to sweep leaves from a low roof, your neighbor twists her arm. She says her elbow hurts, but she can move it. There is some swelling, but no distortion suggesting a fracture or serious sprain. What care do you give?

_____

_____

_____

_____

ADDITIONAL ACTIVITIES AND RESOURCES

If you are in sports, you may be interested in doing Internet research on the value of stretching before, during and after exercise and athletic activity to prevent muscle cramps and injuries. You may find information you were not aware of that has an application in your own exercise or athletic program.

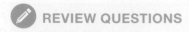

Select the best answers.

1. Steps to help prevent sports and recreational injuries include –

    a. maintaining a healthy weight.

    b. wearing shoes that fit properly.

    c. wearing protective equipment.

    d. All of the above

2. What is true about swelling in most musculoskeletal injuries?

    a. Swelling occurs because of internal bleeding in tissues.

    b. Swelling occurs with all injuries except fractures.

    c. The amount of swelling indicates the seriousness of the injury.

    d. Swelling should be promoted because it aids healing.

3. Cold is best applied to a musculoskeletal injury by –

    a. an ice-water mixture.

    b. a gel pack.

    c. a bag of frozen peas.

    d. All of the above

4. Which statement is generally true of treatment for a musculoskeletal injury?

    a. Apply heat for up to 2 days, then apply cold.

    b. Apply cold for up to 2 days, then apply heat.

    c. Apply cold for the first 12 hours, then apply heat.

    d. Apply cold and heat alternating every 6 hours.

5. The purpose of using a compression bandage on a musculoskeletal injury is to –

    a. dress the injured area.

    b. cut off circulation to the area.

    c. help support injury and prevent swelling.

    d. prevent infection.

6. The most important aspect of fracture care is to –

    a. apply antibiotic ointment to an open fracture.

    b. put the bone ends together in their normal position.

    c. apply traction to prevent shortening of the limb.

    d. immobilize the area.

7. What should *not* be done to a dislocation?

    a. Apply ice or a cold pack on the joint.

    b. Try to move the bone ends back into their normal position in the joint.

    c. Apply a compression bandage over the joint if it is in an extremity.

    d. Prevent the victim from moving the joint.

8. To assess for circulation in the foot when the victim has an ankle injury –

    a. check the toes for color, temperature and sensation.

    b. ask the victim to push against your hand with his or her foot.

    c. determine whether the victim can stand without feeling pain.

    d. have the victim take a few steps and report whether his or her toes tingle.

9. A strain occurs when a muscle –

    a. is bruised by a blunt blow.

    b. is separated from ligaments in a joint.

    c. is stretched too far (overexertion).

    d. becomes dehydrated.

10. First aid for a muscle cramp may include –

    a. returning to activity as soon as possible.

    b. massaging the muscle.

    c. applying a heat pad.

    d. soaking the extremity in icy water.

CHAPTER 15

Extremity Injuries and Splinting

LESSON OBJECTIVES

- Describe the 3 general types of splints and how to improvise splints with common materials.

- List the general guidelines for splinting and use of arm slings.

- Describe how to splint the different areas of the upper and lower extremities.

- Demonstrate how to apply an arm sling.

- Demonstrate how to apply a rigid splint to an injured forearm.

- Demonstrate how to use an anatomic splint for a leg injury.

Your young daughter is playing with two friends on the playground while you watch from a nearby bench. While climbing up a climbing structure, she loses her grip and tumbles to the ground. Although she falls only a couple feet, she lands hard on her arm. When you reach her a few seconds later, she is crying and clutching her arm tightly. What do you do?

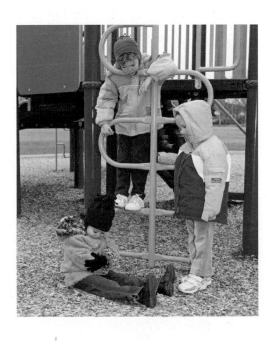

As described in **Chapter 14,** with most musculoskeletal injuries, there is a risk of movement worsening the injury and causing more pain. All such injuries should be stabilized to prevent movement. When a victim has a fracture, dislocation or sprain in an arm or leg, the arm or leg may be splinted if there is a risk for moving the injured area unless help is expected within a few minutes. Always splint an extremity before transporting the victim to a health care provider or the emergency department. Splinting helps prevent further injury, reduces pain and minimizes bleeding and swelling. Splints can be improvised when needed and tied in place with bandages, belts, neckties or strips of cloth torn from clothing.

This chapter describes splinting and other first aid for specific musculoskeletal injuries of the arms and legs. Remember always to first check the victim's breathing and provide care for life-threatening conditions. Consider the forces involved in the injury and whether a spinal injury may be present. If you suspect a spinal injury, the priority is to support the head and neck and prevent spinal movement. Because splinting a fracture may involve moving some part of the victim or may distract from care given for the spinal injury, unless multiple rescuers are present, leave an extremity injury unsplinted while waiting for help to arrive.

Types of Splints

A splint is any object you can use to help keep an injured body area from moving. Various kinds of commercial splints are available and are used by professional rescuers, but splints can also be made from many different materials at hand. There are 3 general types of splints **(Figure 15-1)**:

- **Rigid splints** may be made from a board, a cane or walking stick, a broom handle, a piece of plastic or metal, a rolled newspaper or magazine or thick cardboard.

- **Soft splints** may be made from a pillow, a folded blanket or towel or a triangular bandage folded into a sling.

- **Anatomic splints** involve splinting one part of the body with another part, such as an injured leg to the uninjured leg, or splinting fingers together, or splinting the arm to the chest to immobilize the shoulder.

FIGURE 15-1

Examples of general types of splints.

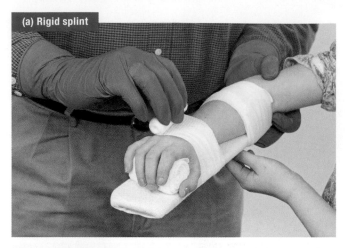
(a) Rigid splint

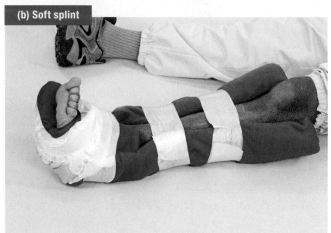
(b) Soft splint

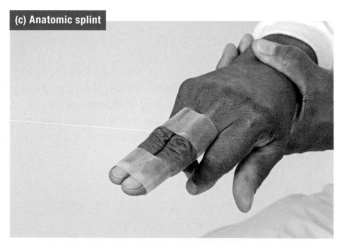
(c) Anatomic splint

The splint is the object to which the injured extremity is secured to prevent movement. The splint is usually secured by wrapping bandages, strips of cloth (often called **cravats**), Velcro straps or other materials around the splint and extremity. Because you may have to loosen or remove a splint if it interferes with circulation to the limb, use knots that can be untied if needed. If tape is used, do not tape to the skin directly. Instead, put a dressing or other material over the skin first, or fold the sticky side back on itself.

In addition to common rigid and soft splints, commercial splints are available that are typically used by rescuers with more training. **Figure 15-2** shows some examples of commercial splints.

FIGURE 15-2

Commercial splints.

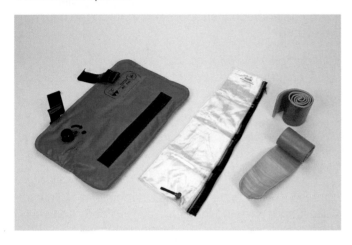

Guidelines for Splinting

Regardless of the specific type of injury and its location, always apply the following general guidelines for splinting. Later sections in this chapter show how to use these guidelines when splinting specific extremity injuries.

- *Put a dressing on any open wound before splinting the area.* This helps protect the wound, control bleeding and prevent infection.

- *Splint an injury only if it does not cause more pain for the victim.* Splinting usually involves touching and perhaps manipulating the injured area, which may cause pain and may worsen the injury. If the victim complains, stop the splinting and have the victim immobilize the area as well as possible until help arrives.

- *Splint the injury in the position in which you find it* **(Figure 15-3).** Trying to straighten out a limb or joint will likely cause pain and could worsen the injury. Blood vessels or nerves near a fracture or dislocation, for example, could be damaged by moving the bone ends. In almost all cases, the injured extremity can be splinted in the position in which you find it, as shown later in this chapter. Only if the victim is in a remote location and will not receive medical attention for a long time, or

if circulation has been cut off in the extremity by the injury, should the limb be straightened (see **Chapter 23**).

FIGURE 15-3

Splint an injury in the position found, such as this knee injury. Do not try to straighten the limb to splint it.

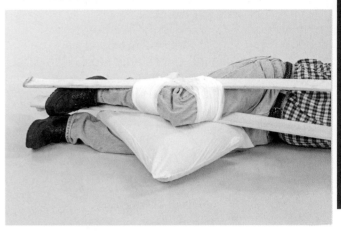

- *Splint to immobilize the entire injured area.* For example, the splint should extend to the joints above and below the injured area. With a bone fracture near a joint, assume that the joint is injured as well, and extend the splint well beyond the joint to keep it and the fracture site immobilized.

- *Put padding such as cloth between the splint and the victim's skin.* This is especially important with rigid splints, which otherwise may press into soft tissues and cause pain and further injury. Use whatever materials are at hand that will conform to the space between the splint and the body part. Pad body hollows, and ensure that the area of the splint close to the injury is well padded.

- *Put splints on both sides of a fractured bone if possible.* If the injury makes this difficult or splinting materials are limited, splint one side.

- *Do not secure the splint on an open wound because the securing bandage or strap could cut into or irritate the wound.* Tie the bandages or other materials used to hold the splint in place on both sides of the wound.

- *Elevate the splinted extremity if possible.* Do not move the injured area to elevate it if it causes the victim pain or may worsen the injury.

- *Apply a cold pack to the injury around the splint.* Because the ice or cold pack must be removed after 20 minutes, it should not be positioned inside the splint. Placing it inside would require removal and repositioning of the splint. This may cause pain and movement in the injured area. Splint the injury first, and then position the cold pack as close to the injury as possible around the splint **(Figure 15-4).**

FIGURE 15-4

Apply a cold pack to the injured area around the splint.

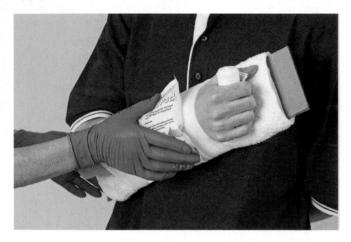

- *With a splinted extremity, do not completely bandage over the fingers or toes, and check them frequently to make sure circulation is not cut off.* To be effective, the splint must be tied firmly enough to the extremity to prevent movement but not so tight that circulation is cut off. Swelling, pale or bluish discoloration, tingling or numbness, and cold skin are signs and symptoms of reduced circulation. If any of these occurs, the splint should be removed or the bandages holding the limb to the splint should be loosened. Periodically check for adequate circulation.

Applying Slings

A **sling** is a device used to support and immobilize the upper extremity. A sling may be used for most upper extremity injuries, including those to the shoulder, upper and lower arm, elbow and wrist. When available, a sling is best made from a large, triangular bandage, but improvised slings can be made from many other materials, such as strips of cloth torn from clothing, neckties and so on. Cloth or soft, flexible material is generally best.

A sling is used to prevent movement of the arm and shoulder, thereby preventing a worsening of the injury, helping to limit pain, and elevating the extremity to help control bleeding and swelling. In some instances, a binder is used along with the sling. A binder (or swathe) is an additional supportive bandage or cloth tied over the sling and around the chest to provide additional support (see Skill: "Applying an Arm Sling and Binder").

Follow these guidelines when using a sling:

- *Splint the injury first, when appropriate.* A fracture of the upper or lower arm or a dislocation of the elbow or wrist should be splinted to prevent movement of the area. Then, a sling is applied to provide additional support and to keep the injury elevated.

- *If you splint the injury in the position found and this position makes the use of a sling impossible or difficult, do not try to use a sling.*

- *Do not move the arm into position for a sling if this causes the victim more pain.* If so, splint the arm in the position found, not using a sling, and have the victim immobilize it until help arrives.

- *A cold pack can be used inside the sling.* Follow the standard guidelines for applying and removing the cold pack and then reapplying it later (see **Chapter 14**).

- *Do not cover the fingers inside the sling.* Ensure circulation in the extremity periodically by checking the fingers for color, temperature and normal sensation.

⚙ SKILL: APPLYING AN ARM SLING AND BINDER

STEP 1
Secure the point of the bandage at the elbow. Use a safety pin or tie the point at the elbow.

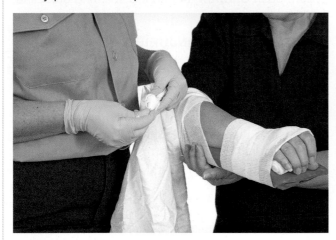

STEP 2
Position the triangular bandage.

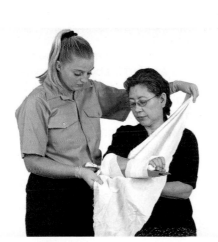

STEP 3
Bring up the lower end of the bandage to the opposite side of the neck.

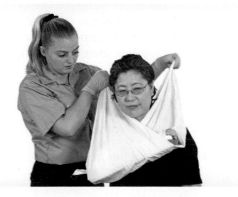

STEP 4
Tie the ends. Pad under the knot.

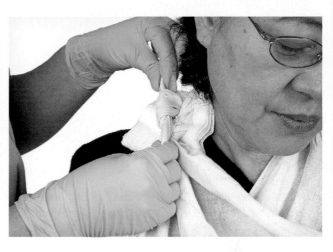

STEP 5
Tie a binder bandage over the sling and around the chest.

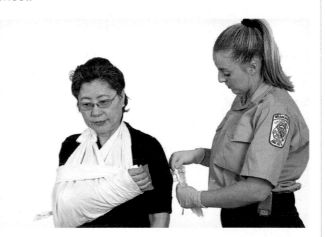

1. You encounter a victim with an obviously fractured forearm. What materials might you be able to find around the home that you can use to make a rigid splint?

   _____

   _____

   _____

   _____

   _____

   _____

2. When using splints, which of the following are actions you should take? (Check all that apply.)

   ☐ Put a heating pad on the area.

   ☐ Straighten out a limb before splinting it.

   ☐ Dress an open wound before splinting.

   ☐ Pad the splint.

   ☐ Put a cold pack around the splint.

   ☐ Splint in the position found.

3. List signs that circulation has been cut off in an extremity below the splint:

   _____

   _____

   _____

   _____

4. Name 2 things you should *not* do when contemplating putting a victim's arm in a sling:

   _____

   _____

   _____

Splinting Extremity Injuries

The following sections describe first aid and splinting techniques for specific bone and joint injuries of the extremities. Remember to follow the RICE acronym described in **Chapter 14** and the splinting guidelines listed earlier.

UPPER EXTREMITY INJURIES

Upper extremity injuries include fractures, dislocations and sprains of the shoulder, upper arm, elbow, lower arm, wrist and hand. Remember the general principle to splint only if help will be delayed and there is a risk of the injured area moving (or a victim with an injured arm or foot is to be transported).

Shoulder Injuries

Shoulder injuries can fracture the clavicle (collar bone), the scapula (shoulder blade) or joint structures. The clavicle is the most frequently fractured bone in the body. Victims have pain and cannot use the shoulder, which often is lower than the opposite shoulder. Swelling and tenderness are present. Fractures of the scapula are very rare. Dislocations of the shoulder are common and cause pain, deformity of the shoulder and an inability to move it.

The goal of splinting the shoulder is to stabilize the area from the trunk to the upper arm with a soft splint. First, check for signs of circulation and sensation in the hand. Have the victim wiggle the fingers and ask whether he or she can feel your light touch on the palm. Then, apply a sling and binder.

1. Use a soft, not rigid, splint for shoulder injuries. Do not move the extremity.

2. Check for signs of circulation and sensation in the hand and fingers. If they are absent, call 9-1-1 for immediate care.

3. Pad the hollow areas between the body and the arm with a small pillow or towels, and apply a sling and binder to support the arm and immobilize it against the chest if this does not cause pain **(Figure 15-5).** If moving the arm closer to the chest causes pain, use a larger pillow between the arm and the trunk.

4. Follow the general guidelines for safe splinting.

5. Check the fingers periodically for circulation.

FIGURE 15-5

Immobilize a shoulder injury with a sling and binder.

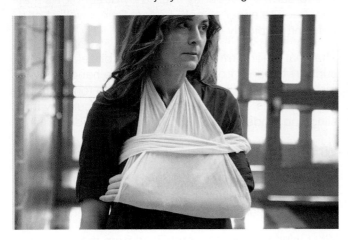

Upper Arm Injuries

Fractures of the **humerus**, the bone of the upper arm, cause pain, swelling and deformity of the arm. Fractures near the shoulder should be treated in a manner identical to shoulder injuries with soft splinting.

The goal of splinting the upper arm is to stabilize the bone between the shoulder and the elbow by using a rigid splint on the outside of the arm and placing the wrist in a sling. The fracture site can then be further secured by applying a wide binder around the arm and chest. Be careful not to apply the binder directly over the fracture site.

1. Check for signs of circulation and sensation in the hand and fingers. If they are absent, call 9-1-1 for immediate care.

2. Apply a rigid splint along the outside of the upper arm, tied above and below the injury.

3. Support the wrist with a sling, and then apply a wide binder to support the arm and immobilize it against the chest **(Figure 15-6).** If it causes pain to raise the wrist for a sling, a long, rigid splint may be used that supports the arm in a straighter position.

4. Follow the general guidelines for safe splinting. Check the fingers periodically for circulation.

FIGURE 15-6

Immobilize an upper arm injury with a splint, sling and binder.

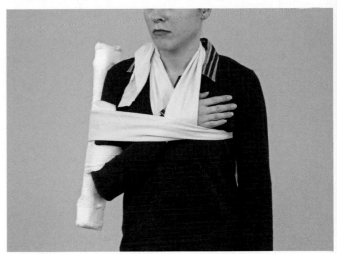

Elbow Injuries

The elbow can be injured by a blow or force that moves the joint beyond its normal limits. Sprains and dislocations are the most common injuries to the joint itself. Fractures of the bones above or below the elbow are also common. Nerves and arteries pass close to the bones of the elbow and may also be injured. Usually, the victim is unable to move the joint and may say the joint is "locked."

The goal of splinting the elbow is to stabilize the joint from the arm to the forearm in the position in which you find it. If the elbow is bent, a soft splint with sling and binder may be sufficient, but a rigid splint provides greater stability. If the elbow is straight, a rigid splint should be applied.

1. Check for signs of circulation and sensation in the hand and fingers. If they are absent, call 9-1-1 for immediate care.

2. If the elbow is bent, apply a rigid splint from the upper arm to the wrist as shown in **Figure 15-7(a).** If more support is needed, use a sling at the wrist and a binder around the chest at the upper arm.

3. If the elbow is straight, apply a rigid splint from the upper arm to the hand as shown in **Figure 15-7(b).** If more support is needed, binders may be used around the chest and upper arm and around the lower arm and waist.

4. Follow the general guidelines for safe splinting. Check the fingers periodically for circulation.

FIGURE 15-7

Immobilize an elbow injury with a rigid splint in the position found. (a) Splinting a bent elbow. (b) Splinting a straight elbow.

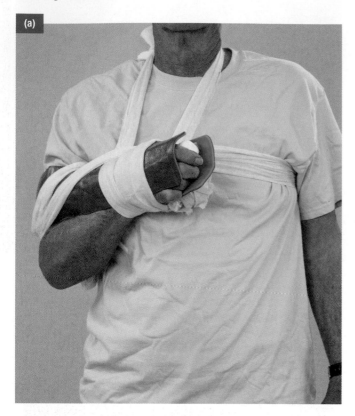

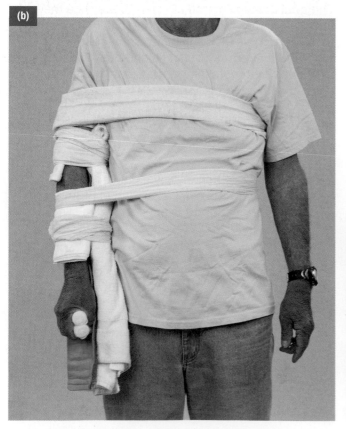

Forearm Injuries

The forearm is frequently injured by direct blows that may fracture either or both bones. Pain, swelling and deformity typically result.

The goal of forearm splinting is to stabilize and support the area from the elbow to the hand. You may use a splint on the palm side of the forearm or on both sides. After splinting the arm, secure it with a sling and binder (see Skill: "Splinting the Forearm").

Wrist Injuries

Common wrist injuries include sprains and fractures. Movement of the wrist produces pain. Swelling, discoloration and deformity may be present.

Wrist injuries should be stabilized from the forearm to the hand. In some cases, a soft splint is sufficient, with the area then elevated and supported with a sling. A rigid splint provides more support, and the joint is stabilized in a manner similar to a forearm injury.

1. Check for signs of circulation and sensation in the hand and fingers. If they are absent, call 9-1-1 for immediate care.

2. Apply a rigid splint on the palm side of the arm from the forearm past the fingertips, tied above and below the wrist. If available, add a roller bandage under the fingers. Leave the fingers uncovered.

3. Support the forearm and wrist with a sling, then apply a binder around the upper arm and chest **(Figure 15-8)**.

4. Follow the general guidelines for safe splinting. Check the fingers periodically for circulation.

FIGURE 15-8

Immobilize an injured wrist with a splint, sling and binder.

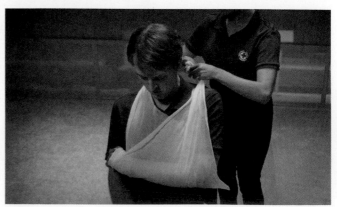

SKILL: SPLINTING THE FOREARM

STEP 1
Support the arm above and below the injury. Check circulation.

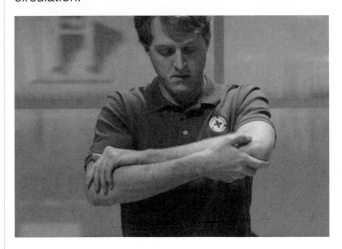

STEP 2
Position the arm on a padded rigid splint. If available, add a roller bandage under the fingers.

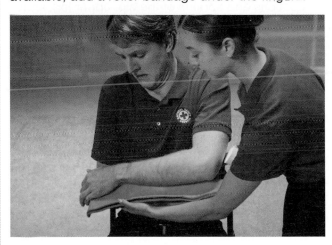

STEP 3
Secure the splint. Check circulation once secured.

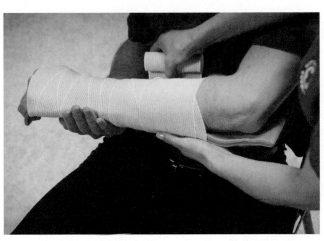

STEP 4
Put the arm in a sling, and tie a binder over the sling and around the chest.

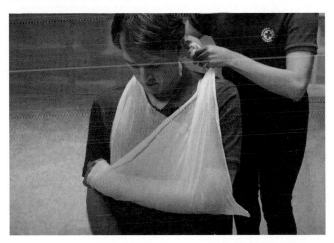

Hand and Finger Injuries

The hand may be injured by a direct blow. Fractures often occur, for example, when the victim punches something with a closed fist. Pain and swelling of the hand typically result.

An injured hand may be immobilized with a soft or rigid splint. First, place a roll of gauze or similar padding in the palm, allowing the fingers to take a naturally curled position. The entire hand is then bandaged, leaving the fingers exposed if possible to check for circulation. Place a rigid splint on the palm side of the hand extending from above the wrist to the fingers, the same as for a wrist injury. Pad the area well between the hand and the splint. Then, support the injury further with a sling and binder.

Finger injuries include fractures and dislocations. Both are common in sports and industrial injuries. Oftentimes, a splint is not required, but victims with a painful injury will benefit from splinting. Use a soft splint if the person cannot straighten the finger without pain. Do not try to manipulate the finger to move a bone into its normal position. Use a rigid splint such as a tongue depressor or ice cream stick secured in place with tape, or make an anatomic splint by taping the finger to an adjoining finger with gauze in between **(Figure 15-9)**.

FIGURE 15-9

Splint a finger injury.

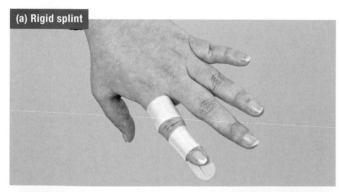

(a) Rigid splint

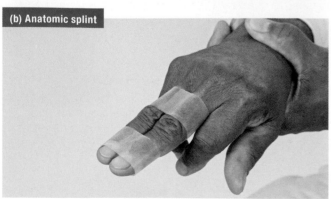

(b) Anatomic splint

Fill in the correct answers for the following statements:

1. For an injured shoulder, use a _____ splint.

2. A splint for a fracture of the forearm should extend from the _____ to the _____ .

3. Why is a binder used over a sling? Select the best answer.

    a. To prevent movement and give additional support

    b. To pull the fractured bone ends back into position

    c. To promote good circulation

    d. All of the above

LOWER EXTREMITY INJURIES

Lower extremity injuries include fractures, dislocations and sprains of the hip, upper leg, knee, lower leg, ankle and foot. Because the bones of the thigh and lower leg are larger than those of the arm, larger forces are typically involved in these injuries. This means that there is a greater risk that a spinal injury may have occurred. Assess the victim carefully, being careful not to move the extremity. A fracture of the femur, the large bone of the thigh, can also damage the large femoral artery and cause life-threatening bleeding. Remember the general principle to splint only if help will be delayed and there is a risk of the injured area moving (or a victim with an injured foot is to be transported).

Hip Injuries

The hip is the joint where the top of the femur meets the pelvis. Hip injuries include fractures, and, less commonly, dislocations. A hip fracture is actually a fracture of the top part of the **femur**. Hip fractures are more common in the elderly, whose bones are often more brittle because **osteoporosis**, a loss of calcium from bones, is common in old age, and because some older people are less stable and more likely to experience a fall. Bleeding and pain may be severe.

Hip dislocations can occur at any age. The victim feels pain and cannot move the joint. Hip dislocations result from falls, vehicular crashes and blows to the body.

First aid is similar to that for a pelvic injury, from which it is often difficult to differentiate a hip injury. Do not move the victim, and immobilize the leg and hip in the position in which you find it. Call 9-1-1 immediately. Immobilize the victim's legs by padding between the legs with a soft pillow or blanket and gently bandaging them together, unless this causes more pain. Treat the victim for shock, but do not elevate the legs.

Upper Leg Injuries

Fractures of the femur are serious because bleeding even with a closed injury can be profuse. The victim experiences severe pain and may be in shock. Swelling and deformity are common.

Call 9-1-1 immediately for a fracture of the femur, and keep the victim from moving. If the victim is lying down with the leg supported by the ground, a rigid splint may be unnecessary. Provide additional support with folded blankets or coats to immobilize the leg in the position found. If help may be delayed, splinting can be used to stabilize the injury. To use an anatomic splint, pad between the legs, move the uninjured leg beside the injured one, and carefully tie the legs together. A rigid splint provides better support if needed:

1. Check for signs of circulation and sensation in the foot and toes.

2. If possible, put a rigid splint on each side of the leg. Pad bony areas and voids between the leg and the splints. The inside splint should extend from the groin past the foot, and the outside from the armpit past the foot.

3. Tie the splints with cravats or bandages **(Figure 15-10).**

4. Follow the general guidelines for safe splinting. Check the toes periodically for circulation.

FIGURE 15-10

Splinting a fractured femur.

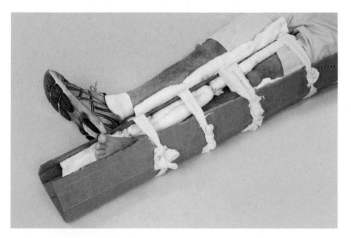

Knee Injuries

The most common knee injuries are sprains, but dislocations also occur. These injuries commonly result from sports injuries, motor vehicle crashes and falls. With large forces, the knee can actually be dislocated, which is a serious emergency because nearby nerves and blood vessels are often injured as well. In addition, fractures of the end of the femur or the tibia or fibula (the bones of the lower leg) can be indistinguishable from other knee injuries. Dislocations of the patella (kneecap) may be mistaken for knee dislocations because they too cause the knee to appear deformed.

Knee injuries cause pain and an inability to move the knee. The knee joint may appear to be "locked." Swelling is usually present with or without bruising. With a dislocation, the knee may be deformed or angulated.

Do not try to transport a victim with a knee injury; instead, call 9-1-1. With any knee injury, the knee should be splinted in the position found. A soft splint can be applied by rolling a blanket or placing a pillow around the knee. If the knee is straight, you can make an anatomical splint by tying the upper and lower leg to the unaffected leg. Rigid splints provide additional support. If the knee is straight, ideally, 2 splints are applied along both sides of the knee. If the knee is bent, splint the joint in the position found.

1. Check for signs of circulation and sensation in the foot and toes.

2. If possible, put a rigid splint on each side of the leg in the position found. Pad bony areas and voids between the leg and the splints.

3. Tie the splints with cravats or bandages.

4. Follow the general guidelines for safe splinting. Check the toes periodically for circulation.

Lower Leg Injuries

Injuries to the lower leg commonly result from sports, motor vehicle crashes and falls. Either or both of the bones of the lower leg can be fractured.

Do not move or transport a victim with a lower leg injury. Call 9-1-1 and immobilize the leg from the knee to the ankle. Either a soft splint or a rigid splint may be used. A rigid splint is applied the same as for a knee injury; a 3-sided cardboard splint can also be used **(Figure 15-11).** Be sure not to tie the splint over the fracture site.

STEP 1

Check circulation. Gently slide 4 or 5 bandages or strips of cloth under both legs. Do not put a bandage over the injury site.

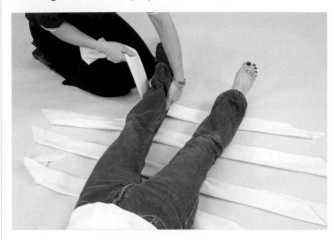

STEP 2

Put padding between the legs. Do not move the injured leg.

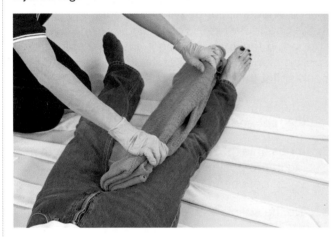

STEP 3

Gently slide the uninjured leg next to the injured leg.

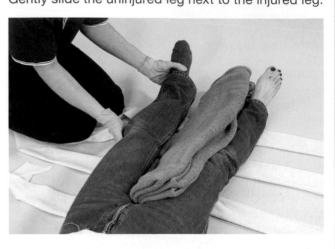

STEP 4

Tie the bandages (snug but not tight), starting in the middle, then at the lower leg and then at the top. Check circulation.

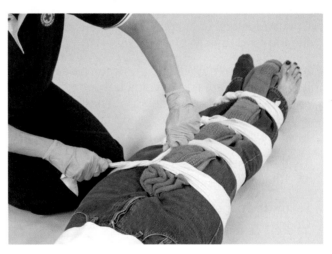

A leg fracture can be splinted using either a rigid splint or an anatomic splint (see Skill: "Anatomic Splinting of Leg"). A similar anatomic splint can be used for an upper leg fracture, with the bandages tied higher (including the hips).

FIGURE 15-11

Rigid splinting of a lower leg fracture using cardboard.

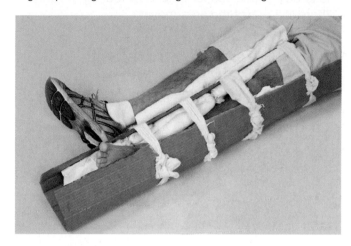

Ankle Injuries

The most common ankle injury is a sprain, which typically occurs when the foot is forcefully twisted to one side. The victim experiences pain and swelling of the ankle. The swelling can be significant, and the victim is unable to put weight on the ankle due to pain. Fracture or dislocation may also occur, often involving torn ligaments and possibly also nerve and blood vessel damage. Usually, a soft splint is best for ankle injuries, along with having the victim avoid the use of the foot and leg:

1. Gently remove the shoe to check for circulation, unless this causes significant pain.

2. Position the foot in the middle of a soft pillow and fold the pillow around the ankle.

3. Using cravats or bandages, tie the pillow around the foot and lower leg **(Figure 15-12).**

4. Check for signs of circulation and sensation in the foot and toes. If they are absent, call 9-1-1 for immediate care.

5. Follow the general guidelines for safe splinting. Check the toes periodically for circulation.

FIGURE 15-12

Soft splint for an ankle injury.

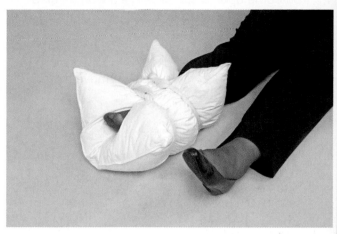

Foot Injuries

Foot injuries most commonly result from direct blows to the foot or from falls. Foot injuries may involve almost any bone or ligament of the foot. Foot injuries should be treated identically to ankle injuries.

Fractures of the toes can be quite painful. The toe often is swollen, tender and discolored. Usually, no splinting is required. If the toe is significantly bent, more than one toe is involved or the foot is very painful, a pillow splint can be used as for an ankle injury.

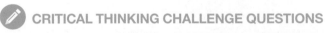

✎ LEARNING CHECKPOINT 3

1. You come upon a scene where a woman on a bicycle apparently ran into a light post. She is lying on the ground and says she has severe pain in her lower leg below the knee. You cannot tell whether the bone is broken, but there is no open wound and she says she cannot move her leg. What should you do?

_____

_____

_____

_____

_____

2. A victim with a fracture of the femur may also experience what other condition? Select the best answer.

   a. Severe bleeding

   b. Open or closed wound

   c. Shock

   d. All of the above

3. Explain when you may use 2 rigid splints.

   _____

   _____

   _____

   _____

   _____

⏱ CONCLUDING THOUGHTS

Although this chapter details how to splint all the different areas of the extremities, it is most important to remember the key principles of splinting for any body area:

- Splint only if help may be delayed (or the victim is to be transported for a hand or foot injury) and there is a risk of the area moving.

- Do not splint if it causes more pain.

- Splint an injury in the position found.

- Splint to immobilize the entire area.

- Check the circulation below the injury and splint.

- Call 9-1-1 or seek medical attention.

✎ CRITICAL THINKING CHALLENGE QUESTIONS

👥 SCENARIO 1

A window washer slips in a soapy water spill and falls to the ground from a second-floor scaffold, landing on his shoulder. He is sitting up, holding his upper arm tight against his body with his good hand, and says his shoulder really hurts and he cannot move it. He will not let you open his shirt to inspect the shoulder, but there does not seem to be any bleeding. What do you do?

_____

_____

_____

_____

_____

_____

SCENARIO 2

At a company picnic at a state park out of town, a child falls from a tree and fractures her forearm. You give appropriate first aid (RICE), and the parents now will take her to the nearest emergency department. Should you splint the arm? If so, describe the steps for doing so.

_____

_____

_____

_____

_____

_____

_____

 REVIEW QUESTIONS

Select the best answers.

1. Which of the following could make an effective rigid splint?
   a. A board
   b. A rolled magazine
   c. A walking stick
   d. All of the above

2. Which statement is true about how splints should be applied?
   a. Tape the splint tightly in place.
   b. For greatest support, tie a cravat directly over the wound.
   c. Straighten the limb as much as possible before splinting.
   d. Dress an open wound before splinting the area.

3. Which is a sign of reduced circulation below an injury?
   a. Cold skin
   b. Hot skin
   c. Red skin
   d. Itching skin

4. Where is a cold pack applied to a splinted open injury?
   a. Outside the dressing but under the bandage and splint
   b. Outside the dressing and bandage but under the splint
   c. Around the splint
   d. Cold packs are not used with splints.

5. How is an injured elbow splinted when you find it in a bent position?
   a. Gently straighten the arm and use a long, rigid splint from shoulder to hand.
   b. Gently bend the elbow to 90 degrees and put it in a sling.
   c. Keep the elbow in its original bent position and use a rigid splint from the upper arm to the hand.
   d. Do not splint the arm, but bind it directly to the chest with bandages.

6. How is an injured hand positioned for splinting?
   a. Let the fingers curl naturally around a soft padding in the palm.
   b. Ask the victim to make a fist before bandaging the hand.
   c. Straighten out the fingers on the surface of a rigid splint.
   d. Keep the fingers spread wide apart with bandaging and padding between them.

7. How can you tell the difference between a hip displacement and a hip fracture?

   a. A fracture is more painful than a displacement.

   b. With a fracture, you can still move the leg, but not with a displacement.

   c. With a displacement, the leg is in an unusual position, but not with a fracture.

   d. You cannot easily tell the difference between a displacement and a fracture.

8. With which of these injuries is it safe for the victim to attempt to walk?

   a. Ankle sprain

   b. Ankle displacement

   c. Ankle fracture

   d. None of the above

CHAPTER 16

Sudden Illness

LESSON OBJECTIVES

- Explain why first aid is needed when someone suddenly becomes ill.

- List the general care steps for any sudden illness.

- Describe the signs and symptoms of, and the first aid for, each of the sudden illnesses described.

Returning to your office after lunch, you find a coworker leaning over her desk looking ill. Her breathing is labored and noisy. You ask her what is wrong, and she says she doesn't know but she feels like she can't breathe. She pauses, gasping between words. Her skin is pale. What do you do?

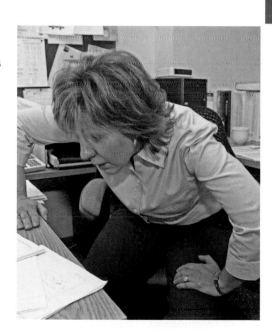

Most chapters in this text involve first aid for injuries. Illness, too can cause an emergency, especially if the person becomes ill suddenly. With most illnesses, a person has time to see a health care provider long before the illness becomes an emergency, but with the specific health problems described in this chapter, the emergency may develop very quickly. Lifesaving action by first aiders and others at the scene is often needed. Because some sudden illnesses, such as a heart attack, may occur with little or no warning and can result in death within minutes if no action is taken, it is important to be aware of the common signs and symptoms and to be prepared to act any time in any place.

General Care for Sudden Illness

Many different illnesses can occur suddenly and become medical emergencies. In some cases you may know or suspect the cause of the problem, such as when a heart attack victim clutches his or her chest and complains of a crushing pressure before collapsing. In other cases, neither you nor the victim may know the cause of the problem. The general first aid principles are the same for all sudden illness emergencies, however, so you do not have to know what the victim's illness is before you give first aid.

Following are common general signs and symptoms of sudden illness:

- Person feels ill, dizzy, confused or weak

- Skin color changes (flushed, pale or ashen), sweating

- Breathing changes

- Nausea or vomiting

Following are the general steps to follow for any sudden illness:

1. Call 9-1-1 for unexplained sudden illness.

2. Help the victim rest and avoid becoming chilled or overheated.

3. Reassure the victim.

4. Do not give the victim anything to eat or drink.

5. Watch for changes, and be prepared to give basic life support (BLS) if needed.

In some cases of sudden illness, the most difficult decision is whether to call 9-1-1. How can you tell if the illness is an emergency? Two key factors can help you decide. First, if the illness is *sudden,* it is more

likely to be an emergency. Many common illnesses come on gradually. For example, with the flu, a person gradually develops a headache or achy joints, fever may begin mildly and slowly rise, respiratory symptoms gradually increase and so on. The illness seldom becomes an emergency before the person seeks health care. Problems that come on suddenly and unexpectedly often become emergencies, however, such as a sudden heart attack or asthma attack.

Second, is the illness *unexplained?* A person suddenly has an excruciating, pounding headache, but this person has never had bad headaches before and nothing special has happened that day that might cause a headache. This headache is likely to be a symptom of a developing emergency. In contrast, a child who develops a "tummy ache" after gobbling down a whole carton of ice cream is unlikely to be having an emergency – unlike some victims with sudden, unexplained severe abdominal pain.

In rare instances, if you cannot decide whether someone's sudden illness might be an emergency, call 9-1-1. Tell the dispatcher exactly what you know and have observed, and let the dispatcher help decide the best course of action.

In addition to these general care principles, when you can identify the specific illness, give first aid as described in the following sections.

Heart Attack

Heart attack, or **acute myocardial infarction (AMI),** involves a sudden reduced blood flow to the heart muscle. It is a medical emergency and often leads to cardiac arrest. Heart attack can occur at any age **(Box 16-1).** Heart attack is caused by reduced blood flow or blockage in the coronary arteries, which supply the heart muscle with blood, usually as a result of atherosclerosis (see **Chapter 5**).

PREVENTION OF HEART ATTACK

Heart attack, angina and stroke are all cardiovascular diseases. **Chapter 5** describes how one can minimize the risk factors for cardiovascular disease by not smoking, eating a healthy diet low in cholesterol and salt, controlling blood pressure, maintaining a normal weight, getting exercise and controlling stress.

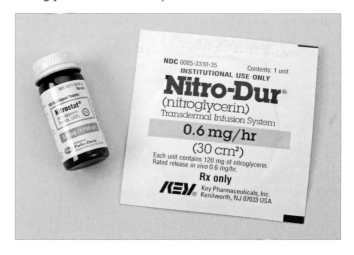

BOX 16-1: FACTS ABOUT HEART ATTACK

- More than 735,000 heart attacks occur a year in the United States, resulting in more than 120,000 deaths.[1] Many of them could have been saved by prompt first aid and medical treatment.

- Heart attack is more likely in those with a family history of heart attack.

- One-fifth of heart attack victims do not have chest pain, but they often have other symptoms. Symptoms may also be somewhat different in women and men.

- Heart attack victims typically deny that they are having a heart attack. Do not let them talk you out of getting help!

[1]*American Heart Association, my.americanheart.org/idc/ groups/ahamah-public/@wcm/@sop/@smd/documents/ downloadable/ucm_470704.pdf Accessed January 2016.*

FIRST AID FOR HEART ATTACK

The signs and symptoms of heart attack vary considerably, from vague chest discomfort (which the victim may confuse with heartburn) to crushing pain, with or without other symptoms. The victim may have no signs and symptoms at all before collapsing suddenly. Sometimes the victim has milder symptoms that come and go for 2 or 3 days before the heart attack occurs. It is important to consider the possibility of heart attack when a wide range of symptoms occurs rather than expecting only a clearly defined situation. Note that some heart attack symptoms are more common in women. Chest pain or discomfort is still the most common symptom, but women are somewhat more likely to have shortness of breath, jaw or back pain, indigestion, nausea and vomiting.

It is important to act quickly when the victim may be having a heart attack, because deaths from heart attack usually occur within an hour or two after symptoms begin. Health care professionals can administer medications to reduce the effects of heart attack and save the victim's life – but only if EMS is involved quickly.

First aid for a heart attack begins with calling 9-1-1 to get help on the way immediately. Then help the victim to rest in the most comfortable position. A sitting position is often easiest for breathing. Loosen any constricting clothing. Try to calm the victim and

reassure him or her that help is on the way. Because heart attack frequently leads to cardiac arrest, be prepared to give BLS if needed (see First Aid: "Heart Attack").

The value of aspirin as a clot-preventing medication is now well-known, and many health care providers advise their patients who are at risk for cardiovascular disease to take 1 low-dose aspirin daily unless they are allergic or experience side effects, such as gastrointestinal bleeding. For victims who do not need to avoid aspirin, chewing 1 adult aspirin or 2-4 low-dose baby aspirin is now recommended when they experience heart attack symptoms. First aiders should never on their own give aspirin or any medication to a victim, but they can encourage the victim to chew an aspirin.

Nitroglycerin is another medication of benefit to a heart attack victim who has been prescribed this drug. Nitroglycerin increases blood flow through partially restricted arteries by dilating them. Nitroglycerin is generally prescribed for angina, a condition of pain in the chest caused by narrowed coronary arteries. If the victim has nitroglycerin, you can help the person use it. Nitroglycerin comes in small tablets that are dissolved under the tongue, tablets that dissolve in the cheek, extended-release capsules, oral sprays and extended-release patches that are applied to the chest, usually daily **(Figure 16-1).** Follow the victim's instructions to help with the drug. The victim should be seated because dizziness or fainting may occur. Do not try to give the drug to the victim yourself if the victim is unresponsive.

FIGURE 16-1

Nitroglycerin tablets and patch.

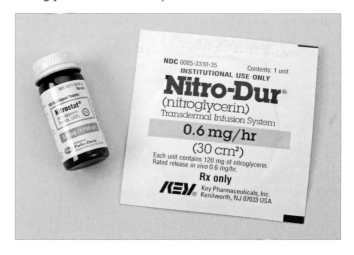

First Aid: Heart Attack

Signs, Symptoms and Care

WHEN YOU SEE

- Complaints of persistent discomfort, pressure, tightness, ache or pain in the chest

- Complaints of pain spreading to neck, shoulders or arms

- Complaints of shortness of breath

- Complaints of dizziness, lightheadedness, feeling of impending doom

- Pale skin or sweating

- In women especially, symptoms include shortness of breath, indigestion, nausea or vomiting and back or jaw pain

- Note that victims having a heart attack may not have all of these signs and symptoms

DO THIS FIRST

1. Call 9-1-1 immediately for any victim experiencing chest discomfort, even if the victim says it is not serious.

2. Help the victim to rest in a comfortable position (often sitting). Loosen any tight clothing. Keep the victim from moving.

3. Ask the victim if he or she is taking heart medication, and help obtain the medication for the victim. Follow the directions on the medication.

4. Encourage the victim to chew and swallow 1 adult (325 mg) or 2-4 low-dose (81 mg each) baby aspirin unless he or she is allergic to aspirin or cannot take aspirin for any other reason.

5. Stay with the victim, and be reassuring and calming.

6. Be prepared to give CPR if the victim becomes unresponsive and normal breathing stops.

ADDITIONAL CARE

- Do not let the victim eat or drink anything.

Angina

Angina pectoris, usually just called angina, is chest pain caused by heart disease that usually happens after intense activity or exertion. Other factors may trigger the pain of angina, such as stress or exposure to extreme heat or cold. The pain is a sign that the heart muscle is not getting as much oxygen as needed, usually because of narrowed or constricted coronary arteries. The pain usually goes away after a few minutes of rest. The pain may also radiate to the jaw, neck or left arm or shoulder. People usually know when they have angina and may carry medication for it, usually nitroglycerin.

Ask if the person has been diagnosed with angina; if so, ask if the pain is like angina pain experienced in the past. If so, help the person take his or her own medication and rest. If the pain persists more than 10 minutes or stops and then returns, or if the victim has other heart attack symptoms not relieved by rest, give first aid for a heart attack.

Stroke

A **stroke,** also called a cerebrovascular accident (CVA) or a brain attack, is an interruption of blood flow to a part of the brain, which kills nerve cells and affects the victim's functioning. Stroke, like heart attack, may be caused by atherosclerosis. A blood clot may form in a brain artery or may be carried there in the blood and lodge in the artery, obstructing flow to that part of the brain. Stroke may also result when an artery in the brain ruptures or other factors impede flow. As noted in **Chapter 5,** about 795,000 people a year have a stroke, resulting in about 130,000 deaths.[1] Strokes are more common in older adults.

[1]*Centers for Disease Control and Prevention. cdc.gov/dhdsp/ data_statistics/fact_sheets/fs_stroke.htm Accessed January 2016.*

Because a stroke victim needs medical help immediately to decrease the chance of permanent damage, it is important to be able to identify the signs and symptoms of stroke. Stroke generally causes a sudden weakness or numbness in the face, arm or leg, especially on one side of the body; drooling; facial droop; slurred speech; and gait problems. Some stroke victims may have a sudden, severe headache, vomiting and loss of consciousness. The exact signs and symptoms vary somewhat, depending on the exact site in the brain where an artery is blocked. First aiders who are not thinking about the possibility of a stroke might attribute the victim's signs and symptoms to some other condition. Because it is so important that medical care begin as soon as possible, screening assessments have been devised to accurately identify strokes **(Box 16-2).**

The most important thing to do for a stroke victim is to call 9-1-1 immediately to access advanced medical care. Drugs can often minimize the effects of a stroke – but only if administered very soon after the stroke. Tell the dispatcher you believe the victim has had a stroke and describe his or her signs and symptoms. Take note of the time that symptoms began, because medical treatment depends, in part, on how much time has passed. With the victim, be calming and reassuring, because often a stroke victim does not understand what has happened and is confused or fearful. Have the victim lay down on their back with head and shoulders slightly raised; this is often called the "stroke position." Monitor the victim and be prepared for vomiting and to give BLS if needed. Move an unresponsive victim into the recovery position, with the affected side down to better maintain the airway (see First Aid: "Stroke").

A first aider who identifies these signs of stroke in a victim and relays that information to EMS speeds the process of quickly getting the most appropriate care to the victim. The chance of survival and recovery is greatest if the victim receives medical treatment as soon as possible after last being seen feeling and acting normally. Call 9-1-1 immediately. The arriving EMS crew can quickly begin medical care at the scene and plan to transport the victim to the best setting for immediate care. Calling ahead helps ensure that resources are mobilized to provide advanced care on arrival.

When gathering SAMPLE history information from a potential stroke victim, as explained in **Chapter 4,** try to learn the time when the signs and symptoms first occurred. Ask family members or others present at the scene as well as the victim. This information is important for the EMS treatment of the victim.

BOX 16-2: THE FAST STROKE ASSESSMENT

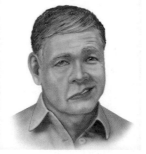

Among EMS professionals, the need to accurately identify a potential stroke victim is well recognized. The more quickly stroke is recognized, the more quickly the victim can be given appropriate prehospital care and rushed to a stroke center or other appropriate treatment center. Several screening processes have proved accurate in the rapid identification of stroke, and most professional rescuers now use a screening process, such as the Cincinnati Prehospital Stroke Scale (CPSS) or the FAST stroke assessment. The screening process can also be used effectively by lay first aiders.

FAST is an acronym standing for Face, Arm, Speech and Time:

F	**Face drooping** – Is one side of the victim's face drooping or is it numb? If you ask the person to smile, is his or her smile uneven?
A	**Arm weakness** – Is one of the victim's arms weak or numb? If you ask him or her to raise both arms, does one drift downward?
S	**Speech difficulty** – Is the victim's speech slurred or is he or she having difficulty speaking or understanding? If you ask the victim to repeat a simple sentence, can he or she do it correctly?
T	**Time to call 9-1-1** – If the victim shows any of these symptoms, call 9-1-1 immediately and note the time when the symptoms first began.

First Aid: Stroke

Signs, Symptoms and Care

WHEN YOU SEE

Most common signs and symptoms:

- Sudden weakness or numbness of face, arm or leg, especially on one side of the body

- Drooling, facial droop or slurred speech

- Gait problems

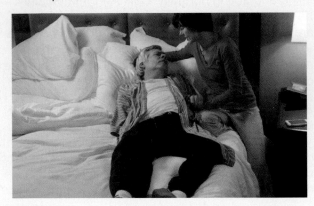

Some stroke victims may have:

- Sudden, severe headache

- Vomiting

- Loss of consciousness

DO THIS FIRST

1. Call 9-1-1.

2. Monitor the victim's breathing and be prepared to give BLS if needed.

3. Have the victim lay on his or her back with head and shoulders slightly raised.

4. Loosen constrictive clothing.

5. If necessary, turn the victim's head to the side to allow drool or vomit to drain.

ADDITIONAL CARE

- Keep the victim warm and quiet until help arrives.

- Put a breathing, unresponsive victim in the recovery position with the affected side down.

ALERT

- Do not let a stroke victim eat or drink anything.

TRANSIENT ISCHEMIC ATTACK

A **transient ischemic attack (TIA),** sometimes called a mini stroke, is a temporary interruption to blood flow in an artery in the brain. A TIA produces signs and symptoms similar to those of a stroke, except they usually disappear within a few minutes. Since a person who experiences a TIA is at high risk for a stroke, you should always call 9-1-1 for a victim who exhibits the signs and symptoms of stroke, even if they seem milder or soon disappear.

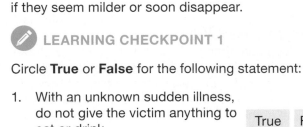 LEARNING CHECKPOINT 1

Circle **True** or **False** for the following statement:

1. With an unknown sudden illness, do not give the victim anything to eat or drink.　　True　False

2. Check off the common signs and symptoms of heart attack:

   ☐ Skin red and flushed

   ☐ Indigestion

   ☐ Tingling in fingers and toes

   ☐ Headache

   ☐ Shortness of breath

   ☐ Pale skin

   ☐ Chest pain or pressure

   ☐ Unusual cheerfulness

   ☐ Sweating

   ☐ Dizziness

3. How do you decide if a victim's chest pain may be a heart attack or angina?

   _____

   _____

4. The immediate first action to take for a heart attack victim is _____ .

5. Select the best answer. It may be important to position a stroke victim such that –

   a. fluids drain from the mouth.

   b. the victim's head is protected from injury during convulsions.

   c. the victim can sit up even if partially paralyzed.

   d. the victim's head is lower than rest of the body.

Respiratory Distress

Respiratory distress, or difficulty breathing, can be caused by many different illnesses and injuries.

PREVENTION OF RESPIRATORY DISTRESS

People with asthma have generally learned what factors may trigger an asthma attack so that they can try to avoid them when possible, and many carry medication with them that can stop an attack when one occurs. People with other chronic respiratory problems, such as chronic obstructive pulmonary disease (COPD), should also learn to avoid situations in which respiratory difficulty may occur and should learn what actions to take if a problem does occur.

CARING FOR RESPIRATORY DISTRESS

A victim in respiratory distress may be gasping for air, panting, breathing faster or slower than normal or making wheezing or other sounds with breathing. Typically, the victim cannot speak a full sentence without pausing to breathe. The victim's skin may look pale or ashen and may be cool and moist; the lips and nail beds may be bluish. Lowered oxygen levels in the blood may make the victim feel dizzy or disoriented **(Figure 16-2).** The victim may be sitting and leaning forward, hands on knees, in what is called the tripod position **(Figure 16-3).**

Because respiratory distress in an infant or child may rapidly progress to respiratory arrest, it is crucial to act quickly when an infant or child is having a problem breathing. In addition to the signs and symptoms just described, with an infant or child you may observe flaring of the nostrils and exaggerated movements of the chest muscles with efforts to breathe.

FIGURE 16-2

Signs and symptoms of distress.

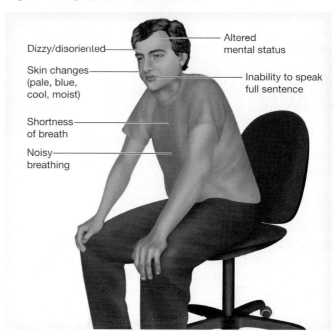

Dizzy/disoriented

Altered mental status

Skin changes (pale, blue, cool, moist)

Inability to speak full sentence

Shortness of breath

Noisy breathing

FIGURE 16-3

The tripod position, commonly assumed by victims in respiratory distress.

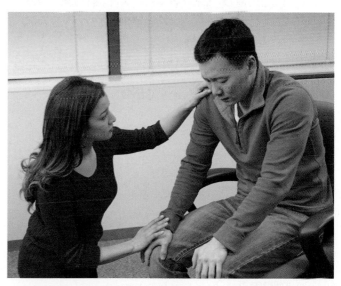

If the cause of a victim's breathing problem is not obvious, look for other signs and symptoms that may reveal the problem. Respiratory distress can be a sign of many of the injuries described in other chapters throughout this text. If you can determine the cause of a victim's breathing difficulty, give first aid for that problem. For example, a victim of a heart attack may have shortness of breath; while it is important to care for this breathing difficulty, it is most crucial to call 9-1-1 immediately for the heart attack and give the first aid described earlier.

Respiratory distress may also result from sudden illness. Asthma and chronic obstructive pulmonary disease (COPD) are two common diseases that may cause episodes of breathing difficulty. These are described in more detail in the following sections along with specific first aid steps.

In some cases, you will not be able to identify the cause of a victim's respiratory distress. In this situation, give the general breathing care described in First Aid: "Respiratory Distress." Call 9-1-1 for a victim of respiratory distress because this condition may progress to respiratory arrest, which is a life-threatening condition.

ASTHMA

Asthma is an increasingly common problem, with about 25 million Americans now having asthma, affecting 1 in 12 adults and 1 in 10 school-age children. Asthma attacks in the United States result in more than 200,000 emergency department visits a year and more than 3,400 deaths.[1] The prevalence of asthma has been increasing gradually in the United States for more than two decades. Asthma is a chronic disease – it cannot be cured, although attacks often become less common as a child becomes older and moves through adulthood. In an asthma attack, the airway becomes narrow, and the person has difficulty breathing. Many asthma victims know they have the condition and carry medication, typically an inhaler, for emergency situations. They also may have learned what situations and factors can trigger an asthma attack and thus they try to avoid these **(Box 16-3)**. When left untreated, a severe asthma attack can be fatal. If a young child who is away from usual caretakers has trouble breathing, always ask if he or she has medication (see First Aid: "Asthma").

[1]*American Academy of Allergy, Asthma & Immunology. aaaai.org/about-the-aaaai/newsroom/asthma-statistics.aspx Accessed January 2016.*

When an asthma attack occurs and the victim has an inhaler, you may assist the victim in using the inhaler under these conditions:

- The victim confirms that an asthma attack is occurring.

- The victim identifies the inhaler as his or her prescribed asthma medication.

- The victim cannot self-administer the medication.

First Aid: Respiratory Distress

Signs, Symptoms and Care

WHEN YOU SEE

- Victim is gasping or unable to catch his or her breath.

- Speaking in shortened sentences

- Breathing is faster or slower, or deeper or shallower than normal.

- Breathing involves sounds such as wheezing or gurgling.

- Victim feels dizzy or lightheaded.

- Pale or ashen skin

DO THIS FIRST

1. Call 9-1-1 for sudden, unexplained breathing problems.

2. Help the victim to rest in the position of easiest breathing (often sitting up).

3. If the victim is hyperventilating, ask him or her to breathe slowly.

4. Ask the victim about any prescribed medicine he or she may have, and help the victim to take it if needed.

5. Stay with the victim and be prepared to give CPR if breathing stops.

ADDITIONAL CARE

- Calm and reassure the victim (anxiety increases breathing distress).

BOX 16-3: ASTHMA TRIGGERS

Asthma attacks are usually triggered by some factor in the person's internal or external environment. Understanding these factors helps prevent or minimize attacks. Common triggers include:

- Respiratory infection, including the common cold (the most common cause of asthma attacks in children under age 5)

- Allergic reaction to pollen, mold, dust mites, animal fur or dander

- Exercise (especially in cold, dry air)

- Certain foods (nuts, eggs, milk)

- Emotional stress

- Medications

- Air pollution caused by things, such as cigarette smoke, vehicle exhaust or fumes from cleaning products

- Temperature extremes

Knowing the specific triggers that provoke asthma can help prevent attacks. A person with asthma may have had a skin test to detect specific allergens that trigger his or her asthma. In addition to avoiding the factors just listed, follow these guidelines:

- Use a damp cloth to dust furniture and surfaces.

- Vacuum rugs frequently and when the person with asthma is not present.

- Avoid fluffy blankets and pillows that collect dust and that contain feathers.

- Enclose mattresses and pillows in plastic covers.

- Do not use air fresheners or products with strong odors.

- Use an air purifier, and stay indoors when pollen counts are high.

Helping with an Asthma Inhaler

Parents and child care providers may need to help a small child with asthma use an inhaler during an asthma attack. An inhaler is a device that contains and delivers the asthma medication in automatically measured doses **(Figure 16-4).** The medication is usually a **bronchodilator,** a drug that relaxes the muscles of the airway, allowing airway passages to open wider (dilate) to make breathing easier. Always follow the health care provider's specific instructions for the inhaler. Use only the child's own prescribed inhaler. Never use an inhaler belonging to another child.

FIGURE 16-4

Many people with asthma use an inhaler.

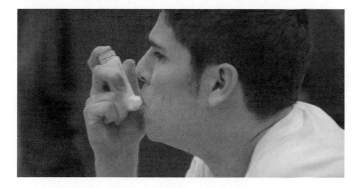

Following are general instructions that may need modification for the specific medication device or for a particular child.

1. Remove the cap, and shake the inhaler several times.

2. If a spacer is used, position it on the inhaler. (A spacer is a tube or chamber that fits between the inhaler and the child's mouth.)

3. Have the child breathe out fully through the mouth.

4. With the child's lips around the inhaler mouthpiece or the spacer, have the child inhale slowly and deeply; press the metal canister down to release one spray of medication as the child inhales. (A face mask is generally used for an infant instead of a mouthpiece.)

5. Have the child hold his or her breath for up to 10 seconds if possible, and then exhale slowly. Follow the directions for the inhaler, or follow the child's treatment plan to repeat doses, if needed.

First Aid: Asthma

Signs, Symptoms and Care

WHEN YOU SEE

- Wheezing and difficulty breathing and speaking

- Dry, persistent cough

- Fear and anxiety

- Gray-blue or ashen skin

- Changing levels of responsiveness

DO THIS FIRST

1. If the victim does not know he or she has asthma (first attack), call 9-1-1 immediately.

2. If the victim identifies the breathing difficulty as an asthma attack and has prescribed medication (usually an inhaler), help them use the prescribed inhaler as directed by his or her health care provider.

   - Remove the cap.

   - Shake the inhaler several times.

   - Connect the spacer (if needed).

   - The victim places the inhaler or spacer end in mouth.

   - The victim presses the metal canister down while slowly inhaling.

   - Remind the victim to hold his or her breath with the medication for about 10 seconds.

3. Help the victim rest in a position for easiest breathing (usually sitting up).

ADDITIONAL CARE

- If needed, the victim may use the inhaler again as prescribed or directed by a medical provider.

- If the breathing difficulty persists after using the inhaler, call 9-1-1.

- Never unnecessarily separate a child from a parent or loved one when providing care.

CHRONIC OBSTRUCTIVE PULMONARY DISEASE

Chronic obstructive pulmonary disease (COPD) includes emphysema, chronic bronchitis and other conditions. More than 12 million people in the United States have been diagnosed with COPD, with an estimated 12 million more who may have COPD but have not been diagnosed. It causes more than 120,000 deaths a year in the United States.[1] These diseases can cause respiratory distress and breathing emergencies.

[1]*National Heart, Lung and Blood Institute nhlbi.nih.gov/health/educational/copd/what-is-copd/index.htm Accessed January 2016.*

Emphysema is a disease that affects the alveoli of the lungs, the tiny sacs where oxygen enters the blood. The alveoli lose elasticity and decrease in number, which reduces oxygen absorption. Chronic bronchitis affects the bronchial tubes in the lungs, causing inflammation and a buildup of mucus. Both diseases are mainly caused by smoking, air pollution and other factors. Both often become worse over time. People with these diseases often get colds and respiratory infections, and they are likely to become short of breath even with mild exertion, such as walking. In advanced cases, the person may need a home oxygen system.

Victims with breathing difficulty related to COPD generally have the same signs and symptoms as described earlier for respiratory distress, and the first aid care is the same. Ask the victim whether he or she has a chronic disease, and give this information to the dispatcher when you call 9-1-1. If the victim has a prescribed medication to help with breathing, you may help the person to take the medication.

HYPERVENTILATION

Hyperventilation is fast, deep breathing usually caused by anxiety or stress, although it may also be caused by some injuries or illnesses. The rapid breathing causes an imbalance in the body's levels of oxygen and carbon dioxide, which may add to the person's anxiety and cause confusion or dizziness. Numbness or tingling of the fingers, toes and lips may occur.

Hyperventilation caused by emotional stress usually does not last long or become an emergency. Help the person to calm down and relax and breathe more slowly. Do not have the person breathe into and out of a bag, which could lower the person's oxygen level too far. Breathing slowly, along with the victim, often helps the victim slow his or her breathing rate.

Because rapid breathing may also be caused by injury or sudden illness, do not assume that the victim is simply hyperventilating. Look for other signs of injury or illness, and ask the victim how the problem started. If there are other signs or symptoms that suggest injury or illness, or if the victim's breathing does not return to normal in a few minutes, call 9-1-1 (see First Aid: "Hyperventilation").

First Aid: Hyperventilation

Signs, Symptoms and Care

WHEN YOU SEE

- Very fast breathing rate
- Dizziness or faintness
- Tingling or numbness in hands, feet and lips
- Muscle twitching or cramping

DO THIS FIRST

1. Make sure there is no other cause for the breathing difficulty that requires care.
2. Reassure the victim and ask him or her to try to breathe slowly.
3. Call 9-1-1 if the victim's breathing does not return to normal within a few minutes.

ADDITIONAL CARE

- A victim who has this problem frequently should seek medical care, because some medical conditions can cause rapid breathing.

ALERT

- Do not ask the victim to breathe into a bag or other container. A victim who repeatedly rebreathes his or her exhaled air will not get enough oxygen.

 LEARNING CHECKPOINT 2

Circle **True** or **False** for the following statement:

1. You cannot give first aid for a person with difficulty breathing unless you know the specific cause of the problem. True   False

2. Select the best answer. To help someone to breathe more easily –

   a. position the victim flat on his or her back.

   b. have the victim stand, and clap him or her on the back with each breath.

   c. have the victim sit and put his or her head between the knees.

   d. let the victim find the position in which he or she can breathe most easily.

3. What is the best thing a victim with asthma can do when having an asthma attack?

   _____

Circle **True** or **False** for the following statement:

4. Have a hyperventilation victim breathe into a bag to start breathing normally again. True   False

5. When should you call 9-1-1 for a victim who seems to be hyperventilating?

   _____

Fainting

Fainting is caused by a temporarily reduced blood flow to the brain. This commonly occurs in hot weather, after a prolonged period of inactivity or from other causes such as fright, emotional shock or lack of food. A temporary drop in blood pressure caused by suddenly standing after prolonged sitting or lying down may cause dizziness or fainting, especially in the elderly. In a young, healthy, non-pregnant adult, fainting is usually not a sign of a more serious problem, unless the person faints often or does not recover quickly. In someone who has heart disease, is pregnant or is older than 65, fainting may be a sign of a serious problem requiring immediate medical attention.

Injury may result if the fainting person falls – try to catch the person and gently lower him or her to the floor. Sometimes a person has signs or symptoms before fainting, including dizziness, sweating, nausea, blurring or dimming of vision and generalized weakness. If fainting is anticipated, have the person sit or lay down (see First Aid: "Fainting").

First Aid: Fainting

Signs, Symptoms and Care

WHEN YOU SEE

- Sudden, brief loss of responsiveness and collapse

- Pale, cool skin; sweating

DO THIS FIRST

1. Monitor the victim's breathing and be ready to give CPR, if needed.

2. Lay the victim down, and raise the legs 6-12 inches. Loosen constricting clothing.

3. Check for possible injuries caused by falling.

4. Reassure the victim as he or she recovers.

ADDITIONAL CARE

- Call 9-1-1 if the victim does not regain responsiveness soon or faints repeatedly. Always call 9-1-1 for all older adults, people with heart disease and pregnant women.

- Place a victim who is breathing normally but remains unresponsive in the recovery position.

ALERT

- Do not pour or splash water on the victim's face; it could be aspirated into the lungs.

Seizures

Seizures, or convulsions, result from a brain disturbance caused by many different conditions, including epilepsy, high fever in infants and young children, head injuries, low blood sugar in a person with diabetes, poisoning or electric shock. The brain's normal electrical activity becomes out of balance, resulting in a sudden altered mental status and uncontrolled muscular contractions that cause jerking or shaking of the body. Most seizures are caused by epilepsy **(Box 16-4)**.

BOX 16-4: FACTS ABOUT EPILEPSY

Epilepsy and seizures affect an estimated 2.2 million people of all ages in the United States.

- Approximately 150,000 new cases of seizures and epilepsy occur each year.

- One in 26 people will develop epilepsy in their lifetime.

- Males are slightly more likely to develop epilepsy than females.

- The incidence is greater in African-American and socially disadvantaged populations.

- In 70% of new cases, no cause is apparent.

- One-third of people with epilepsy live with uncontrollable seizures.

Source: Epilepsy Foundation. epilepsy.com/learn/ epilepsy-statistics Accessed January 2016.

PREVENTION OF SEIZURES

First-time seizures can seldom be prevented, but someone with a diagnosed seizure disorder usually has prescribed medication that will usually prevent most seizures. Sometimes specific factors may increase the risk of a seizure occurring (such as inadequate sleep or flashing lights), and the individual can learn to control these factors. Seizures caused by head injuries can be avoided by preventing injuries (see **Chapter 12**), such as by wearing an appropriate helmet during sports and other activities.

FIRST AID FOR SEIZURES

Seizures generally occur suddenly and without warning. Some victims have an unusual feeling in advance of the seizure called an **aura.** An aura may be a generalized sensation or a hallucinatory sensation involving any of the senses.

Seizures follow a wide variety of patterns, depending in part on the cause. Several different patterns occur in people with epilepsy; some may have only one type of seizure, while others experience different types at different times. Following are some of the more common types of seizures:

- **Complex partial seizures.** These occur in some people with epilepsy. The person is conscious but does not interact normally with others and is not in control of movements or speech. These seizures are called "partial" because only part of the brain is involved. The person seems dazed and may mumble or wander. This type of seizure is often mistaken for a behavioral problem.

- **Absence seizures.** These occur in some people with epilepsy. The person seems to stare blankly into space and does not respond to others; the seizure begins and ends abruptly, often lasting only a few seconds.

- **Generalized tonic-clonic seizures.** These can occur in some people with epilepsy. Other common causes include brain injury, drug overdose and poisoning. This type is also called convulsions or grand mal seizures. The person loses consciousness and falls; the person is at first stiff (tonic), then experiences jerking of muscles (clonic) throughout the body. Breathing may stop momentarily but restarts spontaneously. After the seizure, the person may be confused or agitated.

- **Febrile seizures.** These seizures are not related to epilepsy. Febrile seizures are caused by high fever (usually higher than 102°F) in infants or young children. The convulsions are similar to those of tonic-clonic seizures, and the first aid is the same, followed by measures to bring down the victim's body temperature.

The first aid for all kinds of seizures is primarily directed toward protecting the person until the seizure ends, almost always within seconds or minutes. If the person seems conscious, stay with him or her until it passes. Someone having a complex partial seizure may wander about; if the person is moving into a hazardous situation, gently guide the person away from danger. Look for a medical identification bracelet or necklace if you are unsure why the person is suddenly acting odd. Reassure the person as the seizure ends. If the person seems agitated or angry, stay back but close enough to protect the person from danger. Never try to restrain a person who is having any kind of a seizure.

Do not put anything in the person's mouth because objects may damage teeth or other tissues during the seizure or break and obstruct the airway. Protect the head from injury with a folded jacket or soft padding. Keep track of how long the seizure lasts because 9-1-1 should be called for any seizure lasting longer than 5 minutes. There is nothing you can do to stop or shorten the seizure, but try to keep the person as comfortable as possible during the seizure. Keep bystanders away. Afterward the person is likely to be confused, disoriented, drowsy or agitated; be reassuring and help the person to rest as needed (see First Aid: "Seizures"). Help preserve the victim's privacy and dignity. If incontinence occurs, cover the victim with a blanket or coat. Commonly, the victim is unresponsive for a time after a seizure; place the victim in the recovery position and monitor breathing.

First Aid: Seizures

Signs, Symptoms and Care

WHEN YOU SEE

- Minor seizures: staring blankly ahead; slight twitching of lips, head, or arms and legs; other movements, such as lip smacking or chewing

- Major seizures: crying out and then becoming unresponsive; body becomes rigid and then shakes in convulsions; jaw may clench

- Fever convulsions in young children: hot, flushed skin; violent muscle twitching; arched back; clenched fists

DO THIS FIRST

1. Prevent injury during the seizure by moving dangerous objects and putting soft padding, such as a jacket, under the person's head. Remove eyeglasses.

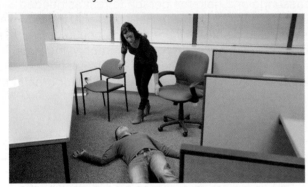

2. Loosen tight clothing around the neck to ease breathing. Check for a medical identification bracelet or necklace.

3. If vomiting occurs, gently turn the person's head to one side to help keep the airway clear.

4. After the seizure, ensure the victim's airway remains open by using the recovery position or head tilt–chin lift, if needed.

5. Be reassuring as the person regains responsiveness.

ADDITIONAL CARE

- Check for a medical identification.

- Call 9-1-1 if the seizure lasts more than 5 minutes, if the person is not known to have epilepsy, if the person recovers very slowly or has trouble breathing or has another seizure, if the person is pregnant or is wearing a medical ID for a condition other than epilepsy or if the person is injured.

- Place an unresponsive victim in the recovery position and monitor breathing.

- For an infant or child with fever convulsions, sponge the body with lukewarm water to help cool the victim, and call 9-1-1.

ALERT

- Do not try to stop the person's movements or restrain the person.

- Do not place any objects in the person's mouth.

SEIZURES IN SPECIAL CIRCUMSTANCES

A person who has a seizure while in the water is at risk of aspirating water into the lungs or even drowning. Because a seizure lasts only a few minutes at most, do not try to move the person from the water. Instead, support him or her with the head tilted to keep water out of the mouth. After the seizure, help the person out of the water. If the person is not responsive, check for breathing, and give CPR if needed.

Another special circumstance is a seizure that occurs in an airplane, motor vehicle or other confined area. If there are empty seats around the person, fold back the armrests so the person can lie on his or her side across the seats with his or her head on a cushion. If there is no room to lay down, use padding or pillows to protect the person's head from striking hard objects around the seat. Try to lean the person to one side to keep the airway open.

Altered Mental Status

Altered mental status is a phrase used to refer to a change from a person's normal responsiveness and awareness. The person may be confused, disoriented, combative, drowsy or partially or wholly unresponsive. Altered mental status is not a condition itself but is a sign or symptom that may result from many different injuries and illnesses. Following are just a few of the many causes of altered mental status:

- Seizures

- Stroke

- Head injury

- Poisoning, drug use or overdose

- High fever

- Diabetic emergencies

- Any condition causing lowered blood oxygen levels

When you encounter someone with altered mental status, determine the nature of the problem, if possible. If the victim is responsive, perform a physical examination and gather a SAMPLE history. Then give first aid for any problems found.

If the person's altered mental status is due to drug or alcohol use, and the person is acting erratically or in a potentially violent manner, the situation may involve a behavioral emergency. In such cases, it is important to ensure your own safety and that of other bystanders. **Chapter 21** describes how to manage behavioral emergencies. Never assume, however, that a person with altered mental status is intoxicated or is using drugs or that someone acting strangely has a mental illness. Certain injuries and sudden illnesses, such as a diabetic emergency, can produce behavior that is easily mistaken for intoxication. Even if the person is intoxicated, he or she may still have an injury or illness that could become an emergency if not cared for.

Altered mental status is often a sign of a deteriorating condition. If you cannot determine a cause for the person's condition or behavior or if you are unsure what to do, call 9-1-1. Describe the situation and the person's signs and symptoms to the dispatcher, who will determine the correct course of action.

Diabetic Emergencies

Diabetes is actually a group of related diseases in which blood sugar (glucose) levels are not well regulated by the body. The hormone insulin, normally produced in the pancreas, is needed for body cells to be able to use glucose. When insulin levels are too low, glucose levels rise too high. A problem results if the body is not producing enough insulin or if the body does not use the insulin well: a condition called insulin resistance. Currently more than 29 million people in the United States have diabetes, about 8 million of whom have not been diagnosed.[1] The disease is chronic and incurable.

[1] *American Diabetes Association, diabetes.org/diabetes-basics/ statistics/?loc=db-slabnav Accessed January 2016.*

There are two primary types of diabetes. In Type 1, formerly called insulin-dependent diabetes or juvenile-onset diabetes, the body does not produce enough or any insulin. The person must receive insulin by injection or a pump. In Type 2 diabetes, formerly called noninsulin-dependent or adult-onset diabetes, body cells do not use insulin well. Eventually, the pancreas may not produce as much insulin. Either way, blood glucose levels may be too high. More than 90% of adults who develop diabetes have Type 2 diabetes, which becomes more common as one grows older or becomes more overweight. Most people with Type 2 diabetes can control the problem with diet, exercise, weight control and oral medication when needed.

Blood glucose levels vary moment by moment in the body as a result of many factors, including what one has eaten, when it was eaten, one's level of activity and other factors. In a person who is not diabetic, insulin maintains a dynamic balance with blood glucose to prevent levels from becoming too high or too low. People with diabetes, however, sometimes have problems maintaining this balance even with careful attention to diet, activity levels and blood glucose monitoring.

PREVENTION OF DIABETES AND DIABETIC EMERGENCIES

Diabetes is a serious and growing problem in the United States. It kills almost 70,000 people yearly, making it the seventh leading cause of death. Diabetes contributes to more than 160,000 additional deaths annually from related causes.[1] In addition, diabetes causes complications throughout the body. Diabetes contributes to heart disease and stroke, is the most common cause of blindness in people ages 20-74, causes severe kidney disease and damages the nervous system. Because of resulting circulation problems, foot infections in diabetics often lead to amputation. An alarming current trend is the increasing numbers of children and adolescents who are developing Type 2 diabetes related to being overweight and lack of exercise.

[1]*American Diabetes Association, http://www.diabetes.org/ diabetes-basics/statistics Accessed January 2016.*

Type 2 diabetes can often be prevented or delayed in people at a high risk for developing the problem. Diet, exercise and weight control are critical for prevention – the same lifestyle factors that can reduce one's risk for cardiovascular disease (see **Chapter 5**). For those with diabetes, careful control of their glucose levels, blood pressure and cholesterol levels, along with preventive care for the eyes, kidneys and feet, can help prevent complications from developing.

Diabetic emergencies can usually be prevented by careful monitoring of blood glucose levels and by controlling diet, medication use and activity levels **(Figure 16-5).**

FIGURE 16-5

People with diabetes often use a blood glucose monitoring system like this one to check their glucose levels using a tiny drop of blood.

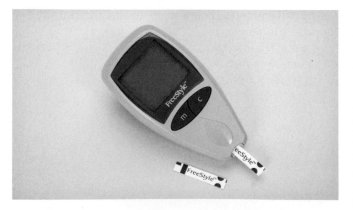

FIRST AID FOR DIABETIC EMERGENCIES

In a person with diabetes, the blood sugar level may become either too low or too high as a result of many interacting factors. Low blood sugar, called **hypoglycemia,** may result if a person takes too much insulin, does not eat enough food or the right kind of food or uses blood sugar too quickly through exercise or emotional stress. High blood sugar, called **hyperglycemia,** may result if a person takes too little insulin, eats too much food or the wrong kind of food or does not use blood sugar through activity **(Figure 16-6).** Other factors can also affect blood sugar levels.

Either hypoglycemia or hyperglycemia can quickly progress to a medical emergency if the person is not treated. In many cases, you may know if a victim experiencing this emergency has diabetes. Both hypoglycemia and hyperglycemia cause altered mental status (drowsiness, disorientation) and a generalized feeling of sickness. When taking the SAMPLE history of any victim who suddenly feels ill, ask about diabetes or other medical conditions, and look for a medical alert ID. If the victim is responsive and alert, he or she may know from experience whether the problem is hypoglycemia or hyperglycemia.

FIGURE 16-6

A diabetic emergency may result if the body's balance of insulin and blood sugar is disrupted.

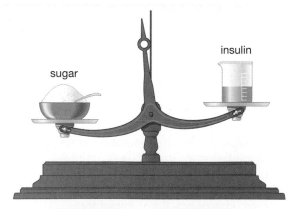

Hypoglycemia	**Hyperglycemia**
• Sudden dizziness	• Frequent urination
• Shakiness	• Drowsiness
• Mood change	• Dry mouth
• Headache	• Thirst
• Confusion	• Shortness of breath
• Pale skin	• Deep, rapid breathing
• Sweating	• Nausea/vomiting
• Hunger	• Fruity-smelling breath

HYPOGLYCEMIA

The signs and symptoms of hypoglycemia include sudden dizziness, shakiness or mood change (even combativeness); headache, confusion and difficulty paying attention; pale or ashen skin or sweating; hunger; and clumsy, jerky movements. A seizure may occur. Although the victim may appear to be intoxicated (slurring words, staggering gait, confusion, etc.), it is important never to dismiss these symptoms without considering the possibility of a diabetic emergency.

First aid for hypoglycemia involves raising the victim's blood sugar level by giving the person food or drink that is high in glucose. Diabetics often carry glucose tablets in case of episodes of low blood sugar **(Figure 16-7).** Glucose is quickly absorbed into the blood, quickly relieving the problem (see First Aid: "Hypoglycemia (Low Blood Sugar)").

FIGURE 16-7

Diabetics often carry glucose tablets in case of low blood sugar.

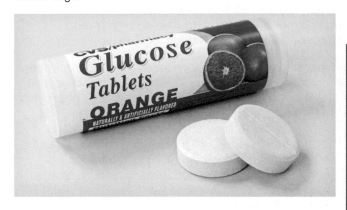

First Aid: Hypoglycemia (Low Blood Sugar)

Signs, Symptoms and Care

WHEN YOU SEE

- Sudden dizziness, shakiness or mood change (even combativeness)

- Headache, confusion, difficulty paying attention

- Pale or ashen skin, sweating

- Hunger

- Clumsy, jerky movements

- Possible seizure

DO THIS FIRST

1. Confirm that the victim has diabetes. Talk to the victim; look for a medical ID tag.

2. Give the victim sugar: preferably 3-5 glucose tablets, or if glucose tablets are unavailable, another source of dietary sugar, such as 8 ounces of orange juice, 5 sugar packets (but not artificial sugar or sweetener packets) or several pieces of candy (such as 15-20 jelly beans or 20-25 Skittles). If the victim still feels ill or has signs and symptoms after 15 minutes, give more sugar.

3. Call 9-1-1 if the victim becomes unresponsive or continues to have significant signs and symptoms.

ADDITIONAL CARE

- If the victim becomes unresponsive or continues to have significant signs and symptoms, call 9-1-1 and monitor breathing.

ALERT

- If a diabetic victim becomes unresponsive, do not try to inject insulin or put food or fluids in his or her mouth.

Hyperglycemia

The signs and symptoms of hyperglycemia include frequent urination, drowsiness, dry mouth and thirst, shortness of breath and deep, rapid breathing, fruity-smelling breath and nausea or vomiting. Unresponsiveness eventually occurs.

Hyperglycemia generally requires medical treatment. Hyperglycemia usually develops gradually over time, allowing the diabetic person to recognize and correct the problem. In an early stage of the problem, the victim may follow the instructions from his or her health care provider. For more significant symptoms, the victim needs medical help. The victim may be taken to an emergency department, or if he or she becomes unresponsive, call 9-1-1 (see First Aid: "Hyperglycemia (High Blood Sugar)").

In some situations, you may know or discover the person has diabetes but not know whether the problem is high or low blood sugar. In this case, if the victim's symptoms are mild, give sugar as for low blood sugar. If it does happen that the victim has high blood sugar, this additional sugar will not worsen the victim's condition, but it could solve the problem if the victim has low blood sugar. If the victim does not improve in 15 minutes, or if signs and symptoms become worse, an emergency is developing, and the victim needs immediate medical attention.

Severe Abdominal Pain

Abdominal injuries were described in **Chapter 13.** Always call 9-1-1 for an abdominal injury. Abdominal pain may also result from illness ranging from minor conditions to serious medical emergencies. Urgent medical care is needed for severe abdominal pain in these situations:

In adults:

- Sudden, severe, intolerable pain or pain that causes awakening from sleep

- Pain that begins in the general area of the central abdomen and later moves to the lower right

- Pain accompanied by fever, sweating, black or bloody stool or blood in urine

- Pain in pregnancy or accompanying abnormal vaginal bleeding

- Pain accompanied by dry mouth, dizziness upon standing or decreased urination

- Pain accompanied by difficulty breathing

- Pain accompanied by vomiting blood or greenish-brown fluid

First Aid: Hyperglycemia (High Blood Sugar)

Signs, Symptoms and Care

WHEN YOU SEE

Early stage signs and symptoms:

- Frequent urination

- Drowsiness

- Dry mouth, thirst

Later stage signs and symptoms:

- Shortness of breath; deep, rapid breathing

- Breath smells fruity

- Nausea or vomiting

- Eventual unresponsiveness

DO THIS FIRST

1. If you suspect high blood sugar, call 9-1-1 and monitor the person.

2. In the early stage, you may not be able to tell whether the victim suffers from high or low blood sugar. In this case:

   - Give glucose tablets or sugar as for hypoglycemia.

   - If the victim does not improve within 15 minutes, or the victim's signs and symptoms become worse, call 9-1-1.

3. In the later stage, high blood sugar is a medical emergency:

   - Call 9-1-1 immediately.

   - Put an unresponsive victim in the recovery position and monitor breathing.

In young children:

- Pain that occurs suddenly, stops and then returns without warning

- Pain accompanied by red or purple jelly-like stool; or with blood or mucus in stool

- Pain accompanied by greenish-brown vomit

- Pain with swollen abdomen that feels hard

- Pain with a hard lump in lower abdomen or groin area

Many different factors and illnesses can result in gastrointestinal distress with or without abdominal pain. Vomiting or diarrhea may also occur from many different causes. Again, seek urgent medical care for the signs and symptoms listed here, and talk with a health care provider for other unexplained or persistent gastrointestinal distress. The following are additional key points:

- Persistent diarrhea or vomiting in an infant or small child or in an elderly or debilitated person can rapidly cause dehydration, which can become an emergency. Seek medical care immediately.

- While awaiting medical help, do not give a person with abdominal pain anything to eat or drink, as this may cause vomiting – except for clear fluids for dehydration.

 LEARNING CHECKPOINT 3

1. When should you call 9-1-1 for a victim who faints?

_____

Circle **True** or **False** for the following statement:

2. When a person has fainted, lay him or her down and raise the head and shoulders 6-12 inches.   True   False

3. Select the best answer. For a victim having seizures –

   a. lay the victim face down on the floor.

   b. ask others to help you hold the victim's head, arms and legs still.

   c. put something flat and soft under the victim's head.

   d. put a wooden object, such as a pencil, between the victim's teeth.

4. Name at least three situations in which you should call 9-1-1 for a seizure victim.

_____

_____

_____

5. What should you do for a young child whose abdomen is swollen and feels hard?

_____

6. Check off common signs and symptoms of a low blood sugar diabetic emergency.

   ☐ Dizziness

   ☐ Red, blotchy skin

   ☐ Hunger

   ☐ Sweating

   ☐ Rapid deep breathing

   ☐ Confusion

   ☐ Clumsiness

   ☐ Swollen legs

7. In the late afternoon, you see a friend at the library who is acting oddly. She is sitting at a table staring into space, and when you ask her if she is OK, she does not seem to understand what you are saying. She looks ill, her skin is pale and she is sweating even though the room is not warm. You know this woman is diabetic, and you suspect that she might have skipped lunch today. You cannot be sure whether she has low or high blood sugar. What should you do?

_____

_____

_____

CONCLUDING THOUGHTS

It can be a frightening experience to be with someone who is suddenly ill, especially if you do not know the cause. Remember the first steps for all first aid situations: Assess the victim and try to find out what happened. If you know the cause of the problem, give appropriate first aid; if you do not know, call 9-1-1 and give supportive care until help arrives. Reassure the victim. Help the victim to rest and avoid getting chilled or overheated, and do not give him or her anything to eat or drink. Stay with the person, watch for changes and be prepared to give BLS if needed.

CRITICAL THINKING CHALLENGE QUESTIONS

SCENARIO 1

You enter your boss's office to find her at her desk looking ill. Her skin is pale, and she is sweating. Her chest hurts, but she says, "It must have been something I ate – it feels like really bad heartburn." She is obviously short of breath. What should you do?

_____

_____

_____

_____

SCENARIO 2

Standing in the checkout line at the supermarket, you see the elderly woman in front of you suddenly stagger and fall over her grocery cart. You help her to sit on the floor. She seems confused and is trying to say something, but you cannot make out her words; one side of her mouth seems frozen. Then she leans back and becomes unresponsive. What do you do?

_____

_____

_____

_____

SCENARIO 3

You encounter a coworker sitting at his desk looking ill. He is having trouble breathing and is gasping and trying to catch his breath. You ask what is wrong and he says he does not know but suddenly he feels dizzy. What do you do?

_____

_____

_____

_____

_____

REVIEW QUESTIONS

Select the best answers.

1. Common general signs and symptoms of sudden illness include –

   a. feeling ill, dizzy, confused or weak.

   b. skin color changes (flushed, pale or ashen) and sweating.

   c. breathing changes.

   d. All of the above

2. Always call 9-1-1 for a victim whose illness –

   a. occurs suddenly and without explanation.

   b. includes a fever.

   c. is chronic.

   d. involves feeling fatigued.

3. The signs and symptoms of heart attack may include –

   a. chest pain, fever and flushed skin.

   b. chest pain, headache and an inability to raise both arms.

   c. chest pain, sweating and shortness of breath.

   d. chest pain, difficulty speaking or swallowing and vision problems.

4. The most crucial aspect of first aid for a stroke victim is –

    a. calling 9-1-1 immediately.

    b. explaining the situation to family members.

    c. elevating the victim's legs.

    d. performing a complete physical examination before calling 9-1-1.

5. Low oxygen blood levels caused by breathing difficulty may cause –

    a. heavy sweating.

    b. dizziness or disorientation.

    c. a reddish coloration of the skin.

    d. hyperactivity.

6. First aid for an asthma attack may include –

    a. calling 9-1-1 if the victim is not better in 30 minutes.

    b. asking the victim to try to breathe slowly.

    c. helping the victim to lay down with feet raised.

    d. helping the victim use an inhaler.

7. To help a person who is hyperventilating –

    a. have the victim breathe into a paper bag.

    b. splash cold water on the victim's face.

    c. ask the victim to try to breathe slowly.

    d. ask the victim to hold his or her breath as long as possible.

8. Help to prevent injury to a person having a seizure by –

    a. putting something flat and soft under the head.

    b. putting a wooden stick between the teeth.

    c. restraining the person by holding the shoulders.

    d. having bystanders help hold the arms and legs still.

9. Altered mental status may result from –

    a. stroke.

    b. poisoning.

    c. head injury.

    d. All of the above

10. If you are unsure whether a diabetic is experiencing hypoglycemia or hyperglycemia –

    a. wait an hour to observe signs and symptoms.

    b. give glucose or sugar and monitor symptoms.

    c. call a family member of the victim to inquire.

    d. give the victim an emergency epinephrine shot in the thigh muscle.

CHAPTER 17

Poisoning

LESSON OBJECTIVES

- Explain different ways poisons can enter the body.

- List things you can do in your own home to prevent poisoning of both children and adults.

- Describe the role of Poison Control Centers in the treatment of poisoning.

- Describe the first aid for swallowed and inhaled poisons.

- List actions to take when exposed to poison ivy, oak or sumac.

With your young son, Danny, you are visiting a friend at her home. Danny has been playing with a toy truck on the floor, which he now pushes down the hallway into the bathroom. You start to get up to bring him back but your friend says, "That's OK, there's nothing in there he can get into." With the normal curiosity of a child, however, Danny starts looking in the bathroom drawers and soon finds a bottle of what looks to him like little candy mints. He puts a handful in his mouth – they don't taste much like mint but he chews and swallows them anyway. You see pills spilled on the floor when you walk into the bathroom. He admits he ate "some" of the pills. What do you do?

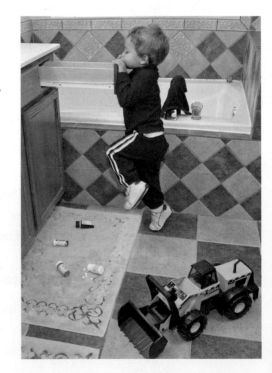

With almost a million emergency department visits for poisoning incidents in the United States every year, resulting in about 38,800 deaths, poisoning is a huge problem in a world where so many products containing toxins are present in the home and workplace. Unintentional poisoning has become the number 1 cause of death from injuries, recently surpassing deaths from motor vehicle crashes as a cause of unintentional injury death.[1] Children younger than 6 comprise nearly half of poison exposures (48%), followed by adults (38%), then teens (7%).[2] Most poisoning deaths are among adults, related to use of drugs.

Most poisonings are unintentional, but some victims take a poison intentionally, either in a suicide attempt or to experience the effects produced by the substance. This chapter focuses primarily on unintentional poisonings. Poisoning caused by the misuse or overdose of alcohol and other drugs, including over-the-counter and prescription medications, is discussed in **Chapter 18.** Behavioral emergencies, such as suicide, are described in **Chapter 21.**

Virtually all poisonings can be prevented. Parents and other caretakers can protect children from poisoning by keeping them safely away from common products that are poisonous. Most adult poisonings involve the careless use or misuse of medications and cleaning products, which can be prevented by following safety guidelines.

[1]*National Safety Council. (2015). Injury Facts®, 2015 Edition. Itasca, IL: Author.*

[2]*National Capital Poison Center, poison.org/poison-statistics-national Accessed January 2016.*

Overview of Poisoning

A **poison** is any substance that enters or touches the body with effects that are injurious to health or are life threatening. Poisons can enter the body by being swallowed, injected (by hypodermic needle or an insect stinger), inhaled or absorbed through the skin or mucous membranes. All too often, people think of the risk of poisoning only in terms of ingesting the substance; however, inhaling fumes from a product or spilling a chemical on unprotected skin can be just as dangerous. **Chapter 11** (Burns) describes the first aid for poisons (chemicals) that contact the skin or eyes. Injected poisons are described in **Chapters 18** (Substance Misuse and Abuse) and **19** (Bites and Stings). This chapter primarily discusses swallowed and inhaled poisons, along with the contact poisons of certain plants, but the prevention guidelines detailed in the next section apply to all forms of poison.

A huge percentage of poisonings occur in the home, most involving common products. The top 25 substances involved in poisonings are listed in **Table 17-1.** These are the most common types of products that contain poisons – a complete list of every product or substance that is poisonous would be many, many pages long. Because there are so many poisons present in so many different products, **the safest thing is to assume that all substances that can be swallowed, injected, breathed in, or put in contact with skin are poisonous unless known to be otherwise.** Note that almost any substance can be poisonous in doses larger than intended, including aspirin, vitamins, herbal supplements and natural remedies and prescribed or over-the-counter medication.

POISON CONTROL CENTERS

A system of **Poison Control Centers (PCCs)** has been developed throughout the United States to provide information and treatment advice for all types of poisonings. Presently there are 55 Poison Control Centers throughout the United States and U.S. territories. All can be reached by dialing the same telephone number: (800) 222-1222, 24 hours a day. Your call will be routed to the regional PCC in your area. This telephone number should be posted by your telephone at home and in your workplace. When you are away from this number, call 9-1-1 and if necessary the dispatcher will contact the Poison Control Center. In almost all cases, it is better to call the PCC in cases of poisoning than a health care provider because the PCC has the most accurate and up-to-date information. Personnel staffing each PCC have information about all known poisons and will advise you what first aid to give in each poisoning case.

The American Association of Poison Control Centers (AAPCC) provides valuable information about how to prevent poisonings, as well as information about specific poisons. On request, the AAPCC will provide a list of poisonous plants in your area to help you identify threats in your yard or in places you may visit (aapcc.org).

TABLE 17-1

Top 25 Substance Categories Involved in Poisoning

Substance (Major Generic Category)	All substances	%
Analgesics	291,062	11.29
Cosmetics/Personal Care Products	199,291	7.73
Cleaning Substances (Household)	198,018	7.68
Sedative/Hypnotics/ Antipsychotics	150,715	5.85
Antidepressants	112,412	4.36
Antihistamines	103,327	4.01
Cardiovascular Drugs	102,170	3.96
Foreign Bodies/Toys/ Miscellaneous	99,835	3.87
Pesticides	83,005	3.22
Topical Preparations	82,819	3.21
Alcohols	68,648	2.66
Vitamins	66,058	2.56
Cold and Cough Preparations	61,288	2.38
Stimulants and Street Drugs	59,869	2.32
Anticonvulsants	56,832	2.20
Hormones and Hormone Antagonists	56,775	2.20
Antimicrobials	56,726	2.20
Bites and Envenomations	55,017	2.13
Gastrointestinal Preparations	48,501	1.88
Plants	44,731	1.74
Dietary Supplements/ Herbals/Homeopathic	42,535	1.65
Chemicals	38,975	1.51
Fumes/Gases/Vapors	33,944	1.32
Other/Unknown Nondrug Substances	32,001	1.24
Hydrocarbons	31,903	1.24

Source: American Association of Poison Control Centers, aapcc.s3.amazonaws.com/pdfs/annual_reports/2014_AAPCC_NPDS_Annual_Report.pdf Accessed January 2016.

Preventing Poisoning

Most poisonings occur unintentionally and can be prevented by following simple guidelines. The safety principles for preventing poisonings in children are based on keeping children away from products and substances that contain poisons and educating children on safe behaviors. Prevention principles for adults, who often use products and medications that can be poisonous, focus on safe and appropriate use and on minimizing or eliminating the risk of unintentional exposure.

PREVENTING POISONING IN CHILDREN

Children younger than 6 are at the highest risk for poisoning. Children are often curious about what things taste like and will put many different substances into their mouths. Colorful product packages may attract a young child who cannot easily distinguish between food products and other products found in the home. Even if they are told to leave certain things alone, young children do not yet have the cognitive skills needed to understand why they should not eat or drink substances they find. Prevention emphasizes keeping all potentially harmful substances where children cannot get to them.

Follow these guidelines provided by the American Association of Poison Control Centers:

Household and Chemical Products

- Use safety locks on all cabinets. Store potential poisons out of reach of small children.

- Store all poisonous household and chemical products out of sight of children.

- If you are using a product and need to answer the telephone or doorbell, take the child with you. Most poisonings occur when the product is in use.

- Store all products in their original containers. *Do not* use food containers, such as milk jugs or soda bottles, to store household and chemical products.

- Store food and household and chemical products in separate areas. Mistaken identity could cause a serious poisoning. Many poisonous products look like and come in containers very similar to those that contain drinks or food – for example, apple juice and pine cleaner.

- Return household and chemical products to safe storage immediately after use.

- Use extra caution during mealtimes or when the family routine is disrupted. Many poisonings take place at these times.

- Pesticides can be absorbed through the skin and can be extremely toxic. Keep children away from areas that have recently been sprayed. Store pesticides in a safe place where children cannot reach them.

- Discard old or outdated household and chemical products.

- Take time to teach children about poisonous substances.

- Keep the Poison Control Center telephone number on or near your telephone.

Medicine

- Keep medicines out of sight, locked up and out of reach of children.

- Make sure all medicines are in child-resistant containers and are labeled properly. Remember that child-resistant does not mean childproof.

- Never leave pills on the counter or in plastic bags. Always store medicines in their original container with a child-resistant cap.

- Keep purses and diaper bags out of reach of children.

- Do not take medicines in front of children. Young children often imitate adult behaviors.

- Do not call medicine "candy." Medicines and candy look alike, and children cannot tell the difference.

- Vitamins are medicine. Vitamins with iron can be especially poisonous. Keep them locked up and out of reach of children.

- Be aware of medicines that visitors may bring into your home. Children are curious and may investigate visitors' purses and suitcases.

Plants

- Contact your local Poison Control Center for more information about toxic plants in your area. **Figure 17-1** shows three common plants that are poisonous when eaten.

- Know the names of the plants in your home and in your yard. Label all of your plants. If you are having difficulty identifying a plant, take a sample to a nursery for identification.

- Keep poisonous plants out of reach of children and pets.

- Teach your children not to eat mushrooms growing in the yard. Some of these mushrooms can be poisonous. Be aware that mushrooms are often abundant after rain.

- Teach your children not to eat leaves and berries that grow in the yard. Do not assume a plant is safe to eat if you see wild animals eating it.

- Keep children and pets away from plants that have recently been sprayed with weed killer, bug killer or fertilizer.

FIGURE 17-1

Examples of plants that are poisonous when eaten.

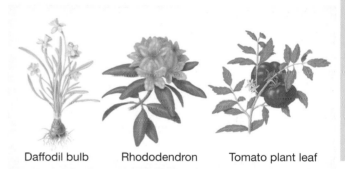

Daffodil bulb   Rhododendron   Tomato plant leaf

Preventing Poisoning in Adults

Follow these guidelines provided by the American Association of Poison Control Centers:

- Keep potential poisons in their original containers. Do not use food containers, such as cups or bottles, to store household and chemical products.

- Store food and household and chemical products in separate areas. Mistaken identity could cause a serious poisoning.

- Read and follow the directions and caution labels on household and chemical products before using them.

- Never mix household and chemical products together. A poisonous gas may be created when mixing chemicals.

- Turn on fans and open windows when using household and chemical products.

- When spraying household and chemical products, make sure the spray nozzle is directed away from your face and other people. Wear protective clothing – long-sleeved shirts, long pants, socks, shoes and gloves – when spraying pesticides and other chemicals.

- Pesticides can be absorbed through the skin and can be extremely poisonous. Stay away from areas that have recently been sprayed.

- Never sniff containers to discover what is inside.

- Discard old or outdated household and chemical products.

- First aid instructions on product containers may be incorrect or outdated. Call the Poison Control Center instead for guidelines to follow if an exposure occurs.

- Keep the Poison Control Center telephone number on or near your telephone.

- Follow the prevention guidelines in **Chapter 18** to prevent unintentional poisoning by the misuse of over-the-counter and prescription medications.

Swallowed Poisons

Most cases of poisoning involve substances that are swallowed. Depending on the poison, effects may begin almost immediately or may be delayed. First aid is most effective if given as soon as possible after the poison is swallowed, and in some cases, the effects can be prevented or minimized by acting quickly. Poisoning is like sudden illness in that often there is no visible injury, and you may not know immediately what happened. The victim may be unresponsive or, even if responsive, may be confused and disoriented and unable to tell you what happened. The most important aspect of first aid for a poisoning often is recognizing that a poisoning has occurred.

As you check the scene and perform your initial assessment of the victim, look around for any sign that the victim may be poisoned. Look for containers nearby or any clue that the person was using a substance or product. Ask others at the scene if anyone saw anything or knows what the person was doing when the problem occurred. If the victim is responsive and identifies a substance to which he or she was exposed, try to learn how much the person may have swallowed and how long ago.

The specific signs and symptoms of poisons depend on the substance and many other factors, although many poisons cause similar general effects:

- The victim may look and feel ill.

- The victim may have abdominal pain, feel nauseated and may vomit or have diarrhea.

- The victim may have altered mental status or become unresponsive.

- There may be burns, stains or odors around the victim's mouth.

- The pupils of the eyes may be dilated or constricted.

- The victim may be breathing abnormally.

Be aware that the condition of a poisoning victim may change rapidly.

First aid for a poisoning depends on the victim's condition. For an unresponsive victim, call 9-1-1 immediately. Check for normal breathing and provide CPR if needed. Because of the risk for vomiting, put a breathing, unresponsive victim in the recovery position, and continue to monitor breathing.

If the victim is responsive, call the Poison Control Center and follow the instructions provided **(Box 17-1).** Depending on the poison, the PCC may direct you to take any of various actions. Some poisons may be diluted by having the victim drink water or milk. For some poisons, the victim may benefit from drinking a solution of activated charcoal, if available, to absorb the poison. Activated charcoal is available in a powder or liquid form without prescription and may be kept in the home medicine cabinet for use only if the PCC advises it **(Figure 17-2).** Because none of these actions is used for all kinds of poisons, *never take any of these actions unless told to do so by the Poison Control Center.* The PCC will also tell you whether to call 9-1-1 or seek other urgent medical care for a poisoning incident (see First Aid: "Swallowed Poisons").

Note that, in the past, syrup of ipecac was used in some situations to induce vomiting in a victim of swallowed poison. Because of problems caused by this and its lack of effectiveness in most cases, PCCs no longer recommend the use of ipecac.

FIGURE 17-2

The Poison Control Center may advise taking activated charcoal in some cases of poisoning.

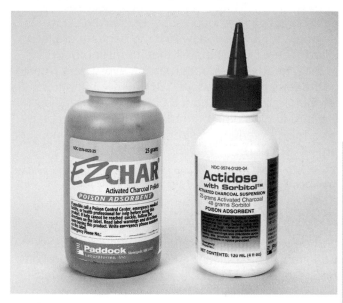

First Aid: Swallowed Poisons

Signs, Symptoms and Care

WHEN YOU SEE

• An open container of a poisonous substance

• Nausea and vomiting; signs of abdominal pain or cramps

• Drowsiness, dizziness, disorientation or other altered mental status

• Changing levels of responsiveness

DO THIS FIRST

1. Determine what was swallowed, when, and how much.

2. For a responsive victim, call the Poison Control Center, (800) 222-1222, immediately and follow the instructions given.

3. For a victim with signs of a life-threatening condition (including sleepiness, seizures, difficulty breathing, vomiting) and for any unresponsive victim, call 9-1-1 and provide basic life support (BLS) as needed.

ADDITIONAL CARE

• Put an unresponsive victim in the recovery position and be prepared for vomiting. Monitor the victim's breathing and be ready to give CPR if needed.

• If a responsive victim's mouth or lips are burned by a corrosive chemical, rinse the mouth with cold water (do not allow the victim to swallow).

ALERT

• Do not give the victim anything to eat or drink unless instructed by the Poison Control Center or health care provider.

• Do not follow first aid instructions present on some household product labels; instead, call the Poison Control Center, (800) 222-1222.

FOOD POISONING

Food poisoning occurs after one eats food that is contaminated with microorganisms, usually bacteria, or their toxins. Most cases of food poisoning are acute infections, although some bacteria make toxins that can poison a food even if the bacteria are later killed. The CDC estimates that 48 million people in the United States become sick every year from pathogens in food. About 128,000 are hospitalized for their illness, and about 3,000 die.[1] Botulism is a life-threatening type of food poisoning produced by a certain bacterium present in improperly canned or preserved food.

[1]*Centers for Disease Control and Prevention, cdc.gov/foodsafety/ foodborne-germs.html Accessed January 2016.*

Contamination can occur at any stage, from growing the food through processing to food preparation and delivery. Food contamination usually results from improper cooking or leaving a cooked food out for more than 2 hours at room temperature. Most bacteria grow rapidly and are undetected because they do not change the odor or taste of the food. Freezing a food will slow or stop bacteria growth but will not kill the bacteria.

Food poisoning symptoms may begin soon after eating or within a day. The most common signs and symptoms are nausea, vomiting, abdominal pain and diarrhea. Talk to your health care provider to see if treatment is needed (see First Aid: "Food Poisoning"). Seek urgent medical care if any of the following signs and symptoms occurs:

- Signs of shock: shallow breathing; cold, clammy, pale or ashen skin; shaking or chills; or chest pain

- Signs of severe dehydration: dry mouth, decreased urine output, dizziness, fatigue or increased breathing rate

- Confusion or difficulty reasoning

BOX 17-2: PREVENTING FOOD POISONING

Follow these guidelines to prevent harmful bacteria from growing in food and causing food poisoning:

- Raw and cooked perishable foods – foods that can spoil – should be refrigerated or frozen promptly. If perishable foods stand at room temperature for more than 2 hours, they may not be safe to eat. Refrigerators should be set at 40 degrees or lower and freezers should be set at 0 degrees.

- Foods should be cooked long enough and at a high enough temperature to kill the harmful bacteria that cause illnesses. A meat thermometer should be used to ensure foods are cooked to the appropriate internal temperature:

  - 145 degrees for roasts, steaks, and chops of beef, veal, pork and lamb, followed by 3 minutes of rest time after the meat is removed from the heat source

  - 160 degrees for ground beef, veal, pork, and lamb

  - 165 degrees for poultry

- Cold foods should be kept cold, and hot foods should be kept hot.

- Fruits and vegetables should be washed under running water just before eating, cutting, or cooking. A produce brush can be used under running water to clean fruits and vegetables with firm skin.

- Raw meat, poultry, seafood, and their juices should be kept away from other foods.

- People should wash their hands for at least 20 seconds with warm, soapy water before and after handling raw meat, poultry, fish, shellfish, produce or eggs. People should also wash their hands after using the bathroom, changing diapers or touching animals.

- Utensils and surfaces should be washed with hot, soapy water before and after they are used to prepare food. Diluted bleach – 1 teaspoon of bleach to 1 quart of hot water – can also be used to sanitize utensils and surfaces.

Source: National Institute of Diabetes and Digestive and Kidney Diseases, niddk.nih.gov/health-information/health-topics/digestive-diseases/foodborne-illnesses/Pages/facts.aspx#10 Accessed January 2016.

First Aid: Food Poisoning

Signs, Symptoms and Care

WHEN YOU SEE

- Nausea and vomiting; signs of abdominal pain or cramps

- Diarrhea, possibly with blood

- Headache or fever

DO THIS FIRST

1. Have the victim rest lying down.

2. Give the victim lots of clear liquids.

3. Seek medical attention.

ADDITIONAL CARE

- Check with others with whom the victim has eaten recently.

Inhaled Poisons

In both home and work settings, various gases and fumes may be present. Products such as paints, thinners and many chemicals give off fumes that can result in a poisoning if there is not enough fresh air or other protection. Some products' fumes are so toxic that a respirator must be worn when working with them, even outdoors where fresh air is plentiful. Always check product labels for health risks and safety precautions.

Inhaled poisons also include gases that may escape from pipelines or tanks being transported. Whenever you smell gas or have other evidence of a leak, stay away from the scene. Remember that not all hazardous gases or fumes can be smelled. Call 9-1-1 and let a specially trained hazardous materials team manage the situation. In such a situation, do not risk your own safety in an attempt to reach a victim. **Chapter 2** describes typical hazardous scenes and the warning placards that may indicate the presence of a poisonous gas.

Smoke and fumes resulting from fires are also poisonous. Fires produce carbon monoxide and, depending on the substances being burned, may produce other highly toxic gases. **Chapter 24** describes actions to take in or near a fire.

The signs and symptoms of inhaled poisons may be similar to those of other poisons. Breathing difficulty with or without chest pain may be present. Altered mental status may include dizziness, disorientation, headache, unresponsiveness or other symptoms.

In most cases, you will not know the specific treatment for an inhaled poison. First, if it is safe for you to go to the victim, try to ensure that the victim is breathing fresh air. Move the victim outdoors or to a well-ventilated area, if possible. If the victim should not be moved because of injuries or other factors, ventilate the area. If the victim is responsive, call the PCC and follow the instructions given. If the victim is unresponsive, call 9-1-1.

The general first aid for an inhaled poison is the same as for carbon monoxide poisoning, described in the next section. Carbon monoxide is the most common gas involved in poisonings.

CARBON MONOXIDE

Carbon monoxide is especially dangerous because it is invisible, odorless, tasteless – and very lethal. This gas results in more fatal unintentional poisonings in the United States than any other poison. Carbon monoxide may be present from motor vehicle or boat exhaust, a faulty furnace, a kerosene heater, industrial equipment, a poorly vented fireplace or a wood stove or fire. Exposure to large amounts causes an immediate poisoning reaction; a small leak may cause gradual poisoning with less dramatic symptoms. To prevent poisoning, carbon monoxide detectors should be installed along with smoke detectors in appropriate locations. If your carbon monoxide detector goes off, do not investigate the problem yourself; instead, leave the premises and call your furnace company or appropriate other professional.

PREVENTING CARBON MONOXIDE POISONING

More than 20,000 cases of carbon monoxide poisoning and more than 400 deaths occur each year in the United States from carbon monoxide poisoning unrelated to fires.[1] The CDC recommends the following strategies to prevent carbon monoxide exposure in the home:[2]

- Do have your heating system, water heater and any other gas, oil or coal burning appliances serviced by a qualified technician every year.

- Do install a battery-operated or battery back-up carbon monoxide detector in your home and check or replace the battery when you change the time on your clocks each spring and fall. If the detector sounds, leave your home immediately and call 9-1-1.

- Do seek prompt medical attention if you suspect carbon monoxide poisoning and are feeling dizzy, light-headed or nauseous.

- Don't use a generator, charcoal grill, camp stove or other gasoline or charcoal-burning device inside your home, basement or garage or near a window.

- Don't run a car or truck inside a garage attached to your house, even if you leave the door open.

- Don't burn anything in a stove or fireplace that isn't vented

- Don't heat your house with a gas oven.

[1]Centers for Disease Control and Prevention, cdc.gov/co/faqs.htm Accessed January 2016.

[2]Centers for Disease Control and Prevention, cdc.gov/co/guidelines.htm Accessed January 2016.

FIRST AID FOR CARBON MONOXIDE POISONING

Carbon monoxide poisoning usually causes altered mental status. Prolonged periods of exposure to carbon monoxide may cause headaches, dizziness, confusion, poor judgment and sleepiness. Continued exposure brings on breathing difficulty, nausea, vomiting and heart palpitations. Exposure to high levels of carbon monoxide for prolonged periods can result in seizures, unresponsiveness and death.

The most important first aid for a victim of carbon monoxide poisoning is to get the victim to fresh air, but do not risk your own health if the scene is dangerous. Call 9-1-1. If it is safe to move the victim, do so quickly. Note that even a victim who seems to recover needs medical care for the poisoning (see First Aid: "Carbon Monoxide and Inhaled Poisons").

First Aid: Carbon Monoxide and Inhaled Poisons

Signs, Symptoms and Care

WHEN YOU SEE

- Headache

- Dizziness, light-headedness, confusion or weakness

- Nausea or vomiting

- Signs of chest pain

- Convulsions

- Changing levels of responsiveness

DO THIS FIRST

1. Immediately move the victim into fresh air.

2. Call 9-1-1 even if the victim starts to recover.

3. Monitor the victim's breathing and be ready to give CPR, if needed.

ADDITIONAL CARE

- Put an unresponsive victim in the recovery position.

- Loosen tight clothing around the neck or chest.

LEARNING CHECKPOINT 1

1. Check off the common signs and symptoms of a swallowed poison.

   ☐ Nausea

   ☐ Red lips

   ☐ Uncontrolled shaking

   ☐ Vomiting

   ☐ Dizziness

   ☐ Unresponsiveness

   ☐ Drowsiness

   ☐ Hyperactivity

2. Name one action you would take for a victim of food poisoning that you would not take for a victim of swallowed poison.

   _____

   _____

3. Select the best answer. The first thing to do for a victim of carbon monoxide poisoning is –

   a. loosen tight clothing around the neck.

   b. call 9-1-1.

   c. move the victim to fresh air.

   d. place the victim in the recovery position.

4. You are in a friend's house when you enter the kitchen and find the friend's child unresponsive on the floor. The cabinet under the sink is open, and the cap is off of a bottle of a cleaning product. Describe what actions you need to take.

   _____

   _____

Poison Ivy, Oak and Sumac

Contact with poison ivy, oak and sumac causes an allergic skin reaction, called **allergic contact dermatitis,** in about half the population. A resin in the leaves of these plants causes the reaction. These plants grow in many areas of the country but can be identified by their distinctive leaves **(Figure 17-3).** The resin can rub off on a person's clothing and shoes and then be transferred to the skin. If someone touches the leaves and gets the resin on the fingers, touching other body areas before washing may transfer the irritating resin to other skin areas, including the face and eyes and even the genitals.

If you know you have made contact with one of these plants, wash the area as soon as possible with soap and water. Also wash clothing and wipe off shoes, because the resin on these can still cause the reaction.

FIGURE 17-3

Common poisonous plants causing rashes.

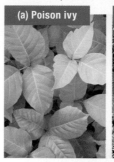 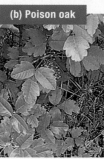 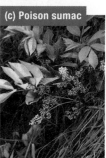

(a) Poison ivy   (b) Poison oak   (c) Poison sumac

The rash may appear within a few hours or up to 2 days after exposure **(Figure 17-4).** The skin is red and often very itchy, and young children must be kept from scratching it because the skin easily breaks and may become infected with bacteria. Once the rash appears on the skin and has been washed, however, it cannot spread to other people. First aid is usually to control the itching, which can be intense and lasts as long as the rash persists (usually less than 2 weeks). Cool, wet compresses applied 4 times a day generally help, along with calamine lotion or a paste of baking soda and water between compresses. Make the baking soda paste just thick enough to cling to the skin without running off. Topical hydrocortisone cream or an oral antihistamine may help in more serious cases. See a health care provider if the reaction is very severe or the rash occurs around the eyes or genitals. Fever or pus oozing from the rash may indicate an infection that should also receive medical treatment (see First Aid: "Poison Ivy, Oak and Sumac").

FIGURE 17-4

Skin rash caused by poison ivy.

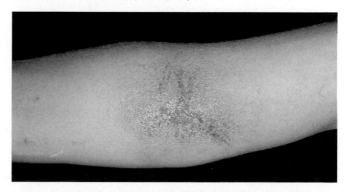

First Aid: Poison Ivy, Oak and Sumac

Signs, Symptoms and Care

WHEN YOU SEE

- Redness and itching occur first
- Rash or blisters (may weep)
- Possible headache and fever

DO THIS FIRST

1. Wash the area thoroughly with soap and water as soon as possible after contact.

2. For severe reactions or swelling on the face or genitals, seek medical attention.

3. Treat itching with colloid oatmeal baths; a paste made of baking soda and water, calamine lotion or topical hydrocortisone cream; and an oral antihistamine (e.g., Benadryl).

ADDITIONAL CARE

- To prevent further spread, wash the victim's hands, clothing and shoes (as well as pets) that came in contact with the plants.

ALERT

- Do not burn these poisonous plants to get rid of them, as smoke also spreads the poisonous resin.

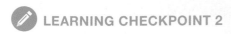 **LEARNING CHECKPOINT 2**

Circle **True** or **False** for the following statement:

1. Never put water on a site of contact with poison ivy because of the risk of spreading the rash further.   True   False

2. When should a person with a poison ivy or oak rash see a health care provider?

_____

3. Which of the following can help reduce the itching of poison ivy? Select the best answer.

    a. Hydrocortisone cream

    b. Rubbing alcohol

    c. A paste made with dishwasher detergent

    d. All of the above

 CONCLUDING THOUGHTS

Remember that a poison is any substance that is injurious to health after it enters the body. In addition to those substances we all think of as obvious poisons, alcohol and drugs can be toxic when misused or abused – prescription and over-the-counter drugs as well as illicit drugs. In fact, poisonings from medications, even everyday aspirin, are more common than poisonings caused by household products. In the next chapter you will learn about the problems of substance abuse and misuse.

CRITICAL THINKING CHALLENGE QUESTIONS

SCENARIO 1

A handyman is working in your garage, stripping old paint using an industrial solvent. When you go to check on his work, you find him leaning against the wall, saying he just feels a bit dizzy. There are strong fumes from the solvent in the garage. What do you do?

_____

_____

_____

SCENARIO 2

In the morning you helped clear away some brush and weeds on a neighbor's property. Now you have developed a red rash on your forearms that is very itchy. What should you do?

_____

_____

ADDITIONAL ACTIVITIES AND RESOURCES

The American Association of Poison Control Centers (AAPCC) website (aapcc.org) provides information on many poisoning prevention topics as well as links to state and regional poison centers that often have websites with additional information. Some poison centers also provide useful written or telephone information, such as lists of poisonous house plants.

 REVIEW QUESTIONS

Select the best answers.

1. Where do most poisonings occur?

   a. Industrial settings

   b. Homes

   c. Farms

   d. Day care centers

2. What group experiences the largest percentage of unintentional poisonings?

   a. Children younger than 6

   b. Children 4-14 years old

   c. The elderly

   d. Construction workers

3. Which of the following types of products may be poisonous?

   a. Cosmetics

   b. Vitamins with iron

   c. Arts and crafts supplies

   d. All of the above

4. The common signs and symptoms of swallowed poisonings often include –

   a. dizziness and aching in the joints.

   b. unresponsiveness and high fever.

   c. nausea and altered mental status.

   d. localized redness and swelling around the joints.

5. For a responsive child who swallowed a substance that might be poisonous, it is best to call –

   a. the Poison Control Center.

   b. the child's pediatrician.

   c. the local hospital emergency department.

   d. the child's school nurse.

6. First aid for most swallowed poisons includes –

   a. giving the victim milk to drink.

   b. inducing vomiting by any means.

   c. having the victim drink as much water as possible.

   d. calling 9-1-1 or the Poison Control Center for help.

7. When should you seek medical care for a victim who feels ill a few hours after eating food that may have been contaminated?

   a. When the victim is experiencing shaking or chills

   b. When the victim feels dizzy

   c. When the victim's skin is cold and clammy

   d. All of the above

8. What should you do for a breathing, unresponsive victim suspected of having swallowed a poison?

   a. Put the victim in the shock position with the feet raised.

   b. Put the victim on his or her back with the head raised.

   c. Put the victim in the recovery position.

   d. Put the victim in the prone position with his or her head lower than the body.

9. Exposure to carbon monoxide may cause –

   a. bleeding at mucous membranes.

   b. dizziness.

   c. dark stains around the mouth.

   d. hyperexcitability.

10. To treat the itching caused by poison ivy, what can be put on the rash?

    a. An oral antihistamine tablet crushed and mixed with water

    b. A paste of baking soda and water

    c. Lemon juice mixed with powdered sugar

    d. Antibiotic cream

CHAPTER 18

Substance Misuse and Abuse

LESSON OBJECTIVES

- Explain actions that can be taken to help prevent youth from abusing drugs and other substances.

- Describe specific steps for preventing someone from accidentally misusing or overdosing on a medication.

- List the steps of first aid for alcohol intoxication and alcohol withdrawal.

- Describe the effects of commonly abused drugs.

- List the steps of first aid for drug abuse or overdose.

- List the steps of first aid for medication overdose.

You are at a friend's holiday party, where some of the guests are drinking rather heavily. At the end of the evening, when most have left, you notice a young woman alone on the sofa, apparently either sleeping or passed out. She seems to be by herself and others are saying to just leave her alone and let her "sleep it off." You are wondering if you should do something – if it could be a more serious problem – but what can you do?

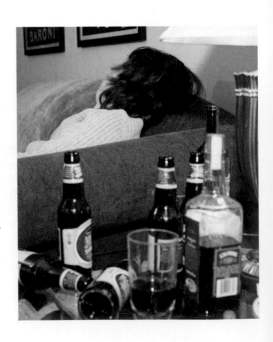

The misuse and abuse of alcohol, illicit drugs, and medications is a huge problem in our society. The effects of alcohol and other drugs may cause a medical or behavioral emergency or may complicate a sudden illness or injury. In either case, first aiders need to understand the effects of alcohol and other drugs and special considerations when giving first aid to victims under their influence.

The Problem of Substance Abuse

Substance abuse is a problem that occurs virtually everywhere in our society. Consider these United States statistics:[1]

- An estimated 24.6 million Americans aged 12 or older—9.4% of the population—used an illicit drug in the past month.

- Most people use drugs for the first time when they are teenagers. There were just over 2.8 million new users of illicit drugs in 2013, or about 7,800 new users per day. Over half (54.1%) were under 18 years of age.

- Drug use is highest among people in their late teens and 20s. In 2013, 22.6% of 18-20-year-olds reported using an illicit drug in the past month.

- About 23% of underage persons (ages 12-20) drink alcohol. Over 14% engage in binge drinking, and about 4% in heavy drinking.

- An estimated 28.7 million people, or 10.9% of persons aged 12 or older, drove under the influence of alcohol at least once in the past year.

Both heavy drinking and binge drinking are most common in the late teen and early adult years and gradually taper off with age, although they remain a common behavior. Although some variations in drinking habits are correlated with ethnic group, socioeconomic status and education levels, studies show alcohol use is a problem at all ages and in all groups.

The popularity of alcohol may be due in part to several common myths that suggest it creates fewer risks than other drugs. Here are some facts about consumption:

- Someone drinking beer is just as likely to become impaired as someone drinking hard liquor. The amount of alcohol in a 12-ounce beer is the same as in a 5-ounce glass of wine or 1.5 ounces of 80-proof spirits.

- Heavier people are no less likely to become impaired by consuming alcohol than lighter people. Many complex factors influence a person's reaction to alcohol and these cannot be easily predicted. It is, therefore, unsafe to drink and drive at any time.

- From the first drink, alcohol impairs motor skills, judgment, reaction time and other abilities needed for safe driving.

The toll of alcohol abuse in society includes automobile death rates, other injuries and huge medical costs spent on alcohol-related health problems such as liver disease and cardiovascular conditions. Millions of victims of alcohol-related injuries and illnesses are brought to hospital emergency departments every year. Over 10,000 people die each year in the United States as the result of alcohol-related crashes, accounting for 31% of all traffic deaths.[2]

[1]*National Institute on Drug Abuse, drugabuse.gov Accessed January 2016.*

[2]*National Highway Traffic Safety Administration nrd.nhtsa.dot. gov/Pubs/812102.pdf Accessed January 2016.*

Illicit drugs include marijuana, cocaine, heroin, hallucinogens, inhalants and the nonmedical use of prescription pain relievers, tranquilizers, stimulants and sedatives. Like alcohol abuse, illicit drug abuse typically begins in the preteen years, peaks in the late teen and early adult years and gradually becomes less common thereafter. Marijuana is the most commonly used illicit drug.

Perhaps most alarming is the increase in drug overdose deaths in the United States. The increasing annual number of overdose deaths continues a decades-long trend for prescription drugs, prescription opioid pain relievers and benzodiazepines (tranquilizers). Most striking is a catastrophic rise in heroin overdose deaths across America **(Figure 18-1)**. In 2014, over 47,000 deaths resulted from all drug overdoses.[1]

[1]*Centers for Disease Control and Prevention, cdc.gov/media/ releases/2015/p1218-drug-overdose.html Accessed January 2016.*

FIGURE 18-1

Number of deaths from heroin overdoses in the United States.

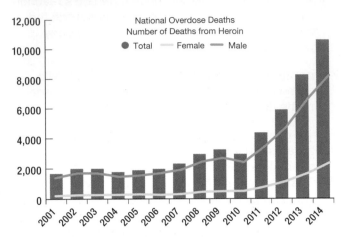

Source: National Institute on Drug Abuse.

Prevention of Substance Abuse

Because alcohol and other drug abuse typically begin at young ages, most prevention efforts focus on children and adolescents. Because the individual and community factors involved in substance abuse are so complex, prevention programs must focus on a wide range of issues if they are to be successful. The National Institute on Drug Abuse has identified 16 principles that should be considered when designing a successful abuse prevention program:

1. Prevention programs should enhance protective factors and reverse or reduce risk factors.

   • The risk of becoming a drug abuser involves the relationship among the number and type of risk factors (e.g., deviant attitudes and behaviors) and protective factors (e.g., parental support).

   • The potential impact of specific risk and protective factors changes with age. For example, risk factors within the family have greater impact on a younger child, while association with drug-abusing peers may be a more significant risk factor for an adolescent.

   • Early intervention with risk factors (e.g., aggressive behavior and poor self-control) often has a greater impact than later intervention by changing a child's life path (trajectory) away from problems and toward positive behaviors.

   • While risk and protective factors can affect people of all groups, these factors can have a different effect depending on a person's age, gender, ethnicity, culture and environment.

2. Prevention programs should address all forms of drug abuse, alone or in combination, including the underage use of legal drugs (e.g., tobacco or alcohol); the use of illegal drugs (e.g., marijuana or heroin); and the inappropriate use of legally obtained substances (e.g., inhalants), prescription medications or over-the-counter drugs.

3. Prevention programs should address the type of drug abuse problem in the local community, target modifiable risk factors and strengthen identified protective factors.

4. Prevention programs should be tailored to address risks specific to population or audience characteristics, such as age, gender and ethnicity, to improve program effectiveness.

5. Family-based prevention programs should enhance family bonding and relationships and include parenting skills; practice in developing, discussing and enforcing family policies on substance abuse; and training in drug education and information.

6. Prevention programs can be designed to intervene as early as preschool to address risk factors for drug abuse, such as aggressive behavior, poor social skills and academic difficulties.

7. Prevention programs for elementary school children should target improving academic and social-emotional learning to address risk factors for drug abuse, such as early aggression, academic failure and school dropout. Education should focus on the following skills:

   • self-control

   • emotional awareness

   • communication

   • social problem-solving

   • academic support, especially in reading

8. Prevention programs for middle or junior high and high school students should increase academic and social competence with the following skills:

    • study habits and academic support

    • communication

    • peer relationships

    • self-efficacy and assertiveness

    • drug resistance skills

    • reinforcement of anti-drug attitudes

    • strengthening of personal commitments against drug abuse

9. Prevention programs aimed at general populations at key transition points, such as the transition to middle school, can produce beneficial effects even among high-risk families and children. Such interventions do not single out risk populations, and therefore, reduce labeling and promote bonding, to school and community.

10. Community prevention programs that combine two or more effective programs, such as family-based and school-based programs, can be more effective than a single program alone.

11. Community prevention programs reaching populations in multiple settings—for example, schools, clubs, faith-based organizations and the media—are most effective when they present consistent, community-wide messages in each setting.

12. When communities adapt programs to match their needs, community norms or differing cultural requirements, they should retain core elements of the original research-based intervention which include:

    • Structure (how the program is organized and constructed);

    • Content (the information, skills and strategies of the program); and

    • Delivery (how the program is adapted, implemented and evaluated).

13. Prevention programs should be long term with repeated interventions (i.e., booster programs) to reinforce the original prevention goals. Research shows that the benefits from middle school prevention programs diminish without follow-up programs in high school.

14. Prevention programs should include teacher training on good classroom management practices, such as rewarding appropriate student behavior. Such techniques help to foster students' positive behavior, achievement, academic motivation and school bonding.

15. Prevention programs are most effective when they employ interactive techniques, such as peer discussion groups and parent role-playing, that allow for active involvement in learning about drug abuse and reinforcing skills.

16. Research-based prevention programs can be cost effective. Similar to earlier research, recent research shows that for each dollar invested in prevention, a savings of up to $10 in treatment for alcohol or other substance abuse can be seen.

[1]*National Institute on Drug Abuse, drugabuse.gov/publications/ preventing-drug-abuse-among-children-adolescents-in-brief/ prevention-principles Accessed January 2016.*

Studies have shown that many prevention programs are having a positive effect. Youths exposed to substance abuse prevention messages in or outside of school, who have talked with their parents about the dangers of drug and alcohol use and who have participated in various special programs are all less likely to use or abuse alcohol and other drugs. But as the earlier statistics show, abuse remains a huge problem, and clearly, more efforts are needed both to understand the many complex factors involved in substance abuse behavior and to develop prevention strategies to successfully counter those factors.

Prevention of Drug Misuse and Overdose

Substance abuse is the intentional and often frequent nonmedical use of a substance for its effects, typically without regard for potential negative health effects. **Substance misuse,** in contrast, may involve using a drug for an unintended purpose or using it in larger amounts than prescribed, including unintentional misuse. Misuse may occur, for example, if a person takes more of a medication than prescribed either by mistake or from a false belief that more of the medication is better.

Because misuse, like abuse, can lead to a drug **overdose,** it is important to take steps to prevent it:

- Use medications only as prescribed and read product information.

- Keep all medications in their original, clearly labeled containers. Check the label before taking the medication. (Never take a medication in the dark.) Help the elderly organize their medications to prevent accidental overdose.

- If a person's judgment may be diminished by a medical or other condition, make sure that the person cannot unintentionally use too much of any prescribed or over-the-counter medication.

- Read and follow the directions and warnings on the label before taking any medicine.

- If you have any questions about the intended use of your medicine, contact your doctor.

- Some medicines are dangerous when mixed with alcohol. Consult your doctor or pharmacist.

- Be aware of potential drug interactions. Some medicines interact dangerously with food or other medicines. Your doctor should be made aware of all medicines, prescription or over-the-counter, you are currently taking. Talk to your doctor before taking any natural or herbal supplements.

- Dispose of old and outdated medicines. Some medications can become dangerous or ineffective over time.

- Never share prescription medicines. Medicines should be taken by the person to whom they are prescribed and for the reason prescribed.

- Remember that any over-the-counter drug, including herbal supplements, vitamins and natural remedies, can be toxic in doses larger than recommended in the product information.

 LEARNING CHECKPOINT 1

1. Select the best answer. The most commonly abused drugs in the United States are –

   a. alcohol and marijuana.

   b. marijuana and cocaine.

   c. cocaine and pain relievers.

   d. heroin and hallucinogens.

2. Substance abuse prevention efforts should focus on people in what age group(s)?

   _____

3. Put a check mark next to all actions that are appropriate for helping to prevent the misuse of prescribed drugs.

   ☐ Take medications only when you feel the symptoms for which the medication is prescribed.

   ☐ Read product information that comes with prescription medications.

   ☐ Keep medications in their original labeled containers.

   ☐ Use medications prescribed for someone else only when you are certain you have the same condition as the person with the medication.

   ☐ Ensure that a person with diminished judgment cannot unintentionally take too much medication.

Intoxication

Excessive alcohol consumption causes problems that may lead to a medical emergency. In addition to the problems caused by intoxication, the person may have an injury or sudden illness requiring care. Remember to not assume that a victim is experiencing signs and symptoms only as a result of intoxication. In some cases, someone who behaves as if intoxicated may not have consumed alcohol at all but may be experiencing a problem such as a diabetic emergency that causes altered mental status.

Drinking a large amount of alcohol in a short period of time can lead to alcohol poisoning, which may result in unresponsiveness, seizures or death. Alcohol has depressant effects on the respiratory

---

First Aid: Intoxication

Signs, Symptoms and Care

WHEN YOU SEE

- Smell of alcohol about the person
- Flushed, moist face
- Vomiting
- Slurred speech or staggering
- Rapid heart rate
- Impaired judgment and motor skills
- Agitated or combative behavior
- Changing levels of responsiveness, coma

DO THIS FIRST

1. Check for injuries or illness. Do not assume alcohol is the factor, or the only factor, involved.

2. For a responsive, intoxicated person:

   a. Stay with the person and protect him or her from injury (take away car keys).

   b. Do not let the person lie down on his or her back.

   c. Care for any injuries.

   d. Calm and reassure the person.

   e. If you have any doubt about whether the person may be injured or ill, may have consumed a dangerous amount of alcohol or may injure his- or herself or others, call 9-1-1 and let the dispatcher decide what help is needed.

3. For an unresponsive, intoxicated person:

   a. Position the victim in the recovery position; be prepared for vomiting.

   b. Monitor the victim's breathing and be prepared to provide BLS if necessary.

   c. Call 9-1-1 if the victim's breathing is irregular, if seizures occur or if the victim cannot be roused (coma).

4. For an injured, intoxicated person:

   a. Because alcohol may keep the person from feeling pain, do not rely on the victim's perception of an injury to guide your care.

   b. Give first aid as you would if the victim were unresponsive, based on your assessment of the signs of injury or illness rather than reported symptoms.

   c. If the mechanism of injury suggests the victim could have a spinal injury, do not move the victim; instead, keep the head aligned with the body.

ADDITIONAL CARE

- In a cold environment, an intoxicated person is likely to experience hypothermia because dilated, peripheral blood vessels allow the body's heat to escape more easily. Take steps to keep the victim warm (see **Chapter 20**).

ALERT

- Intoxication makes some people hostile and violent. Stay a distance away and call law enforcement if the person threatens violence.

system and can cause an overdose similar to that of depressant drugs. First aid focuses on ensuring that the person receives medical care if needed and protecting the person from injury due to the intoxication (see First Aid: "Intoxication").

ALCOHOL WITHDRAWAL

Someone who drinks heavily for a long time may develop a physical **dependence** on alcohol. **Withdrawal** from alcohol dependence may then cause delirium tremens (sometimes called "the DTs"), an altered mental status characterized by confusion, disorientation, agitation and altered perception such as hallucinations or illusions (see First Aid: "Alcohol Withdrawal").

First Aid: Alcohol Withdrawal

Signs, Symptoms and Care

WHEN YOU SEE

- Hand trembling, head shaking

- Nausea or vomiting

- Seizures

- Hallucination, irrational fears or extreme confusion

- Unusual behavior

DO THIS FIRST

1. Call 9-1-1.

2. Give first aid as for an intoxicated victim, including the use of the recovery position for an unresponsive victim and monitoring breathing.

ADDITIONAL CARE

- Stay with the victim and protect him or her from injury until help arrives.

Drug Abuse

Illicit drugs and prescription drugs used for non-medical purposes cause a wide variety of effects, depending on the type of drug and the amount used **(Figure 18-2).** The primary effects of drugs commonly abused are described in **Table 18-2.** In most cases, you do not need to know the type of drug taken in order to care for the victim. Consider the possibility of drug abuse or overdose whenever a victim's behavior or signs and symptoms cannot otherwise be explained. Observe the scene for drug paraphernalia, such as needles and syringes; eyedroppers; burnt spoons; straws or rolled-up dollar bills used for snorting; pipes; glass bulbs; razor blades; paper or plastic bags reeking of inhalants; or bottles of pills, powder or liquid **(Figure 18-3).**

FIGURE 18-2

Illicit drugs.

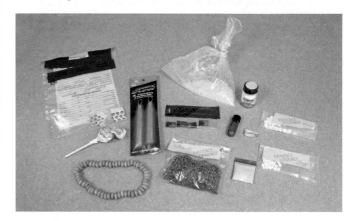

FIGURE 18-3

Drug paraphernalia.

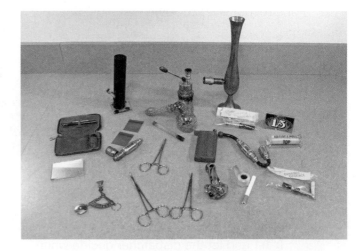

FIRST AID FOR DRUG ABUSE OR OVERDOSE

The signs and symptoms of drug abuse and overdose vary widely, depending on the type and amount of the substance taken, but first aid follows the same general principles (see **Table 18-2**). Remember that a drug overdose is a type of poisoning. If you know the drug or other substance taken, call the Poison Control Center (PCC) and follow the instructions given (see **Chapter 17**). Otherwise, call 9-1-1 and provide supportive care and give first aid for any injuries until help arrives (see First Aid: "Drug Abuse or Overdose").

The first aid for an opioid drug overdose may be different from other drug overdose emergencies because an emergency medication may be available to counteract the effects of the opioid drug. This special situation is described in the later section "Opioid Drug Overdose."

In some cases, an overdose victim may become violent or suicidal or may act bizarrely under the influence of the drug. Remember the general rule to never enter a scene that is dangerous; withdraw from the scene if a victim's behavior becomes threatening. Note that when illegal drugs are involved, this is also a crime scene: be very careful to avoid potential dangers. **Chapter 21**, "Behavioral Emergencies," provides more information about dealing with victims who act in unusual or unpredictable ways.

TABLE 18-2

Effects Of Commonly Abused Drugs

Drug Class or Type	Septic Drugs	Examples of Street Names	Common Effects
Marijuana	Marijuana, hashish	Grass, pot, dope, weed, bamba, ganja, joint	Elation, relaxation, dizziness, distorted perceptions, hunger, fast pulse
Opioid narcotics	Heroin, morphine, codeine, oxycodone (OxyContin, Percocet, Percodan)	H, horse, junk, stuff, smack, scag, poppy, ox, OCs, perc	Euphoria or stupor, depressant effects, dizziness, pain relief, muscle relaxation, impaired judgment, slowed respiration, coughing and sniffing, contracted pupils, slurred speech
Hallucinogens	LSD, PCP, mescaline, psilocybin	Acid, purple hearts, angel dust, peyote mushrooms	Stimulant effects, hallucinations, disorientation, anxiety, paranoia, trance-like state, euphoria, dilated pupils, fast pulse
Inhalants	Amyl nitrite, butyl nitrite, nitrous oxide, many solvents and common household products	Sniffing, huffing, snorting, bagging	Mood alterations, depressant or stimulant effects, nausea, excitability, slurred speech, impaired coordination
Stimulants	Amphetamine, methamphetamine, dextroamphetamine, cocaine and crack cocaine, designer drugs such as "ecstasy"	Speed, bennies, uppers, pep pills, white crosses, dex, ice, crank, rock, coke, snow, flake	Increased mental alertness, physical energy, talkativeness, restlessness, irritability or aggressive behavior, dilated pupils, increased respiration and blood pressure
Sedatives, depressants, tranquilizers	Barbiturates, benzodiazepines, muscle relaxants	Downers, goofballs, reds, ludes	Decreased mental alertness, relaxation, dizziness, slurred speech, dilated pupils, nausea and vomiting, delusions, slowed respiration and pulse

First Aid: Drug Abuse or Overdose

Signs, Symptoms and Care

WHEN YOU SEE

- Unusual or erratic behavior

- The signs and symptoms of drug abuse

- Drug paraphernalia

DO THIS FIRST

1. Call 9-1-1 for serious signs and symptoms or call the Poison Control Center for instructions if you know the substance taken and the symptoms are not serious.

2. Some drugs cause violent behavior. If the victim demonstrates a potential for violent behavior, withdraw and wait for help to arrive.

3. Put an unresponsive victim in the recovery position (if no suspected trauma, especially a neck, back, hip or pelvic injury); monitor breathing and give BLS as needed.

4. Check the victim for any injuries requiring care, and provide care for any condition that occurs (seizures, shock, cardiac arrest, etc.).

5. Try to keep the victim awake and talking.

6. Keep the victim from harming himself or herself or others.

7. Question the victim and others present at the scene about the drug or substance used, the amount used and when it was used. Give this information to arriving EMS personnel. For an opioid drug overdose, check the scene for an emergency overdose kit (see First Aid: "Opioid Drug Overdose").

ADDITIONAL CARE

- Try to keep the victim calm.

ALERT

- Do not try to induce vomiting, which may cause further harm and is unlikely to help the victim.

- Some drugs make people hostile and violent. Stay a safe distance away and call law enforcement if you feel threatened.

Opioid Drug Overdose

Because opioid drug overdose emergencies have become increasingly common, many first aiders may encounter this special resuscitation situation. Opioid drugs include heroin, morphine, oxycodone (such as OxyContin), methadone, hydrocodone (such as Vicodin), codeine and some other prescription pain medications. If a victim is unresponsive despite efforts to wake him or her, and no other cause is apparent, you should consider an opioid overdose as a possible cause. This is especially important when the person is known to use prescription pain medications or recreational opioids.

Because of their effects on the part of the brain that regulates breathing, opioids in high doses can cause respiratory depression leading to cardiac arrest and death. Combining an opioid with alcohol or a sedative medication increases the risk of respiratory depression and death, and such combinations are often present in fatal drug overdoses.

An opioid overdose can be identified by a combination of three signs often called the "opioid overdose triad."

These signs are pinpoint pupils that do not react to light, unresponsiveness despite your best efforts to wake the victim and respiratory depression. The victim may be breathing at a rate of only 2-4 breaths a minute, and breathing may sound like snoring or choking. In severe cases, the victim may have become hypoxic due to the respiratory depression, manifesting the signs that are common in near-death situations: The victim's skin may look dusky, the lips and nail beds may turn bluish or ashen, and the pulse may be slow and erratic or so weak that it is undetectable. Seizures may occur.

In addition, it is important to examine the scene for evidence of drug use, such as the presence of a pill bottle or drug paraphernalia, and to talk to others at the scene. Family members or friends may identify the victim's drug use, or unacquainted bystanders may be able to provide information about how the victim was behaving before becoming unresponsive.

To care for a victim who is unresponsive due to a suspected opioid drug overdose, first try to learn what drug was taken and call 9-1-1. As usual, call immediately for an unresponsive victim. Perform the initial assessment and be prepared to provide basic life support until help arrives.

In addition, if possible, administer naloxone to the victim to counteract the opioid drug's effects. Naloxone is the drug in an emergency overdose kit (such as Narcan). A naloxone emergency kit may be present at the scene, or the victim's family may have or know of a nearby emergency kit. Naloxone may be administered intramuscularly via an auto-injector (like an emergency epinephrine auto-injector for a severe allergic reaction) or intranasally via a nasal device. To administer the drug, always follow the instructions on the kit. Additional doses may be required if the victim's signs do not improve before emergency personnel arrive. Note that you do not have to be absolutely certain that the victim has taken an opioid drug, because naloxone will not harm a victim with these signs and symptoms due to some other cause (see First Aid: "Opioid Drug Overdose").

First Aid: Opioid Drug Overdose

Signs, Symptoms and Care

WHEN YOU SEE

- Pinpoint pupils

- Unresponsiveness

- Slow, shallow breathing

- In severe cases, victim's lips and nail beds may turn bluish or ashen, seizures may occur

DO THIS FIRST

1. If the victim is unresponsive despite efforts to wake him or her, consider opioid overdose a possible cause, especially when the person is known to use prescription pain medications or recreational opioid drugs.

2. Try to find out what drug was taken and call 9-1-1.

3. Check for an emergency overdose kit at the scene (naloxone or Narcan) in either nasal administration or auto-injector. Ask others at the scene if they know if an overdose kit is available.

4. Administer the emergency overdose medication to the victim, following the manufacturer's directions on the kit.

ADDITIONAL CARE

- Put a breathing, unresponsive victim in the recovery position (if no suspected trauma, especially a neck, back, hip or pelvic injury), and be ready to give basic life support if needed.

Following are the general steps for using an auto-injector for an opioid drug overdose. Be sure to follow the instructions on the specific product.

1. Prepare the auto-injector for use. Remove it from its case and remove the safety guard.

2. To administer the medication, press the auto-injector firmly against the victim's outer thigh. Follow the manufacturer's instructions for how long to hold the device in place to ensure all of the medication has been delivered.

3. Ensure 9-1-1 has been called. Monitor the victim's symptoms and be prepared to give basic life support as needed.

4. If the victim's symptoms continue or return after the first dose, administer a second dose using a second auto-injector, if EMS personnel have not arrived. Follow the instructions on the package.

Following are the steps for CPR and AED in opioid drug overdose:

1. For an unresponsive victim who is not breathing or only gasps occasionally, send someone to call 9-1-1 (or your local emergency number) and get an AED and naloxone. If alone with the victim, first give 2 minutes of CPR and then call 9-1-1 and get naloxone and an AED if available.

2. Administer naloxone as soon as available; may repeat after 4 minutes.

3. If the victim does not respond or begin breathing regularly, continue CPR and use the AED as soon as available.

4. Continue to check for responsiveness and normal breathing until EMS personnel arrive. If the victim responds or begins breathing regularly, continue to monitor and be prepared to renew CPR and repeat naloxone if the victim stops responding.

Medication Overdose

Although many drug overdoses occur in people intentionally abusing drugs, overdose may also result from drug misuse, including unintentional drug poisoning caused by taking too much of a prescription or over-the-counter medication. A person having an overdose of a prescription medication may experience a wide range of behaviors and symptoms, depending on the drug. Drug withdrawal can also be an emergency. In some cases, it is impossible to know whether behaviors or symptoms are caused by drugs or by an injury or sudden illness. While caring for the victim, try to determine what drug the person may have taken: Ask family members or others present at the scene, and look for pill bottles or other evidence of medications taken (see First Aid: "Medication Overdose").

First Aid: Medication Overdose

Signs, Symptoms and Care

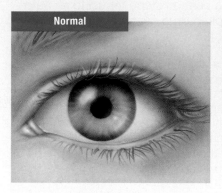
Normal

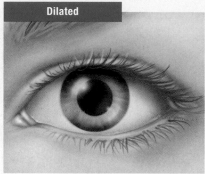
Dilated

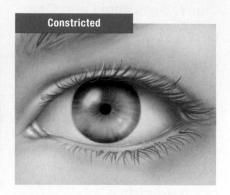
Constricted

WHEN YOU SEE

- Very small or large pupils of the eye

- Stumbling, clumsiness, drowsiness or incoherent speech

- Difficulty breathing (very slow or fast)

- Irrational or violent behavior

- Changing levels of responsiveness

DO THIS FIRST

1. Put an unresponsive victim in the recovery position, monitor breathing and be prepared to give BLS as needed. Call 9-1-1.

2. For a responsive victim, first, be sure that it is safe to approach the person. If the victim's behavior is erratic or violent, call 9-1-1 and stay a safe distance away.

3. Try to find out what drug the victim took. If there is evidence of an overdose, call 9-1-1.

4. If symptoms are minor and you know the substance taken, call the Poison Control Center and follow the instructions given.

5. If the victim vomits, save a sample for arriving medical personnel. Do not try to induce vomiting, which may cause further harm and is unlikely to help the victim.

ADDITIONAL CARE

- Monitor the victim's condition while waiting for help.

- Provide care for any condition that occurs (seizures, shock, cardiac arrest. etc.).

LEARNING CHECKPOINT 2

1. Describe what to do for an intoxicated person who "passes out."

   _____

   _____

   _____

   _____

2. How is alcohol similar to narcotic drugs in high doses? Select the best answer.

   a. Both stimulate the user to increased mental alertness.

   b. Both are depressants and can lead to impaired respiration or coma.

   c. Both can cause dangerously high blood pressure and internal bleeding.

   d. All of the above

3. Check off appropriate actions to take for a person with a drug or medication overdose.

   ☐ Position an unresponsive victim on the back with legs raised (shock position).

   ☐ Call 9-1-1 or the Poison Control Center.

   ☐ Restrain a potentially violent person to prevent self-injury.

   ☐ Check for injuries that may require first aid.

   ☐ Induce vomiting if the person is responsive.

   ☐ Try to keep the person awake and talking.

   ☐ Try to find out what the person took.

CONCLUDING THOUGHTS

Although substance abuse is a huge problem in our society, do not jump to the conclusion that someone who is behaving oddly must be on drugs. Remember that many illnesses and injuries also cause altered mental status that may lead to unusual behaviors. Take the time to assess the victim and situation and to call for help and give first aid when needed. Whenever giving first aid, it is important not to be judgmental – a state of mind that could lead to not providing the best care for a person in need.

CRITICAL THINKING CHALLENGE QUESTIONS

SCENARIO 1

You enter a room where your Aunt is closing a medication container, saying she has just taken her prescribed daily pills. Then, she admits she was interrupted by a telephone call, and in her confusion, may have taken too many. Now she is feeling a little drowsy. Is there reason to be concerned? What should you do?

   _____

   _____

   _____

SCENARIO 2

You are at a party on campus where some of the students are drinking excessively and you suspect a few may be using drugs. A man bursts into the room from the hallway leading to the bedrooms, looking very distraught, and says, "Man, Sandra's really out of it! She's really sick." No one else seems to be paying attention, so you ask him what is wrong. He is incoherent, however, repeating over and over in a slurred voice that she's sick, and you notice that the pupils of his eyes are very dilated.

a. You go to the bedroom and find a woman on the bed, who has just vomited. You ask if she needs help, and she seems unable to focus on you. She says nothing. What should you do?

   _____

   _____

   _____

b. You ask again if you can help and she shakes her head violently. A moment later, her eyes close and she seems to have passed out. Her breathing is slow. You try to rouse her, but cannot. Now what should you do?

   _____

   _____

ADDITIONAL ACTIVITIES AND RESOURCES

Patterns of alcohol and drug abuse vary widely in different regions of the country (and even within specific regions). Research the most significant abuse problems in your particular area or even on your own campus. Sources of information may include the student health center, local law enforcement authorities and the Internet. Specific topics for research can include statistics related to problems of abuse and current preventive programs. National-level research may include Internet searches for prevention programs that have been successful in other regions or states and the potential for their success in your area.

 REVIEW QUESTIONS

Select the best answers.

1. To help prevent drug misuse or overdose in an elderly person who is taking prescription medications –

   a. consult with a health care provider or pharmacist before allowing the person to drink alcohol while using the drug.

   b. always have the person take all medications at the same time.

   c. have the person drink lots of water while taking the medications.

   d. monitor the person continually for 2 hours after each dose.

2. Substance abuse prevention programs involve –

   a. youths at risk.

   b. parents and families.

   c. schools and communities.

   d. All of the above

3. Alcohol poisoning may cause –

   a. diabetes.

   b. seizures.

   c. heart attack.

   d. anaphylaxis.

4. Assessment of an intoxicated victim's injuries depends mostly on –

   a. the visible signs of injury.

   b. the victim's mental status when first encountered.

   c. the victim's reported symptoms.

   d. how much alcohol the victim drank.

5. Alcohol withdrawal in a dependent person may cause –

   a. anaphylaxis.

   b. permanent psychosis.

   c. hallucinations.

   d. circulation problems.

6. You are giving first aid to a man who seems mildly "high." He tells you he took two "percs." To determine how best to treat him, whom should you call for more information?

   a. Law enforcement personnel

   b. A family member

   c. The Poison Control Center

   d. The federal drug information website

7. First aid for a drug overdose is generally the same as first aid for –

   a. poisoning.

   b. stroke.

   c. diabetic coma.

   d. hypothermia.

8. A drug overdose may occur with –

   a. illicit drugs.

   b. non-prescription medication.

   c. small amounts of some substances.

   d. All of the above

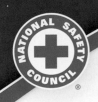

CHAPTER 19

Bites and Stings

LESSON OBJECTIVES

- List guidelines for preventing common bites and stings.

- Explain the risk of infection from common types of bites and stings.

- Describe the first aid to give in cases of bites and stings not involving severe symptoms or an allergic reaction.

- List signs and symptoms for which you should call 9-1-1 after a bite or sting.

- Describe how to remove an embedded tick and the stinger from a bee or wasp.

You are at the beach boardwalk with your family on a bright summer day. The girls are thirsty, so Mom opens a carton of juice and pours it into cups, trying to ignore a wasp that has appeared and is buzzing around the juice. As the toddler takes her first sip, she slaps at the wasp, which stings her lip. Her juice spills everywhere, she is screaming with pain and the wasp is now nowhere to be seen. What, if anything, should you do?

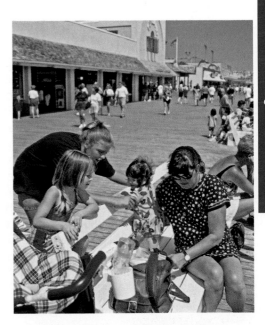

Every year, millions of people are bitten or stung by animals, snakes, spiders, insects and marine life, making this a significant first aid issue. Fortunately, the majority of cases are not medical emergencies, but oftentimes, medical treatment is needed for bleeding, wound care or to treat infection or a reaction to an injected poison. In some cases, particularly when the victim is allergic, a medical emergency does occur, and appropriate, timely first aid is needed.

Animal Bites

Millions of people are bitten by dogs in the United States every year, followed by a large number of cat bites and a much lower number of bites from other domestic or wild animals. More than 32,000 dog bites are serious enough to require emergency department treatment and, on average, about 34 people a year die from dog bites.[1] Most victims are young children who often have not learned how to act around dogs and other animals. With an estimated 77 million pet dogs in the United States,[2] it is crucial that children as well as adults learn how to safely interact with dogs and other animals kept as pets **(Box 19-1)**. In general, most bites occur to the arm or hand, followed by the leg or foot, but in children younger than 4, many sustain injury to the head or neck – an often dangerous injury.

[1]*National Safety Council. Injury Facts®, 2015 Edition. Itasca, IL: Author.*

[2]*Humane Society of the United States, humanesociety.org/ issues/pet_overpopulation/facts/pet_ownership_statistics.html Accessed January 2016.*

Animal bites can be serious for 3 reasons. Depending on the location and depth of the bite injury, bleeding can be serious. Control bleeding from an animal bite as you would bleeding caused by other injuries (see **Chapter 8**). Second, because bacteria are present in animals' mouths, there is a risk that the wound will become infected. Even a small wound from a dog bite can become infected; the bites of cats have an even higher risk. Give wound care to prevent infection (see **Chapter 10**) and consult with your health care provider to see if additional measures may be needed. Finally, the bite of any animal, even a house pet, carries the risk of **rabies.** This risk is much higher with wild animals, as most pets are vaccinated against rabies, but the risk is present with all animals.

In many other countries, dog bites are the most common source of rabies, and any dog bite should immediately be examined by a health care provider. Caused by a virus that can be transmitted by saliva into the blood of a bite victim, rabies remains a major threat in all areas of the United States even though vaccinations and other precautions have made it very rare in humans. Because rabies is fatal unless vaccination injections are given early, every bite from a mammal, domestic or wild, must be considered serious. Unless the bite occurs from your own pet and you are certain the animal's rabies vaccination is current, all dog and other animal bites should be reported to your local public health department or animal control office. Because the threat of rabies is so serious, many states have laws that require quarantining or observing any biting animal – even one with a current vaccination – to ensure that there is no risk for the bite victim. In most locations, any wild animal that bites a person is assumed to have rabies, unless the animal can be caught or killed and have its brain examined for the virus.

First aid for the bite of any animal focuses on controlling bleeding and on wound care to prevent infection. Wash the wound well and apply a sterile dressing (see **Chapter 10**). Seek medical attention immediately for a puncture wound, a wound to the head or neck and any bite wound from an animal that is not your own pet. Even with a superficial wound caused by the bite of your own pet, it is a good idea to contact your health care provider to see whether medical treatment may be needed. In all cases, observe the wound carefully over the next few days for any signs of infection (see First Aid: "Animal Bites").

BOX 19-1: PREVENTING DOG BITES

The CDC recommends the following to prevent dog bites and rabies:[2]

Before you bring a dog into your household:

- Consult with a professional (e.g., veterinarian, animal behaviorist or responsible breeder) to learn what breeds of dogs are the best fit for your household.

- Dogs with histories of aggression are not suitable for households with children.

- Be sensitive to cues that a child is fearful or apprehensive about a dog. If a child seems frightened by dogs, wait before bringing a dog into your household.

- Spend time with a dog before buying or adopting it. Use caution when bringing a dog into a household with an infant or toddler.

If you decide to bring a dog into your home:

- Spay/neuter your dog (this often reduces aggressive tendencies).

- Never leave infants or young children alone with a dog.

- Don't play aggressive games with your dog (e.g., wrestling).

- Properly socialize and train any dog entering your household. Teach the dog submissive behaviors (e.g., rolling over to expose the abdomen and giving up food without growling).

- Immediately seek professional advice (e.g., from veterinarians, animal behaviorists or responsible breeders) if the dog develops aggressive or undesirable behaviors.

To help prevent children from being bitten by dogs, teach the following basic safety tips and review them regularly:

Do:

- Remain motionless (e.g., "be still like a tree") when approached by an unfamiliar dog.

- Curl into a ball with your head tucked and your hands over your ears and neck if a dog knocks you over.

- Immediately let an adult know about stray dogs or dogs that are behaving strangely.

Don't:

- Approach an unfamiliar dog.

- Run from a dog.

- Panic or make loud noises.

- Disturb a dog that is sleeping, eating or caring for puppies.

- Pet a dog without allowing it to see and sniff you first.

- Encourage your dog to play aggressively.

- Let small children play with a dog unsupervised.

If approached by an unfamiliar dog:

- Stop! Stay still and be calm.

- Do not panic or make loud noises.

- Avoid direct eye contact with the dog.

- Say "No" or "Go Home" in a firm, deep voice.

- Stand with the side of your body facing the dog. Facing a dog directly can appear aggressive to the dog. Instead, keep your body turned partially or completely to the side.

- Slowly raise your hands to your neck, with your elbows in.

- Wait for the dog to pass or slowly back away.

Source: Centers for Disease Control and Prevention, cdc.gov/features/dog-bite-prevention/index.html Accessed January 2016.

First Aid: Animal Bites

Signs, Symptoms and Care

WHEN YOU SEE

- Any animal bite

DO THIS FIRST

1. Clean the wound with large amounts of warm or room-temperature water with or without soap (except when bleeding is severe).

2. Control bleeding.

3. Cover the wound with a sterile dressing and bandage (see **Chapter 10**).

4. The victim should see a health care provider or go to the emergency department right away.

ADDITIONAL CARE

- Report all animal bites to local animal control officers or police. The law requires certain procedures to be followed when rabies is a risk.

- An antibiotic ointment may be applied to a shallow wound (but not a puncture) before dressing it, if the victim is not allergic to the antibiotic.

ALERT

- Do not try to catch any animal that may have rabies, but note its appearance and describe it to the health care provider.

Human Bites

Small children often bite others when angry or acting out. Human bites are rarer among adults, but the same result may occur in a fight if someone's knuckles strike another person's teeth and break the skin. Because our mouths harbor many bacteria, a bite from a human can cause an infection the same as an animal bite. Because many of the pathogens that are harmless in the mouth can cause serious infection if they enter the blood, all human bites should be seen by a health care provider (see First Aid: "Human Bites").

First Aid: Human Bites

Signs, Symptoms and Care

WHEN YOU SEE

- A human bite

- Open puncture wound

- Bleeding

DO THIS FIRST

1. Clean the wound with large amounts of warm or room-temperature water with or without soap (except when bleeding is severe).

2. Control bleeding.

3. Cover the wound with a sterile dressing and bandage (see **Chapter 10**).

4. The victim should see a health care provider or go to the emergency department right away.

ADDITIONAL CARE

- If any tissue has been bitten off, bring it with the victim to the emergency department.

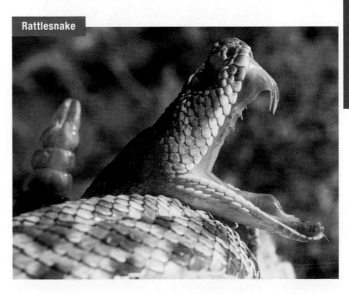

LEARNING CHECKPOINT 1

1. Select the best answer. To minimize the risk of rabies from an animal bite, you should take which action?

   a. See a health care provider immediately.

   b. See a health care provider if you experience heavy salivation 5-7 days after the bite.

   c. Capture the animal and take it to a veterinarian for examination.

   d. Soak the wound area with rubbing alcohol.

2. Why can a human bite lead to a serious medical condition?

   _____

   _____

   _____

   _____

Snake Bites

Poisonous snakes in North America include rattlesnakes, copperheads, water moccasins (cottonmouths), coral snakes and exotic species kept in captivity **(Figure 19-1).** An estimated 7,000-8,000 bites from venomous snakes occur every year in the United States, causing an average of 5 deaths annually.[1] World travelers should be aware, however, that snake bites in many other countries are more common and more lethal, causing about 30,000 deaths annually worldwide.

[1]Centers for Disease Control and Prevention, cdc.gov/niosh/ topics/snakes/default.html Accessed January 2016.

Snake bite statistics in the United States reveal an interesting pattern. Most venomous snake bites occur in adolescent and young adult males, and most of these occur on the hands and arms. Alcohol is often involved, and many of these victims were trying to impress their friends by handling or molesting the snake. Clearly, the first step in preventing a snake bite is to avoid a snake when one is seen **(Box 19-2).**

Even with venomous snakes, in about half of bite cases, the snake does not inject venom. In all, the risk of a lethal snake bite is very low. Nonetheless, people who live or work in areas where venomous snakes are common should take preventive steps and know what first aid to give in case a bite occurs. Venomous snakes are most common in the Southeast and the Southwest United States. Rattlesnake bites cause the most snake bite deaths.

Unless you are absolutely certain that a victim's snake bite was from a nonpoisonous snake, treat all snake bites as potentially dangerous. First, calm the victim and have the victim remain still. Anything that increases the heart rate, including strong emotions and physical movement, will speed the spread of the venom. Try to identify the snake species or be able to describe it to responding EMS personnel, because **antivenin** (antidote to the poison) is available in many areas where snake bites are common. Call 9-1-1. Wash the bite area and remove any constrictive jewelry or clothing from the limb, which will likely swell (see First Aid: "Snake Bites").

Many of the traditional myths and techniques for managing snake bites do not, in fact, improve the victim's condition or minimize the risk. Do not try to suck out the venom, do not cut across the fang holes in an attempt to remove the venom and do not put a tourniquet on the limb. In addition, do not put ice on the bite because of the potential for injuring tissue further with the cold.

For venomous snake bites, it is now recommended that a bitten extremity be wrapped snugly but not tightly with an elastic bandage; you should be able to insert one finger under the bandage. Wrap the entire length of the extremity, wrapping away from the body toward the end of the limb, to reduce the spread of the venom by slowing lymph flow. The extremity should also be immobilized, and the victim should receive medical attention as soon as possible.

FIGURE 19-1

Examples of poisonous snakes.

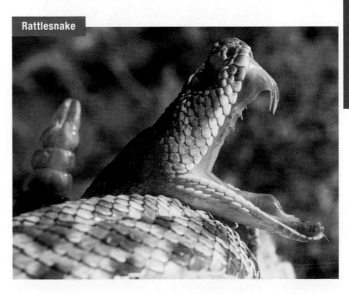

Rattlesnake

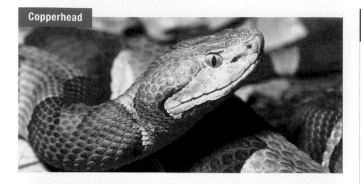

Copperhead

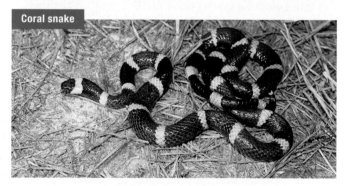

Yellow eyelash pit viper

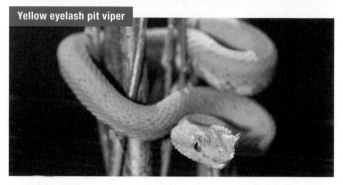

Coral snake

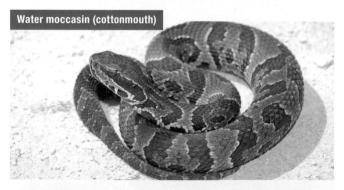

Water moccasin (cottonmouth)

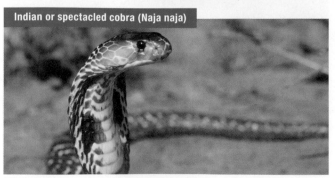

Indian or spectacled cobra (Naja naja)

BOX 19-2: PREVENTING SNAKE BITES

- Stay away from areas known to have snakes.

- If you see a snake, reverse your direction and retrace your steps, watching for other snakes.

- Stay away from underbrush areas, fallen trees and other areas where snakes may live.

The Arizona Poison and Drug Information Center (APDIC)[3] makes these additional recommendations for preventing snake bites in areas where venomous snakes are common:

- Leave wild animals alone. 50%-70% of reptile bites managed by the APDIC were provoked by the person who was bitten – that is, someone was trying to kill, capture or harass the animal.

- Be aware of peak movement times. During the hottest months, snakes will be most active at night. They may be encountered during the day in spring and fall or during a warm day in winter.

- Watch where you put your hands and feet. Try to keep your hands and feet out of crevices in rocks, wood piles and deep grass. Always carry a flashlight and wear shoes or boots when walking after dark.

- Dead snakes can bite. Never handle a venomous reptile, even after it is dead. Reflex strikes with injected venom can occur for several hours after death.

- Install outdoor lighting for yards, porches and sidewalks. If you see a venomous reptile in your yard, it is probably just "passing through." However, if you are concerned about a dangerous animal in your yard, seek professional assistance in removing it.

[3]*Arizona Poison and Drug Information Center, azpoison.com/venom/rattlesnakes Accessed January 2016.*

First Aid: Snake Bites

Signs, Symptoms and Care

WHEN YOU SEE

- Puncture marks on skin

- Complaint of pain or burning at bite site

- Redness and swelling

- Depending on species: difficulty breathing, numbness or muscle paralysis, nausea and vomiting, blurred vision, drowsiness or confusion, weakness

DO THIS FIRST

1. Have the victim lie down and stay calm. (Do not move the victim unless absolutely necessary.) Keep the bitten area immobile and below the level of the heart.

2. Call 9-1-1.

3. Wash the bite wound with large amounts of warm or room-temperature water with or without soap.

4. Wrap the extremity with a snug but not tight elastic bandage. Wrap away from the body toward the end of the limb. The pressure is sufficient if the bandage is snug but a finger can be slipped under it.

5. Remove jewelry or tight clothing before swelling begins.

ADDITIONAL CARE

- Do not try to catch the snake, but note its appearance and describe it to the health care provider.

- Monitor the victim's breathing and be ready to give CPR if needed.

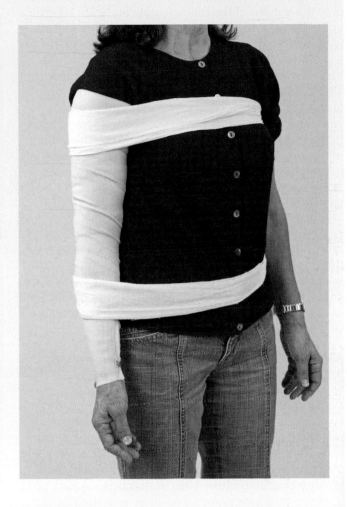

ALERT

- Do not put a tourniquet on the victim.

- Do not cut open the wound to try to drain out the venom or try to suck out the venom.

- Do not put ice on the bite.

Spider Bites

Many types of spiders bite, but in the United States, only the venom of the black widow and brown recluse spiders is serious and sometimes fatal. The black widow often has a red hourglass-shaped marking on the underside of the abdomen. The brown recluse has a violin-shaped marking on its back **(Figure 19-2).** Reliable statistics are not available for how many spider bites occur every year, but in recent years, only 3-7 deaths have resulted from venomous bites, mostly from black widow spiders.[1] The venom of the brown recluse spider can cause severe tissue damage, but rarely causes death.

Both species are more common in warm climates and generally live in areas that are dry and undisturbed. Outside the home, they are often found in woodpiles, sheds or debris. Inside the home, they may live in closets, rarely used cabinets, attics, crawl spaces and similar areas. Although these spiders are small and usually not seen before the bite occurs, preventive steps are important in areas where these spiders are known to live **(Box 19-3).**

Although the signs and symptoms of the bites of these 2 spiders vary, the first aid is generally the same. A black widow bite causes immediate pain, swelling and redness at the site, followed later by sweating, nausea, stomach and muscle cramps, headache, dizziness or weakness and possible difficulty breathing. A brown recluse bite causes more slowly developing pain or stinging at the site, followed later by blistering at the site, fever, chills, nausea or vomiting and joint pain; an open sore at the site will continue to grow without medical treatment.

With either bite, the victim needs emergency medical care. An antivenin is available for black widow spider bites. Wash the wound with soap and water to help prevent infection and apply an ice or a cold pack. Keep the bite area below the level of the heart (see First Aid: "Spider Bites").

[1]*National Safety Council. Injury Facts®, 2015 Edition. Itasca, IL: Author.*

FIGURE 19-2

Poisonous spiders.

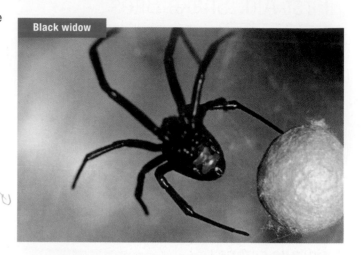

Black widow

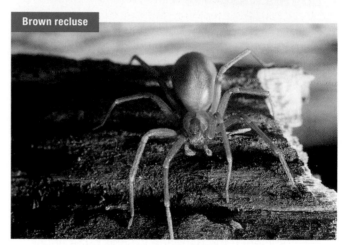

Brown recluse

BOX 19-3: PREVENTING SPIDER BITES

Neither black widow nor brown recluse spiders attack humans: they bite defensively when someone comes too close. Preventing these and other spider bites involves 2 types of actions: avoiding bites in places where spiders are likely and controlling spider populations.

AVOIDING SPIDER BITES

- Wear gloves and a long-sleeved shirt when cleaning basement or attic areas, seldom-used closets, sheds or garages and similar areas where spiders may live. Wear gloves when gathering wood from a woodpile.

- Before putting on long clothing or shoes that have been unused for a time, shake them out. Consider storing clothing and shoes in sealed plastic bags or boxes.

- Check inside tents, sleeping bags and other seldom-used equipment before using.

- Before sleeping in a bed that has not been used in a while, carefully check between the covers.

CONTROLLING SPIDER POPULATIONS

- Use appropriate pesticides or spider traps (glue traps) in areas where spiders or their nests have been identified.

- Thorough, routine housecleaning helps control spider populations. Vacuum up webs and egg sacs when they are seen and dispose of the vacuum bag.

- Reduce clutter in storage areas.

- Repair or seal off openings in screens, windows, chimneys and other openings through which spiders may enter the home.

- Clean up any debris around the home where spiders may breed.

First Aid: Spider Bites

Signs, Symptoms and Care

WHEN YOU SEE

For black widow bite:

- Complaint of pain or burning at bite site

- Red skin at site

- After 15 minutes and up to several hours: sweating, nausea, stomach and muscle cramps, increased pain at site, dizziness or weakness and difficulty breathing

For brown recluse bite:

- Stinging sensation at site

- Over 8-48 hours: increasing pain, blistering at site, fever, chills, nausea or vomiting, joint pain, open sore at site

DO THIS FIRST

1. If the victim has difficulty breathing, call 9-1-1 and be prepared to give CPR if needed. Call 9-1-1 immediately for a brown recluse spider bite.

2. Keep the bite area below the level of the heart.

3. Wash the area with soap and water.

4. Put ice or a cold pack on the bite area (with a damp cloth or paper towel between the cold pack and the skin). Apply the cold for 20 minutes (or 10 minutes if it produces discomfort), then remove it for 30 minutes; reapply for 20 (or 10) minutes, then remove again for 30 minutes.

ADDITIONAL CARE

- Try to safely identify the spider for the health care provider.

- If 9-1-1 was not called, the victim should go to the emergency department.

Tick Bites

Tick bites are not poisonous, but can transmit serious diseases, such as Rocky Mountain Spotted Fever or **Lyme disease (Figure 19-3).** Ticks cannot fly but will crawl up clothing or body areas that touch the ground or will fall off vegetation that one brushes against. Ticks may also be brought into the home in the fur of a dog or other pet that has picked up a tick outside. For guidelines to prevent tick bites, see **Box 19-4.**

FIGURE 19-3

Common types of ticks found in the United States. Only the blacklegged tick carries Lyme disease in the United States.

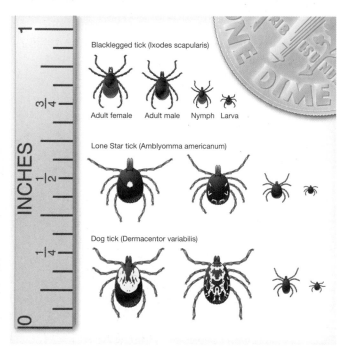

The tick usually crawls to an unexposed part of the body and bites into the skin, embedding its mouthparts in the skin to avoid being brushed off **(Figure 19-4).** Because ticks are very small and often seek unexposed areas to bite, such as the scalp, an embedded tick may not be found unless you search diligently. If not detected and removed, the tick may remain in the skin for days. A careless attempt to remove a tick may result in breaking off its body and leaving the head or mouthparts embedded in the skin, which could lead to infection. Remove a tick correctly by pulling gently but steadily with fine-tipped tweezers until the tick lets go. Then, wash the area well and apply an antibiotic cream.

FIGURE 19-4

Tick bite.

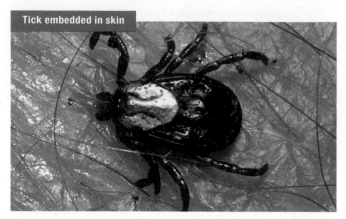

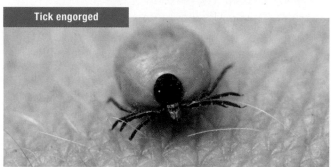

Medical treatment is not usually needed for tick bites. In areas where Lyme disease occurs frequently **(Box 19-4),** talk with your health care provider about whether treatment may be beneficial. Most importantly, after a tick bite, you should watch for the development of the signs and symptoms of Lyme disease. Lyme disease often produces a characteristic "bull's-eye" rash **(Figure 19-5),** typically 7-14 days after the bite, but sometimes as soon as 3 or as long as 30 days later. Other nonspecific symptoms include fever, headache, fatigue, muscle and joint pain or other flu-like symptoms (see First Aid: "Tick Bites").

FIGURE 19-5

Bull's-eye rash characteristic of Lyme disease.

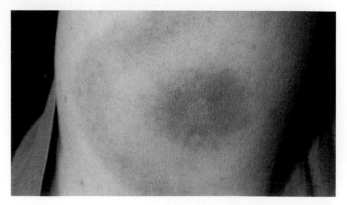

BOX 19-4: LYME DISEASE

Lyme disease, spread by ticks, is a potentially serious bacterial infection that has become a serious problem in many parts of the United States. Of the over 27,000 reported cases in 2013[1], most were in the Northeast or Upper Midwest, although as the map shows, people living in many other areas are at some risk. Lyme disease is a bacterial infectious disease that first causes fever, chills and other flu-like symptoms, and oftentimes, much later, causes heart and neurological problems. The longer the tick remains on the body, the greater the chance of transmitting the disease. Look for a bull's-eye rash that appears around the bite site 3-30 days later. Get medical attention if you have this rash or flu-like symptoms, or joint pain after a tick bite.

Preventing Tick Bites

- Keep lawns mowed, brush cleaned up and woodpiles stacked off the ground.

- Wear socks with shoes or boots. Tuck long pants into socks.

- Wear light-colored clothing, which makes it easier to see ticks before they reach your skin. Tuck your shirt into your pants.

- Do not lay clothing or towels on the ground.

- Walk in the middle of paths, away from tall grass and underbrush.

- Comb or brush your hair after being in an infested area.

- Check your body everywhere when bathing or showering, including your neck and scalp.

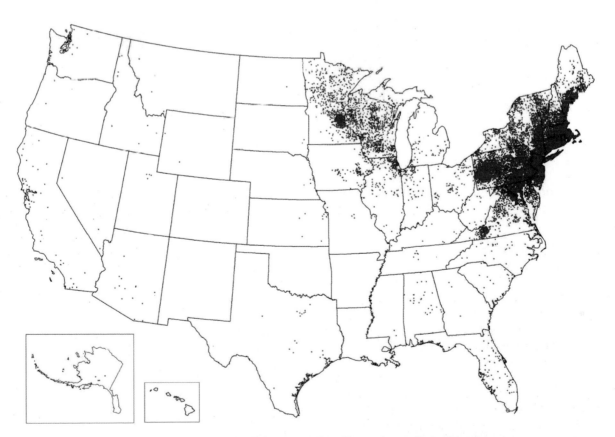

1 dot placed randomly within county of residence for each confirmed case

[1]*Centers for Disease Control and Prevention, cdc.gov/lyme/stats/tables.html Accessed January 2016.*

19 • Bites and Stings

First Aid: Tick Bites

Signs, Symptoms and Care

WHEN YOU SEE

• Tick embedded in skin

DO THIS FIRST

1. Remove the tick by grasping it close to the skin with tweezers and pulling very gently to "tent" the skin until the tick lets go. Avoid pulling hard or jerking, which may leave part of the tick embedded in the skin. Keep the tick for later identification.

2. Wash the area with soap and water.

3. Put an antiseptic on the site, such as rubbing alcohol or antibiotic cream, if the victim is not allergic to the antibiotic.

ADDITIONAL CARE

• Seek medical attention if a rash appears around the site or the victim later experiences fever, headache, chills, muscle and joint pain or other flu-like symptoms.

ALERT

• Do not try to remove an embedded tick by covering it with petroleum jelly, soaking it with bleach, burning it away with a hot pin or other object or similar methods. These methods may result in part of the tick remaining embedded in the skin.

✏ LEARNING CHECKPOINT 2

1. List 3 key actions to take for a victim of a snake bite.

   _____

   _____

   _____

   _____

2. Check off situations in which you should call 9-1-1 for a spider bite.

   ☐ All spider bites

   ☐ Any spider bite in a diabetic victim

   ☐ Any brown recluse spider bite

   ☐ If there is any pain at the bite site

   ☐ If the victim has trouble breathing

   ☐ If you have no ice to put on the bite

3. Fill in the correct answer: A tick is best removed from the skin using _____.

4. Select the best answer. A prominent initial sign of Lyme disease following a tick bite is –

   a. pain and burning at the site.

   b. a "bull's-eye" rash.

   c. high fever within 24 hours.

   d. All of the above

Mosquito Bites

With the spread of **West Nile virus (WNV)** throughout the United States, mosquitoes are now a greater public health issue. WNV is a bloodborne disease that is a seasonal epidemic in many parts of North America **(Figure 19-6)**. According to the Centers for Disease Control and Prevention, 2,205 human cases were reported nationwide in 2014, causing 97 deaths.[2] A low percentage of people infected with WNV develop severe illness, however, and more than half have no signs and symptoms at all. WNV is spread mostly by the bite of infected mosquitoes, which often transmit the virus from infected birds.

In the eastern United States, eastern equine encephalitis (EEE) is another serious mosquito-borne infection that is fatal in 33% of those infected. Fortunately, there are only a few human cases of EEE annually in the United States.[3] EEE transmission is prevented the same as WNV – by preventing mosquito bites.

[2]*Centers for Disease Control and Prevention, cdc.gov/westnile/ resources/pdfs/data/wnv-disease-cases-and-pvds-by-state-2014_06052015.pdf Accessed January 2016.*

[3]*Centers for Disease Control and Prevention, cdc.gov/EasternEquineEncephalitis Accessed January 2016.*

FIGURE 19-6

2014 Reported West Nile virus activity in the United States.

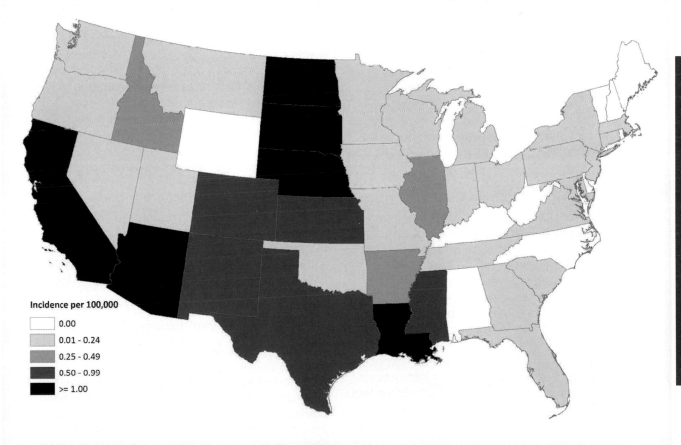

Incidence per 100,000

	0.00
	0.01 - 0.24
	0.25 - 0.49
	0.50 - 0.99
	>= 1.00

Source: cdc.gov/westnile/resources/pdfs/data/wnv-neuro-incidence-by-state-map_2014_06052015.pdf Accessed January 2016.

Many affected states and communities have expanded mosquito control programs, but in many areas, people still need to take precautions to prevent mosquito bites. The best way to avoid WNV is to prevent mosquito bites in these ways:

- Wear long-sleeved shirts and pants.

- Use an insect repellent when outside in areas where mosquitoes are common **(Box 19-5).**

- Be aware of peak mosquito hours (from dusk to dawn).

- Mosquito-proof your home by draining standing water around your home and installing or repairing screens.

- Report dead birds to local authorities.

- Support local mosquito control programs.

Bee and Wasp Stings

Bee, wasp and other insect stings are not poisonous but can cause life-threatening allergic reactions, called anaphylaxis, in victims who have severe allergies to them. Venomous insects include honeybees, bumblebees, hornets, wasps, yellow jackets and fire ants. There are no reliable statistics about how many stings occur every year, but 3% of adults and 0.4%-0.8% of children are allergic to stinging insects to the extent that a life-threatening reaction could occur.[4] Many people have very serious or life-threatening reactions, and about 50-70 people die every year from allergic reactions to insect stings.[5]

[4]*American Academy of Allergy, Asthma & Immunology. aaaai.org/media/statistics/allergy-statistics.asp Accessed March 5, 2011.*

[5]*National Safety Council (2015). Injury Facts®, 2015 Edition. Itasca, IL: Author.*

Chapter 9 discusses anaphylactic shock and the first aid to give. Oftentimes, someone who knows he or she is allergic to bee or wasp stings carries an EpiPen or other emergency medication to take if stung. **Chapter 9** also describes steps you can take to prevent insect stings.

In most cases, a bee or wasp sting causes pain but is not an emergency or serious problem. If present in the skin after the sting, the stinger can be scraped away with a rigid piece of plastic, such as a credit card. The area is washed to prevent infection, and a cold pack is applied to reduce the pain and swelling. Always observe for the signs of an allergic reaction, and if they appear, call 9-1-1 immediately and prepare to treat anaphylactic shock. Some sting victims who do not have allergic reactions may have other delayed symptoms that include fever, rash, joint pain and swollen glands (see First Aid: "Bee and Wasp Stings").

BOX 19-5: CDC RECOMMENDS MOSQUITO REPELLENTS

The Centers for Disease Control and Prevention recommends using products that have been shown to work in scientific trials and that contain active ingredients that have been registered with the United States Environmental Protection Agency (EPA) for use as insect repellents on skin or clothing. When the EPA registers a repellent, it evaluates the product for efficacy and potential effects on human beings and the environment. EPA registration means that the EPA does not expect a product, when used according to the instructions on the label, to cause unreasonable adverse effects to human health or the environment.

Of the active ingredients registered with the EPA, CDC believes that 2 have demonstrated a higher degree of efficacy in the peer-reviewed, scientific literature. Products containing these active ingredients typically provide longer-lasting protection than others.

- DEET (N,N-diethyl-m-toluamide)

- Picaridin (KBR 3023)

Oil of lemon eucalyptus, a plant-based repellent, is also registered with EPA. In some recent scientific publications, when oil of lemon eucalyptus was tested against mosquitoes found in the United States, it provided protection similar to repellents with low concentrations of DEET.

Source: cdc.gov/westnile/faq/repellent.html Accessed January 2016.

First Aid: Bee and Wasp Stings

Signs, Symptoms and Care

WHEN YOU SEE

- Complaints of pain, burning or itching at sting site

- Redness or swelling

- Stinger possibly still in skin

DO THIS FIRST

1. Remove the stinger from the skin by scraping it away gently with a piece of plastic, such as a credit card (not a knife blade). Call 9-1-1 if the victim has a known allergy to stings.

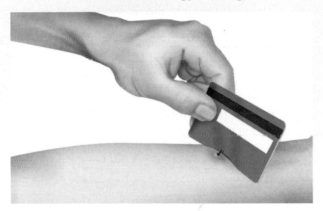

2. Wash the area with soap and water.

3. Put ice or a cold pack on the sting site (with a damp cloth or paper towel between the cold pack and the skin). Apply the cold for 20 minutes (or 10 minutes if it produces discomfort), then remove it for 30 minutes; reapply for 20 (or 10) minutes, then remove again for 30 minutes.

4. Watch the victim for 30 minutes for any signs or symptoms of allergic reaction (difficulty breathing, swelling in other areas, anxiety, nausea or vomiting); if any of these occur, call 9-1-1 and treat for anaphylactic shock.

ADDITIONAL CARE

- An over-the-counter oral antihistamine may help reduce discomfort.

- For an insect sting in the mouth, have the victim suck on ice to reduce swelling. Call 9-1-1 if breathing becomes difficult.

- Do not let the victim scratch the sting; this increases swelling and itching, along with the risk of infection.

Scorpion Stings

In Southwestern and Southern states, thousands of scorpion stings occur every year, but few become emergencies **(Figure 19-7)**. The great majority of scorpion species are not venomous. Even the sting of the poisonous bark scorpion, found in the Southwest, fortunately, is seldom fatal. In one report, only 4 deaths resulted from scorpion stings in an 11-year period in the United States. In other countries, stings are more common; in Mexico, for example, as many as 1,000 people are believed to die every year from scorpion stings.[6] Scorpions are more active at night, and most stings occur during the warm summer months. People can avoid scorpions in areas where they are common by not walking barefoot or in sandals, and by shaking out clothing and shoes before putting them on.

[6]*Medscape. emedicine.medscape.com/article/168230-overview Accessed January 2016.*

Scorpion stings are most dangerous for infants, young children and the elderly. When death does occur, it is usually the result of anaphylactic shock caused by the victim's reaction to the venom. The victim of a sting should always be observed for this potential reaction. The more usual symptoms, however, consist of pain at the site along with numbness and tingling. More serious symptoms include nausea and vomiting, breathing difficulty, fever, convulsions and in children, hyperactivity.

The first aid for a scorpion sting is similar to the first aid for a wasp or bee sting.

The Arizona Poison and Drug Information Center, which manages thousands of stings a year, says most stings in healthy adults can be managed safely at home. Wash the area and apply a cold pack. Monitor the victim's symptoms and seek medical attention for signs and symptoms beyond those at the sting site. Seek urgent medical attention for a sting in a child or elderly person. Antivenin for scorpion stings may be available in some areas (see First Aid: "Scorpion Stings").

FIGURE 19-7

Scorpion.

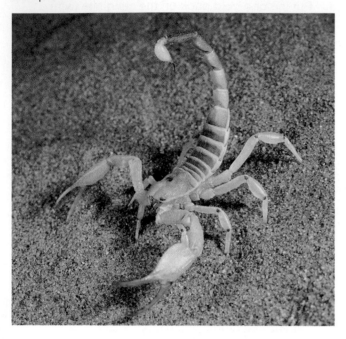

Marine Bites and Stings

Biting marine animals include sharks, barracudas and eels, although such bites are generally rare. The first aid for marine bites is essentially the same as for bleeding and wound care. For a bite that causes severe bleeding:

1. Stop the bleeding.

2. Care for shock.

3. Summon help from lifeguards.

4. Call 9-1-1.

Stings from marine life are much more common than bites. Stinging marine life include jellyfish, Portuguese man-of-war, corals, spiny sea urchins, anemones and stingrays. Most stings are like bee or wasp stings: painful but not dangerous, except in the very rare few people who may experience an allergic reaction or severe toxic reaction. Even the venomous sting of the Portuguese man-of-war, although it can be very painful and cause other symptoms, is rarely an emergency or life threatening.

Most marine stings can be prevented by paying attention to your environment. Warnings are generally posted on public beaches when Portuguese man-of-

First Aid: Scorpion Stings

Signs, Symptoms and Care

WHEN YOU SEE

- The scorpion sting with its tail

- Complaints of severe burning pain at sting site, later numbness, tingling

- Possible nausea, vomiting

- Hyperactivity in a child

- Possible signs of shock, breathing difficulties

DO THIS FIRST

1. Call 9-1-1 if the victim has a problem breathing or severe symptoms.

2. Monitor the victim's breathing and be prepared to give CPR if needed.

3. Carefully wash the sting area.

4. Put ice or a cold pack on the area (with a damp cloth or paper towel between the cold pack and the skin). Apply the cold for 20 minutes (or 10 minutes if it produces discomfort), then remove it for 30 minutes; reapply for 20 (or 10) minutes, then remove again for 30 minutes.

5. Seek urgent medical attention unless the symptoms are very mild.

ADDITIONAL CARE

- Keep the victim still.

wars are present in the water, or you may see their blue floats washed up on the beach or floating in the water **(Figure 19-8).** Long tentacles streaming from the floating body are the source of stings; these tentacles can break off and continue to cause stings in the water or on the beach. Do not touch a jellyfish or Portuguese man-of-war on the beach. In more isolated areas, check the water around you frequently, and if there are known risks, wear a wetsuit for skin protection. Do not swim or snorkel in shallow water where you may bump into coral, urchins or anemones. Watch the area in front of you when walking in shallow water where stingrays may be present and shuffle your feet to scare them away. Do not let small children play in such areas. If you have ever had an allergic reaction to any marine sting, talk with your health care provider about having an allergy kit.

FIGURE 19-8

Portuguese man-of-war.

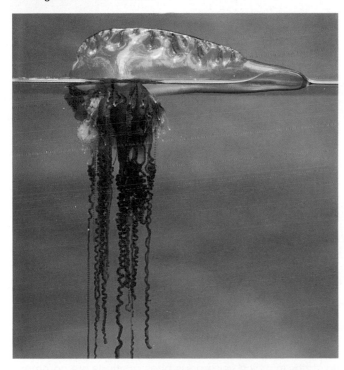

Jellyfish or Portuguese man-of-war stings cause an immediate intense pain and burning that may last for hours. The stinging may continue after the initial contact; the application of vinegar has been shown to inactivate the venom. Red welts usually appear on the skin, often in a row caused by a tentacle. In most cases, these are the only symptoms. If a severe toxic or allergic reaction occurs after any marine sting, however, the victim may experience difficulty breathing, swelling of the throat, signs of shock, muscle paralysis, seizures or unresponsiveness. If

any of these signs and symptoms occurs, or if the victim is a young child or is stung on the face or eyes, call 9-1-1.

Give this first aid for jellyfish and Portuguese man-of-war stings:

1. Wash the sting area with lots of vinegar (4%-6% acetic acid) as soon as possible, for at least 30 seconds or longer, to inactivate the venom. Remove any remaining tentacles with a gloved hand.

2. If vinegar is unavailable, use a mix of baking soda and water.

3. To reduce pain, immerse the area in water as hot as can be tolerated (113°F or 45°C) for at least 20 minutes or as long as pain is felt. If pain returns on removal from the hot water, immerse the area again.

4. If hot water is unavailable, use a dry hot pack (preferable) or a dry cold pack to reduce pain.

5. Do not use meat tenderizer, a fresh water wash, commercial aerosol products or a pressure bandage.

6. Call 9-1-1 if –

   • The victim is very young or very old.

   • A sting near the mouth is causing swelling.

   • The sting involves a large area of the body, the face or genitals.

   • The victim experiences serious signs and symptoms, such as difficulty breathing or swallowing or chest pain.

   • The sting is from a box jellyfish (rare in United States).

To care for urchin or stingray puncture wounds:

1. Relieve the pain by immersing the injured part in hot water for 30 minutes. Make sure the water is not so hot that it causes a burn.

2. Wash the wound with soap and water, and apply a dressing.

3. Seek medical attention.

19 • Bites and Stings

LEARNING CHECKPOINT 3

1. Fill in the correct answer: A bee's stinger can be removed from the skin using _____.

2. A coworker was stung by a honeybee near the flower garden by the office building's entrance. As she tells you about this, you see that her face is turning red, the skin around her eyes and mouth looks puffy, and she seems short of breath. What are the most important actions to take first? Why?

   _____

   _____

   _____

   _____

3. Select the best answer. What substance should be put on a jellyfish sting?

   a. Boiling water

   b. Ketchup or mayonnaise

   c. Vinegar or baking soda

   d. Any of the above

 CONCLUDING THOUGHTS

Bites and stings are common occurrences, but fortunately, they seldom become emergencies. First aid, in most cases, is as simple as pain relief and wound care, along with observing for more serious signs and symptoms and then seeking medical care. For those who are often outdoors where most bites and stings occur, prevention is important. Most importantly, people who are known to be allergic to bee or other insect stings or bites, should carry an emergency epinephrine kit and follow precautions when in areas where stings or bites are likely.

 CRITICAL THINKING CHALLENGE QUESTIONS

SCENARIO 1

A friend is bitten by a dog, which then runs off. The wound is minor, but the skin is broken. What should you advise him to do?

_____

_____

_____

_____

SCENARIO 2

You are visiting another student, who tells you she was just bitten by a spider in her basement. She saw it only momentarily, but thinks it may have been a black widow spider. What do you do?

_____

_____

_____

_____

 ADDITIONAL ACTIVITIES AND RESOURCES

In states in which venomous bites or stings are common, the regional Poison Control Center (PCC) often has additional information related to the prevention or first aid treatment of bites and stings. Do an Internet search for a state PCC website, and report your findings to the class.

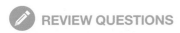

Select the best answers.

1. Possible rabies infection should be a consideration with –

    a. only wild animal bites.

    b. only dog bites if you do not know the owner.

    c. snake bites.

    d. all animal bites from mammals.

2. Seek immediate medical attention for –

    a. a puncture wound from an animal bite.

    b. a bite to the head or neck.

    c. a bite wound from an animal that is not your own pet.

    d. All of the above

3. Why should all bites from a human be seen by a health care provider?

    a. Many pathogens in the mouth can cause serious infection.

    b. Later bleeding is likely even if it is controlled at first.

    c. Many humans are carriers of the rabies virus.

    d. Saliva is acidic and may cause tissue damage.

4. First aid for snake bite includes –

    a. sucking the venom from the bite holes.

    b. applying a tourniquet.

    c. washing the wound with soap and water.

    d. applying a hot compress on the area.

5. When should you seek urgent medical care for a brown recluse spider bite?

    a. Only if the victim is known to be allergic

    b. With all victims bitten

    c. Only if the victim develops a breathing problem

    d. Only if the victim develops fever and chills

6. The best way to remove a tick embedded in the skin is to –

    a. pull it out with tweezers.

    b. burn it with a needle sterilized in a flame.

    c. cover it with petroleum jelly.

    d. cover it with an alcohol-saturated dressing.

7. Which of the following is the most important reason to prevent mosquito bites?

    a. Mosquito bites always cause infections when scratched.

    b. Many people have allergic reactions to mosquito bites.

    c. Mosquito bites can cause infection with West Nile virus.

    d. Multiple mosquito bites can add up to cause toxic effects.

8. When should 9-1-1 be called for a bee sting?

    a. Always

    b. When a child younger than 8 is stung

    c. When the victim has a known allergy

    d. When the bee was particularly aggressive before the sting

9. Which statement is true about scorpion stings?

    a. Almost all scorpion species are venomous.

    b. Scorpion stings are very rarely fatal.

    c. Scorpion stings are likely to cause anaphylaxis.

    d. The venom from a scorpion sting is easily washed out of the bite.

10. When can the tentacles of a Portuguese man-of-war sting?

    a. When the Portuguese man-of-war is floating in the water

    b. When the Portuguese man-of-war is washed up on the sand

    c. When the tentacles are detached from the body

    d. All of the above

CHAPTER 20

Cold and Heat Emergencies

LESSON OBJECTIVES

- Describe the different types of cold and heat emergencies and what you can do to prevent them.

- Explain factors that may make a person more susceptible to a cold or heat emergency.

- List the signs and symptoms and first aid for:
  - Frostbite
  - Hypothermia
  - Heat cramps
  - Heat exhaustion
  - Heat stroke

After several days of bitterly cold weather, you wonder how your elderly neighbor is coping with the cold, so you stop by his house. You have to ring the door several times before he answers, and when you step inside, it feels very cold inside his house. You ask why it is so cold, and he mumbles that with rising fuel prices, he can't afford to turn the thermostat any higher. You follow him into the living room where he stumbles before sitting on the sofa. You notice that he is shivering. You ask if you can get him a blanket. He is slow to respond, and his words are slurred. Is he experiencing a problem? What should you do?

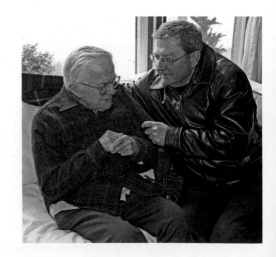

In temperature extremes or as a result of injury or illness, the body may not be able to successfully maintain its normal temperature, which can lead to medical problems. Oftentimes, cold- and heat-related injuries begin gradually, but if a person remains exposed to an extreme temperature or engaged in strenuous activity, an emergency can develop. Untreated, either a cold or a heat emergency can lead to serious injury or death.

Body Temperature

A fairly constant internal body temperature is necessary for body systems to function. The body has several mechanisms to create heat or to lose heat when necessary. In most environments, these mechanisms, along with protective clothing and shelter from temperature extremes, work well, and body temperature is not a health issue. When exposed to environmental temperature extremes for an extended time, however, these mechanisms cannot maintain a constant internal temperature indefinitely, particularly if the victim is injured or in poor health. Infants and the elderly are also more susceptible to temperature extremes.

MECHANISMS FOR STAYING WARM

Most of the body's heat is produced by metabolic processes that break down nutrients to release energy for use by the body. About 60% of the energy in the food we eat is released as heat within the body, and this heat energy in most environments is sufficient to keep the body at the optimal temperature, averaging 98.6°F. The contraction of muscle tissue also produces heat. Shivering is an involuntary movement of muscles to produce additional heat when the body needs it.

The body also has mechanisms to conserve heat when needed. Much of the body's heat is lost to a cooler environment through the process of radiation – heat radiates out from the skin in the same way that you can feel heat radiating from a hot surface. Skin temperature is normally much cooler than the body's internal temperature. If the body is losing too much heat by radiation, blood vessels in the skin contract (**vasoconstriction**) so that less internal heat is brought by the blood to the skin to radiate away. Minimizing heat loss helps the body to conserve its heat when necessary. We have also learned behaviors to minimize heat loss, such as putting on more clothing or moving to a warmer environment.

MECHANISMS FOR STAYING COOL

Cold is the absence of heat, not a positive quality in itself – the body cannot *make* cold to cool itself when a very hot environment or prolonged exertion threatens to raise body temperature. Nor can the body shut down its own heat-producing processes, as cells continue to need energy to survive and function. Therefore, the body must lose internal heat when necessary to prevent overheating. A primary heat loss mechanism is dilation of blood vessels (**vasodilation**) to bring more blood to the skin. The skin becomes warmer as the blood carries heat out from the body's core, and more heat is then radiated from the body. Sweating is a second mechanism. Sweat evaporates from the skin's surface, cooling the skin and helping to dissipate the heat brought to the surface by the blood. We also have learned behaviors to promote heat loss when needed, such as removing clothing to allow more heat to radiate away, getting out of the sun to avoid absorbing more radiated heat, spraying or wiping the body with water to help cool the skin by evaporation or moving inside to a cooler environment where we can radiate heat more effectively.

THE BODY IN TEMPERATURE EXTREMES

The body's normal heat production, heat conservation and heat loss mechanisms, regulated by the nervous system, usually cope well with changes in environmental temperatures to maintain a constant internal temperature. With extended exposure to temperature extremes, however, these mechanisms are not enough to maintain a normal body temperature.

With prolonged exposure to cold, especially when wet (because water conducts heat away from the body much faster than does air), not enough heat can be conserved in the body, and shivering cannot produce enough extra heat to keep the body warm. The person develops hypothermia, a potentially life-threatening condition. Because some cellular processes cannot occur at too low a temperature, organ systems gradually begin to fail, leading eventually to death.

With prolonged exposure to heat, the body eventually cannot lose enough heat to maintain a normal temperature. Profuse sweating in an attempt to cool the body frequently leads to dehydration, which reduces blood volume and blood pressure. Even when the environment is not very hot, a long period of physical exertion, such as that which accompanies endurance sports, can lead to dehydration caused by prolonged sweating. Without sufficient fluid, the body cannot cool itself adequately. Heat stroke occurs when the body temperature rises; sweating stops as the body tries to conserve its remaining fluid. Without treatment, organ damage eventually occurs, followed by death.

Hypothermia and heat stroke are the most dangerous temperature injuries. Because both develop gradually and worsen with continued exposure, the signs and symptoms of a developing problem must be recognized early and the condition corrected before it becomes life threatening. The first aid for these and other cold and heat emergencies is described in this chapter.

Hypothermia and heat stroke can happen to anyone in certain conditions. Generally, a healthy adult is most at risk after prolonged exposure to significant temperature extremes, such as being immersed in cold water or engaging in strenuous activities in the heat without drinking enough fluid. A number of factors, however, increase the risk for cold and heat injuries **(Box 20-1)**.

BOX 20-1: RISK FACTORS FOR COLD AND HEAT INJURIES

- **Age:** Young children and the elderly are at greatest risk. Young children are at risk because their shivering produces less heat due to smaller muscle mass. They also have less body fat than others, making them more likely to lose heat. Older people are at a greater risk because their lower metabolic rate can result in a failure to maintain a normal body temperature, even indoors, when the air temperature falls under 64°F. It is also believed that older people may not perceive cold as well as younger people do, and they may be slower to act to compensate for the cold. Older adults are also more likely to have a chronic illness, such as diabetes, that increases the risk for hypothermia.

- **Illness or injury:** Many injuries and chronic health problems, particularly those affecting circulation or the heart, increase one's susceptibility to heat and cold injuries. For example, a victim in shock often produces insufficient body heat; for this reason, shock treatment usually includes keeping the victim warm. The body responds less well to heat and cold with diabetes, infection, burns, head injuries and other conditions.

- **Mental impairment:** People with cognitive disabilities are less likely to take action to prevent hypothermia when they are exposed to cold.

- **Dehydration:** Not drinking enough fluid makes one more susceptible to both heat and cold emergencies.

- **Body type:** People with little body fat have a greater risk of hypothermia, as body fat has an insulating effect to slow environmental cooling. People with a large amount of body fat have a greater risk of experiencing a heat emergency.

- **Activity:** Those who work outdoors in hot environments, such as construction workers or athletes in training, are more likely to experience a heat emergency if they do not take precautions, such as resting and drinking fluids. People who work or participate in outdoor recreation in extreme cold are at greater risk for hypothermia, especially if they are not dressed properly, or are in situations where they may not be able to reach shelter.

- **Drugs and medications:** Many medications and drugs increase the risk for heat and cold injuries. Alcohol dilates blood vessels, making hypothermia more likely because heat is lost more quickly; alcohol is also a diuretic (increases urination), so the person becomes dehydrated more quickly and is more susceptible to heat stroke. Caffeine is also a diuretic. Alcohol and some other abused drugs can suppress shivering, thereby reducing heat production, and can prevent surface blood vessels from constricting, thereby allowing more heat loss than normal. Many prescription medications also can increase a person's susceptibility to either heat or cold emergencies. Commonly used psychiatric medications, for example, predispose people to heat and cold emergencies because of the drug's physiological mechanisms. Finally, alcohol and drugs that affect the user's judgment and reasoning often lead to the person taking risks or entering situations where a heat or cold emergency is more likely, such as falling into cold water or going into a freezing environment without adequate protection.

- **Environmental variables:** The risk of hypothermia is increased by becoming wet from rain or immersion in water. Water conducts heat away from the body much more quickly than heat can be radiated into the air. Wind also increases heat loss through the "wind chill" effect. The wind chill chart in **Figure 20-1** shows how the effects of cold increase with wind; for example, a temperature of 0°F with a wind of 20 mph has a wind chill effect of -22°F. High humidity increases the risk of heat emergencies because sweat evaporates more slowly and provides less cooling effect, as shown in the heat index chart **(Figure 20-2)**. For example, an air temperature of 90°F with a humidity of 90% has the same effect on the body as an air temperature of 122°F.

FIGURE 20-1

Wind chill. (National Weather Service)

National Weather Service, nws.noaa.gov/om/winter/windchill.shtml Accessed January 2016.

TEMPERATURE (°F)

WIND (MPH) \ Temp	40	35	30	25	20	15	10	5	0	-5	-10	-15	-20	-25	-30	-35	-40	-45
5	36	31	25	19	13	7	1	-5	-11	-16	-22	-28	-34	-40	-46	-52	-57	-63
10	34	27	21	15	9	3	-4	-10	-16	-22	-28	-35	-41	-47	-53	-59	-66	-72
15	32	25	19	13	6	0	-7	-13	-19	-26	-32	-39	-45	-51	-58	-64	-71	-77
20	30	24	17	11	4	-2	-9	-15	-22	-29	-35	-42	-48	-55	-61	-68	-74	-81
25	29	23	16	9	3	-4	-11	-17	-24	-31	-37	-44	-51	-58	-64	-71	-78	-84
30	28	22	15	8	1	-5	-12	-19	-26	-33	-39	-46	-53	-60	-67	-73	-80	-87
35	28	21	14	7	0	-7	-14	-21	-27	-34	-41	-48	-55	-62	-69	-76	-82	-89
40	27	20	13	6	-1	-8	-15	-22	-29	-36	-43	-50	-57	-64	-71	-78	-84	-91
45	26	19	12	5	-2	-9	-16	-23	-30	-37	-44	-51	-58	-65	-72	-79	-86	-93
50	26	19	12	4	-3	-10	-17	-24	-31	-38	-45	-52	-60	-67	-74	-81	-88	-95
55	25	18	11	4	-3	-11	-18	-25	-32	-39	-46	-54	-61	-68	-75	-82	-89	-97
60	25	17	10	3	-4	-11	-19	-26	-33	-40	-48	-55	-62	-69	-76	-84	-91	-98

Wind Chill (F) = 35.74 + 0.6215T − 35.75(V^0.16) + 0.4275T(V^0.16)
Where, T = Air temperature (F) V = Wind speed (mph)

Frostbite times: 30 minutes | 10 minutes | Danger

FIGURE 20-2

Heat index. (National Weather Service)

Source: National Weather Service, nws.noaa.gov/om/heat/heat index.shtml Accessed January 2016.

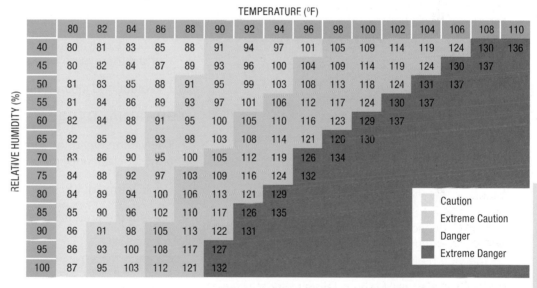

TEMPERATURE (°F)

RELATIVE HUMIDITY (%) \ Temp	80	82	84	86	88	90	92	94	96	98	100	102	104	106	108	110
40	80	81	83	85	88	91	94	97	101	105	109	114	119	124	130	136
45	80	82	84	87	89	93	96	100	104	109	114	119	124	130	137	
50	81	83	85	88	91	95	99	103	108	113	118	124	131	137		
55	81	84	86	89	93	97	101	106	112	117	124	130	137			
60	82	84	88	91	95	100	105	110	116	123	129	137				
65	82	85	89	93	98	103	108	114	121	126	130					
70	83	86	90	95	100	105	112	119	126	134						
75	84	88	92	97	103	109	116	124	132							
80	84	89	94	100	106	113	121	129								
85	85	90	96	102	110	117	126	135								
90	86	91	98	105	113	122	131									
95	86	93	100	108	117	127										
100	87	95	103	112	121	132										

Caution | Extreme Caution | Danger | Extreme Danger

Cold Emergencies

Exposure to cold temperatures can cause either **frostbite,** which is localized freezing of skin and other tissues, or **hypothermia,** which is lowering of the whole body's temperature.

FROSTBITE

Frostbite is the freezing of skin or deeper tissues. Frostbite occurs when the temperature is 32°F or colder. It usually happens to exposed skin areas on the head or face, hands or feet. Wind chill increases the risk of frostbite. Severe frostbite kills tissue and can result in gangrene and having to amputate the body part.

The first aid for frostbite involves removing the affected area from the cold as soon as possible, and protecting the area until the victim receives medical treatment. In special circumstances, the body part may be rewarmed – but only under certain conditions. If the frostbitten area is at any risk of being refrozen, it should not be rewarmed, because warming followed by freezing increases the tissue damage. If the extrication, rescue or transport of a frostbite victim may subject the area to cold again, do not warm it, but let health care or EMS professionals treat the frostbite. In a situation where help will be delayed, and only if refreezing can be prevented, then severe frostbite can be rewarmed by immersing the area in lukewarm – not hot – water for 20-30 minutes. Never apply a direct heat source to frostbitten skin, such as heat lamp, hot water bottle or heating pad, because of the risk of additional tissue damage (see First Aid: "Frostbite").

First Aid: Frostbite

Signs, Symptoms and Care

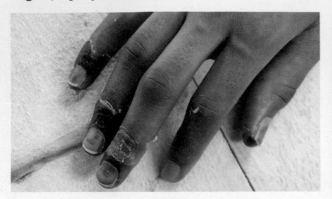

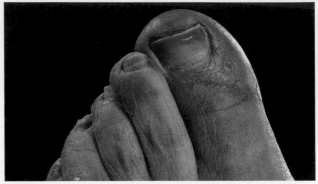

WHEN YOU SEE

- Skin looks waxy and white, gray, yellow or bluish.
- The area is numb or feels tingly or aching.

Severe frostbite:

- Area feels hard.
- May become painless.
- After warming, area becomes swollen and may blister.

DO THIS FIRST

1. Move the victim to a warm environment. Do not let the victim walk on frostbitten feet. Check the victim also for hypothermia.

2. Remove wet clothing and constricting items, such as jewelry.

3. Protect between fingers and toes with dry gauze. Protect the area from being touched or rubbed by clothing or objects.

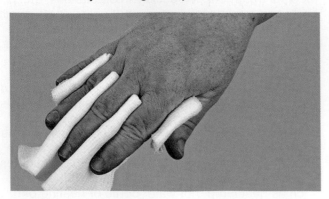

4. Seek medical attention as soon as possible.

5. Warm the frostbitten area in lukewarm water (99°F to 104°F or 37°C to 40°C) for 20-30 minutes *only* if medical care will be delayed, and if there is no danger of the skin refreezing.

6. Protect and elevate the frostbitten area.

ADDITIONAL CARE

- The victim may choose to take aspirin (adults only), acetaminophen or ibuprofen for pain.
- Drink warm liquids, but not alcohol.
- Prevent the area from refreezing.

ALERT

- Do not rub frostbitten skin because this can damage the skin.
- Do not rewarm frostbitten skin if it may freeze again, which could worsen the injury.
- Do not use a fire, heat lamp, hot water bottle, chemical warmers or heating pad to warm the area.
- After rewarming, be careful not to break blisters.

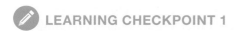

Circle **True** or **False** for the following statement:

1. Rubbing *frostbitten* fingers is the best way to warm them.   True   False

2. Frostbitten skin usually has what color(s)?

_____

3. A friend stops by your house after being outside for some time, complaining of being very cold. He has lost his hat, and his ears are white and hard and he says he has no feeling in them. Describe 3 actions to take for this man's frostbite.

_____

_____

HYPOTHERMIA

When the body cannot make heat as fast as it loses it in a cold environment, hypothermia develops. In hypothermia, body temperature drops below 95°F. It does not have to be freezing cold for hypothermia to occur. Hypothermia can occur at almost any cool temperature if the body is unprotected, especially if the victim is wet, exposed a long time, or unable to restore body heat because of a medical condition. An average of about 1,300 individuals die each year in the United States of hypothermia, and about half of them are older than 65.[1] Because hypothermia alters a person's mental status, an affected victim may not take corrective actions to avoid continued exposure to cold **(Box 20-2).**

Hypothermia is a progressive problem, as the victim transitions from simply feeling cold to mild hypothermia and, without the condition being relieved, to more serious symptoms and possibly to death. This progression may occur gradually, over hours or even days or very quickly, especially with a wind chill or if the victim is wet.

[1]*Centers for Disease Control and Prevention, cdc.gov/mmwr/ preview/mmwrhtml/mm6151a6.htm Accessed January 2016.*

Preventing Hypothermia

When planning to be outdoors for a long time, be prepared for a cold emergency:

- Check the weather forecast before going outdoors for an extended period.

- Take along extra clothing, socks, a sleeping bag or survival bag (see hypothermia blanket in **Chapter 23**).

- Have high-energy food bars and warm drinks.

- Do not use tobacco or consume alcohol or caffeine, which increase heat loss.

In addition, dress for the cold:

- Wear layers of clothing that do not retain moisture (wool or polypropylene).

- Choose a coat with a wind- and waterproof outer layer.

- Wear a hat (up to 50% of body heat is lost from the head).

- Use rain gear to avoid becoming wet.

During cold periods, check on people who are at risk for hypothermia:

- Check on older family members, friends and neighbors to ensure that the home is kept warm.

- Be familiar with the signs and symptoms of early hypothermia so you can recognize the problem and seek treatment.

- Employees of public health facilities, detoxification centers, shelters for the homeless and similar facilities should be educated to recognize hypothermia so that victims receive appropriate treatment early.

BOX 20-2: FACTS ABOUT HYPOTHERMIA

- Hypothermia occurs more easily in elderly or ill people.

- People under the influence of alcohol or drugs are at greater risk for hypothermia.

- A person immersed in cold water cools 30 times faster than in cool air.

- Victims in cold water are more likely to die from hypothermia than to drown.

- Victims in cardiac arrest after immersion in cold water have been resuscitated after a long time underwater – don't give up!

FIRST AID FOR HYPOTHERMIA

Since hypothermia may begin gradually, it is crucial to recognize the first signs and symptoms in order to take early action. Shivering, numbness, lethargy, poor coordination and slurred speech are early manifestations. Victims of early or mild hypothermia often experience the "umbles": mumbles, fumbles, stumbles. Infants may have bright red skin and little energy. As body temperature drops, hypothermia progresses and becomes more serious. Shivering typically stops and the victim may not even feel cold. Check the victim's skin temperature under clothing at the abdomen; cool skin here often indicates hypothermia. Breathing becomes shallow and

mental status continues to deteriorate. In severe cases, the victim becomes unresponsive and may stop breathing.

First aid for hypothermia begins with removing the victim from the cold. Remove wet clothing and cover the victim with blankets or warm clothing. Call 9-1-1, and in severe cases, be prepared to give basic life support. Do not try to actively warm the victim with a heat source except when far from medical care, because a heart rhythm disturbance may result.

A hypothermia victim who is not breathing may still be resuscitated. Handle the victim gently, but provide CPR or other care as needed while waiting for help to arrive (see First Aid: "Hypothermia").

First Aid: Hypothermia

Signs, Symptoms and Care

WHEN YOU SEE

- Shivering; may be uncontrollable (but stops in severe hypothermia)

- Victim seems apathetic, confused or irrational; may be belligerent

- Lethargy, clumsy movements, drowsiness

- Pale, cool skin – even under clothing (check abdomen)

- Slow breathing

- Changing levels of responsiveness

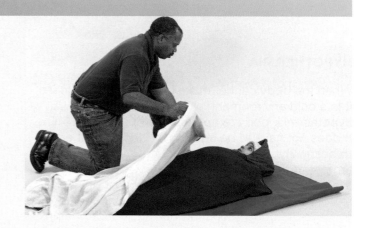

DO THIS FIRST

1. Check for responsiveness and normal breathing and call 9-1-1. Except in mild cases, the victim needs immediate medical care.

2. Provide CPR if the victim is unresponsive and not breathing normally.

3. Quickly move the victim out of the cold. Remove any wet clothing.

4. Warm the victim with blankets or warm clothing.

5. Only if the victim is far from medical care, use active rewarming by putting the victim near a heat source and putting warm (but not hot) water in containers against the skin.

6. Monitor breathing and be ready to give CPR if needed.

ADDITIONAL CARE

- Give warm (not hot) drinks to an alert victim who can easily swallow, but not alcohol or caffeine.

- Stay with the victim until he or she reaches a health care provider or help arrives.

ALERT

- Do not immerse a victim of hypothermia in hot water because warming him or her too rapidly can cause heart problems.

- Do not rub or massage the victim's skin. Be very gentle when handling the victim.

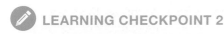

Circle **True** or **False** for each of the following statements:

1. Hypothermia occurs only when the air temperature is below freezing.

   True   False

2. A hypothermia victim who is generating heat by shivering still needs first aid and warming.

   True   False

3. Select the best answer. A hypothermic victim is brought into a ski lodge to be warmed. It will help to –

   a. give him a warm rum drink.

   b. have him take off his outer clothes and sit close to the fire.

   c. send him to a hot shower.

   d. remove his damp clothing and warm him with a blanket.

4. You are on a backpacking camping trip in the mountains and are caught in an unexpected snowstorm. On the way back down the mountain, about 4 miles from your car, you encounter a teenager sitting in the snow. His clothes are snowy and damp. He is lethargic and seems very confused. You call for help on your cell phone, but it will be at least 2 hours before the rescue team arrives. Using typical camping gear, what first aid can you give this victim?

   _____

   _____

   _____

   _____

Heat Emergencies

Heat illnesses can result when people become overheated in a hot environment. Generally, there are 4 types of heat illnesses:

- **Heat cramps** are the least serious and usually first to occur.

- **Exertional dehydration** occurs when the body loses more fluid than it takes in due to excessive sweating.

- **Heat exhaustion** develops when the body becomes dehydrated in a hot environment.

- **Heat stroke,** occurring with a seriously high body temperature, may develop from heat exhaustion. It is a medical emergency and, if untreated, usually causes death.

Most heat stroke deaths occur from exposure to a high temperature for a sustained period. Most heat-related deaths occur during hot weather, but heat stroke also affects people in settings where heat is generated, such as furnace rooms, factories or vehicles. Over the last decade, an average of 618 heat-related deaths a year have occurred in the United States. About half of these are related to hot weather.[1] Extreme heat is defined as temperatures that rise 10 degrees or more above the normal high temperature for the region, and last several days to several weeks. As noted earlier in this chapter, many factors can increase the risk for developing a heat illness, including old age and infancy, obesity, certain medical conditions, such as heart disease, the use of certain medications, drinking alcohol, not drinking enough fluid and strenuous activity in a hot environment.

[1]*Centers for Disease Control and Prevention, cdc.gov/mmwr/ preview/mmwrhtml/mm6136a6.htm Accessed January 2016.*

Like hypothermia, heat stroke is a progressive disease. In the mild stage (heat exhaustion), the victim is becoming dehydrated and the body is unable to cool itself. If the condition is not corrected, with continuing exposure to heat, the victim's body temperature begins to rise and more serious symptoms occur, potentially leading to death. Prevention of life-threatening heat stroke depends on recognizing the early signs and symptoms, and providing care before the condition becomes more serious.

PREVENTING HEAT EMERGENCIES

Follow these guidelines to help prevent heat emergencies:

- In hot environments, wear loose, lightweight clothing.

- Rest frequently in shady or cool areas.

- Drink adequate fluids before, during and after activity, but avoid alcohol and caffeine. Prehydrating is especially important before an endurance sport activity.

- For sports and endurance activities that may last longer than short periods of time, carbohydrate-electrolyte drinks, such as sports drinks, are generally better than water, but in most other situations, adequate water consumption will prevent heat exhaustion.

- Avoid exertion if you are overweight or elderly.

- When new to a hot area, take several days (up to a week to 10 days) to gradually acclimate to heat and humidity before engaging in strenuous activity.

- During heat waves, check on elderly friends, family and neighbors, particularly those who live alone or have mental impairment, and if necessary, move them to an air-conditioned area.

- Do not leave children alone in a vehicle. Make sure they cannot lock themselves into an enclosed space.

- Use sunscreen because sunburn causes a loss of body fluid as well as skin damage.

HEAT CRAMPS

Activity in a hot environment may cause painful cramps in muscles, called **heat cramps,** often in the lower legs or abdominal muscles. The muscle cramps result when sweating lowers the body's sodium levels. Heat cramps may occur along with heat exhaustion and heat stroke (see First Aid: "Heat Cramps").

EXERTIONAL DEHYDRATION

Exertional dehydration occurs when the body loses more fluid than it takes in due to excessive sweating.

Vigorous physical activity can lead to dehydration, especially in hot and humid weather.

First Aid: Heat Cramps

Signs, Symptoms and Care

WHEN YOU SEE

- Signs of muscle pain, cramping, spasms

- Heavy sweating

DO THIS FIRST

1. Have the person stop the activity and sit quietly in a cool place.

2. Give the victim a carbohydrate-electrolyte drink, such as a sports drink, to promote rehydration. (Other beverages, such as 2% milk and coconut water, are also effective.) If a carbohydrate-electrolyte drink is not available, give the victim water.

3. Have the person avoid strenuous activity for a few hours to prevent progression to heat exhaustion or heat stroke.

ADDITIONAL CARE

- For abdominal cramps, continue resting in a comfortable position.

- For leg cramps, stretch the muscle by extending the leg and flexing the ankle. Massage and ice the muscle.

- Seek medical attention for a victim who has heart problems or is on a low-sodium diet, or if the cramps do not subside within an hour.

First Aid: Exertional Dehydration

Signs, Symptoms and Care

WHEN YOU SEE

- Dry mouth
- Muscle cramps

- Increased thirst
- Lightheadedness

- Headache
- Fatigue

DO THIS FIRST

1. Have the victim rest, in a cool environment if possible.

2. Give the victim a carbohydrate-electrolyte drink, such as a sports drink, to promote rehydration. (Other beverages, such as 2% milk and coconut water, are also effective.) If a carbohydrate-electrolyte drink is not available, give the victim water.

HEAT EXHAUSTION

Activity in a hot environment usually causes heavy sweating, which may lead to dehydration and depletion of salt and electrolytes in the body if the person does not get enough fluids. This dehydration can lead to **heat exhaustion.**

A victim of heat exhaustion is usually sweating and the skin is pale or ashen, moist and often cool. Other signs and symptoms include thirst, fatigue and muscle cramps. Late signs and symptoms include headache or dizziness; fainting; nausea or vomiting; and fast, shallow breathing.

First, move the victim from the heat to rest in a cool place. Loosen or remove unnecessary clothing and help cool the victim's body with wet cloths, sponging the skin with cool water or spraying the skin with water and fanning the area. Give the victim a carbohydrate-electrolyte drink or water to drink. The victim's condition should improve within 30 minutes. If it does not, or if the victim has a heart condition or high blood pressure, seek medical attention immediately. Remember that if unrelieved, heat exhaustion may develop into heat stroke, a life-threatening emergency (see First Aid: "Heat Exhaustion").

First Aid: Heat Exhaustion

Signs, Symptoms and Care

WHEN YOU SEE

- Sweating, pale or ashen, moist skin (often cool)

- Thirst

- Fatigue

- Muscle cramps

Later signs and symptoms:

- Headache, dizziness, fainting

- Nausea or vomiting

- Fast, shallow breathing

DO THIS FIRST

1. Move the victim from the heat to rest in a cool place. Loosen or remove outer clothing.

2. Cool the victim with one of these methods:

    - Put wet cloths on the forehead and body.

    - Sponge the skin with cool water.

    - Spray the skin with water from a spray bottle and then fan the area.

3. Give the victim a carbohydrate-electrolyte drink, such as a sports drink, to promote rehydration. (Other beverages, such as 2% milk and coconut water, are also effective.) If a carbohydrate-electrolyte drink is not available, give the victim water.

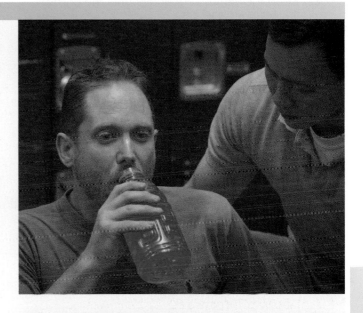

ALERT

- Do not give salt tablets to a heat exhaustion or heat stroke victim. Use a carbohydrate-electrolyte drink instead (if the victim is awake and alert).

- Do not give liquids containing caffeine or alcohol.

- If the victim is lethargic, nauseous or vomiting, do not give any liquids.

ADDITIONAL CARE

- Seek medical care if the victim's condition worsens or does not improve within 30 minutes.

- Seek urgent medical attention if the victim has a heart condition or high blood pressure.

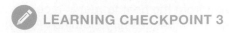
Circle **True** or **False** for the following statement:

1. For abdominal heat cramps, the best care is vigorous massage and stomach kneading.   True   False

2. Select the best answer. To treat heat cramps:

    a. Immerse the victim in a bathtub of cold water.

    b. Give a carbohydrate-electrolyte drink or water to drink.

    c. Keep the victim very active until the cramp works itself out.

    d. Do not let the victim eat or drink anything.

Circle **True** or **False** for the following statement:

3. Give salt tablets to victims who have both heat cramps and heat exhaustion.   True   False

4. Fill in the correct answer: Heat exhaustion begins when a person in a hot environment is not getting enough _____ .

5. List 3 possible ways to cool a victim who has heat exhaustion.

    _____

    _____

    _____

    _____

6. On a hot day, you join a friend on the athletic field who has been working out for a couple of hours. He is sitting on the grass in the sun. He is sweating heavily and says he has a headache and feels nauseated. Someone has already given him a sports drink. What should you do now? List in correct order the first 4 actions you would take.

    _____

    _____

    _____

    _____

HEAT STROKE

Heat stroke is a life-threatening emergency that is more common during hot summer periods. It occurs when the body can no longer effectively cool itself and results in a seriously high body temperature. It may develop slowly over several days or more rapidly when engaged in strenuous activity in the heat. The victim may be dehydrated and not sweating when heat stroke gradually develops, or he or she may be sweating heavily from exertion. Heat stroke causes a body temperature of 104°F or higher and is different from heat exhaustion, although it may develop from untreated heat exhaustion (see First Aid: "Heat Stroke"):

*   In heat stroke, the victim's skin is flushed and feels very hot to the touch; in heat exhaustion, the skin may be pale or ashen and clammy.

*   In heat stroke, the victim becomes very confused and irrational, and may become unresponsive or have convulsions; in heat exhaustion, the victim is dizzy or tired, or may be irritable or have a headache.

First Aid: Heat Stroke

Signs, Symptoms and Care

WHEN YOU SEE

- Skin is flushed, dry and hot to the touch; sweating usually has stopped

- Fast breathing

- Headache, dizziness, confusion

- Irrational behavior

- Possible convulsions or unresponsiveness

DO THIS FIRST

1. Call 9-1-1.

2. Move the victim to a cool place.

3. Remove outer clothing.

4. Immediately cool the victim with any means at hand, preferably by immersing the victim up to the neck in cold water (with the help of a second rescuer). If immersion in ice cold water is not possible, place the victim in a cold shower or move to a cool area and cover as much of the body as possible with cold, wet towels.

ADDITIONAL CARE

- Monitor the victim's breathing and be ready to give CPR if needed.

- Put an unresponsive victim in the recovery position and monitor breathing.

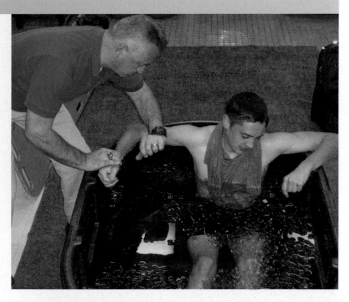

- Protect a victim having convulsions from injury (see **Chapter 16**).

ALERT

- Do not apply rubbing alcohol to the victim's skin.

- The victim should not take pain relievers or salt tablets.

- Do not try to force the victim to drink liquids.

✎ **LEARNING CHECKPOINT 4**

Circle **True** or **False** for the following statement:

1. It is safe to drive a heat stroke victim home after you have given first aid and cooled his or her body down to 100°F, as long as the victim is feeling better.   True   False

2. In what situation should you call 9-1-1 for a heat stroke victim?

   _____

3. Describe how a heat stroke victim's behavior may be different from the way in which that person usually behaves.

   _____

   _____

   _____

   _____

4. Your softball game happens to fall on the hottest day of the year. Your coach knows you have first aid training, and asks you to help out to make sure none of the students have problems with heat exhaustion or heat stroke.

a. To be prepared for these possibilities, what things should you make sure are present at the ball field?

_____

b. You decide to give a safety talk to your team before the game begins. What would you tell them about how to prevent heat emergencies? What signs and symptoms of a potential problem should players watch out for in others on their team?

_____

c. Despite these precautions, by the seventh inning, the center fielder seems to be showing signs and symptoms of heat stroke. What is the first step you should take?

_____

 CONCLUDING THOUGHTS

Heat and cold emergencies can be prevented by following common sense guidelines and taking steps in extreme temperatures to maintain normal body temperature. Recognizing the early signs and symptoms of both heat and cold emergencies is important to keep these conditions from worsening. When heat or cold illness does occur, act quickly to get medical attention before the emergency becomes life threatening. Be sure to take special precautions when engaged in activities in rural or wilderness areas where a victim cannot be easily or quickly reached by EMS professionals. **Chapter 23** describes these extra preparations to prevent these emergencies from occurring in such situations.

 CRITICAL THINKING CHALLENGE QUESTIONS

SCENARIO 1

You are working outside on a bitterly cold day. Your coworker is wearing only thin, cotton gloves, and after a few hours, he says his fingers have become numb. You look at them and the skin looks waxy and white. What should you do?

_____

_____

_____

_____

SCENARIO 2

A worker broke through the ice in a shallow pond, and it was some time before he could be pulled out. His head did not go below the surface, but he is shivering uncontrollably and seems very lethargic. What steps should you take?

_____

_____

_____

_____

SCENARIO 3

You are driving through a road construction area on a hot day when you see 2 men standing around a coworker who is lying on the ground. They do not know what happened to her or what to do. She is unresponsive and breathing fast. Her skin is flushed, dry and hot to your touch. What should you do?

_____

_____

_____

_____

 ADDITIONAL ACTIVITIES AND RESOURCES

1. Athletes who train for or compete in endurance sports, particularly those outdoors in warm weather, are particularly at risk for heat exhaustion and heat stroke. Considerable research has been conducted into the most effective strategies for prevention, hydration strategies, etc. **The National Athletic Trainers' Association (nata.org)** is a good source of additional information on heat stroke prevention.

2. If you live in an area frequently subject to extreme heat or cold, research your state's incidence of deaths resulting from heat stroke or hypothermia in recent years. What were causative factors in specific incidents that resulted in death? How could the problem have been prevented?

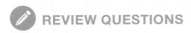

Select the best answers.

1. Muscle contraction produces –

    a. heat.

    b. heat loss.

    c. vasoconstriction.

    d. vasodilation.

2. Heat and cold emergencies are more likely to occur in –

    a. the elderly.

    b. people with certain chronic diseases.

    c. infants.

    d. All of the above

3. First aid for frostbite includes –

    a. rapid rewarming using a heat lamp or heating pad.

    b. protecting the area from rubbing or constricting jewelry.

    c. vigorously rubbing the area.

    d. running very hot water over the affected area for 10 minutes.

4. To help prevent hypothermia when outdoors in frigid temperatures –

    a. drink lots of coffee or hot tea.

    b. wear thick boots, because most heat loss is through the feet.

    c. try to stay dry.

    d. drink alcohol to stay warm.

5. The signs and symptoms of hypothermia include –

    a. apathy or confusion.

    b. red, blotchy skin.

    c. talkativeness.

    d. perceptions of being overly warm.

6. First aid for severe hypothermia includes –

    a. putting the victim in a hot shower.

    b. massaging the victim all over.

    c. calling 9-1-1.

    d. giving CPR regardless of whether the victim is breathing.

7. In what order do heat illnesses typically progress with continued activity in a hot environment?

    a. Heat cramps -> heat stroke -> heat exhaustion

    b. Heat cramps -> heat exhaustion -> heat stroke

    c. Heat exhaustion -> heat cramps -> heat stroke

    d. Can occur in any order

8. First aid for heat cramps includes –

    a. vigorously exercising the muscle.

    b. drinking a sports drink or water.

    c. applying a compression bandage.

    d. splinting the extremity until the cramps pass.

9. The late signs and symptoms of heat exhaustion include –

    a. headache, dizziness, fainting.

    b. constipation or diarrhea.

    c. extreme excitability.

    d. cold, tingling fingers or toes.

10. How can you cool down someone who is experiencing heat stroke?

    a. Immerse the victim up to the neck in cold water.

    b. Place the victim in a cold shower.

    c. Cover as much of the body as possible with cold, wet towels.

    d. Any of the above

CHAPTER 21

Behavioral Emergencies

LESSON OBJECTIVES

- Describe common emotional and behavioral responses to injury and illness.

- Explain how to reassure and calm an emotional victim.

- Describe how to interact with a victim experiencing anxiety or depression.

- List actions to take when dealing with a suicidal or potentially violent victim.

- Describe appropriate care for victims of child abuse, spousal abuse, elder abuse and sexual assault and rape.

Your boss has asked to meet with you and another employee, Meg, the woman in charge of order fulfillment. There have been several problems with important orders lately, and as the meeting explores ways to prevent future problems, Meg becomes increasingly emotional and defensive. You know she has been experiencing a lot of stress lately, and you've overheard gossip that she has some personal problems, but that doesn't seem to account for how worked up she is becoming in this meeting. Finally, when the boss asks if she will be able to solve the order problems, Meg seems to explode, rising from her chair with her hands in fists. You are alarmed and wonder what you can do before the situation is completely out of control or becomes violent.

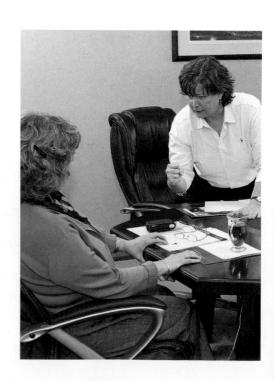

The process of giving first aid is sometimes complicated by the victim's behavior. Many injuries and medical emergencies may cause altered mental status, which can lead to a victim acting in unusual or unpredictable ways. Injury and illness also typically cause emotional responses that may affect how first aid must be given. Other victims may have emotional problems, such as panic reactions or depression that also must be addressed when giving first aid. **Behavioral emergencies** involve situations in which the victim's behavior, whether caused by injury, illness, personality or mental health factors, results in or complicates an emergency situation. Abuse and rape are additional behavioral situations.

Emotional and Behavioral Responses to Injury and Illness

Injury, sudden illness and other emergencies typically lead to strong emotional reactions in those involved. Normal reactions in these situations include fear, anxiety and apprehensiveness. In addition to the physical effects of the injury or illness itself, which may include altered mental status, normal emotional reactions may cause other stress-related physical signs and symptoms, such as trembling or shakiness, feelings of nausea, a fast heartbeat and breathing and perspiration.

Victims with preexisting emotional problems or mental illness are more likely to have more severe reactions. They may overreact, panic and act wildly, speak incoherently, become argumentative or withdrawn or become violent.

There is no clear-cut line between "normal" and "abnormal" responses to injury and sudden illness. Think of these responses as a continuum from normal to abnormal with a wide range of behaviors in the middle. It is important not to judge a victim's behavior too quickly but rather to assess the situation first. For example, a person who is usually calm and rational may become seemingly irrational and act inappropriately when in great pain. In such a case, accept the victim's emotional state and address his or her concerns while providing first aid. At the other extreme, a person who is usually quick to anger and aggressive may respond to the stress of an injury with violent behavior. In this case, it may become more important to protect yourself and others at the scene.

Your decision on how to approach a victim in a potential behavioral emergency depends on understanding normal versus abnormal reactions and an assessment of the victim's emotional and mental condition. Always remember your own safety: Do not approach a victim who may become violent. Call 9-1-1, and stay at a safe distance until help arrives.

ALTERED MENTAL STATUS

As noted in previous chapters, altered mental status or altered responsiveness may result from many different injuries and illnesses. The brain requires a steady level of oxygen for normal functioning, and any injury or illness that affects oxygenation may affect the victim's mental status – and therefore his or her behavior. Lowered levels of responsiveness may result from significantly reduced oxygen levels. Mental status may suddenly or gradually diminish. The victim may first feel dizzy, drowsy, disoriented or confused. The victim may suddenly or eventually become completely unresponsive. Often in such cases, the appropriate first aid is to care for the underlying cause of the altered mental status **(Box 21-1).**

Even small oxygen reductions can cause other reactions. A victim may respond to reduced brain oxygen with extreme anxiety and panic and potentially violence. In such cases, in addition to providing first aid, you also need to calm the victim to help prevent possible further injury caused by the victim's behavior. You may need to protect yourself as well. For example, near-drowning victims who are panicking as they desperately fight for air often behave irrationally and may grab onto a rescuer so forcefully that both lives are threatened.

TYPICAL EMOTIONAL REACTIONS

As noted earlier, typical reactions to injury, sudden illness and other emergencies include fear, anxiety and apprehensiveness. Sometimes people panic at the sight of their own blood. It is difficult to think clearly when in great pain. A victim with a serious injury may overreact and become fearful of dying. A victim may be unable to act, seemingly frozen by emotional shock, or may be acting irrationally and out of control. Any of these reactions can complicate the process of giving first aid for the victim's injury or illness.

Because emotional stress can have negative physical effects on the body, it may be just as important to address the victim's emotional reaction as it is to care for the physical injury or illness. The victim needs to be calmed and reassured.

REASSURING AND CALMING VICTIMS

How you act in the face of the victim's emergency can dramatically affect how the victim responds. If you react negatively, your words, gestures or facial expressions may increase the victim's stressful response rather than diminish it. You may show your own concern or fear about the emergency. You may act impatiently if the victim is not immediately cooperative. If you show a lack of self-confidence in your ability to manage the emergency and provide first aid, the victim's level of stress may increase.

Instead, take steps to calm and reassure the victim, following these guidelines (**Figure 21-1**):

1. Tell the victim who you are, and explain that you are there to help. Avoid seeming judgmental.

2. Do not assume the victim is intoxicated, using drugs or otherwise impaired, as the victim's behavior may result from a medical condition. Even if you smell alcohol on the victim's breath, do not assume a problem is due only to intoxication – you could overlook a serious injury.

3. Reassure the victim that help is on the way (after 9-1-1 has been called).

4. Ask the victim his or her name, and use it when speaking with him or her.

5. If possible, try to involve friends or family of the victim if present at the scene.

6. Let the victim tell you what he or she thinks is wrong.

7. Let the victim know you understand his or her concerns.

8. Make eye contact with the victim, and stay at the victim's eye level.

9. Speak in a caring, reassuring voice, but do not give false assurances or lie about the victim's condition.

10. Do not argue with the victim. Show that you understand the victim's concerns by repeating or rephrasing what the victim tells you.

11. If the victim seems irrational or delusional, do not make statements to support their false beliefs, but do not challenge them either.

12. Stay a safe distance away from the victim until your help is accepted. If the victim does not accept your help, do not try to restrain or force care on him or her. Withdraw if the scene seems unsafe or if you sense that the victim may become violent.

13. Tell the victim what you plan to do before doing it.

14. Move calmly and slowly, touching the victim only as necessary.

BOX 21-1: CAUSES OF ALTERED MENTAL STATUS

*   Respiratory emergencies
*   Cardiac emergencies
*   Poisoning
*   Head injuries
*   Seizures
*   Diabetic emergencies
*   Stroke
*   High fever
*   Substance abuse
*   Drug overdose
*   Heat or cold emergencies

FIGURE 21-1

When trying to calm an emotional victim, be careful not to assume a position that may seem threatening. Stay a comfortable distance away and use accepting, non-threatening body language.

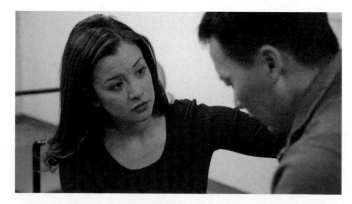

Victims with Emotional Problems

Some victims have preexisting emotional problems that may present greater challenges than the emotions normally provoked by emergencies. Two common problems are anxiety/panic and depression.

ANXIETY AND PANIC

Although it is normal to feel fear and apprehension when injured or suddenly ill, some people are prone to extreme **anxiety** and may have a **panic attack.** A panic attack is a sudden, overwhelming fear that is excessive for the situation. Signs and symptoms of extreme anxiety include:

- Agitation, inability to hold still, rapid movements, pacing

- Speaking very fast or not making sense

- Inability to judge the situation accurately

- Rapid emotional changes: crying, hysteria, anger

- A desire to leave the scene or not wait for medical help

- Fast heartbeat and breathing

- Difficulty breathing, dizziness, trembling

With a victim exhibiting signs and symptoms of extreme anxiety or panic, it is important to remain calm and patient at all times. Any attempt you make to restrain the person or to shock the person out of this behavior will likely worsen the situation. Often the panic will begin to ease in a few minutes because the physiological response of the body is self-limiting.

Follow the guidelines given earlier for calming and reassuring victims. Recognize that an individual prone to extreme anxiety or panic may need more time to calm down and may suddenly experience renewed anxiety. Continue to use the calming techniques while providing first aid. Be empathetic and gentle, and always explain what you are doing. Avoid touching the victim without first explaining what you are about to do and why. Allow victims to keep talking about what they are feeling and to express their concerns.

DEPRESSION

Victims who experience depression also require special attention. Major **depression** is a common psychological illness. In 2014, an estimated 15.7 million adults 18 and older (6.7%) in the United States had at least one major depressive episode in the past year. It occurs in people of all ages, is most prevalent in relatively young people and is about three times as common in women as in men.[1] Common signs and symptoms of depression include:

- Frequent feelings of sadness

- Loss of energy

- Feelings of hopelessness or worthlessness

- Difficulty concentrating

- Difficulty making decisions

- Physical symptoms, such as abdominal pain, insomnia, appetite loss or recurrent headaches

- Thoughts of death or suicide

[1]*National Institute of Mental Health, nimh.nih.gov/health/ statistics/prevalence/major-depression-among-adults.shtml Accessed January 2016.*

Someone experiencing depression often acts withdrawn, apathetic and subdued. Although the person may not resist your first aid care, he or she may not cooperate and may not offer information that would help you assess the situation. Therefore, it is important to make an effort to communicate with a victim who seems depressed. Follow these guidelines:

1. Encourage the victim to talk. Acknowledge that the person seems sad and ask why.

2. Be reassuring and sympathetic.

3. Show the victim that you care about him or her as a person. Helping to make the person comfortable, such as offering a drink of water or a blanket and providing other comforts, can encourage the victim to open up and talk about the problem.

4. If the victim is crying, do not try to make him or her stop. Allow the person to work through the emotion.

5. If the victim complains about something in his or her life, listen sympathetically but do not offer false reassurances such as saying, "Everything will be just fine," or "I'm sure that problem won't last long." Instead, talk about resources you are aware of that help people with problems such as the victim's.

6. Be alert to the possibility of suicide (see later section on "Suicide").

Behavioral Emergencies

The previous sections have focused on interacting with victims of injury or sudden illness who are experiencing normal or abnormal emotional reactions. In most cases, those reactions complicate the first aid problem but are not the primary problem. In some cases, however, the person's behavior is the emergency. Behavioral emergencies include situations in which victims have suicidal feelings or the potential to act violently in a way that may harm themselves or others.

When a victim's behavior becomes obviously abnormal, remember not to assume simply that the person is intoxicated or under the influence of a drug. Many different factors can radically change a person's behavior, including:

- The stress of the situation

- Illnesses or injuries causing altered mental status

- Mental illnesses

BOX 21-2: SUICIDE RISK FACTORS AND WARNING SIGNS

Risk Factors

- Mental disorders, including depression

- History of substance abuse

- Feelings of hopelessness

- Recent emotional crisis or painful illness

- Impulsive or aggressive tendencies

- Past suicide attempts

Warning Signs

- Talking about suicide (it is a myth that people who talk about it rarely act on the threat)

- Comments about feeling hopeless or worthless

- Taking risks that could cause death, such as driving too fast

- Loss of interest in one's past activities.

- Suddenly and unexpectedly seeming calm or happy after being sad.

SUICIDE

More than 39,000 individuals committed suicide in the United States in a recent year. Suicide is the second leading cause of death among people 15-24 years old. Men are about 4 times more likely to commit suicide than women, although women report attempting suicide 3 times more often than men. Overall, suicide is the tenth leading cause of death among people 10 and older.[2] Drug overdose (see **Chapter 18**) is the most common method used by females, and firearms is the method used most by men.

[2]*National Safety Council [NSC]. (2015). Injury Facts®, 2015 Edition. Itasca, IL: Author.*

The risk factors and signs of potential suicides are listed in **Box 21-2.** Research has shown that most people who commit suicide communicated their desire to others, although not always in an obvious way. Anyone who makes comments suggestive of suicidal feelings should be taken seriously.

Follow these guidelines if you are caring for a person who may be suicidal or whose injury may have been self-inflicted:

1. Take the person seriously and listen to what he or she is saying. Ask what the person is planning to do. Talk calmly and supportively.

2. Do not try to argue the person out of committing suicide, but let him or her know that you understand and care. Do not give false reassurances.

3. Seek help. Call 9-1-1 if appropriate, and involve friends or family members, if possible, in any care given.

4. Do not leave the person alone unless your own safety is threatened.

5. Remove any weapons, drugs or medications that might be used in a suicide attempt. Do not let the person drive.

6. If the person has a firearm and is threatening violence, withdraw, call 9-1-1 and wait for help to arrive and handle the situation. (See following section on "Violent Behavior.")

7. Give first aid and other care as appropriate.

VIOLENT BEHAVIOR

In any behavioral emergency, consider the potential for violence. The person may threaten violence to him- or herself or others on the scene. Following are signs that violent behavior may occur:

- The person is holding a weapon or any object that might be used as a weapon.

- The person is in a threatening or bullying posture, has his or her hands in fists, or is pacing and waving his or her arms around **(Figure 21-2).**

- The person is threatening, verbally abusing or yelling at you or someone else.

- The person is uncontrollably angry, kicking or throwing things.

- The person seems to be hallucinating or yelling at someone not present.

- The person is known to have committed violent acts in the past.

If you think the person may commit an act of violence, follow these guidelines:

1. Do not enter the scene if your safety is at risk. Encourage others at the scene to withdraw.

2. Call 9-1-1.

3. Do not try to restrain the person unless you have had special training and have assistance from others. Monitor the situation from a safe distance and wait for help to arrive.

4. While waiting for help, do the following if it is safe to remain with the person:

    - Talk to the person calmly and quietly and listen to what he or she has to say. Do not argue or be falsely reassuring, which the person may perceive as condescending or patronizing behavior. Try to divert the person from any violent action by keeping him or her talking.

    - Do not move about or do anything the person may perceive as threatening.

    - Offer to give first aid if the person calms down, but do not try to do anything without the person's consent.

    - Maintain an open exit from the room or scene; do not let a potentially violent person get between you and the door.

FIGURE 21-2

An emotional person is potentially violent.

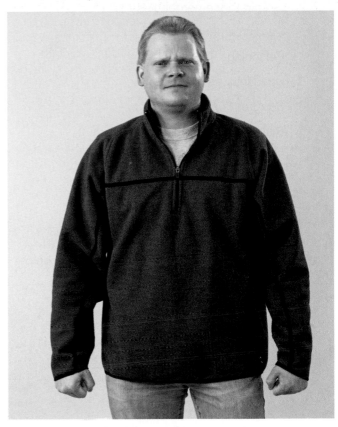

✏ LEARNING CHECKPOINT 1

1. Select the best answer. Normal responses to many injuries and sudden illnesses include –

    a. trembling or shakiness.

    b. altered mental status.

    c. fear and anxiety.

    d. All of the above

2. Check off any of the following conditions that may cause altered mental status:

    ☐ Respiratory emergencies

    ☐ Cardiac emergencies

    ☐ Poisoning

    ☐ Head injuries

    ☐ Seizures

    ☐ Diabetic emergencies

    ☐ Stroke

    ☐ High fever

    ☐ Drug overdose

    ☐ Heat or cold emergencies

3. Describe at least five things you can do to help calm an emotional victim.

    _____

    _____

    _____

    _____

    _____

Circle **True** or **False** for each of the following statements:

4. Never acknowledge that a depressed person seems sad, but be cheerful and pretend nothing is wrong.   True   False

5. People who talk about committing suicide rarely act on the threat.   True   False

6. You see an injured victim who is shouting and making threatening gestures, and you realize he is potentially violent. Number the following actions in the order in which you should take them:

    ____ Talk to the person calmly and quietly, and try to divert the person from any violent action by keeping him or her talking.

    ____ Call 9-1-1.

    ____ Do not enter the scene if your safety is at risk. Encourage others at the scene to withdraw.

Abuse

Abuse is the intentional inflicting of injury or suffering on someone under the abuser's power, such as a child, spouse or elderly parent. In some cases, a victim needs first aid for injuries sustained in an abuse incident. In other cases, abuse may become apparent when a victim is being treated for another injury or sudden illness. In still other cases, you may encounter a victim of abuse who does not have a present injury requiring first aid. In all situations, and in incidents of sexual abuse or rape, you need to be sensitive to the victim's emotional status and aware of special issues for handling the situation.

PREVENTION OF ABUSE

Many individual and cultural factors are involved in the causes of abuse. Tension, anger and frustration can grow to the point where the person in a rage commits an act of violence. In most cases, this leads to a cycle of regret and promises to change, but the cycle repeats as stresses again build and lead to often increasingly violent acts.

What originally causes a person to become an abuser? Many abusers were abused themselves as children or observed abuse in their homes. Some people never develop ways to manage stress and control their feelings. Many different psychological factors are involved in why some people easily lose their temper and become violent. Unfortunately, there is no simple way to predict who may become an abuser and, therefore, no simple way to prevent abuse from happening the first time. The cycle of repeated abuse, however, can be broken. Laws have become more protective of victims, shelters and hotlines are increasingly available for victims to break away from their abusers and programs have been developed to help abusers learn to control impulses toward violence. Preventing abuse, therefore, begins with recognizing and acknowledging it when it occurs and understanding that resources are available for both victims and abusers. The following sections on child abuse, domestic violence, elder abuse and rape include telephone hotline numbers for finding such resources throughout the United States.

CHILD ABUSE[1]

Consider these annual statistics for the United States:

- Almost 700,000 children are found to be victims of child abuse (about 20%) or neglect (about 80%).

- About 1,500 children die of child abuse or neglect.

- Nearly ¾ of all child fatalities are younger than 3.

- Four-fifths of child fatalities were caused by one or both parents.

[1]*The information in this section on child abuse comes from the Children's Bureau in the Administration on Children, Youth and Families, the Administration for Children and Families within the U.S. Department of Health and Human Services (HHS). Additional information is available at this agency's website: acf.hhs.gov/programs/cb/resource/child-maltreatment-2013 Accessed December 2015.*

Why Abuse Occurs

All the causes of child abuse and neglect are not fully understood, but several risk factors have been identified. When there are multiple risk factors present, the risk is greater. These risk factors include:

- Lack of preparation for or knowledge about parenting

- Financial or other environmental stressors

- Difficulty in relationships

- Depression or other mental health problems

Parents may lack an understanding of their children's developmental stages and hold unreasonable expectations for their abilities. They may also be unaware of alternatives to corporal punishment or how to discipline their children most effectively at each age. Parents also may lack knowledge of the health, hygiene and nutritional needs of their children. These circumstances, combined with the challenges of raising children, can result in otherwise well-intentioned parents causing their children harm or neglecting their needs.

Abuse may also result from uncontrolled emotional states. A particular problem is **shaken baby syndrome,** in which a parent or caregiver, including babysitters and child care workers, becomes frustrated with a crying infant and shakes the infant. Such shaking causes the infant's head to flop around and can cause severe brain injury, spinal injury or

death. Everyone who cares for infants needs to understand this problem and to learn to control their emotions when frustrated by the crying of a child.

Who Is Abused

Any child may be abused. Boys and girls are almost equally likely to experience neglect and physical abuse. Girls are about 4 times more likely to experience sexual abuse. Children of all races and ethnicities and all socio-economic levels experience abuse. Children of all ages are susceptible to experiencing abuse and neglect, but younger children are most vulnerable.

In more than 90% of cases of abuse and neglect, one or both parents are involved. In about 80% of cases of sexual abuse, the perpetrator is known by the child. Sexual abuse often occurs in a repeating pattern rather than as a single incident.

TYPES OF ABUSE AND NEGLECT

The **Federal Child Abuse Prevention and Treatment Act,** as amended by the CAPTA Reauthorization Act of 2010, defines child abuse and neglect as, at minimum:

- Any recent act or failure to act on the part of a parent or caretaker that results in death, serious physical or emotional harm, sexual abuse or exploitation, or an act or failure to act that presents an imminent risk of serious harm.

- Each state, however, has its own laws and exact definitions of child abuse and neglect, which are typically based on the national standard. Most states recognize four major types of maltreatment: neglect, physical abuse, sexual abuse and psychological or emotional abuse. The specific types of neglect are often defined differently, using different terms, by different states. Nationally, for the most recent year reported, 79.5% of victims were neglected, 18% were physically abused, 9% were sexually abused and 8.7% were psychologically maltreated.

Although any of these types may occur separately, most often they are combined. For example, a physically abused child is often emotionally abused as well, and a sexually abused child may also be neglected.

Neglect

Neglect is failure to provide for a child's basic needs, including these forms of neglect:

- *Physical neglect.* Failure to provide necessary food or shelter or lack of appropriate supervision.

- *Medical neglect.* Failure to provide necessary medical or mental health treatment.

- *Educational neglect.* Failure to educate a child or attend to special education needs.

- *Emotional neglect.* Inattention to a child's emotional needs, failure to provide psychological care or permitting the child to use alcohol or other drugs.

These situations do not always mean a child is willfully neglected, however. Sometimes cultural values, community standards and poverty are contributing factors. The family may need information or assistance. When a family fails to use information and resources, and the child's health or safety is at risk, child welfare intervention may be required.

Physical Abuse

Physical abuse is physical injury (ranging from minor bruises to severe fractures or death) as a result of punching, beating, kicking, biting, shaking, throwing, stabbing, choking, hitting (with a hand, stick, strap or other object), burning or otherwise harming a child. These injuries are considered abuse regardless of whether the caretaker intended to hurt the child.

Sexual Abuse

Sexual abuse includes any kind of sexual activity by a parent or caretaker, such as fondling a child's genitals, penetration, incest, rape, sodomy, indecent exposure or exploitation through prostitution or the production of pornographic materials.

Emotional Abuse

Emotional abuse is a pattern of behavior that impairs a child's emotional development or sense of self-worth. This may include constant criticism, threats or rejection, as well as withholding love, support or guidance. Emotional abuse is often difficult to prove, and government agencies often cannot intervene without evidence of harm to the child. Emotional abuse is almost always present when other types of abuse occur.

Results of Abuse and Neglect

Abuse and neglect have short- and long-term consequences that may include brain damage, developmental delays, learning disorders, problems forming relationships, aggressive behavior and depression. Survivors of child abuse and neglect may also be at greater risk for problems later in life, such as low academic achievement, drug use, teen pregnancy and criminal behavior.

SIGNS OF ABUSE AND NEGLECT

The first step in helping abused or neglected children is learning to recognize the signs of abuse and neglect. A single sign does not prove child abuse is occurring, but when signs appear repeatedly or in combination, you should consider the possibility of child abuse.

General Signs of Abuse

Behavioral signs may signal abuse or neglect long before any physical changes occur in a child. The following behaviors may suggest the possibility of child abuse or neglect:

The child:

- Has sudden changes in behavior or school performance

- Has not received help for physical or medical problems brought to the parents' attention

- Has learning problems or difficulty concentrating unrelated to specific physical or psychological causes

- Is always watchful, as though preparing for something bad to happen

- Lacks adult supervision

- Is overly compliant, passive or withdrawn

- Comes to school or other activities early, stays late or does not want to go home

The parent:

- Shows little concern for the child

- Denies the existence of, or blames the child for, the child's problems in school or at home

- Asks teachers or other caretakers to use harsh physical discipline if the child misbehaves

- Sees the child as entirely bad, worthless or burdensome

- Demands a level of physical or academic performance the child cannot achieve

- Looks primarily to the child for care, attention and satisfaction of emotional needs

The parent and child:

- Rarely touch or look at each other

- Consider their relationship entirely negative

- Say they do not like each other

Signs of Neglect

The child:

- Is frequently absent from school

- Begs or steals food or money

- Lacks needed medical or dental care, immunizations or glasses

- Is consistently dirty and has severe body odor

- Lacks sufficient clothing for the weather

- Abuses alcohol or other drugs

- Says there is no one at home to provide care

The parent or other adult caregiver:

- Appears indifferent to the child

- Seems apathetic or depressed

- Behaves irrationally or in a bizarre manner

- Is abusing alcohol or other drugs

See **Box 21-3** for specific signs of the different types of abuse.

Helping an Abused Child

Parents or other caregivers who abuse or neglect a child need help. Programs are available in most communities to provide professional help. Child care workers, teachers and other caregivers should not, however, try to talk to suspected abusers in an effort to get them to seek help. The abuser will almost always deny the problem, and the situation may become worse than if you had said nothing. Instead, the single most important thing you can do if you suspect a child is being abused or neglected, is report it to the proper authorities. Your report will help protect the child and get help for the family.

REPORTING ABUSE

If you work with children as part of your job, you may be legally required to report suspected cases of child abuse or neglect. State laws vary in the specifics of who must make a report and to what agency. If this is required in your job, follow your employer's policy. For example, you may be required to speak to your supervisor about your suspicion before making a report.

The law provides ways for private citizens to report suspected abuse or neglect as well, and it is important for the child's welfare that you do this even if not required to do so by your employer. Contact your local child protective services agency or police department.

For more information about where and how to file a report, call the Childhelp National Child Abuse Hotline (1-800-4-A-Child).

When you call to report child abuse, you will be asked for specific information, which may include:

- The child's name

- The suspected perpetrator's name (if known)

- A description of what you have seen or heard

- The names of any other people having knowledge of the abuse

- Your name and phone number

Your name will not be given to the family of the child you suspect is being abused or neglected. If you are making the report as a private citizen, you may request to make the report anonymously, but your report may be considered more credible and can be more helpful to the child protective services agency if you give your name.

BOX 21-3: SIGNS OF CHILD ABUSE

SIGNS OF PHYSICAL ABUSE

The child:

- Has unexplained scalding or burns, rope burns, lacerations, bites, bruises, broken bones or black eyes

- Has fading bruises or other marks after an absence from school or child care

- Seems frightened of parents and protests or cries when it is time to go home

- Shrinks at the approach of adults

- Reports being injured by a parent or another adult caregiver

- Appears withdrawn or depressed and cries often – or is aggressive and disruptive

- Seems tired often and complains of frequent nightmares

The parent or other adult caregiver:

- Offers conflicting, unconvincing or no explanation for the child's injury

- Describes the child with words such as "evil" or other negative terms

- Uses harsh physical discipline with the child

- Is known to have a history of abuse as a child

SIGNS OF SEXUAL ABUSE

The child:

- Has difficulty walking or sitting

- Suddenly refuses to change clothing when necessary or to participate in physical activities

- Reports nightmares or bed-wetting

- Experiences a sudden change in appetite

- Demonstrates bizarre, sophisticated or unusual sexual knowledge or behavior

- Becomes pregnant or contracts a venereal disease, particularly if under age 14

- Runs away from home

- Reports sexual abuse by a parent or other adult caregiver

- Seems afraid of a particular person or being alone with that person

The parent or other adult caregiver:

- Is unduly protective of the child or severely limits the child's contact with other children, especially of the opposite sex

- Is secretive and isolated

- Is jealous or controlling with family members

SIGNS OF EMOTIONAL ABUSE

The child:

- Is extreme in behavior, such as overly compliant or demanding or extremely passive or aggressive

- Acts either inappropriately like an adult (such as parenting other children) or inappropriately like an infant (such as frequently rocking or banging head)

- Has delayed physical or emotional development

- Has attempted suicide

- Demonstrates a lack of attachment to the parent

The parent or other adult caregiver:

- Constantly blames, belittles or berates the child

- Seems unconcerned about the child and refuses to consider offers of help for the child's problems

- Overtly rejects the child

Remember: Your suspicion of child abuse or neglect is enough to make a report. You do not have to provide proof. Almost every state has a law to protect people who make good-faith reports of child abuse from prosecution or liability.

What Happens When a Report Is Made

When a report is made, it will first be screened by the agency. If the agency determines there is enough credible information to indicate that maltreatment may have occurred or is at risk of occurring, an investigation will be conducted. Depending on the potential severity of the situation, investigators may respond within hours or days. They may speak with the child, the parents and other people who have contact with the child, such as health care providers, teachers or child care providers.

If the investigator feels the child is at risk of harm, the family may be referred to various programs to reduce the risk of future maltreatment. These may include mental health care, medical care, parenting skills classes, employment assistance and support services, such as financial or housing assistance. In rare cases where the child's safety cannot be ensured, the child may be removed from the home.

The best way to prevent child abuse and neglect is to support families and provide parents with the skills and resources they need. Prevention efforts build on family strengths. Through activities such as parent education, home visitation and parent support groups, many families are able to find the support they need to stay together and care for their children in their homes and communities. Prevention efforts help parents develop their parenting skills, understand the benefits of nonviolent discipline techniques, and understand and meet their child's emotional, physical and developmental needs.

FIRST AID FOR AN APPARENTLY ABUSED CHILD

If you suspect a child in your care is being abused or neglected, do not confront the parents or ask the child direct questions about abuse. If the child needs first aid for an illness or injury, provide it as you would for any child, following the standard guidelines for providing care. Follow your facility's guidelines for documenting the care and any additional actions. If the child tells you an injury was caused by a parent or other adult, include this information when making your report.

SPOUSE ABUSE

Like child abuse, spouse abuse – or domestic violence, also called intimate partner violence (IPV) – is a major problem in our society:[1]

- On average, 24 people per minute are victims of rape, physical violence or stalking by an intimate partner in the United States, which is more than 12 million women and men over the course of a year.

- Nearly 3 in 10 women (29%) and 1 in 10 men (10%) in the United States have experienced rape, physical violence and/or stalking by a partner and report a related impact on their functioning.

- Nearly 15% of women (14.8%) and 4% of men have been injured as a result of IPV that included rape, physical violence and/or stalking by an intimate partner in their lifetime.

- 1 in 4 women (24.3%) and 1 in 7 men (13.8%) 18 and older in the United States have been the victim of severe physical violence by an intimate partner in their lifetime.

- More than 1 in 3 women (35.6%) and more than 1 in 4 men (28.5%) in the United States have experienced rape, physical violence and/or stalking by an intimate partner in their lifetime.

- Nearly half of all women and men in the United States have experienced psychological aggression by an intimate partner in their lifetime (48.4% and 48.8%, respectively).

- Females in age groups 18-24 and 25-34 generally experienced the highest rates of intimate partner violence.

- From 1994 to 2010, about 4 in 5 victims of intimate partner violence were female.

- Most female victims of intimate partner violence were previously victimized by the same offender, including 77% of females 18-24; 76% of females 25-34; and 81% of females 35-49.

[1]*Domestic Violence Resource Center, dvrc-or.org/Dv-facts-stats Accessed January 2016.*

Domestic violence and spouse abuse affect people of all races, nationalities, economic levels and religions. The primary types of domestic violence are physical abuse, sexual abuse/rape and verbal/emotional abuse. Physical abuse may involve hitting, slapping, punching, kicking, choking, biting and assault with objects.

Many abusive relationships continue for some time without the victim reporting the abuse to authorities. Commonly, the victim stays with the abusing spouse or partner for several reasons:

- They love their partner – they just want the abuse to stop.

- They are afraid of their partner.

- They feel guilty and may blame themselves for the violence.

- They often have low self-esteem.

- They are isolated from family and friends.

- They depend emotionally and/or financially on their partner.

- They do not know their rights or that help is available.

Care for a Victim of Domestic Violence

It is seldom obvious that a victim's injuries resulted from physical abuse. Because there is often a history of abuse and physical injury, the victim may be experienced in covering up the cause of injuries. Certain signs, however, may raise a suspicion of domestic violence:

- The victim seems unusually fearful.

- The victim's account of the injury seems inconsistent or unlikely.

- The victim is uneasy in the presence of a spouse or partner.

- The victim's spouse or partner aggressively blames the woman for being injured.

If these or other signs of possible domestic violence are present, consider the possibility that the injury resulted from abuse. Follow these guidelines:

1. Provide first aid as usual for the injury. Call 9-1-1 for significant injuries and tell responding EMS personnel in private about your suspicions; they will know the correct steps to take.

2. Ensure privacy for the victim while providing care.

3. Do not directly confront the victim with your suspicions, especially if the victim's spouse or partner is present.

4. Try to involve a friend or family member of the victim in your care giving.

5. If you are giving first aid as part of your employment responsibilities, you may be required to report suspected cases of domestic violence to authorities. Many health care workers are generally required by law to report suspected abuse. Check with your supervisor.

6. If the victim communicates information to you that suggests abuse, or if it is appropriate in your relationship with the victim to raise the issue yourself, you may choose to tell the victim that domestic violence is against the law and that help is available.

7. If you see physical abuse occurring or are certain a crime has been committed, or if the victim's partner is threatening and potentially violent, call law enforcement personnel. Withdraw from the scene to ensure your own safety. Local and state agencies are present in all 50 states to assist victims of domestic violence in many ways. Often help can be provided to the abuser so that the relationship can continue if that is the wish of both partners. Many support groups are available to help both victims and abusers. Other assistance is available for spouses who choose to end the relationship. Victims should never feel they have no choice but to remain in an abusive relationship.

The National Domestic Violence Hotline can provide information and local contacts for those seeking help: Call 1-800-799-SAFE or visit thehotline.org.

ELDER ABUSE

Elder abuse is another common type of domestic violence. Typically elder abuse refers to physical, emotional or financial abuse or neglect inflicted on someone older than 60. The National Center on Elder Abuse estimates that more than 1 in 10 elders may experience some type of abuse, but only 1 in 23 cases are reported; this means that very few seniors who have been abused get the help they need.[1] This problem has become more common as the elderly population grows and as more elderly people live with and are often cared for by family members. In the great majority of cases, the abuser is a family member, usually an adult child or spouse of the victim. Generally, the older a person is, the greater the risk of elder abuse. An older adult who needs help with daily activities, who has lost bladder control or who behaves unusually because of altered mental status is more likely to be abused or neglected.

[1]*National Center on Elder Abuse, ncea.aoa.gov/Resources/ Publication/docs/NCEA_WhyCare_508.pdf Accessed January 2016.*

There are seven types of elder abuse[2]:

- *Physical abuse:* use of force to threaten or physically injure an elder

- *Emotional abuse:* verbal attacks, threats, rejection, isolation or belittling acts that cause or could cause mental anguish, pain or distress to a senior

- *Sexual abuse:* sexual contact that is forced, tricked, threatened or otherwise coerced upon an elder, including anyone who is unable to grant consent

- *Exploitation:* theft, fraud, misuse or neglect of authority and use of undue influence as leverage to gain control over an older person's money or property

- *Neglect:* a caregiver's failure or refusal to provide for a vulnerable elder's safety or physical or emotional needs

- *Abandonment:* desertion of a frail or vulnerable elder by anyone with a duty of care

- *Self-neglect:* an inability to understand the consequences of one's own actions or inaction that leads to, or may lead to, harm or endangerment

[2]*National Center on Elder Abuse, ncea.aoa.gov/Resources/ Publication/docs/NCEA_WhyCare_508.pdf Accessed January 2016.*

Because older adults are often frail, physical abuse is more likely to result in injury. Physical elder abuse is defined as the willful infliction of physical pain or injury, such as slapping, hitting with an object, shoving, shaking, kicking, burning, sexually molesting, force-feeding, administering of unwanted drugs or restraining the person.

The most important signs of elder maltreatment are:

- Frequent, unexplained crying

- Unexplained fear of or suspicion of a particular person(s) in the home

The signs and symptoms of elder abuse are listed in **Box 21-4.**

CARE FOR A VICTIM OF ELDER ABUSE

If the signs of possible elder abuse are present, consider the possibility that the injury resulted from abuse. Follow the same general guidelines as for a victim of spouse abuse or other domestic violence. All 50 states have specific elder abuse laws. Suspected elder abuse should be reported to your state's adult protective services agency. As with reports of suspected child abuse, the information you report will be kept confidential. The state agency will investigate the case and will provide services as needed for the elder and family members.

BOX 21-4: SIGNS AND SYMPTOMS OF ELDER ABUSE AND NEGLECT

PHYSICAL ABUSE

- Bruises, black eyes, welts, lacerations and rope marks

- Bone or skull fractures

- Open wounds, cuts, punctures, untreated injuries and injuries in various stages of healing

- Strains, dislocations and internal injuries/bleeding

- Broken eyeglasses, physical signs of being subjected to punishment and signs of being restrained

- Laboratory findings of medication overdose or underutilization of prescribed drugs

- An elder's report of being hit, slapped, kicked or mistreated

- An elder's sudden change in behavior

- A caregiver's refusal to allow visitors to see an elder alone

SEXUAL ABUSE

- Bruises around the breasts or genital area

- Unexplained venereal disease or genital infections

- Unexplained vaginal or anal bleeding

- Torn, stained or bloody underclothing

- An elder's report of being sexually assaulted or raped

EMOTIONAL/PSYCHOLOGICAL ABUSE

- Emotional upset or agitation

- Extreme withdrawal, lack of communication and responsiveness

- An elder's report of being verbally or emotionally mistreated

NEGLECT

- Dehydration, malnutrition, untreated bedsores and poor personal hygiene

- Unattended or untreated health problems

- Hazardous or unsafe living conditions (e.g., improper wiring, no heat or no running water)

- Unsanitary or unclean living conditions (e.g., dirt, fleas, lice on person, soiled bedding, fecal/urine smell, inadequate clothing)

- An elder's report of being neglected

ABANDONMENT

- The desertion of an elder at a hospital, nursing facility or other similar institution

- The desertion of an elder at a shopping center or other public location.

- An elder's own report of being abandoned

SELF-NEGLECT

- Dehydration, malnutrition, untreated or improperly attended medical conditions and poor personal hygiene

- Hazardous or unsafe living conditions (e.g., improper wiring, no indoor plumbing, no heat or no running water)

- Unsanitary or unclean living quarters (e.g., animal/insect infestation, no functioning toilet, fecal/urine smell)

- Inappropriate and/or inadequate clothing, lack of necessary medical aids (e.g., eyeglasses, hearing aid, dentures)

- Grossly inadequate housing or homelessness

Source: "The National Elder Abuse Incidence Study," The Administration on Aging, U.S. Department of Health and Human Services, aoa.gov/AoA_Programs/Elder_Rights/Elder_Abuse/docs/ABuseReport_Full.pdf. Accessed January 2016.

Sexual Assault and Rape

The following definitions of rape and sexual assault are from the U.S. Department of Justice[1]:

Rape is forced sexual intercourse including both psychological coercion as well as physical force. Forced sexual intercourse means penetration by the offender(s). It includes attempted rape, male as well as female victims, and both heterosexual and homosexual rape. Attempted rape includes verbal threats of rape.

Sexual assault includes a wide range of victimizations, separate from rape or attempted rape. These crimes include attacks or attempted attacks generally involving unwanted sexual contact between victim and offender. Sexual assaults may or may not involve force and include such things as grabbing or fondling. It also includes verbal threats.

[1]bjs.gov/index.cfm?ty=tp&tid=317 Accessed January 2016.

Rape and sexual assault are serious problems in our society:[2]

- 1 out of every 6 American women has been the victim of an attempted or completed rape in her lifetime (14.8% completed rape; 2.8% attempted rape).

- 17.7 million American women have been victims of attempted or completed rape.

- 2.78 million men in the United States have been victims of sexual assault or rape.

- 9 of every 10 rape victims are female.

- 15% of sexual assault and rape victims are younger than 12. 80% are younger than 30. 12-34 are the highest risk years.

- Victims of sexual assault are:

  - 3 times more likely to suffer from depression.

  - 6 times more likely to suffer from post-traumatic stress disorder (PTSD).

  - 13 times more likely to abuse alcohol.

  - 26 times more likely to abuse drugs.

  - 4 times more likely to contemplate suicide.

[2]Rape, Abuse & Incest National Network (RAINN) rainn.org/ get-information/statistics/sexual-assault-victims Accessed January 2016.

PREVENTION OF RAPE AND SEXUAL ASSAULT

To reduce the risk of rape and sexual assault, the Rape, Abuse & Incest National Network (RAINN) recommends these precautions:

- In a social setting, do not leave your beverage unattended or accept a drink from an open container because the drink may be drugged.

- When you go to a party, go with a group of friends. Arrive together, watch out for each other and leave together.

- Be aware of your surroundings at all times.

- Don't allow yourself to be isolated with someone you do not know or trust.

- Think about the level of intimacy you want in a relationship, and clearly state your limits.

CARE FOR A VICTIM OF RAPE OR SEXUAL ASSAULT

1. Be sensitive to the victim's psychological trauma. After a rape, the victim may be hysterical, crying, hyperventilating or in a dazed, unresponsive state. Provide emotional support as appropriate.

2. Ensure that 9-1-1 has been called. Rape requires a coordinated response of law enforcement and EMS personnel.

3. Ensure privacy for the victim.

4. Try to involve a friend or family member of the victim in your care giving. A first aider of the same sex may be more comforting.

5. Provide first aid as needed for any injury. Someone should stay with the victim until help arrives.

6. For legal reasons, it is important to preserve evidence of a rape. Ask the victim not to urinate, bathe or wash any area involved in the rape or assault before EMS personnel arrive. Follow-up care of rape victims usually includes a full physical examination as well as possible later testing for sexually transmitted diseases and pregnancy.

Because rape can lead to later traumatic stress and psychological problems, victims may benefit from counseling provided by rape crisis centers and support groups. To find a center in your area, call the National Sexual Assault Hotline at 1-800-656-HOPE, or visit the RAINN website: rainn.org.

1. Select the best answer. If you suspect a child is being abused by a parent, the most important thing to do is –

    a. talk to the parent so he or she can get help.

    b. remove the child from the home.

    c. report the situation to authorities.

    d. talk to the spouse of the abusing parent and let him or her decide what to do.

2. Check off common characteristics of victims of domestic violence.

    ☐ They love their partners.

    ☐ They are not afraid of their partners.

    ☐ They feel guilty and may blame themselves for the violence.

    ☐ They often have low self-esteem.

    ☐ They feel close to family and friends.

    ☐ They depend emotionally and/or financially on their partners.

3. Select the best answer. Elder abuse includes –

    a. sexual abuse.

    b. abandonment.

    c. neglect.

    d. All of the above

4. List six important first aid actions for a victim injured during a rape.

    _____

    _____

    _____

 CONCLUDING THOUGHTS

Behavioral emergencies and abuse situations are generally stressful for first aiders because of the unpredictable behavior and difficult emotions of those involved. Remember that in most cases these situations last only a few minutes before EMS professionals, or sometimes law enforcement personnel, arrive and take over. These professionals have the training to manage the situation safely and appropriately. For the few minutes

you may be with a victim, be sensitive to the situation and alert for your own safety. In almost all cases, you can use common sense and the general guidelines in this chapter to avoid a confrontation while providing first aid.

 CRITICAL THINKING CHALLENGE QUESTIONS

SCENARIO 1

You are walking across campus when you notice a student seated alone on a bench, holding his head in his hands, immobile. You recognize him from one of your classes and say hello as you walk by. He looks up, a vacant look in his eyes, but doesn't say anything. Because he is acting oddly, you stop and ask him if he feels OK. He stares at you, then holds his forehead with one hand as if experiencing an intense pain. You ask if he needs help and he abruptly shouts at you, "I'm OK! Leave me alone!"

a. Should you do anything or just walk away?

    _____

    _____

b. You decide to try to talk to him to see if he may be experiencing a medical problem. You take care not to seem to challenge him but express your concern that perhaps he is not feeling well and you may be able to help him. You follow the general guidelines for calming and reassuring a victim in a behavioral emergency.

    He listens a moment, still not saying anything, then jumps to his feet and stares you in the face, scowling. His hands are clenched into fists. What do you do?

    _____

    _____

c. You walk away. When you look back, he is again seated and holding his head. Is there anything you can do now?

    _____

    _____

ADDITIONAL ACTIVITIES AND RESOURCES

1. In recent decades, suicide has become more common among college students. Research student suicides, and learn the causative factors involved as well as local resources to help students who feel depressed or suicidal. Talk with the student health center. If suicide is a significant problem on your campus, ask a mental health professional associated with the student health center to offer information.

2. Rape and sexual assaults are also increasing on many campuses, particularly "date rape." If this is a significant problem on your campus, research preventive programs in the area and gather tips on preventing the problem.

 REVIEW QUESTIONS

Select the best answers.

1. Normal physical signs and symptoms of injury-related stress include –

    a. dry skin.

    b. nausea.

    c. slow breathing.

    d. drowsiness.

2. Altered mental status may result from any injury that causes –

    a. reduced oxygen levels.

    b. increased oxygen levels.

    c. faster heartbeat.

    d. fluid loss.

3. Why is it important to calm and reassure an emotional victim?

    a. Emotional stress has negative physical effects on the body.

    b. It is difficult to give first aid to an emotional, uncooperative victim.

    c. Calming may help prevent a victim from becoming violent.

    d. All of the above

Circle **True** or **False** for the following statement:

4. Making eye contact with a victim who is irrational, delusional or potentially violent will likely upset the person and make the situation worse.   True   False

5. You should try to reassure an injured victim who is depressed by saying things such as, –

    a. "Don't worry, everything will be just fine."

    b. "Don't cry. Let's talk about more positive things in your life."

    c. "There are programs available to help you deal with problems like this."

    d. "I'm sure this problem won't last long."

6. Call 9-1-1 for –

    a. a potentially violent victim of any kind of injury.

    b. someone talking about suicide who has a bottle of pills.

    c. an injured person who is shouting at a hallucination.

    d. All of the above

7. A parent who abuses his or her child, when confronted with an accusation, is most likely to –

    a. deny the problem.

    b. admit the problem and feel relief that now he or she will get treatment.

    c. become violent and attack the accuser.

    d. blame his or her spouse for the problem.

8. Which of these statements is true?

    a. Authorities want proof of child abuse before they will take your report.

    b. A reasonable suspicion of child abuse is sufficient grounds to report to the authorities.

    c. After you report suspected child abuse, the authorities will ask you to help them "trap" the abuser to get a confession.

    d. You may be sued for making a report if your accusation turns out to be false.

9. Suspected cases of child abuse or domestic violence should be reported only by –

    a. people who have cause to suspect abuse or violence.

    b. people whose jobs require it.

    c. the victims.

    d. family members of the victims.

10. Preserving evidence of a rape includes –

    a. asking the victim not to wash until examined by a health care provider.

    b. asking the victim to avoid talking until examined by a health care provider.

    c. not allowing the victim to move at all from the position in which he or she was found.

    d. not touching the victim when giving first aid for any injuries.

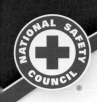

CHAPTER 22

Pregnancy and Childbirth

LESSON OBJECTIVES

- List healthy behaviors during pregnancy to prevent problems for the woman and fetus.

- Describe the stages of pregnancy and the stages of labor and delivery.

- Explain the first aid for vaginal bleeding during pregnancy and for possible miscarriage.

- Describe how to assist during childbirth and care for the mother and newborn after the birth.

- Explain actions to take in case of complications: breech presentation, prolapsed cord, the cord wrapped around the infant's head and bleeding after delivery.

Melanie is almost 9 months pregnant with her first baby, but still a week away from her due date. You have just trimmed her hair and are blowing it dry when she suddenly gets a funny look on her face and says, "Oh, no!" Then she tells you, "My water just broke." What do you do?

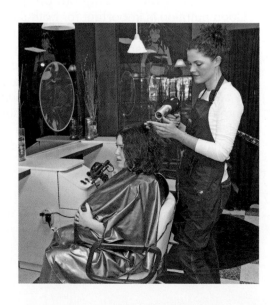

Although rare, certain health problems may occur during pregnancy that require first aid. In addition, childbirth sometimes occurs outside a planned setting. Because no one can predict in every case when labor will begin or how long it will last before the infant is delivered, a pregnant woman may find herself unable to reach the planned setting for childbirth, and without the attendance of a doctor, midwife or other person trained in childbirth. In such a situation, a first aider may be called upon to assist. This is very rarely a medical emergency, because childbirth is a normal, natural process that usually takes place without problems or complications – and with only minimal assistance from others.

Prevention of Problems in Pregnancy

Preventing problems in pregnancy and maintaining good health for both the woman and the fetus begin with regular **prenatal** (before birth) care. Health care practitioners generally recommend that a woman see her health care provider as soon as she knows or suspects that she is pregnant.

The health care provider thereafter will schedule a series of regular visits to ensure the pregnancy is progressing well and to treat any complications that may arise.

Following are general guidelines many health care practitioners will recommend for pregnant women. *With any guideline, however, always follow the health care provider's specific instructions, because all guidelines do not automatically apply to all pregnant women.*

- **Eat a healthy diet throughout pregnancy.** Good nutrition is important for both the woman and the developing fetus. A higher-than-usual caloric intake is usually advised, along with specific recommendations for balanced nutrition and daily supplements. Most pregnant women are advised to take folic acid (vitamin B) and iron supplements and to ensure that their diet contains sufficient calcium, protein, carbohydrates, fluids and other vitamins as well as moderate salt. Follow the health care provider's guidelines.

- **Accept normal weight gain.** Pregnant women should follow their health care provider's recommendations, but generally a woman of normal prepregnancy weight should gain 25-35 pounds gradually during pregnancy. Attempts to diet or exercise too much in an attempt to prevent weight gain are generally unhealthy for the fetus.

- **Minimize caffeine from coffee, tea and soft drinks.** Although studies do not clearly show exactly how much caffeine is safe, it has been demonstrated that high levels of caffeine are associated with higher rates of **miscarriage** and can cause other problems for the fetus.

- **Avoid alcohol entirely.** Even very small amounts of alcohol have been shown to affect fetal growth, and higher levels can cause **fetal alcohol syndrome,** which causes growth deficiencies, mental retardation and other problems.

- **Stop smoking.** Cigarette smoking in pregnancy has been associated with lowered birth weight and preterm delivery.

- **Do not use illicit drugs.** Some studies suggest that marijuana use in pregnancy may have harmful effects on the fetus, and drugs such as crack cocaine are known to have serious, detrimental effects.

- **Get exercise.** The American Congress of Obstetricians and Gynecologists generally recommends 30 minutes of moderate exercise a day for most healthy pregnant women.[1] The health care provider can recommend the most effective and safest types of exercise.

- **Get enough rest.** Sufficient sleep is important during pregnancy, as are frequent rest breaks during the day. The health care practitioner may also recommend avoidance of certain kinds of activities.

- **Prevent injury.** Avoid situations that may lead to falls, such as when climbing a ladder or standing on a chair to reach a high shelf. Get help when needed, such as getting out of a bathtub during the last weeks of pregnancy. Avoid risky sports and recreational activities.

[1]acog.org/Patients/FAQs/Exercise-During-Pregnancy Accessed January 2016.

Pregnancy and Labor

Pregnancy begins with fertilization of the woman's ovum (egg cell), by a sperm cell in a process often called conception. Growth and development proceed in an orderly manner for about 40 weeks at which time childbirth typically occurs. Pregnancy is usually composed of 3 trimesters, followed by labor and delivery.

STAGES OF PREGNANCY

Pregnancy is often divided into 3 trimesters of roughly 3 months each. Within the first few days, the single cell that results from fertilization divides into a mass of many cells. After it implants in the uterus at 5-7 days, and thereafter for the first 8 weeks, the developing human is called an **embryo;** thereafter it is called a **fetus.** The embryo develops inside the **amniotic sac,** which contains **amniotic fluid** (often called "water"). The embryo is attached to the woman's **placenta,** an organ that develops in pregnancy to supply the embryo and fetus with oxygen and nutrients, via the **umbilical cord (Figure 22-1).** By 8 weeks, the embryo has developed all major organ systems. Throughout the rest of the pregnancy, it continues to grow and develop to the point where the infant can live independently outside the mother's body.

FIGURE 22-1

The fetus at 8 months.

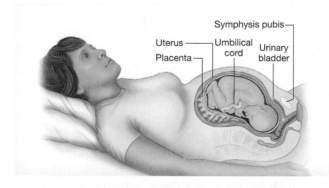

During the first trimester, although the fetus has recognizable human features and is about 2½ inches long, the pregnant woman experiences few visible changes. Her heart rate has increased by about 8 beats per minute, and she may experience some normal results of hormonal changes in her body, such as nausea **(morning sickness)** and breast tenderness.

During the second trimester, weeks 13-28, the fetus grows to a length of 12 inches. At about 18-20 weeks, the woman may feel it moving. The woman's abdomen gradually swells, and she may experience

discharge from the nipples caused by changes in the milk-producing glands.

In the third trimester, weeks 29-40, the fetus grows rapidly. By week 36, it is fully formed, weighs about 6½ pounds and can live outside the mother without advanced medical intervention. The head of the fetus is positioned downward in the woman's pelvis. The woman's uterus has expanded high into the abdomen and presses on the lungs, possibly causing a slight shortness of breath. The pregnant woman may also experience backache, heartburn, constipation and frequent urination.

STAGES OF LABOR AND DELIVERY

Labor and delivery occur in 3 stages, beginning with the first uterine contractions. Up to 10 days before the beginning of contractions, the mucus plug from the cervix, which had blocked the uterus from possible infection from the vagina, is released; this is sometimes called "the show," or "bloody show," but it often goes unnoticed. Uterine contractions begin and eventually push the infant's head into the **cervix,** which is dilating (opening). The cervix is the lower part of the uterus opening into the vagina. Contractions gradually become stronger and more frequent. The amniotic sac ruptures either shortly before or during the first stage of labor, causing the fluid to either rush or trickle out of the vaginal opening; this is often called the "water breaking." The first stage may last from a few hours to a day in a woman who has not given birth before, but sometimes occurs in only a few minutes in a woman who has given birth previously. At first, contractions are usually 10-15 minutes apart, and shortly before childbirth, they may be only 2-3 minutes apart.

In the second stage, the infant is delivered. This stage typically lasts 1-2 hours, but may happen more quickly in women who have given birth previously. The cervix has fully dilated, and contractions are powerful and often painful. The infant's head presses on the floor of the pelvis and the woman feels a strong urge to push down. The vagina, or birth canal, stretches open as the infant's head moves out of the uterus, and the top of the infant's head can now be seen; this is called **crowning (Figure 22-2).** The vagina stretches more as the head emerges, often quickly, and the rest of the infant's body is typically pushed out very quickly **(Figure 22-3).** The person assisting with the delivery supports the infant's head as it emerges and ensures that the umbilical cord is not wrapped around the infant's neck.

In the third stage, the placenta separates from the uterus and is delivered, usually within 30 minutes after childbirth. The uterus then contracts and seals off bleeding vessels.

FIGURE 22-2

Crowning: The infant's head begins to show.

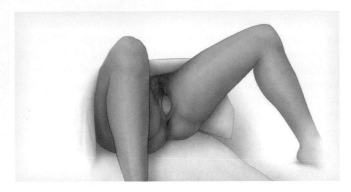

FIGURE 22-3

The infant moves through the birth canal.

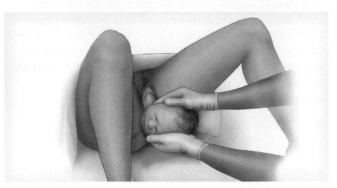

✎ LEARNING CHECKPOINT 1

1. Put a check mark before the accepted guidelines for a healthy pregnancy:

   ☐ Walk at least a mile a day.

   ☐ Eliminate salt from the diet.

   ☐ Minimize caffeine and alcohol consumption.

   ☐ Take dietary supplements as recommended.

   ☐ Exercise to prevent weight gain.

   ☐ Adopt a low-carbohydrate diet.

2. Select the best answer. The first stage of labor begins with –

   a. crowning.

   b. uterine contractions.

   c. cervical dilation.

   d. rupture of the amniotic sac.

3. Select the best answer. Shortly before birth occurs, contractions usually occur –

   a. every 30 seconds.

   b. every 2-3 minutes.

   c. every 5-10 minutes.

   d. between 1-10 minutes.

First Aid in Pregnancy

Most pregnant women receive regular care and are advised by their health care providers about potential problems to watch for. Although rare, problems may occur that require emergency care, and possibly first aid, before the woman receives medical attention.

VAGINAL BLEEDING

Vaginal bleeding during pregnancy is abnormal. Bleeding may be caused by cervical growths or erosion, by a problem with the placenta or by miscarriage. In the third trimester, vaginal bleeding may be a sign of potential preterm birth. The woman should see her health care provider immediately. Call 9-1-1 for heavy bleeding. While waiting for help, calm the woman, and help her into a comfortable position. Have a female assistant present if possible. Give the woman a towel or sanitary napkins to absorb the blood, but do not try to pack the vagina. Save the blood and any expelled material to give to arriving EMS personnel.

MISCARRIAGE

Miscarriage, also called spontaneous abortion, is loss of the embryo or fetus, usually during the first 14 weeks of pregnancy. An estimated 10%-25% of all pregnancies end in miscarriage,[1] which is a natural way that the body manages a potential problem in the pregnancy. It may result from a genetic disorder or fetal abnormality, some factor related to the woman's health or to no known cause. Smoking and the use of alcohol or drugs are also risk factors. Most women who have a miscarriage do not have problems with later pregnancies.

[1]American Pregnancy Association, americanpregnancy.org/ pregnancy-complications/miscarriage Accessed January 2016.

The early signs of a possible miscarriage are vaginal bleeding and abdominal pain or cramping. The woman needs immediate medical attention. Give first aid for bleeding, and call 9-1-1 if the bleeding is heavy.

Take steps to minimize shock if bleeding is heavy (see **Chapter 9**). Because the possibility of miscarriage is usually very distressing, be calm and reassuring.

OTHER SIGNS OF POSSIBLE PROBLEMS

Bleeding is one of the most serious problems during pregnancy, but other signs and symptoms may also indicate a problem. The woman should see her health care provider if she experiences any of the following:

- **Abdominal pain,** which may result from miscarriage or a problem with the placenta. The woman should rest until she receives medical advice.

- **Persistent or severe headache,** especially in the last trimester, which may be a sign of a serious condition called **toxemia.** Toxemia may also cause unusual weight gain, blurred vision and swollen fingers or face.

- **Sudden leaking of water from the vagina,** unless the woman is close to the time of labor, which may indicate premature rupture of the amniotic sac. If this happens, the woman should see her health care provider.

- **Other serious signs and symptoms include persistent vomiting, chills and fever, convulsions and difficulty breathing.** All should be reported immediately to a health care provider.

 LEARNING CHECKPOINT 2

1. Describe first aid to give a pregnant woman who has heavy vaginal bleeding.

_____

_____

_____

_____

2. Select the best answer. The early signs of a possible miscarriage include –

   a. vaginal bleeding.

   b. high fever.

   c. altered mental status.

   d. All of the above

3. Check off the signs and symptoms that may indicate a possible problem during pregnancy:

   ☐ Abdominal pain

   ☐ Persistent headache

   ☐ Chills and fever

   ☐ Convulsions

   ☐ Difficulty breathing

   ☐ Water leaking from vagina in week 20

CHOKING CARE FOR A PREGNANT WOMAN

Do not use abdominal thrusts on a responsive pregnant woman who is choking. Instead, give chest thrusts as described in **Chapter 7.**

Childbirth

In our society, childbirth has occurred predominantly in hospitals for so long that people may assume it is so difficult or dangerous that hospitals are always needed. In reality, childbirth is a natural process that seldom involves complications or requires elaborate medical care. It is true that some complications are possible and that medical steps are then necessary for the health of the mother or infant. But if a woman is unable to reach medical care when contractions suggest childbirth may be imminent, this should not be a cause for panic. *The childbirth itself is not an emergency.* Nonetheless, a pregnant woman who realizes she may have her baby before reaching her planned location, and perhaps without health care providers present, is likely to be fearful and distressed. If you are helping the woman and realize that it may be you who helps deliver the infant, you are likely to experience similar emotions. Coping with these stresses may be more difficult than assisting with the childbirth itself.

Remember that once you have called 9-1-1, help is usually only minutes away. It is very unlikely that a woman close to childbirth will actually give birth before advanced care personnel arrive. Remember also that even if help is delayed or her labor advances very quickly to childbirth, in the great majority of cases, there are no complications, and you will be able to assist her through this process for the short time that help is needed. It is crucial that you remain calm in order to reassure and assist the woman. Although you may be concerned about doing something wrong, try to relax and focus on the woman's need for your calm guidance to help manage her fears and the pain of labor.

IS DELIVERY IMMINENT?

Depending on how the woman's labor is progressing and how soon EMS personnel are expected to arrive, you may be assisting the woman only with labor or also with delivery. An important initial step in first aid, therefore, is assessing whether delivery may occur soon.

Remember that labor usually lasts for several hours, allowing plenty of time for the woman to be transported to the hospital or other planned childbirth location or for other assistance to arrive. In rare cases, however, labor may proceed very quickly, or transportation may be delayed. Even an expert cannot predict exactly when childbirth will occur, but the following assessments can help determine whether delivery may be imminent. If so, do not try to transport the woman; instead, prepare for childbirth.

- **Assess the contractions**. How close together are they, and how long does each last? When timing contractions, time from the beginning of one contraction to the beginning of the next contraction, not the time between them. Contractions generally become stronger, last longer and come more frequently as labor progresses. If contractions are less than 5 minutes apart and each lasts 45-60 seconds, delivery may occur soon, and you should be making preparations. When contractions are about 2 minutes apart, delivery will likely occur soon.

- **Ask the woman if she has given birth before.** First childbirths usually take longer than later ones. If she has given birth in the past, labor is likely to proceed more quickly this time. Also, ask if she knows whether she may be having twins or triplets – most women have learned this during their prenatal care.

- **Check whether the amniotic sac has ruptured.** Ask the woman if her water has broken. Because this often occurs hours before delivery, however, it is not a reliable sign that childbirth is imminent.

- **Ask whether the woman feels a strong urge to push.** This may mean delivery is approaching. Similarly, a feeling that she needs to have a bowel movement may indicate the infant's head has moved to a position close to delivery.

- **If other signs are suggestive of delivery, check whether the infant's head is crowning.** If possible, ask another woman present to check this. Once the top of the head is visible through the vaginal opening during a contraction, be prepared for delivery to occur very soon. At this point, you should not be preparing the woman for transport.

Note that labor may begin potentially many weeks before the woman is due, resulting in a premature birth. Because a premature infant is more likely to need medical care after birth, it is important to recognize the first signs of labor at any point in the pregnancy and take appropriate action.

ASSISTING DURING LABOR

If labor has begun but delivery is not imminent, give supportive care to the expectant mother. Follow these guidelines:

- Ensure that a plan is in place for the woman's transport to the planned childbirth location or for the arrival of the planned attendant.

- Help the woman to rest in whatever position is most comfortable for her.

- Provide any desired comfort measures, such as massaging the lower back (which may help reduce pain). Although the woman should not eat or drink, she may suck on small ice chips or have her lips moistened if her mouth is dry.

- Do not let the woman have a bath if the amniotic sac has ruptured, because of the risk of infection.

- Time the length of contractions and the interval between them and write down this information.

- Help remind the woman to control her breathing: short, quick breaths (panting) during contractions and deep, slow breaths between.

- Continue to help the woman stay calm and provide reassurance. Anxiety and fear will only add to her pain. Regular, deep breathing in through the nose and out through the mouth may help her to relax. (Using the same technique yourself, in sync along with the woman, may help you to relax, too. If you are tense and nervous, this will make the woman more fearful.)

ASSISTING WITH DELIVERY

If signs are present that delivery may be imminent, prepare to assist with the delivery. Remember that childbirth is a natural process that will essentially occur by itself. Your role is simply to prepare the environment to maintain cleanliness for the mother and child and to support both of them during and after the birth.

PREPARATIONS

Ensure that someone stays with the woman while preparations are being made. If you do not have a sterile delivery kit, you can gather household items to prepare. If possible, another woman should be present, preferably a friend or family member.

First, gather the items needed or helpful for the delivery:

- A clean blanket or coverlet

- Several pillows

- A plastic sheet (or shower curtain) or a stack of newspapers

- Clean towels and washcloths

- Sanitary napkins or pads made of clean, folded cloth

- Medical examination gloves (use clean kitchen gloves or plastic bags on your hands if gloves are unavailable)

- Plastic bags (for afterbirth and cleanup)

- Bowl of hot water (for washing)

- Empty bowl or bucket (in case of vomiting)

- Clean handkerchief (to wear as a face mask)

- Eye and face protection for yourself, if available.

- Clean, soft towel, sheet or blanket (to wrap the newborn)

- Bulb syringe, if available (to suction infant's nose and mouth) or sterile gauze

- If help may be delayed: clean, strong string, shoelaces or cloth strips to tie the cord

- If help may be delayed:

  - Sharp scissors or knife sterilized in boiling water for 5 minutes, or held over a flame for 30 seconds, to cut the cord.

  - Prepare the birthing bed with clean sheets over a rubber or plastic sheet (or shower curtain or several sheets of newspaper) to protect the mattress. If a bed is not present, prepare a clean place on the floor or ground, making a padded area of newspapers, cloths or blankets.

  - Roll up your sleeves, wash your hands thoroughly for 5 minutes and put on medical examination gloves.

  - If possible, protect your eyes, mouth and nose from likely splashes of blood and other fluids; a handkerchief can be tied over your mouth and nose.

When childbirth seems imminent, follow the steps listed in First Aid: "Assisting with Delivery." If a telephone is available at the scene, have someone call the woman's health care provider or 9-1-1 so additional instructions can be given over the phone during or after the childbirth, if necessary.

First Aid: Assisting with Delivery

Signs, Symptoms and Care

WHEN YOU SEE

- Contractions occurring 2-3 minutes apart.

- The woman feels a strong urge to push.

- Crowning of the infant's head.

DO THIS FIRST

1. Help the woman lie on her back with knees bent and apart and feet flat on the bed. Note that she may have been trained already in other birthing positions, which are acceptable. Ensure that she is not wearing undergarments or other clothing that may get in the way. If she prefers, cover her above the knees with a blanket or sheet. Have folded towels or a blanket under her buttocks.

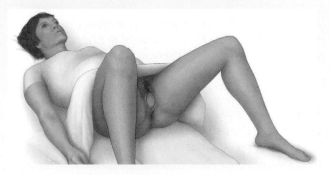

2. As the infant's head appears, have your gloved hands ready to receive and support the head, which may emerge very quickly. Check that the head is not covered by the amniotic sac; if so, pull it away as the mouth and nose emerge.

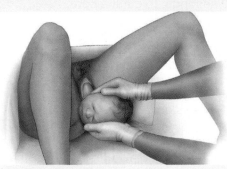

3. As the head emerges (usually face down), support the head. Check that the umbilical cord is not wrapped around the infant's neck; if it is, see if it is loose enough to slip over the head or shoulder to prevent strangulation, but avoid putting pressure on the cord or pulling it. Use a bulb syringe to gently suck secretions from the mouth and nose, or wipe both with sterile gauze. Compress the bulb syringe before insertion.

4. After the head is out, have the woman stop pushing and breathe in a panting manner. Do not attempt to pull the infant out, but support it as its body emerges, often very quickly after the head. Usually, the infant turns to the side as the shoulder emerges. Newborns are usually very slippery and should be handled carefully. Grasp the infant's feet as they emerge. If the mother is having multiple births, prepare for the delivery of the second infant. Note the time of delivery to tell medical personnel later.

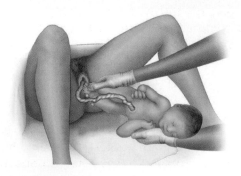

5. The newborn normally begins to cry. Hold it at the level of the woman's vagina with head lower than the feet to allow secretions to drain from the nose and mouth. Use a bulb syringe to gently suck secretions from the mouth and then the nose or wipe both with sterile gauze. If you don't have a bulb syringe, gently stroke downward on the baby's nose to help expel excess mucus and amniotic fluid. If the infant is not crying, gently flick the bottom of its feet with a finger or gently rub its back. If he or she is still not crying, check for breathing, and start CPR if needed (see **Chapter 5**).

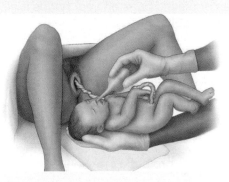

6. Gently dry and wrap the infant in a towel or blanket to prevent heat loss, keeping the cord loose and free of compression and kinks. Place the infant on the mother's abdomen, on its side with its head low for the nose and mouth to drain. The position on the mother's stomach provides warmth. If you cannot place the newborn here for any reason, keep it warm and above the level of the mother's heart. Only if the infant must be separated from the mother in order to provide emergency care should the cord be cut.

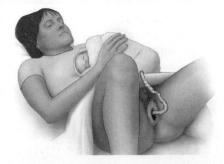

7. Stay with the mother and infant while waiting for the delivery of the afterbirth, the placenta and umbilical cord, which usually occurs with milder contractions in 10-30 minutes. Typically,

there will be a gush of blood as the placenta detaches from the uterus. Save the placenta in a plastic bag or towel because it is important for health care providers to examine it.

8. In most situations, it is not necessary to tie or cut the umbilical cord, even after the placenta has been delivered, because medical help will be arriving very soon. Keep the placenta at the same level as the infant while waiting for help to arrive. If help may be delayed in a remote location, tie and cut the cord before delivery of the afterbirth. Wait until the cord stops pulsating. Then, tie a tight knot around the cord about 10 inches from the infant, using string, clean shoelaces or thin strips of cloth. Tie a second knot about 7 inches from the infant, and cut the cord between the 2 ties with sterilized scissors or knife.

ADDITIONAL CARE

• The mother may continue to bleed for a time, normally up to a pint following delivery. Place sanitary napkins or folded clean cloths against the vaginal opening but do not push. Gently massage the mother's abdomen with a circular motion just below the navel to help the uterus contract to stop the bleeding.

• Ensure that the infant stays warm and continues to breathe. Skin-to-skin contact between mother and infant helps the infant stay warm. The

mother can begin nursing the infant immediately, which will help the uterus to contract and stop bleeding.

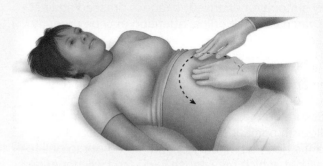

ALERT

• Do not try to delay the birth by having the woman hold her legs together or any other maneuver.

• Do not place your hands or anything else in the woman's vagina.

• Do not interfere with the childbirth or touch the infant until the head is completely out.

• Do not pull on the head or shoulders.

• Do not try to wash the infant's skin, eyes or ears.

• Do not pull on the umbilical cord in an effort to pull out the afterbirth.

CARE OF THE MOTHER AFTER DELIVERY

After the delivery, continue to support and comfort the mother. Ensure that she is warm and comfortable. She may drink water now and may find it comforting to have her face wiped with cool water. Even with a successful delivery, she and the infant should still see a health care provider because problems sometimes occur within the first 24 hours.

CARE OF THE NEWBORN

Once you have determined that the newborn is breathing well, little specific care is needed. A normal newborn respiratory rate is 40 breaths per minute or more. Dry but do not try to wash the newborn, whose skin may be covered with a white, cheesy protective coating called vernix. Ensure that the infant stays

wrapped, including the head, to stay warm. Support the newborn's head if it must be moved for any reason. Continue to check the newborn's breathing.

A very small or premature infant born a significant time before the mother's due date is at greater risk for complications after birth. It is crucial to keep a small newborn warm. There is also a greater likelihood that resuscitation may be needed.

CHILDBIRTH PROBLEMS

Most deliveries occur without problems or complications, but you should be prepared to manage a problem if one does occur. The most common problems involve the **presentation** of the infant (its position at emergence) or maternal bleeding after delivery.

Breech Birth

A **breech presentation** occurs when the infant's buttocks or feet appear first in the birth canal rather than the head **(Figure 22-4)**. This can become an emergency because as the head enters the birth canal, the umbilical cord is squeezed and blood flow may stop. Also, if the infant's head becomes lodged in the birth canal and the infant tries to breathe, it may suffocate because the face is pressed against the vaginal wall. Medical attention may be urgently needed.

When you first see a breech presentation, move the woman to a kneeling position with her head and chest down **(Figure 22-5)**. This helps to minimize pressure on the cord and is generally the preferred childbirth position in this situation. Support the infant's body as it emerges, but do not try to pull the head out, which may cause injury and will not speed up the birth. If the head does not emerge soon after the body, you may need to open a breathing space for the infant. Carefully insert one hand alongside the infant's head, palm against the face and make a V with 2 fingers positioned on each side of the infant's nose. Press against the birth canal to allow air to reach the infant's nose while waiting for the head to be delivered. Check the infant immediately, and be prepared to give CPR if needed.

FIGURE 22-4

Breech presentation.

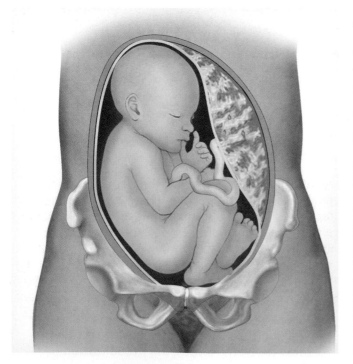

FIGURE 22-5

Position for breech presentation.

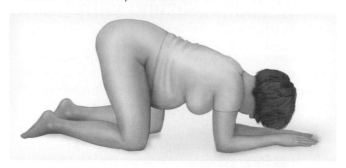

Limb Presentation

Very rarely one arm or leg may emerge first from the birth canal. This is an emergency requiring immediate medical assistance. Position the woman in the same knee-chest position as for a breech birth while waiting for help. Do not try to pull the infant out or push the arm or leg back inside the woman.

Prolapsed Cord

The umbilical cord is said to be **prolapsed** when a segment of it protrudes through the birth canal before childbirth **(Figure 22-6)**. This is an emergency because the cord will be compressed as the infant begins to move through the birth canal, cutting off blood flow. Position the woman in the knee-chest position to reduce pressure on the cord. Do not try to push the cord back inside the mother. If medical personnel have not arrived when the infant presents and begins to emerge, carefully insert your hand into the birth canal and try to separate the cord and the presenting body part while allowing the birth to continue. Check the infant immediately, and be prepared to give CPR if needed.

FIGURE 22-6

Prolapsed cord.

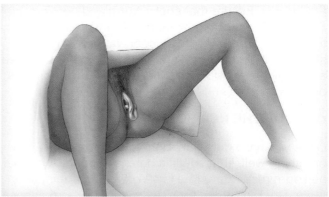

Cord Around Neck

If the umbilical cord is wrapped around the infant's neck when the head emerges, you can slip it over the head or shoulder to allow the infant to emerge without strangling on the cord. Rarely, it may be wrapped so tight that you cannot release the infant's head and the cord will strangle the infant, preventing emergence of the body. This is a life-threatening emergency. If medical personnel are not present, you must tie off the cord in two places and cut the cord between the two.

Bleeding After Delivery

It is normal for bleeding to occur with childbirth and with delivery of the placenta. Use sanitary pads or clean, folded cloths to absorb the blood. Bleeding usually stops soon after the placenta is delivered. As described earlier, massage the mother's abdomen below the level of the navel, where you should feel the uterus as a mass about the size of a softball. Massage with your palms using a kneading motion. Continue massaging gently until bleeding stops.

Bleeding that persists can become an emergency. Keep the mother still, and try to calm her while waiting for help to arrive. Give first aid to treat shock (see **Chapter 9**).

 LEARNING CHECKPOINT 3

Circle **True** or **False** for the following statement:

1. Childbirth is a difficult process that frequently involves complications and the need for medical treatment.   True   False

2. Put a check mark next to signs and symptoms that childbirth may occur soon:

   ☐ Contractions every 10 minutes

   ☐ Woman feels urge to push

   ☐ Amniotic sac has ruptured

   ☐ Infant's head is crowning

   ☐ Cervix is starting to dilate

   ☐ Contractions are painful

3. Select the best answer. Assisting a woman with childbirth may include –

   a. helping position the woman.

   b. supporting the infant as it emerges from the birth canal.

   c. helping secretions drain from the infant's nose and mouth.

   d. All of the above

4. List at least 3 things you should *not* do when assisting with childbirth.

   _____

   _____

   _____

   _____

5. When the umbilical cord can be seen protruding from the birth canal before childbirth occurs, what should you do? Select the best answer.

   a. Cut the cord and wait for childbirth.

   b. Push the cord back inside the mother.

   c. Position the mother to reduce pressure on the cord.

   d. Pull on the cord to speed up the birth.

Circle **True** or **False** for the following statement:

6. Some bleeding normally occurs with childbirth and delivery of the placenta.   True   False

 CONCLUDING THOUGHTS

Although problems sometimes do occur during childbirth, and in such cases it is important to know what to do, remember that the overwhelming majority of births occur naturally and without problems, even outside health care settings. Countless numbers of healthy infants have been born in taxis caught in traffic en route to hospitals and other similar places. Should you ever find yourself in such a situation, stay calm and remember the simple basics of supporting the mother and newborn through this natural process.

ADDITIONAL ACTIVITIES AND RESOURCES

Do some online research on childbirths that have occurred in unexpected places away from health care facilities. Analyze the individual stories to see how rarely medical problems occur. Such stories may also reveal how materials and supplies at hand can be used in unexpected situations.

 REVIEW QUESTIONS

Select the best answers.

1. During pregnancy, a woman should avoid or minimize the consumption of –

    a. unsaturated fats.

    b. alcohol.

    c. artificial sweeteners.

    d. beta carotene.

2. Which sign or symptom is abnormal during pregnancy?

    a. Backache

    b. Vaginal bleeding

    c. Heartburn

    d. More frequent urination

3. When the amniotic sac ruptures after contractions begin, which of these statements is true?

    a. Childbirth may occur soon.

    b. The infant must be delivered immediately before suffocation occurs.

    c. The infant's lungs are likely to become infected if childbirth does not occur soon.

    d. The mother needs care to prevent dehydration.

4. Crowning occurs –

    a. in breech presentations.

    b. when the cord is prolapsed.

    c. when the woman pushes too hard before the delivery begins.

    d. in all normal head-first births.

5. First aid for a pregnant woman with vaginal bleeding includes –

    a. massaging the abdomen with a kneading motion.

    b. packing the vagina with a pad made from sterile dressings.

    c. absorbing the blood with a towel or sanitary napkin.

    d. controlling the bleeding with direct pressure on the abdomen.

6. A pregnant woman should see her health care provider for which of these signs and symptoms?

    a. Severe headache

    b. Difficulty breathing

    c. Abdominal pain

    d. All of the above

7. Choking care for a pregnant woman includes –

    a. abdominal thrusts.

    b. chest thrusts.

    c. back blows.

    d. abdominal thrusts and back blows.

8. During labor, you can support the woman by –

    a. urging her to push with each contraction.

    b. massaging her uterus.

    c. helping her to control her breathing.

    d. holding an ice pack against her abdomen.

9. If the newborn is not crying or breathing after birth –

    a. start care for an airway obstruction.

    b. blow air into his or her mouth using the bulb syringe.

    c. flick the bottom of his or her feet with your finger.

    d. give back blows.

10. Care of the newborn includes –

    a. supporting the head when holding or moving the newborn.

    b. keeping the newborn warm.

    c. monitoring the newborn's breathing.

    d. All of the above

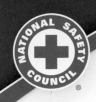

CHAPTER 23

Remote Location First Aid

LESSON OBJECTIVES

- Explain what is different about first aid principles when help may be delayed.

- Describe common situations when help is likely to be delayed.

- List actions to take to be prepared for injury and illness emergencies in remote locations.

- Describe methods by which EMS can be contacted from isolated areas.

- Explain how to protect a victim until help arrives or how to safely transport a victim if help cannot reach the victim.

- Describe special care for victims with common injuries and illnesses when help will be delayed.

- Explain what to do in special wilderness emergencies, such as avalanche or ice rescue, lightning strikes, altitude sickness and scuba diving illness.

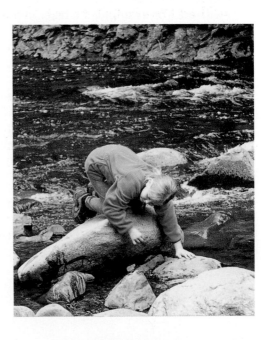

You are on a hike with several friends and family members. About 5 miles along the trail you stop for lunch beside a river, where a friend's daughter is climbing on rocks at the water's edge. Her foot slips on a mossy patch and she falls and strikes her head on a rock. Immediately an adult in the party helps her away from the water. Her head did not go under water, but she has a welt on her forehead and she seems groggy and mildly confused. A few minutes later she seems better, although she has a slight headache. You allow her to rest, but now you face the decision whether it is safe for her to hike back out. Unfortunately you have no means to call for help, and the terrain is too steep and rough to consider carrying her out. What should you do?

The principles of first aid described earlier in this text are based on the fact that in most locations in the United States medical help will arrive in 10-20 minutes or sooner, after a call is made to 9-1-1 or the local emergency number. That means that the care first aiders give in emergencies is intended primarily to meet *short-term* goals until advanced medical personnel arrive and take over. In remote locations, however, advanced medical care may not be available for many hours or longer. In such situations you should be prepared to give additional care and, when necessary, to make decisions regarding evacuating and transporting the victim, going for help and preparing to assist in special rescues.

Remote Locations

Being prepared for the possibility of injury or illness in a remote location is crucial. It is important to plan ahead to prevent emergencies from occurring, to be able to communicate the need for help, to have additional first aid supplies when needed and to know how to care for a victim with common injuries and illness when more advanced medical help may be delayed. First aiders should also be prepared to manage certain types of emergencies that are more likely in remote locations, often involving extreme environmental conditions such as cold, heat or other special circumstances.

The specific issues involved in seeking medical care and caring for the victim depend on the setting where the emergency occurs, but the same general principles apply in most situations. This chapter cannot detail all procedures to follow in every possible emergency, as so many different variables are involved. For example, if a hiker in the mountains breaks his leg 20 miles from the nearest road and his only companion discovers his cell phone has no signal, the situation is different from that of an electrical power line worker who falls and breaks his leg on a rural road 40 miles from the nearest town with his partner nearby. First aiders who live, work or engage in recreational activities in remote areas should take a special remote location or wilderness first aid course and prepare for the situations in which they may find themselves.

This chapter focuses on how general principles of first aid may need to be modified when help is delayed and on other issues first aiders face in remote locations.

Situations When Help May Be Delayed

RURAL AREAS

Rural areas include open countryside, isolated farms and ranches and even some very small towns at a distance from medical services. The primary issue is usually only the length of time before help arrives, as roads and telephones are typically present. Any type of emergency may occur, although those working with certain types of farm equipment or in other specialized activities may face special risks. Injury prevention is especially important because an injury that may be more easily cared for in an urban area where help can be expected to arrive within minutes may become life-threatening if it takes an hour or more for help to arrive.

HIKING, CAMPING AND BOATING

Millions of people enjoy a wide range of recreational activities in natural settings far from roads, landline telephones and shelter. If an emergency occurs in such a wilderness area, you may not be able to contact EMS immediately and rescue vehicles may not be able to reach the victim. In addition to providing first aid for what may be an extended time, you may need to decide how best to shelter the victim from harsh weather and whether to send someone for help or to evacuate the victim. Again, being prepared for emergencies is crucial, but psychological and emotional issues may also become important.

Emergencies that occur when boating on remote lakes and rivers present issues similar to hiking and camping emergencies. Transportation and communication problems are likely. Boating in the ocean offshore or in remote coastal areas often involves different communication and rescue issues, generally involving the Coast Guard in addition to land-based EMS agencies. Like others entering remote areas, boaters need to think and plan ahead for possible emergencies and carry the appropriate first aid, communication and signaling equipment.

NATURAL AND OTHER DISASTERS

People who live in areas that are prone to natural disasters, such as hurricanes or earthquakes, are generally aware of the need to be prepared. But other types of natural disasters can strike many other places, such as wildfires, floods, tornadoes and unanticipated ice storms that may close roads and cut off electricity for days. Because many natural disasters cause widespread damage and injuries, even if a hospital is not far away, you may need to provide first aid in an emergency when help will be delayed. Widespread injuries may stretch emergency resources thin, increasing the time before a victim receives care. An airliner crash, industrial explosion or terrorist act may have similar effects (see **Chapter 25**).

 LEARNING CHECKPOINT 1

1. Name at least three different emergency situations in which rescue and medical help may be delayed.

   _____

   _____

   _____

2. Select the best answer. Being prepared for emergencies in remote locations includes –

   a. knowing how to give first aid for an extended period.

   b. planning how to contact EMS if needed.

   c. having appropriate first aid supplies at hand.

   d. All of the above

General Principles When Help Is Delayed

Preventing injury and illness when help may be delayed is especially important. This book has emphasized specific actions and guidelines for prevention and all of these apply in remote locations. People who live or work in rural areas, and those entering remote locations for recreational or other purposes, should be thinking about safety issues at all times because of the risk that serious problems may develop if EMS cannot respond within minutes.

Regardless of the specific rural or remote location, five general principles apply whenever medical help may be delayed:

1. Be prepared for the situation. Plan for emergencies and have the right equipment and supplies.

2. Understand the psychological and emotional issues involved in a remote location emergency, and be prepared to use leadership skills.

3. Know how to contact EMS or call for help by alternative means, or know how to use distress signals.

4. Know how to decide when to send someone for help, versus evacuating the victim.

5. Know how to protect the victim until help arrives.

The following sections discuss these principles as they apply in different situations.

BEING PREPARED FOR THE SITUATION

Like people who live or work in rural or remote locations, those planning a trip to remote locations should be prepared for emergencies. What will you do if someone in your group is injured and you are unable to telephone for help? Will you have the right equipment and supplies with you? Anticipating problems not only can help prevent them but also can help to ensure that you are ready to act if they do occur.

Being prepared involves several guidelines that should be followed in all situations, as well as making specific preparations for the location.

1. **Do not enter remote locations alone.** All wilderness agencies and experts advise against this. Even a simple injury, such as a sprained ankle that prevents walking, can become life threatening if you are unable to reach help. Do not assume your cell telephone will bring help instantly. You may not have a signal, or rescuers may not be able to find you or reach you in time. Even a small wound can bleed severely, for example, and if you are unresponsive or unable to stop the bleeding, you may go into shock rapidly and die before help arrives. Ideally, go in a group of three or more; if there are only two of you and one is injured, no one is left to help the injured person if the other has to go for help.

2. **Tell someone where you are going and when you plan to return.** If an emergency develops and you are unable to call for help, your contact person should be able to send help to you if you do not return as scheduled.

3. **Take a first aid kit equipped for possible emergencies you may face. Chapter 1** describes a general first aid kit. If you anticipate other types of injuries or illness because of the location you are entering, you should include additional items in your kit, including survival supplies and signaling devices.

4. **Take more food and water than you expect to need.** Any kind of emergency may delay your return, and running out of food or water would only worsen the situation. Although most people can survive a long time without food, becoming weak with hunger complicates the emergency. Anyone can rapidly become dehydrated without adequate water intake, and this can become an emergency within hours, depending on the environment and the person's health status. Severe fluid loss caused by the injury, vomiting, diarrhea, excessive sweating or other conditions is a medical emergency.

5. **Expect weather emergencies.** Take extra clothing and some means to stay dry. Remember that being wet greatly increases heat loss from the body, making hypothermia a risk even at temperatures you do not consider "cold."

6. **Know where you are at all times.** Take a map along and know where you are on it. A **GPS,** a handheld location device using the satellite-based global positioning system, can show you where you are on a topographical map or water chart. If you can call for help in an emergency, you will need to be able to tell rescuers exactly where you are.

7. **Do not use alcohol or other drugs.** Alcohol and other drugs affect your physical performance and judgment, increasing the risk of injury and other emergencies.

8. **Study the location.** Be sure you are not trying to do something beyond your physical abilities. Becoming fatigued puts you at a greater risk for injury. Learn the conditions of the trail, find out whether any dangerous animals may be present and so on. Talk to local recreational groups, park rangers, the Coast Guard or other appropriate agencies.

In addition to these general principles, being prepared involves trip planning and having the right equipment and supplies, as described in the next sections.

TRIP PLANNING

Trip planning begins with the eight general principles described in the previous section. The following are additional suggestions that depend on the specific locale.

1. Ensure that you are in good physical condition for the trip.

2. Choose the equipment you need for the setting.

3. Plan an appropriate menu with enough nutritious foods.

4. Learn the specifics of the area you plan to enter, including weather, presence of water, fire history and conditions.

5. Obtain maps and guidebooks for the route you plan to take.

6. Refresh your first aid and CPR skills, if needed.

7. Plan for communications needs.

ESSENTIAL WILDERNESS EQUIPMENT

The Wilderness Medical Society recommends a list of "10 Essentials for Outdoor Adventures."[1] For people traveling through very isolated areas, these items should also be kept in your vehicle.

1. Topographic map and magnetic compass

2. Flashlight (with extra batteries and bulb)

3. Extra clothing (including mittens, hat, jacket and rain gear)

4. Sunglasses

5. Extra food and water

6. Waterproof matches in waterproof container

7. Candle/fire starter

8. Pocket knife

9. First aid kit

10. Space blanket or two large heavy-duty trash bags (for shelter)

[1]*wms.org Accessed January 2016.*

Additional items that may prove useful when driving through isolated areas, especially in temperature extremes, include:

- Emergency flares or bright orange "help" sign

- Sleeping bag

- Cell phone or CB radio

- Extra engine oil

- Toolkit

- Jumper cables

- Tire chains

- Shovel

- Sand (for tire traction)

- De-icer for fuel line

REMOTE LOCATION FIRST AID KIT

If an emergency occurs in a remote location, despite the best planning and having all the appropriate equipment, the single most important item may be your first aid kit. In addition to the items listed in **Chapter 1** for a standard first aid kit, a kit carried into remote locations should have the items listed in **Box 23-1.** These should be kept also in rural location first aid kits.

WATER DISINFECTION

Always take more water than you anticipate needing in a remote location. If you are a long distance from help or in an emergency situation where you may have to wait for some time, you may still run out of water. You should be prepared to disinfect the water found at your location. Surface water is often contaminated with bacteria, viruses or protozoa that may cause serious or life-threatening illness.

The three most common methods of disinfecting water for drinking are boiling, filtering and treating with chemicals. Boiling water effectively kills bacteria, viruses and protozoa and is often the best solution, but boiling is not always possible or practical. Many different filters are now sold in camping and specialty stores for filtering surface water. Most remove bacteria and protozoa from water but do not remove viruses. Viruses are generally rare in water that is found in wilderness areas.

Several different chemical treatments are available for disinfecting water, commonly using iodine or chlorine in tablet or liquid form. Both are generally effective for killing bacteria, viruses and some protozoa. These products must be used as directed. Before planning to use any product to obtain drinking water, it is best to learn about the characteristics of the surface water you are likely to find where you are going **(Figure 23-1).**

In an emergency, if you have no method of disinfecting water, a difficult decision may have to be made between the risk of drinking untreated water and the risk of dehydration. Certainly it is better to be prepared and to have a disinfecting method along with other supplies and first aid items.

BOX 23-1: FIRST AID KIT FOR REMOTE LOCATIONS

- First aid guide

- Pain/anti-inflammatory medication

- Antihistamine

- Laxative

- Anti-diarrhea tablets

- Ibuprofen

- Safety pins

- Calamine lotion

- Oral decongestant

- Eye drops

- Motion sickness/anti-nausea medication

- Antifungal cream

- Antacid tablets

- Oral rehydration solution (especially for small children)

- Moleskin or Spenco 2nd Skin (for burns or open blisters)

- Oral hypothermia thermometer (to 85°F)

- Oil of cloves or other product for dental pain

- Temporary dental filling kit

- Throat lozenges

- Sunscreen and lip protection

- Sunburn lotion (aloe vera)

- Insect repellent

- Lightweight, flexible splint (such as a SAM splint)

- Sanitary napkins or tampons for bulky wound dressings

- Penlight

- Irrigation syringe

- Water purification tablets

- Sports drink containing sodium for endurance activities

PSYCHOLOGICAL ISSUES

Emergencies are always stressful, and in remote locations, mental and emotional issues can become much more significant. The victim may not receive advanced care for many hours or days, and many decisions may be required about how best to care for the victim: whether to attempt **evacuation** or wait for help, how to provide shelter and so on. An outdoor environment often adds further stresses, such as coping with weather, temperature extremes, shortages of food or water and other problems and uncertainties. The victim or other members of the party may not be able to cope with such stresses and may experience panic attacks, depression, denial, emotional shock or other problems that worsen the situation. In a worst-case scenario, just when cool heads and clear thinking are needed to address the emergency and first aid needs, there is a risk of the situation deteriorating because of panic, fear, confusion or indecision. Experts in wilderness survival and crisis management emphasize the importance of mental preparedness and leadership skills to be ready to act effectively in an emergency.

FIGURE 23-1

Commercially available water purification kit and filter.

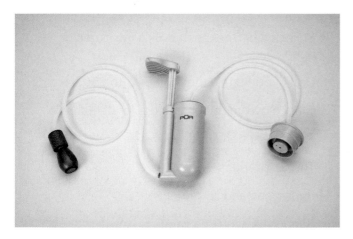

BOX 23-2: PRESCRIPTION MEDICATIONS IN REMOTE LOCATION FIRST AID

Experts debate whether first aiders should have prescription medications for use in remote locations. One side argues that when medical help may be one or several days away, prescription medications, such as a narcotic pain medication or systemic antibiotics have great value for a victim's health and well-being and may even save a life. A responsible adult can be instructed in the safe use of certain prescription medications and trusted not to misuse or abuse them. On the other side, others argue that the situations in which such medications are genuinely needed are rare and do not justify the potential for misuse or abuse.

Those planning long trips to remote locations that involve activities that put them at risk for medical emergencies are advised to talk with their health care provider about this issue. Medications that have been prescribed in such situations include cardiac emergency medications, pain medications, antibiotics, treatments for gastrointestinal infections, allergic reaction medications and others. When such prescribed medications are added to the first aid kit for remote locations, care must be taken to ensure that they are used only as directed and only in controlled circumstances.

MENTAL PREPAREDNESS

Being mentally prepared for an emergency in a remote location begins with first aid training and learning how best to provide care when help will be delayed. Self-confidence is important, but so is a realistic attitude about what you can and cannot do. When a life-threatening injury or illness occurs far from help, you may need to accept that you do not have the tools needed to give the victim all the help he or she needs. Yet it is equally important to not give up hope and fail to take actions that may help a victim.

Six aspects of mental preparedness are important for wilderness survival situations. They also apply in many other emergency situations.

1. Stay confident and remember your training.

2. Do not deny the seriousness of the situation, but calmly think through what you need to do.

3. Consider all your equipment and supplies as well as human resources. Be creative and improvise as necessary.

4. Stay focused on the goal and not on the hardships of the situation. Help others in the group to stay calm and act productively.

5. Remain positive but realistic.

6. Keep the faith – in yourself and in your beliefs.

Staying calm can be difficult in an emergency but is one of the most important actions one can take. If necessary, take time to control your own stress before beginning to act. Breathe deeply and slowly, and try to relax. Help others to control their fears to prevent panic, and then use your leadership skills to develop and carry out a plan.

LEADERSHIP SKILLS

Whenever two or more people are with a victim in an emergency, someone needs to be in charge. Often one person has more experience or training and naturally assumes leadership. In other situations, such as a group of friends going on a week-long backpacking trip, the group should discuss this before the trip begins. Who is packing the first aid kit? Who has thought about emergency communications? Advance conversations about emergency preparedness often naturally lead to consensus about who should take charge.

The most important leadership skill involves mental preparedness. Be confident and calm and help others to focus on the goal. Other leadership strategies include calmly talking through all actions with other members of the group and asking for suggestions when appropriate. Remember that you are caring not only for the victim but for other group members. Avoid rushing into decisions, but first assess the situation and the victim's needs. Make a plan for first aid and rescue steps. Delegate responsibilities to others as needed; everyone should participate in some useful way. Then reassess the situation and change the plan when needed, with the focus on helping the victim. At the same time, work to keep up morale and prevent panic.

CALLING FOR HELP

In any emergency, one of the highest priorities is to call for help. With serious injuries or illness, medical care is needed beyond first aid. In remote locations or wilderness areas it may be more difficult to contact EMS, but with advanced planning and the appropriate equipment, help can be summoned in most situations. Communication options include cellular or satellite telephones, radios and emergency rescue beacons.

Cell Phones

Some hikers and other users of wilderness areas refuse to carry a cell phone, preferring to "get away from it all." Others take their cell phones along and assume they can simply call for help if they get lost or have any problems. Many forest rangers and park officials have received calls from hikers who were tired and lost and who expected instant help even though they had no idea where they were.

Between these two extremes, cell phones obviously have value in emergencies, although because of their limitations, no one should depend entirely on a cell phone in an emergency. Cell phones are relatively fragile devices that may stop working due to temperature extremes, moisture, physical shocks or simply a dead battery. Many remote areas lack a signal. Follow these guidelines for using a cell phone in a remote area:

- Protect the phone from extreme cold, moisture and shocks.

- Pack the phone in a way that it cannot accidentally turn on and discharge the battery.

- Ensure that the battery is strong by saving the phone for emergency use.

- If you need the phone in an emergency and do not have a signal, try to get to a higher location, such as a ridge top; even climbing a tree may help. Move the phone around your body, as even your own body can block a weak signal. Switch the phone from digital to analog, if you have this choice.

- Be sure you know where you are before making the call. Inexpensive handheld GPS units can provide exact longitude and latitude coordinates for rescuers.

Satellite Phones

Although still relatively expensive, satellite telephones are available for communication anywhere in the world and can be rented for special trips to very remote locations. Their use is similar to using cell phones, but signal strength is not usually an issue.

Radios

Different types of radios are available for various specialized or general uses **(Figure 23-2).** In some areas, a handheld citizen's band (CB) radio may be able to reach authorities or other CB users, although cell phones have led to the declining use of CBs. Channel 9 is the emergency frequency for calling for help. Be aware of the limited range of CB radios (typically under 4 miles).

FIGURE 23-2

Devices for summoning help.

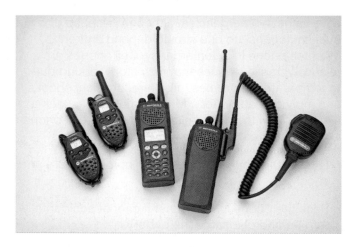

Family radio service (FRS) is a citizen's band frequency used by inexpensive handheld radios. Even in the best conditions, however, these radios generally transmit less than 3 miles, giving them limited use in remote locations. In areas where numbers of people are likely to be close by, however, such as ski areas, FRS radios may allow contact with others for help. They may also be useful for staying in touch when members of a group split up.

Amateur (ham) radio is another option. Portable units generally reach a significantly wider area and more people are likely to monitor common frequencies. An FCC license is required to use ham equipment, which is also generally more expensive.

VHF radios are used on boats. Because of the lack of signal obstructions on the water, high-power VHF (very high frequency) radios can cover up to 30 miles. Most U.S. coastal areas have coverage by Coast Guard towers. The Coast Guard monitors Channel 16 and can send a rescue ship or helicopter in an emergency. The Coast Guard recommends boaters use VHF radio rather than a cell phone to call for help in an emergency, because their triangulation equipment can help them better determine the location of the vessel in distress and because nearby boaters also can hear the call for help and may

render assistance. Although less powerful, handheld VHF radios used in smaller watercraft have enough power to summon help from the Coast Guard or other boaters in the vicinity. VHF radios equipped with digital selective calling (DSC) and GPS can report your emergency and exact location to the Coast Guard and other DSC-equipped mariners nearby, with the single press of a button. Larger boats often use single sideband (SSB) radio. These units use a frequency that travels greater distances beyond coastal areas.

Rescue Beacons

Emergency beacons send out a signal that is picked up by an international system of satellites. All commercial and most civil airplanes carry these beacons, known as emergency locator transmitters (ELTs), which automatically send out a signal if the aircraft crashes or has an emergency landing.

Using the same system, marine rescue beacons called **emergency position indicating radio beacons (EPIRBs)** are available for boats that leave coastal areas and cannot depend on radio transmission in an emergency. Some units are manually operated, while others automatically begin sending rescue signals upon being immersed if the boat capsizes.

In 2003, the FCC authorized the use of **personal locator beacons (PLBs).** Hikers and other wilderness users now have the same ability to summon help from any remote location. These units have become more widely available and less expensive.

Most rescue beacons are one-way communication devices – they function only to send an emergency signal that is received by satellites. Typically only the device's location is communicated, although some new services include a short text message with appropriate devices. With most PLBs, no information is sent about the nature of the emergency, nor can the user know for certain that the signal is being received. Rescue beacons must be used only in a true emergency requiring rescue. In addition, users must register beacons, each of which sends out a unique signal, to help rescuers determine if an emergency has occurred when a signal is received.

EPIRBs and PLBs have led to more than 37,000 rescues worldwide, including 7,492 in the United States.[1] These included stranded hikers, shipwrecked boaters and downed pilots.

[1]*National Oceanic and Atmospheric Administration, noaanews. noaa.gov/stories2015/20150129_sarsatrescues_2014.html Accessed January 2016.*

Distress Signals

If help cannot be summoned by telephone, radio, rescue beacon or other means when rescue is required, distress signals may be used to catch the attention of passing aircraft. The following are recognized distress signals for different situations:

- At night, build three small campfires in a triangle up to 100 feet apart. Three flares can also be used or a series of three flashes from a flashlight.

- In the daytime, make a large campfire and put green branches or leaves on it to create smoke. Do this in a clearing or on a hilltop.

A standard signal is to create three puffs of smoke in a row by covering and uncovering a campfire by any means available.

- Make a large X of markings in the snow or on clear ground. Green branches or bright clothing may be used. Use any material available that will contrast with the ground.

- If a passing aircraft is close enough to see you, raise both (not just one) arms above your head.

- If you have a firearm, fire three shots in a row or try three whistle blasts.

- In sunlight, use a signal mirror to flash light at a passing aircraft. The reflected beam can be aimed at the aircraft by sighting the beam past a nearby object or your own hand **(Figure 23-3)**. If you do not have a mirror, use any shiny object, such as the lid from a can or a piece of glass with mud coating the back side.

Many commercial distress signals are available, including such things as flares and aerial flare guns, strobe lights, signal flags and banners and orange smoke signals.

FIGURE 23-3

To send a distress signal to an aircraft, aim the mirror's reflected sunlight past your fingers or a stationary object.

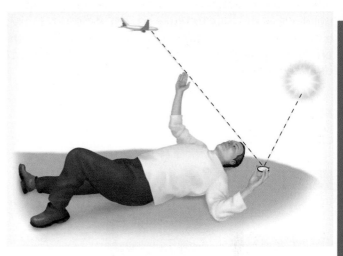

SENDING SOMEONE FOR HELP

In a situation in which an injured or ill victim cannot easily be transported to medical care and it is impossible to call for help, one or more people may need to go for help while others remain with the victim. Difficult decisions are involved, particularly in small groups with only one leader experienced in the area. Should that person be the one to go for help if he or she may get there faster or more safely, or is he or she better equipped to deal with building a camp and caring for the victim? There are no simple rules that apply in all situations, as so many different variables are involved. Most important, before decisions are made, the group should talk through the issues so that everyone understands what may be involved in both staying and going.

The person going for help must be able to communicate the group's location to rescuers. This information should be written down and carried. Unless this location is a well-known place, the person going for help must also be confident about his or her ability to lead rescuers back to the victim.

SHELTERING THE VICTIM

While awaiting rescuers, a victim of injury or sudden illness needs to be protected from the environment. Unless you have camping equipment with you, you need to create an emergency shelter to keep the victim (and yourself) warm and dry. The type of shelter depends on the characteristics of the area and what materials you have with you. Look for natural shelters, such as a cave or rock overhang. If you need to make a shelter, use a poncho or tarp hung over a rope or pole to make a lean-to or tent **(Figure 23-4a and b).** If you have no waterproof material, make a lean-to from branches or poles and cover the framework with leaves, grass or other material **(Figure 23-4c).** In swampy areas, where the victim must be elevated to stay dry, cut saplings to build a "swamp bed" **(Figure 23-4d).** A "debris hut," a tent-like structure made of branches piled over with brush, twigs and leaves, can keep you and the victim dry and warm **(Figure 23-4e).** In a heavy snowfall, dig a pit in the snow around the base of an evergreen tree with low boughs, piling boughs against the trunk to form a snow roof as more snow falls **(Figure 23-4f).** In a desert or on a shadeless beach, where the victim needs to be sheltered from the sun and heat, construct a shade shelter by digging a trench in cooler sand, stretching clothing or other material between mounds on each side and anchoring the material with more sand on top at its edges **(Figure 23-4g).**

FIGURE 23-4

Emergency shelters.

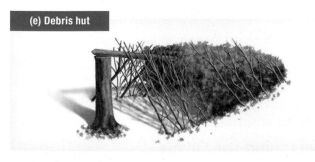

(a) Poncho lean-to

Wind

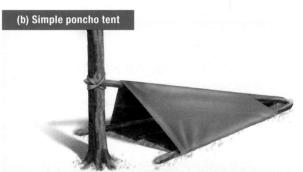

(b) Simple poncho tent

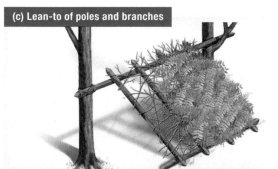

(c) Lean-to of poles and branches

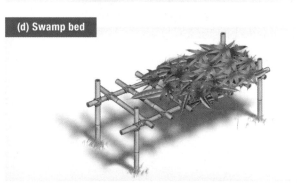

(d) Swamp bed

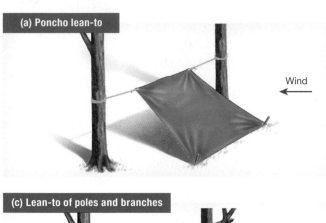

(e) Debris hut

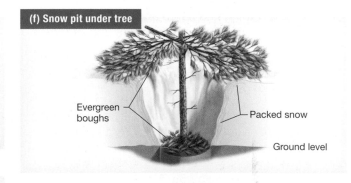

(f) Snow pit under tree

Evergreen boughs

Packed snow

Ground level

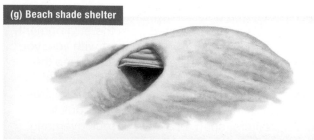

(g) Beach shade shelter

LEAVING THE VICTIM ALONE

Consider leaving a victim alone to go for help only if you are alone, if you cannot communicate your need for help and if it is unlikely that someone will pass your location. Because a victim's condition may deteriorate without further care, take this action only if there is no alternative. Prepare the victim as well as possible before leaving, attending to shelter and food and water needs. Leave a written note with the victim explaining when you anticipate returning with help. Carry a note on your own person also, stating the location and condition of the victim as well as your destination, in case something happens to you before you reach help.

With three or more in the group, never leave the victim alone, even when you feel sure the victim will be okay – and even if the victim agrees. Conditions may change or unanticipated things may happen.

PREPARING FOR RESCUE

Once an emergency has been communicated from the remote location to authorities such as EMS, search and rescue operations or the Coast Guard, it is critical to remain in the same location until help arrives. You may need to help rescuers find you as they approach the area, by signaling with a fire or flashlight, smoke or a whistle. Depending on the urgency of the situation and the terrain, rescuers may arrive by vehicle, on foot or by other means.

Helicopter rescues are often used in remote areas to get a victim to advanced medical care quickly. Following are safety principles when a helicopter is arriving at your location (**Figure 23-5**):

- A large, clear area is needed for a safe landing. Stay far back from any clearing where the helicopter is likely to land.

- The "rotor wash" wind from the helicopter typically exceeds 100 mph. Protect your face and the victim from injury caused by flying debris.

- Once the helicopter has landed, do not approach it until signaled to do so. The spinning tail rotor cannot be seen and you may inadvertently walk into it. Approach only in a crouch and never from an uphill side where the blade is closer to the ground.

- When making a rescue at sea or in a wilderness area where landing is impossible, the helicopter may lower a basket on a cable. Sometimes the helicopter crew lower a two-way radio first to enable communication and give instructions for the rescue.

FIGURE 23-5

Rescue helicopter.

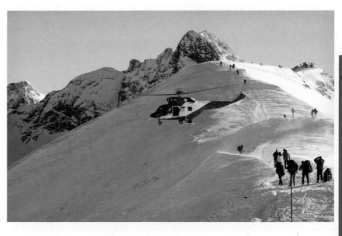

EVACUATION OF VICTIM

Generally it is better to wait for help to come to you rather than to try to evacuate the victim yourself from a remote location. Moving the victim may worsen the victim's condition and is likely to cause additional pain. The decision to evacuate a victim depends on several key factors:

- The length of time before help can be expected to arrive

- Whether the victim's condition will be aggravated more by waiting for help than by moving the victim

- The number of people present and their ability to safely carry the victim out

- How much daylight remains and whether the weather may deteriorate

- Whether it is possible to continue giving first aid during evacuation

According to the Wilderness Medical Society, victims with the following conditions may be evacuated if help will be delayed and group members can safely carry the victim:

- A worsening condition, such as a breathing problem, deteriorating mental status, shock or recurring diarrhea or vomiting

- Severe pain

- Inability to walk

- Persistent bleeding

- Severe altitude sickness

- An infection getting worse

- Chest pain symptomatic of a cardiac condition

- Mental or behavioral disorder that threatens the safety of the victim or others

- Near-drowning

- Severe burns or wounds

- Severe traumatic injury

If enough people are present, someone should be sent ahead for help, as those carrying the victim will travel more slowly.

Four or six people can carry the victim on an improvised stretcher or litter. Cut two poles from saplings and create a litter from a blanket or sleeping bag, or even two jackets or shirts as shown in **Figure 23-6.** Use other clothing to pad the litter under the victim. Use belts or rope to secure the victim in the litter and support the head and neck. During the evacuation, monitor the victim's condition and stay alert for vomiting, which can threaten the airway of a victim lying on his or her back.

Other emergency carries, such as the hammock, carry (see **Chapter 24**) are ineffective for the distances typically involved in remote location evacuations. In certain circumstances, the two-person walking assist may be appropriate for a short distance.

FIGURE 23-6

Emergency litters for evacuating an injured victim.

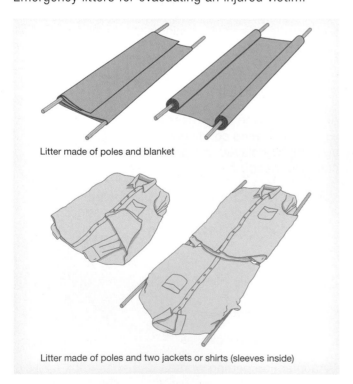

Litter made of poles and blanket

Litter made of poles and two jackets or shirts (sleeves inside)

✏ **LEARNING CHECKPOINT 2**

1. Check off important principles for planning a trip into a wilderness location:

   ☐ Do not go alone.

   ☐ Do not go longer than 3-4 days.

   ☐ Tell someone where you are going and when you will return.

   ☐ Take more food and water than you expect to need.

   ☐ Split up the first aid kit among 3-4 people in the group in case someone gets lost.

   ☐ Do not drink more alcohol than usual.

Circle **True** or **False** for the following statement:

2. When dealing with a complex emergency in a remote location, the group's leader must set the plan and resist any temptation to change it along the way.   True   False

3. Name three reasons why you should not depend on a cell phone in a wilderness location.

   _____

   _____

   _____

   _____

4. Select the best answer. Never leave a victim alone to go for help when –

   a. you cannot communicate your need for help.

   b. it is unlikely that someone will pass by your location.

   c. there are three or more people in the group.

   d. All of the above

Special Care for Emergencies When Help Is Delayed

Earlier chapters describe the standard first aid for injuries and sudden illness. **This chapter describes only special considerations when help may be delayed.**

BLEEDING, WOUNDS AND SHOCK

Special care for bleeding may be needed in a remote location for these reasons:

- Bleeding can soon become life threatening if it is not stopped and medical care will not be provided soon.

- A contaminated wound that a first aider may leave for medical personnel in normal situations can become seriously infected if medical care is not provided soon.

- A victim in shock caused by blood loss requires special care if medical attention is delayed, such as providing fluids if possible.

Special remote location care for bleeding, wounds and shock includes the following steps *in addition to the care described in earlier chapters.*

1. Control external bleeding as soon as possible. Maintain direct pressure as long as needed with a pressure bandage, but check for circulation below the bleeding site to avoid cutting off circulation to the limb unless absolutely necessary to control bleeding.

2. A **tourniquet** can be used to stop bleeding from an arm or leg to save the victim's life when medical attention will be delayed. The tourniquet will cut off most circulation to the limb, however, which over a longer period of time will likely necessitate later amputation of the limb. In usual circumstances, tourniquets should be used only by rescuers trained in their use, but a wilderness setting may necessitate a decision between losing the limb or losing the person's life. See **Chapter 8** for steps to apply a tourniquet. To improvise a tourniquet:

   - Wrap a wide belt or bandage around the limb just above the bleeding site and knot it.

   - Knot a metal rod or strong stick over the first knot and twist it to tighten the constricting band until bleeding stops **(Figure 23-7)**. Note that considerable pressure may be necessary to squeeze closed the bleeding artery deep within the limb.

   - Tape or fasten the rod in place to hold the pressure.

   - Note the time of application to inform medical personnel.

3. After stopping bleeding from a wound, you should clean the wound to prevent infection. Wash the wound with large amounts of water, if possible; then apply a sterile dressing and bandage over the wound to keep out dirt. For a deeper wound or one visibly contaminated with dirt or foreign matter, use an irrigation syringe to forcefully rinse the wound clean; if necessary, part the wound edges to allow the water to reach the bottom of the wound. Then apply a sterile dressing and bandage, applying pressure again, if necessary, to stop bleeding. For gaping wounds, use "butterfly" bandage strips or strips of clean tape to hold the wound closed or pack a deep wound that will not close with a dressing.

4. There is one exception to the usual care for shock caused by bleeding as described in **Chapter 9.** Normally a shock victim is not given anything to drink in the brief time before medical help arrives, but when help is delayed, the victim needs fluid. If the victim is responsive and can swallow, give water, a clear fluid or an oral rehydration solution in small amounts, frequently but only as tolerated. If the victim vomits, wait awhile before giving another drink.

5. If the victim's shock resulted from dehydration, keep giving fluids slowly but steadily.

FIGURE 23-7

An emergency tourniquet is used only as a last resort to stop bleeding.

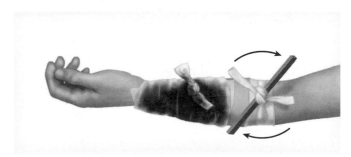

MUSCULOSKELETAL INJURIES

As explained in **Chapter 15,** an injured extremity normally is splinted only if the victim is at risk for moving the injured area before help arrives. When help is delayed, especially if the victim is to be evacuated, splinting is often necessary. You may need to improvise the splint with materials at hand, such as a ski pole or a sturdy piece of wood broken from a tree branch **(Figure 23-8).** Ideally, a first aid kit used in remote locations should include a SAM splint. When the splint will be in place for an extended time, it is essential to check circulation below the injury and to periodically loosen the splint to improve blood flow.

FIGURE 23-8

Improvising a splint with materials at hand.

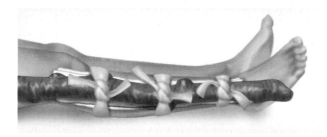

In very rare cases of an extremity fracture, circulation may be cut off below the injury site. If medical care is hours away and you are certain there is no circulation in the extremity below the injury, then you may try to carefully straighten the extremity to restore circulation unless this would increase bleeding. Never try to straighten a fractured limb if the victim may receive medical care within 30 minutes or if there is some circulation below the injury site.

In some cases, a dislocation may impair circulation to an extremity. If you have been trained to reduce a dislocation (return bones to their normal position in the joint), and if you are sure that circulation to the extremity is cut off and the victim will not receive medical care within 30 minutes, you may then try to reduce the dislocation.

Spinal Injuries

In remote locations, three aspects of first aid in cases of suspected spinal injuries are somewhat different from the usual care described in **Chapter 12.** First, if the victim is thought to have a possible spinal injury, it may be difficult to keep the spine immobilized for an extended time. You may need to improvise with materials at hand, such as using large pieces of wood or stones padded with clothing positioned on both sides of the head to immobilize the spine of a victim who is lying down. If the victim is on the ground, you may need to put clothing or other material under the victim's body to prevent heat loss; do this by holding the head in line with the body as others roll the body to one side long enough for an insulated material to be put under the victim's body. A victim with a spinal injury should not be evacuated.

Second, although it is generally best to immobilize a victim in the position found when help will arrive soon, in remote locations it is generally better to gently place the victim in a normal position with head straight and eyes forward to prevent further injury to the spine. Do not move the victim's head, however, if it causes more pain or you feel resistance to movement.

Finally, great care is needed in assessing a possible spinal injury. When help will arrive soon, it is better to be safe than sorry, and a conservative approach is generally advised: immobilize the victim's head and neck in line with the body, keep the victim still and wait for advanced medical personnel to determine how best to manage the possible spinal injury. In a remote location, however, other risks may be involved in waiting a long time for help, and in such cases if the presence of a spinal injury is not obvious, the victim may be further assessed to determine whether immobilization is in fact necessary. The Wilderness Medical Associates have developed a protocol for spinal injuries in which a spine injury can be ruled out if all of the following criteria are met:

1. The victim is alert, sober and cooperative.

2. The victim does not feel neck or back tenderness when you press your fingers along the spine.

3. The victim does not have other injuries that mask or distract him or her from feeling the pain or tenderness of a spinal injury.

4. The victim has normal function in all four limbs:

   • The fingers of both hands can be opened and closed and the wrist moved up and down.

   • Both feet can be moved up and down and the big toe moved up and down.

   • The victim has no tingling sensation but has normal sensation in all four limbs, as determined by being able to feel a light touch and a painful pinch in all areas. One specific area may have reduced function if the cause is clearly not related to a spinal injury, such as occurs with a sprained wrist.

HEAD INJURIES

Chapter 12 describes how when help is expected to arrive soon, it is generally best to call 9-1-1 and give supportive care while waiting for help. In a delayed help situation, especially if you cannot communicate with EMS to ask advice, you may need to make difficult decisions about whether to evacuate the victim.

A victim with a concussion caused by a blow to the head may be able to safely walk out of a remote location. The victim should be closely monitored for the signs and symptoms of a more serious brain injury, however, and should be awakened and checked every 2-3 hours.

A victim with a more serious head injury may have swelling or bleeding in the brain, a potentially life-threatening condition. The signs and symptoms of a brain injury are described in **Chapter 12.** A serious brain injury is unlikely to improve by itself; the victim needs immediate medical attention. If possible, call for emergency evacuation, by helicopter if available. If communication is impossible, you may face the difficult decision of whether to attempt to evacuate the victim yourself. The sooner the victim receives medical care, the better his or her chances for survival, but moving the victim over difficult terrain may worsen the condition. Either way, the victim may die. Evacuate the victim only if necessary to prevent a dangerous delay and if you can do so safely.

ABDOMINAL INJURY OR ILLNESS

A victim with an abdominal injury or severe abdominal pain needs to receive medical attention as soon as possible. As with a head injury, if communication with EMS is impossible, you must balance the risk of the victim's condition being worsened by evacuation with the risk of waiting for delayed help. A closed or open abdominal wound may progress to life-threatening shock, and abdominal pain may be a sign of appendicitis, which can rapidly become an emergency.

BURNS

The care for burns when help is delayed is similar to standard burn care. In addition, because a severe or large burn may cause a significant loss of body fluids, a victim who is alert should be given large amounts of water or clear fluids slowly and a little at a time to minimize shock.

Burn prevention is especially important in outdoor recreational activities, such as camping. Fire is a greater risk with an outdoor campfire because of the risk of windblown sparks and the flammability of tents, sleeping bags and other camp gear. Because many of the synthetic fabrics used in such camping equipment and clothing melt when on fire, causing deeper and more serious burns when in contact with skin, water should be immediately available for dousing flames.

SUDDEN ILLNESS

Special considerations may be necessary for diabetic emergencies or anaphylactic shock when help may be delayed.

A diabetic who regularly self-injects insulin or takes medication should inform others in the remote environment how to administer insulin or medication in an emergency. It is especially important that diabetics monitor their blood sugar levels and inform others of the signs and symptoms of hypoglycemia and hyperglycemia as well as what to do. Prevention is critical, but others should be prepared to take action by giving a sugar substance. If diabetic shock develops, give water and other shock care. Evacuate a victim in a diabetic crisis as quickly as possible.

Similarly, someone who has severe allergies should inform others in the group and the first aid kit should contain emergency epinephrine, such as an EpiPen, if possible. Someone with severe allergies entering a wilderness location may carry up to three emergency epinephrine doses. Be sure others know where the EpiPen is kept and how to use it. A victim who develops anaphylaxis should be evacuated as quickly as possible. The protocol of the Wilderness Medical Associates calls for administering epinephrine to victims with a definite reaction marked by difficulty breathing and generalized skin redness or swelling. Although usually only one dose is needed, up to three doses may be administered if required, every 5 minutes if the condition is worsening or every 15 minutes if the victim's condition does not change.

HYPOTHERMIA

Hypothermia is more likely to occur during outdoor activities in cold environments, especially if one is wet or a wind is blowing. Because the body loses heat 25-30 times faster when immersed in cold water, hypothermia is even more likely if a victim falls into cold water.

A responsive victim of mild hypothermia, with a body temperature higher than 90°F may recover with adequate warming. Follow the standard guidelines to warm the victim. With sufficient rest and warming, in time this person may be able to walk out of the remote location.

A body temperature below 90°F indicates severe hypothermia. At this point the victim is usually no longer shivering and often has changing levels of responsiveness. This is a life-threatening emergency. It is unlikely that you will be able to fully rewarm the victim in the remote location, but make every effort to prevent further heat loss and to warm the victim as much as possible while waiting for help. Do not try to evacuate the victim by foot, as it will be difficult or impossible to keep the victim warm while being transported through a cold environment. Send someone for help immediately. Put the victim in dry clothing and inside a sleeping bag protected by shelter. The victim should be wrapped fully to prevent heat loss, including the use of a space blanket if available **(Figure 23-9)**. Avoid rough handling. Add heat with bodily contact, heating pads or warm water bottles beside the neck, armpits or groin. Whereas a hypothermia victim should not be actively rewarmed with heat sources when close to medical care, in a remote location you may actively warm the victim with a heat source and by putting containers of warm (not hot) water against the victim's skin.

FIGURE 23-9

Hypothermia wrap.

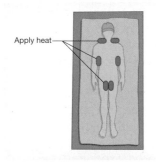
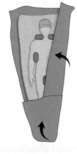
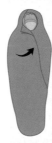

Apply heat

A victim in very severe hypothermia may seem to be dead. The skin is cold and blue and the victim is totally unresponsive. The internal body temperature may be lower than 85°F. Do not rush to provide CPR, however, which can lead to a life-threatening heart dysrhythmia if the victim still has a heartbeat. Assess the victim carefully. The victim may be breathing only once every 30 seconds or so. Rewarm the victim as described previously and provide CPR if the victim is not breathing.

Hypothermia caused by immersion in cold water may occur very rapidly and is often severe. These victims generally need both rewarming and CPR. Because the body's need for oxygen decreases when very cold, resuscitation may occur even after significant time in the water. Although CPR is generally not given

for longer than 30 minutes in normal temperatures, victims with severe hypothermia have been given CPR for as long as 3 hours and recovered fully. The saying "a victim is never cold and dead, only warm and dead" reminds us to not assume a victim is dead until rewarming has occurred, because severe hypothermic victims often survive.

HEAT EMERGENCIES

Like cold emergencies, heat emergencies, such as heat stroke, are more common during outdoor activities in remote locations where no relief may be possible from extreme temperatures. Prevent heat emergencies by staying out of direct sunlight, minimizing activity and staying well hydrated.

For heat exhaustion or heat stroke, cool the victim as soon as possible. If the victim is alert and not vomiting, give water or a sports drink a little at a time. A victim with heat exhaustion may be able to travel from the location after cooling and resting. The victim may remain in a weakened condition, however, and walking in continued heat may renew the problem and lead to an emergency.

Heat stroke is a life-threatening emergency. Cool the victim and evacuate, if possible, rather than waiting for delayed medical attention. Even if the victim seems to recover, there may be damage to internal organs.

SNAKE BITES

Unless you are certain the bite was from a non-poisonous snake, assume a snake bite is poisonous. Splint the limb to reduce movement and keep the area below the level of the heart.

Check the fingers or toes periodically to ensure that circulation is not impeded. Evacuate the victim as soon as possible. To be effective, antivenin must be administered within 4-6 hours after the bite. Other medical care may be needed.

CPR

Chapter 5 describes the standard procedures for CPR. Follow the same approach for a victim in cardiac arrest in a remote location, although in some cases the victim has smaller chances for recovery when advanced medical care cannot be given soon. CPR was developed as a short-term treatment to keep the victim alive until treated by medical professionals. Depending on the cause of the cardiac arrest, resuscitation in a remote location may be unlikely, as when cardiac arrest is caused by a heart attack or traumatic injuries. Nonetheless, always give CPR for 30 minutes. If the victim is far from medical care and does not revive within 30 minutes, except in certain special situations, you can stop CPR after 30 minutes.[1]

[1]*Wilderness Medical Associates, "Wilderness Medicine Field Protocols," wildmed.com/wp-content/uploads/2013/10/wma-field-protocols.pdf Accessed January 2016.*

In three types of situations, victims have been successfully resuscitated after CPR was over for longer than 30 minutes: hypothermia, drowning and lightning strike. As noted earlier, victims with severe hypothermia have survived after hours of CPR. In these cases, follow the standard protocol to give CPR until another trained rescuer takes over or you are too exhausted to continue.

 LEARNING CHECKPOINT 3

1. What is important about first aid for bleeding in a remote location? Select the best answer.

   a. Control bleeding as quickly as possible.

   b. Use a tourniquet only as a last resort.

   c. A responsive victim in shock can drink water.

   d. All of the above

Circle **True** or **False** for each of the following statements:

2. If you suspect a victim in a remote location may have a spinal injury, do not move him or her no matter how long you may have to wait for help. True False

3. In a remote location, the best thing to do for a victim believed to have a brain injury is to wait and see if the victim's condition improves. True False

4. On a cold day, a hiker in your group of four falls into an icy stream about a 3-hour walk from the car. After being pulled out, he develops the signs and symptoms of severe hypothermia. Which is the best action to take? Select the best answer.

   a. Immediately start hiking out – keep the person moving and he'll be okay.

   b. Send someone to get help while rest of the group works to warm the victim.

   c. Put the victim in a hypothermia wrap and carry him out.

   d. None of the above

5. Fill in the correct answer: Except in cases of hypothermia, drowning and lightning strike, CPR in a remote location can be stopped if the victim does not revive within _____ minutes.

Special Wilderness Emergencies

In addition to being prepared for an emergency in a remote location and knowing what first aid to give when help will be delayed, people entering wilderness locations where there is a risk of certain kinds of emergencies need special preparations. These special situations include:

• Ice rescue

• Snow emergencies

• Desert survival

• Lightning strikes

• Altitude sickness

• Scuba diving incidents

This text only introduces the issues involved in these situations. Special training programs are available for people planning a trip into locations where these emergencies may occur, including preparations, equipment and first aid and survival techniques.

ICE RESCUE

In circumstances where EMS can be called and trained rescuers can arrive within minutes, you should never go onto ice yourself to rescue a victim. In a remote location, however, a rescuer may choose to go onto the ice as a last resort.

Lie flat with arms and legs spread to distribute your weight and push a tree limb or other object ahead of you for the victim to grab. If at all possible, others should hold onto your legs or use clothing to fashion a rescue line if rope is not available, in case the ice breaks under you.

SNOW EMERGENCIES

Avalanches

Avalanches are a risk for backcountry trekkers and skiers. Try to avoid areas that are prone to avalanches, and talk with local officials before entering the area. Avalanche transceivers (beacons) are available that emit signals from a trapped person to transceivers carried by others in the group to help them to locate the victim. Most avalanche deaths occur by suffocation; the snow packs tightly around the victim, preventing breathing or digging out. The victim's chances of survival rapidly diminish as time passes after burial. An avalanche airbag pack is an effective safety item that can self-inflate and "float" an avalanche victim to the top of the sliding snow to prevent burial.

Call for help if someone in your group is buried by an avalanche, but time is critical and those present should begin searching for the person immediately. Start at the point where the victim was last seen and work down the slope, using an avalanche probe, a ski pole or tree branch to probe into the snow. CPR will likely be necessary.

Snow Blindness

Snow blindness is a burn on the cornea of the eyes caused by intense sunlight reflected from snow. It can be prevented by wearing dark sunglasses or goggles with UV protection. At first the eyes feel scratchy or burning sensations and become more sensitive to light. Headache may develop. Eventually the victim loses vision. First aid involves bandaging the eyes to prevent any further exposure to light. Cold compresses may ease the pain. The victim usually recovers sight in 12-18 hours, but if symptoms linger, medical care should be sought.

DESERT SURVIVAL

Desert hiking and trekking have become more popular, exposing more people to the risks of very harsh climates. As when entering very cold climates, preparation and training are essential. Appropriate clothing is necessary for sun and heat protection, as are the right camping equipment and first aid supplies. Perhaps most important is water. Few people realize that the daily intake of water can increase to up to 3-5 gallons per person in extreme dry heat. Because water weighs 8 pounds per gallon, it is impractical to carry enough to sustain life for days in an emergency. Desert survival training, therefore, includes skills in finding and purifying water as well as techniques for building shelter, sending communications and distress signals, finding

direction and traveling at night to avoid the worst heat.

LIGHTNING STRIKES

Chapter 11 lists tips to avoid being struck by lightning. About ⅓ of victims of lightning strike die, usually as a result of cardiac arrest. Immediate CPR is therefore critical to increase the victim's chances for survival. Remember that lightning strikes are one of the three situations (along with drowning and hypothermia) in which CPR should be continued past the 30-minute limit.

ALTITUDE SICKNESS

Hikers at altitudes above 8,000-10,000 feet are at risk for different forms of **altitude sickness** caused by the lower concentration of oxygen. Know what symptoms to watch for and what actions to take. As many as ¼ of people may experience altitude sickness, and it is impossible to predict in advance whether one is susceptible.

Acute mountain sickness (AMS) is common, and up to 75% of people will have mild symptoms after spending 1 or 2 days above 10,000 feet. Others may experience more severe symptoms at as low as 8,000 feet. Symptoms include headache, dizziness, fatigue, shortness of breath, nausea and lack of appetite and general malaise. Moderate AMS causes more severe headaches not relieved by medication, nausea and vomiting, decreased coordination and worsening of the mild symptoms. Severe AMS causes shortness of breath even at rest, decreasing mental status and inability to walk. Mild AMS may be overcome with acclimatization, but descent to lower altitude is the only cure for more severe symptoms. To assess the seriousness of AMS, a person experiencing AMS symptoms can try to walk a straight line heel to toe (like a sobriety test). Someone who has difficulty doing this should start the descent immediately before symptoms worsen.

Medication is available to treat mild to moderate symptoms in people who have experienced AMS in the past. Hikers should also maintain good hydration, since body fluid is lost more rapidly at high altitudes. New research also suggests that a high-carbohydrate diet before and during the high-altitude period may reduce the symptoms of AMS.

Two other types of altitude sickness, **high altitude pulmonary edema (HAPE)** and **high altitude cerebral edema (HACE),** are rare but more serious. Both occur after more time at altitude and involve a fluid buildup – in the lungs in HAPE or the brain in HACE – that becomes life-threatening. A victim of HAPE experiences shortness of breath even at rest; a feeling of tightness in the chest, significant fatigue and weakness, a persistent, productive cough; and confusion or irrational behavior. A victim of HACE has significant mental signs and symptoms including headache, loss of coordination, memory loss, possible hallucinations, psychotic confusion and coma. Any victim thought to be experiencing HAPE or HACE must be evacuated immediately down the mountain to a medical facility.

SCUBA DIVING

Underwater divers, as part of their scuba training and certification, learn about the risks of staying down too long or surfacing too quickly. Operators of dive boats and facilities know what signs and symptoms to look for and typically have the communications equipment and resources needed to call for professional medical help when necessary. Some divers, however, may dive on their own or accompanied by others without this training. EMS should be contacted immediately for any diver experiencing breathing difficulty, pain in joints or extremities, feelings of paralysis, tingling or numbness, significant fatigue and generalized weakness, convulsions, coma or nonresponsiveness. Decompression treatment and other specialized care may be needed.

 LEARNING CHECKPOINT 4

1. Fill in the correct answer: In a desert or other extremely dry, hot environment, a person's daily intake of water may increase to _____ gallons.

2. Put a check mark next to the typical signs and symptoms of acute mountain sickness:

   ☐ Headache

   ☐ Dizziness

   ☐ Diarrhea

   ☐ Cold, dry skin

   ☐ Fatigue

   ☐ Nausea

 CONCLUDING THOUGHTS

For people living or working in rural areas or visiting remote locations for any reason, the most important thing is to be aware that if an injury or sudden illness strikes, you may be on your own for a time before being rescued or reaching advanced care. This makes injury and illness prevention crucial, as is being prepared for the kinds of emergencies that are more likely to occur in the specific setting. With preparation and a healthy attitude toward minimizing the risks, you will likely be among the millions who live in remote locations or visit wilderness areas every year without incident.

SCENARIO 1

You are 1 of a group of 5 backpackers hiking high in the mountains in October when you experience a snow squall. The group, believing the snow will not accumulate much, has decided to push on, and starts a single-file ascent up a steep, narrow stretch of trail. The woman at the end of the line loses her footing in the snow and slides over the edge of a rocky embankment. She tumbles and slides down to a flat ledge.

a. When you reach her, she is responsive but groggy. She has minor bleeding in several places and a large gash across her forehead. As you begin your assessment, what condition should you be watching for?

b. You assess her head injury and check for a spinal injury. She has very diminished sensation in her hands and feet and cannot squeeze your hand with hers. What are your first priorities for her care?

c. Because you have established that she has a likely spinal injury, you know she needs emergency care. You are about 10 miles from the trailhead where your vehicles are parked. Although you have a cell phone, it does not have a signal in this remote area. With 4 of you to help, should you try to carry her back down the trail on an improvised stretcher?

d. After a quick discussion, your group decides that 2 will go for help and 2 will stay with the victim. What are the priorities of each group? What planning should be done before the 2 leave to go for help?

e. The 2 hikers have left to summon help. What are the priorities for the 2 hikers remaining with the victim? What else can they do to improve their chances for timely rescue?

ADDITIONAL ACTIVITIES AND RESOURCES

Several of the wilderness associations have websites that provide additional information about preparedness and training for emergencies in remote locations. If you plan to enter any remote area where help would be delayed in an emergency, conduct further research and consider taking a special wilderness survival or emergency training course.

 REVIEW QUESTIONS

Select the best answers.

1. If you will be in the wilderness for several days, consider bringing along –

    a. more water than you expect to need.

    b. special medications you might need.

    c. a device for emergency communication.

    d. All of the above

2. If you need to use your cell phone to call for help while in a remote location and the signal is weak, what can you try in order to get a stronger signal?

    a. Point the antenna directly at the horizon.

    b. Move the phone around your body.

    c. Try to get near a body of water.

    d. Wrap a damp cloth around the antenna.

3. Standard distress signals involve making what number of sounds, lights or visual signals that may be heard or seen by others?

    a. 2

    b. 3

    c. 4

    d. As many as possible

4. In a remote location, leave a victim alone to go for help only if –

    a. you are alone with the victim.

    b. you cannot communicate your need for help.

    c. it is unlikely someone will pass your location soon.

    d. All of the above

5. Your group in a wilderness area decides to use a litter to carry an unresponsive injured victim back to safety. Which of the following is the most dangerous possibility to stay alert for as you carry the victim?

    a. Vomiting

    b. Heat exhaustion

    c. Pain caused by jiggling the litter

    d. Dehydration

6. What is different about wound care if medical attention may be delayed a day or two?

    a. Try to insert antibiotic cream into a puncture wound by any method, even cutting open the wound if necessary.

    b. Rather than covering the wound with a dressing, leave it open to "breathe" and to be able to check it frequently for signs of infection.

    c. Clean the wound after the bleeding stops, even at the risk of bleeding starting again.

    d. Use your sewing kit, if available, to stitch closed any wound.

7. A hiker in your group has experienced a blow to the head. The group cannot decide whether to send someone immediately to call for emergency evacuation or to wait and see if the victim is well enough to walk out in a few hours. Which of the following signs and symptoms may indicate a more serious brain injury requiring medical treatment as soon as possible?

    a. Unequal pupils not responding to light

    b. Headache

    c. Warm, flushed skin

    d. Bleeding of the scalp

8. Guidelines for burn prevention when camping are based in part on which of the following?

    a. Lightning strikes are very common at campsites.

    b. Tents, sleeping bags and other camping gear are often highly flammable.

    c. Campfires usually flare up several hours after going "out."

    d. Burns from boiling water are more likely when cooking over a campfire.

9. A person with diabetes who is in a group of campers in a remote location should –

    a. tell others the signs and symptoms of a diabetic emergency and what to do.

    b. bring glucose or a sugar substance to take in case of hypoglycemia.

    c. monitor his or her blood sugar levels carefully.

    d. All of the above

10. Which of these types of cardiac arrest victims have been revived when CPR lasts longer than 30 minutes?

    a. Heart attack victims

    b. Trauma victims

    c. Drowning victims

    d. Stroke victims

CHAPTER 24

CHAPTER 24

Rescuing and Moving Victims

LESSON OBJECTIVES

- Describe how to rescue or care for a victim in each of the following emergencies:

  - Fire scene

  - Hazardous materials incident

  - Vehicle crash

  - Potential drowning situation

  - Broken ice

- Describe how to prioritize care for multiple victims with different types of injuries.

- Explain when it may be necessary to move a victim.

- Demonstrate the following emergency moves:

  - Shoulder drag

  - Clothes drag

  - Ankle drag

  - Blanket drag

  - Walking assist

  - Packstrap carry

  - Cradle carry

  - Piggyback carry

  - 2-handed seat carry

  - Hammock carry with multiple rescuers

You are called to the equipment room where an employee has been found unresponsive. He is lying on the floor beneath a rack of electrical equipment that he apparently was working on. Thinking he may have been electrocuted, you first make sure the power to this equipment is turned off, and then you check him and determine he is not breathing normally. Because he is lying on his side beneath overhanging equipment, however, you cannot give him chest compressions. Given the risk of a spinal injury, you know that normally you should not move him. What should you do?

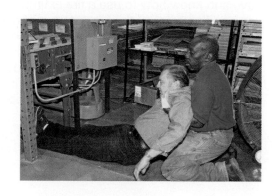

Before you can give first aid and basic life support (BLS), you have to reach the victim. If the scene is dangerous, you must stay away or take special precautions. Sometimes there is more than 1 victim, and you have to decide whom to care for first. Sometimes, the victim must be moved, if it is safe to do so, before you can give first aid. Never attempt any rescue or move a victim unless it is safe for both you and the victim.

Rescuing a Victim

Common situations involving victim rescue are fires, hazardous materials incidents, motor vehicle crashes and water rescues. Before entering any of these situations, however, be sure that it is safe to do so. If the scene is dangerous and you cannot safely approach the victim, *stay away and call for help*. The 9-1-1 dispatcher will send a crew with the appropriate training and equipment to safely reach and care for the victim. **Chapter 2** discusses scene safety in more detail. Safe rescues in most situations described in this chapter require specialized training and gear. It is essential that you do only what you have been trained to do, because otherwise, you may become another victim that others will have to rescue.

FIRE

If a victim needs rescue from a fire scene, do not approach him or her unless you are certain it is safe to do so. Smoke or fumes are usually present in fire situations and can easily overcome anyone entering the scene. Invisible gases resulting from fire pose a threat in both indoor and outdoor locations.

If a fire breaks out in your location, quick action is essential. Most importantly, evacuate others present, and call 9-1-1. Do not enter an area of smoke or flames to search for victims, however, because of the high risk that you will be overcome by smoke or fumes. Do not remain in the area in an attempt to fight the fire unless the fire is very small, you have and know how to use a fire extinguisher, and you can flee safely if the fire gets out of control. If caught indoors in a smoky area, take action to avoid the smoke as much as possible by staying close to the floor (smoke rises), not opening doors and preventing the entry of smoke through vents or door cracks (**Figure 24-1** and First Aid: "Fire"). See other guidelines in **Chapter 11**.

FIGURE 24-1

If trapped in a building where there is a fire, take precautions to avoid smoke inhalation.

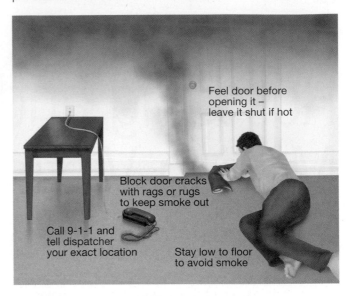

Feel door before opening it – leave it shut if hot

Block door cracks with rags or rugs to keep smoke out

Call 9-1-1 and tell dispatcher your exact location

Stay low to floor to avoid smoke

HAZARDOUS MATERIALS

Chapter 2 describes precautions to take around a spill of hazardous materials. Treat any unknown substance you see spilled as a hazard until proven otherwise. Avoid any spilled liquid or powder as well as possible fumes. Because the cleanup of hazardous materials takes special training, knowledge and equipment, leave this to Hazardous Materials (HAZMAT) professionals. Do not enter a scene contaminated by hazardous materials to reach a victim. If a victim emerges from the spill area with potentially hazardous substances on clothing or skin, do not touch the victim because of the risk of contaminating yourself as well. If possible, use a water hose to wash the victim's skin and clothing before providing first aid. **Chapter 11** describes the first aid for chemicals on the skin. While waiting for help to arrive, cover a wet victim with a blanket or coats to preserve body warmth. Do not let anyone who has had contact with a potentially hazardous material leave the area before Emergency Medical Service (EMS) professionals arrive (see First Aid: "Hazardous Materials").

First Aid: Fire

Signs, Symptoms and Care

WHEN YOU SEE

- Flames or smoke

- A fire alarm sounding

DO THIS FIRST

1. Remove everyone from the area. Close doors behind you as you leave.

2. Call 9-1-1, set off alarms or follow other workplace protocols.

3. Use a fire extinguisher to combat a fire only if:

   - The fire is small.

   - You can easily and quickly escape the area.

   - You know how to use the fire extinguisher.

   - You can stay between the exit and the fire, so you can always get out safely.

4. Do not enter an area of flames and smoke in an attempt to rescue others.

5. If trapped inside:

   - In a smoky room, crawl along the floor, where there is breathable air.

   - Do not open a door that feels hot.

6. Do not use elevators.

   - If stuck inside, turn off the ventilation system, stuff towels or rags (wet if possible) into door cracks and vents, and use a phone to report your location.

ALERT

- Never put yourself at risk to rescue a victim.

- When hazards are present, leave the rescue to the professionals.

- Never try to perform any rescue technique you have not been trained to do.

First Aid: Hazardous Materials

Signs, Symptoms and Care

WHEN YOU SEE

- Warning signs or placards (with "flammable" or other warning terms) (see **Chapter 2**)

- Any spilled substance

- Visible vapors or fumes you can smell

DO THIS FIRST

1. Stay out of the area, and keep bystanders away.

2. Outside, stay upwind of the area to avoid possible fumes.

3. Call 9-1-1.

4. Approach the victim only if you are sure it is safe to do so. For a large exposure to hazardous materials, guide the victim to an emergency shower, or rinse skin and clothing with a hose. Do only what you have been trained to do.

ADDITIONAL CARE

- If it is safe to reach the victim, move him or her away from the hazard, and give first aid for a chemical burn or smoke inhalation (see **Chapter 11**).

VEHICLE CRASHES

Vehicle crash scenes can be extremely dangerous for rescuers because of the risks of passing traffic, fire, vehicle instability and other factors. Rescuers have been injured by unintentionally setting off an automatic air bag while trying to reach a victim. For all of these reasons, it is crucial to ensure that the scene is safe before approaching the vehicle and providing care for the victim.

If it is safe to reach the vehicle, do not try to remove a victim unless fire or another threat to life is likely. Call 9-1-1 as soon as you recognize a victim is present, and describe the circumstances to the dispatcher so the appropriate rescue team is sent. Crash victims often have spinal or other injuries that could be made worse by moving the victim unnecessarily. Provide needed first aid through the door or window or from behind the driver's seat if the vehicle is stable and it is safe to approach (see First Aid: "Vehicle Crashes"). Since an unresponsive victim is likely to have a spinal injury, support the head and neck with your hands while waiting for help to arrive (see **Chapter 12**).

First Aid: Vehicle Crashes

Signs, Symptoms and Care

WHEN YOU SEE

- A victim inside a motor vehicle after a crash

DO THIS FIRST

1. Stop a safe distance past the crash, and turn on your vehicle's hazard lights.

2. Call 9-1-1 if you have a cell phone, or ask someone else to call.

3. If available, set up warning triangles far back from the scene to warn oncoming traffic. Flares should be used only when there are no spilled chemicals and no chance of a grass fire.

4. Ensure that the scene is safe before you approach the crashed vehicle. Stay away if there are risks from passing traffic, downed electrical wires, fire or vehicle instability. Do not try to stabilize the vehicle unless you have special training.

5. If the vehicle is still running, ask the driver to turn off the ignition. If the driver is unresponsive and you can do so safely, reach in and turn off the ignition.

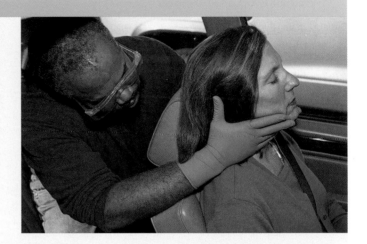

6. Do not try to remove a victim trapped inside a vehicle; wait for professional rescuers.

7. Assume that an unresponsive victim may have a neck injury. If the scene is safe, support the victim's head and neck with your hands in the position found.

8. Do not move the victim unless there is an immediate threat of fire. If there is, get several bystanders to help move the victim while you support the victim's head in line with the body the entire time.

9. Provide BLS and care for any serious injuries while waiting for help.

WATER RESCUES

Water rescues are often needed to prevent drowning. A non-swimmer may have gotten into deep water, or a swimmer may have sustained an injury or sudden illness, such as a heart attack or seizure, that prevents the person from reaching safety. Regardless of the reason, if someone in deep water cannot reach safety, immediate rescue may be required.

Preventing Drownings

As discussed in **Chapter 5,** drowning is a common cause of unintentional death in the United States, resulting in 3,900 deaths in a recent year and about 5 times that many visits to emergency departments for treatment of near-drowning victims. Near-drowning can result in brain damage and other permanent disabilities.[1] Drowning is the first or second leading cause of injury-related death for children in ages 1-14.[2] The Centers for Disease Control and Prevention (CDC) reports that the following are the most common risk factors for drowning:[3]

- Lack of swimming ability: Many adults and children report that they can't swim. Research has shown that participation in formal swimming lessons can reduce the risk of drowning among children ages 1-4

- Lack of barriers: Barriers, such as pool fencing, prevent young children from gaining access to the pool area without caregivers' awareness. A 4-sided isolation fence (separating the pool area from the house and yard) reduces a child's risk of drowning by 83% compared to 3-sided property-line fencing.

- Lack of close supervision: Drowning can happen quickly and quietly anywhere there is water (such as in bathtubs, swimming pools, buckets) even in the presence of lifeguards.

- Location: People of different ages drown in different locations. For example, most children ages 1-4 drown in home swimming pools. The percentage of drownings in natural-water settings, including lakes, rivers and oceans, increases with age. More than half of fatal and nonfatal drownings among those 15 years and older (57% and 57%, respectively) occurred in natural-water settings.

- Failure to wear life jackets: In 2010, the United States Coast Guard received reports for 4,604 boating incidents; 3,153 boaters were reported injured; and 672 died. Most (72%) boating deaths that occurred during 2010 were caused by drowning with 88% of victims not wearing life jackets.

- Alcohol use: Among adolescents and adults, alcohol use is involved in up to 70% of deaths associated with water recreation, almost a quarter of emergency department visits for drowning, and about 1 in 5 reported boating deaths. Alcohol influences balance, coordination and judgment, and its effects are heightened by sun exposure and heat.

[1]*Centers for Disease Control and Prevention, www.cdc.gov/ HomeandRecreationalSafety/Water-Safety/waterinjuries-factsheet.html Accessed January 2016.*

[2]*National Safety Council. (2015). Injury Facts®, 2015 Edition. Itasca, IL: Author.*

[3]*Centers for Disease Control and Prevention, www.cdc.gov/ HomeandRecreationalSafety/Water-Safety/waterinjuries-factsheet.html Accessed January 2016.*

Following are guidelines to help prevent children from drowning:

- Never leave children alone near water. Do not leave small children alone in a bathtub or wading pool.

- Do not let children dive into shallow, murky or unknown water.

- At open waterfronts, keep children away from areas with big waves, undertows and boats.

- Both children and adults should use personal flotation devices (PFDs) on boats and around water.

- In public swimming areas, let children enter the water only where lifeguards are present.

- Make sure rescue floats and other devices are present at pools and other water areas.

- At appropriate ages, children should learn how to swim and be safe in the water from a qualified instructor.

- Adult supervisors should realize that even children who can swim are not "drown-proof."

- Do not let older siblings or babysitters supervise children in the water.

- Most importantly, when supervising children in or near water, avoid all distractions. Do not read, eat or socialize with others. Most children drown when being "supervised" by someone who is not paying close attention.

- Childproof home pools with appropriate fencing, gates, floating pool alarms and other safety devices **(Figure 24-2).**

Adults also should practice water safety principles to prevent drowning:

- Never drink or use other drugs when in or on the water. This includes when boating.

- Always wear a PFD when boating, even when in calm water and well away from the edge of the boat. No one ever plans to fall into the water – drowning usually occurs when the victim feels sure that a PFD is not needed.

- Dive into water only in depths of 9 feet or more when the water is clear and no obstructions are present.

- Do not swim alone.

- Consider your swimming ability before attempting to swim out to a float or boat to ensure that you are not exhausted before reaching safety. Consider waves and other conditions.

- Be aware that swimming in cold water can lead to hypothermia, which may lead to drowning.

- Be prepared for an emergency. Keep CPR skills fresh, and have a telephone handy when supervising others in the water.

FIGURE 24-2

Make a residential swimming pool safe for children with preventive devices.

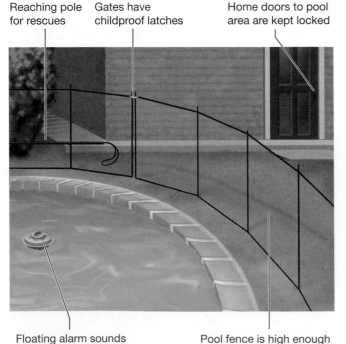

Reaching pole for rescues

Gates have childproof latches

Home doors to pool area are kept locked

Floating alarm sounds if someone falls in pool

Pool fence is high enough to keep children out

Safe Techniques for Water Rescue

Rescuing someone at risk of drowning in deep water first requires recognizing that the person needs help. There are common misconceptions about how drowning victims act. You should not expect the victim to shout for help, nor is it true that "going down for the third time" is a prelude to drowning.

Recognizing a drowning situation depends on understanding 3 general scenarios of how people drown:

- **People who can swim,** "dog paddle" or float well enough to keep their head above water at least for a time, may gradually or suddenly be at risk of drowning. A swimmer may become too tired to keep swimming, or hypothermia may set in and weaken the victim. If the problem develops gradually, the person may be in trouble but not yet actively drowning. This type of victim may call for help in some circumstances or may be able to keep his or her head above water but unable to make progress toward safety. Because it can sometimes be difficult to know whether someone in this situation needs help, it is better to offer assistance than to wait until it is obvious that the person is drowning.

- **A responsive drowning victim** cannot swim, float or tread water effectively and is at immediate risk of drowning. This victim is struggling just to keep his or her head out of the water and is in a panicked state. This victim is very unlikely to call or wave for help. You may see the victim's face just above the surface or bobbing in and out, and his or her arms may be flailing. The victim is clearly struggling, however, rather than treading water or moving forward.

- **An unresponsive drowning victim** is no longer breathing. This victim may be a swimmer who became too exhausted to tread water, or even float; a non-swimmer who can no longer keep his or her face up to breathe and has stopped struggling; or a swimmer or non-swimmer who has experienced an injury or sudden illness (such as a heart attack or seizure) that prevents him or her from swimming or staying at the surface, resulting in submersion and respiratory arrest. Breathing stops either when water enters the lungs or when water in the larynx causes a spasm that closes the airway. When breathing stops, the victim soon becomes unresponsive. Depending on the victim's body composition and the presence or absence of air in the lungs, the victim may be floating face down at the surface or may be underwater.

When you recognize any of these scenarios, quick action is needed to rescue the victim. Your choice of rescue technique depends on the type of situation, the equipment or objects at hand, and the circumstances. Resist the temptation to jump immediately into the water to save the victim. An actively drowning victim is in a state of panic that often leads to the victim grabbing you so forcefully and desperately that you may become a drowning victim yourself. The victim may grab your head or arms in a way that you can neither swim back to safety nor tread water to keep both of you afloat. Lifeguards receive special training on how to manage such victims. They are trained to keep a rescue tube between themselves and the victim to avoid being grabbed and also to break a victim's hold underwater should it become necessary.

Even a tired swimmer who is not yet struggling and panicking may become panicked before you reach him or her. Therefore, it is a poor choice to swim out to assist this kind of victim as well.

It may be appropriate to swim to an unresponsive victim, however, if you have no other means to get the victim quickly out of the water so that you can give CPR if needed. Similarly, a responsive small child may be rescued by an adult who is a good swimmer – although even children may cling tenaciously to one's head or arms when panicked, making a swimming rescue difficult or dangerous for the adult.

The safest and oftentimes most effective rescue technique is to reach to the victim with some object that the victim can grasp while you pull him or her to safety. The second most safe and effective technique is to throw something that floats to the victim, preferably with a rope attached for pulling the victim to safety. Third, and least safe and effective, is to go to the victim yourself. This is called the **reach-throw-go** priority, which emphasizes which techniques to try first.

"Reach" Rescue

Most public and some private pools have a rescue pole, which often has a hook at the end (called a **shepherd's crook**). This pole is usually long enough to reach a victim from the edge of the pool. Let a responsive victim hold on to it while you slowly pull the victim to the edge **(Figure 24-3)**. If the victim is unresponsive, you can hook the victim's body to pull the victim to the edge or shallow water. Unless the unresponsive victim is a small child, pulling an unresponsive victim to the edge will be faster than jumping in to tow the victim to the pool's edge.

Use anything available to reach to the victim. A residential pool may not have a reaching pole, but a broom or rake handle may work just as well. In open-water settings, you may use a fishing pole, a boat's oar or even a long branch. If the victim is close enough to the pool's edge, a dock or the shore, you may also reach with your own body; for example, you could hold on to something secure with your arms and extend your legs on the surface to the victim.

In a natural-water setting in which the water gradually gets deeper farther from the shore, you may be able to reach to the victim with an object after wading a short distance into the water. If possible, stay in water shallow enough for you to stand on the bottom while reaching to the victim.

FIGURE 24-3

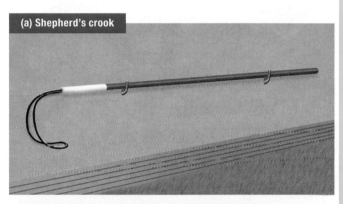
(a) Shepherd's crook

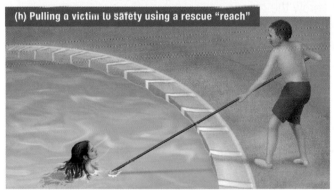
(b) Pulling a victim to safety using a rescue "reach"

"Throw" Rescue

If you cannot reach to the victim, look for anything that floats that you can throw. Swimming pool or boating equipment may include a life ring, rescue tube, life jacket or other device **(Figure 24-4)**. Some boats carry a "throw bag," which has a coiled rope inside that uncoils when the bag is thrown to a victim while you hold the other end. If no throwable rescue device is available, look around for anything that will float – such as a buoyant seat cushion, a water jug that can be mostly emptied (keep some water inside to give it weight for throwing) or even an empty beverage cooler.

If a rope is already attached to the throwable device (or can quickly be tied on), hold it in 1 hand, coil the rope loosely and throw with your stronger arm. Try to throw it over the victim so that the line comes down beside the person and can be easily grasped **(Figure 24-5).**

FIGURE 24-4

Rescue devices and objects that can be thrown to a drowning victim.

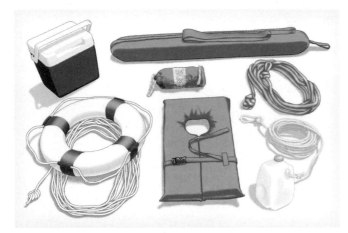

FIGURE 24-5

Throw the rescue device where the victim can grab it or the rope.

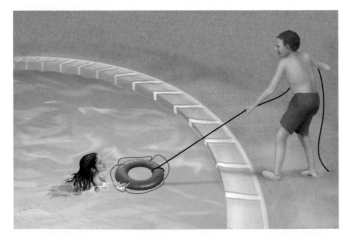

If you have no rope handy for the rescue device, throw it to the victim anyway if it is buoyant enough to help the victim keep his or her head above water. A victim who can float by holding on to something can breathe more easily and may have the strength to kick to shore while holding the object. Even if the victim is too weak to do anything but just hold on, the thrown object can keep the victim safely afloat while you find a rope or something to reach with. Even if

you must enter the water to go to the victim, a victim who is holding on to something that floats is much less likely to panic and grab you, and you can more easily tow the object and victim to safety.

In a natural-water setting in which the water gradually gets deeper farther from the shore, you may be better able to throw a rope or floating object to the victim after wading out into the water to get closer to the victim. If possible, stay in water shallow enough for you to stand on the bottom while throwing to the victim.

"Go" Rescue

As noted earlier, swimming to rescue a responsive victim is very dangerous – so much so that unless you have training, you should not attempt this except with a small child or unresponsive victim. Look for other ways to go to the victim. At a waterfront, you may find a surfboard, kayak or other watercraft in which to go to the victim. Even if it is too small to support both of you, it likely has enough buoyancy to keep you both afloat until help arrives, or the victim may be able to hold on to it for buoyancy while you tow him or her to shore. Wear a life jacket when entering the water or going in a boat to the victim. Remember that the victim is likely panicking, and keep the object between you and the victim so you cannot be grabbed and pulled underwater. The same is true if you decide to swim to a responsive victim. If at all possible, take something with you that the victim can hold on to and that you can release if the victim tries to grab you, keeping the object between you and the victim. Note: If an unresponsive victim in the water may have a spinal injury (e.g., a diving incident), take care to stabilize the head and neck before removing the victim from the water if possible.

Walking Assist

Many natural bodies of water gradually get deeper away from the shore. If a responsive victim in the water is at a depth where he or she can stand, or if you can assist the victim to that depth, you can help the victim to exit the water with a **walking assist (Figure 24-6).** Put the victim's arm around your shoulder, and hold it at the wrist with your hand. Put your other arm around the victim's waist, and support the victim as you walk the person out of the water.

FIGURE 24-6

Walking assist.

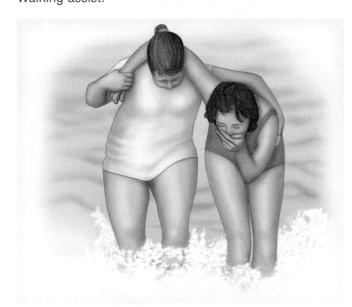

BEACH DRAG

An unresponsive victim who is in or can be brought to shallow water that has a gradual shoreline can be taken from the water using a **beach drag (Figure 24-7).** Reach under the victim's shoulders and hold the victim at the armpits, resting the victim's head on your forearms (and preventing head or neck movement in case of a possible spinal injury). Then, slowly back out of the water, dragging the victim out. This rescue technique is similar to the shoulder drag used to move an unresponsive victim on land from a hazardous scene shown later in this chapter.

FIGURE 24-7

Beach drag.

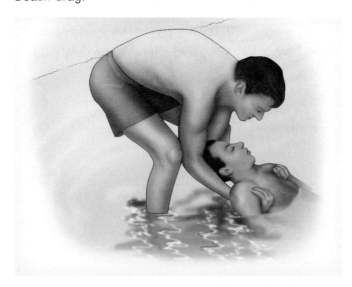

If Stranded in Cold Water

If you are immersed in cold water and cannot swim to safety or climb out of the water on to an overturned boat or other floating object, try to minimize heat loss from your body while awaiting rescue. If alone, use the "heat escape lessening position" (HELP). Hold your arms close to your sides and raise your knees to your chest, remaining as still as possible **(Figure 24-8).**

Two or more people together in cold water should use the "huddle position" to conserve heat: Everyone puts arms around each others' shoulders to bring the sides of their chests together (if 3 or more) in a tight circle **(Figure 24-9).** Children should be sandwiched between adults.

FIGURE 24-8

The "HELP" position.

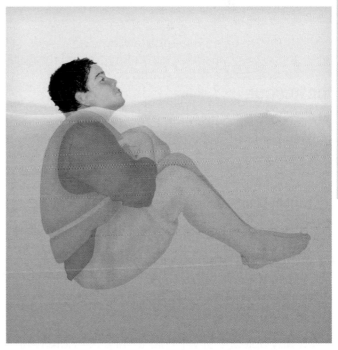

FIGURE 24-9

The "huddle" position.

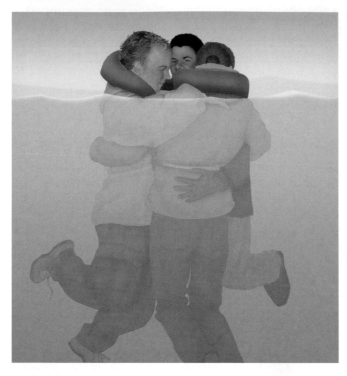

ICE RESCUE

As described in **Chapter 2,** ice rescues are very dangerous. Cold-water immersion is very serious and can quickly doom even the best swimmers. Ice rescue should be left to specially trained personnel who have the necessary safety equipment. Call 9-1-1 immediately to summon emergency personnel.

If it is safe to do so and emergency personnel will not arrive in time, you may attempt an ice rescue using the same priorities as a water rescue: reach-throw-go. Try first to reach to a victim who has broken through ice using a pole or tree limb **(Figure 24-10).** If you cannot reach to the victim, throw a rope or any buoyant object tied to a rope. As a last resort, throw any object that will float to help the victim stay afloat, but be aware that in icy water, hypothermia sets in very quickly, and the victim will not be able to hold on to an object very long. Only as an extreme last resort should you try to go to the victim yourself. Realize that the ice may not hold your weight and that you too may become a victim. If you must go on the ice, lie down to distribute your weight over a larger surface area. Another person should hold your feet and be prepared to pull you out if the ice under you breaks. If possible, push a branch or other object ahead of you to the victim to minimize the distance you must go on to the ice.

Following an ice rescue, the victim is likely to need treatment for hypothermia **(Chapter 20).**

FIGURE 24-10

Try to reach to a victim who has fallen through ice with a pole or tree limb.

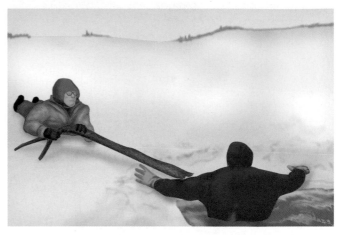

✏️ **LEARNING CHECKPOINT 1**

1. Select the best answer. During a fire, the first action to take is –

    a. get everyone out.

    b. throw water on the fire immediately.

    c. use a fire extinguisher.

    d. close all doors and windows.

2. Select the best answer. If you are caught in a building that is on fire –

    a. stay low to the floor.

    b. feel doors before opening them.

    c. use stairs, not the elevator.

    d. All of the above

Circle **True** or **False** for each of the following statements.

3. OSHA requires fire prevention and safety guidelines in the workplace.　　True　False

4. The first action to take for a spilled, dry chemical is to vacuum it up.　　True　False

5. Spilled liquids may produce poisonous fumes.　　True　False

6. You are the first on the scene where a car has crashed into a telephone pole. After you make sure that the scene is safe, you approach the car and find the driver alone, slumped forward against the steering wheel and unresponsive. What can you do to help?

_____

_____

_____

_____

7. Select the best answer. The safest order in which to attempt a water rescue is -

   a. throw-reach-go.

   b. go-throw-reach.

   c. reach-throw-go.

   d. reach-go-throw.

Multiple Victims

An incident such as a car crash or a workplace explosion may involve multiple victims who need first aid. In such a case, the first thing you must do after calling 9-1-1 to get help on the way, is decide who needs your care most and who can wait until others can help. This process of setting priorities is called **triage (Figure 24-11).**

FIGURE 24-11

In an emergency with multiple victims, first determine which victim is the highest priority for first aid.

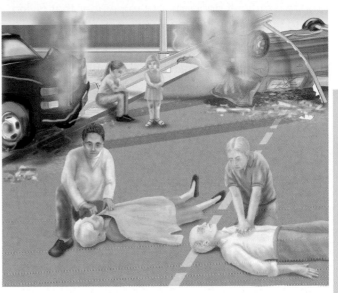

Triage systems usually put each victim into 1 of 4 categories **(Table 24-1).** Because the goal of triage is to determine which victim(s) require immediate care, this process should be done very quickly. As you check the scene for safety and approach, ask who can walk. Have these victims move to one side – they are the third priority. Try to assess each of the

TABLE 24-1

Triage Priorities For Multiple Victims

Priority	Victim's Condition	Severity	Examples
First	Critical	Victims with life-threatening injuries who cannot wait for help	• Breathing problems • Severe bleeding • Shock • Severe burn
Second	Serious	Victims with injuries that need care very soon but may be able to wait for help	• Burns • Broken bones • Other injuries not severely bleeding
Third	Stable	Victims who can wait for some time	• Minor injuries • Victims who can walk
Fourth	Obviously dead or dying	Victims who cannot be saved	• Not breathing with massive head or chest trauma with severe blood loss

remaining victims in less than a minute by checking for responsiveness, breathing and severe bleeding; do not start to give care to any victim until you have quickly checked all victims. If a victim is very severely injured and is not breathing, and other victims require your immediate care, you should attend to others whom you judge can be saved. This situation can require a difficult decision, but remember that giving BLS to an obviously dying victim may mean that someone who could have been saved may not be.

Because a victim's condition may change during the process of triage or giving care, you may have to change priorities. For example, if you are treating a second-priority victim with a fracture, another victim who at first seemed to have only minor injuries (third priority) may suddenly become unresponsive and require your immediate attention (first priority) to maintain an open airway (see First Aid: "Multiple Victims").

First Aid: Multiple Victims

Signs, Symptoms and Care

WHEN YOU SEE

- 2 or more victims needing care

DO THIS FIRST

1. Call 9-1-1 immediately. Tell the dispatcher there are multiple victims.

2. Ask any victims who can walk (third priority) to move to one side. These victims do not have immediate life-threatening problems.

3. For the remaining victims, starting with unresponsive victims, quickly check for normal breathing and severe bleeding, looking for life-threatening injuries in victims who can be saved (first priority). Spend a minute or less with each victim, and do not start giving care until you have checked all victims.

4. Start providing BLS to first-priority victims first. Move to second-priority victims only when the first-priority victims are stable. Ask any bystanders with first aid training to help you with other victims.

5. When help arrives, quickly tell the EMS professionals about the victims present. Offer to help them care for victims.

 LEARNING CHECKPOINT 2

Circle **True** or **False** for each of the following statements:

1. A victim with a broken arm is a second priority in a multiple-victim incident.

    True   False

2. Victims with life-threatening injuries are first priority in a multiple-victim incident.

    True   False

3. You are the lone responder at a construction site where a collapsed wall has injured 4 workers. Using standard triage priorities, rank these 4 in terms of who gets care first, second, third and fourth:

    _____A woman with a bruised face and abrasions on her arms who is walking around holding her bleeding forehead

    _____A man on the ground with no apparent external injuries but who is unresponsive

    _____A man who is not breathing, whose chest has caved in under a steel beam and who is surrounded by a pool of blood

    _____A man sitting up and leaning against the rubble, looking very pale, who says he feels nauseated

Moving Victims

Moving an injured victim is more likely to cause further injury than not. In most cases, you should wait for professionals who have training and equipment to transport the victim to advanced medical care.

In some instances, however, you must move a victim to protect him or her from a danger at the scene, such as a spreading fire, the chance of an explosion, or a structure at risk of collapse **(Figure 24-12)**. *Remember: Never enter a scene unless you can do so safely.* You may have to move 1 victim to reach another victim who has a life-threatening condition. You may also have to move a victim to a firm, flat surface to provide CPR. If you decide to move a victim, several factors are involved in choosing the best method (see First Aid: "Moving Victims"):

- How quickly must the victim be moved?

- Does the victim's condition affect the move (nature of injury, responsiveness, potential spinal injury, etc.)?

- Are others present who can help with the move?

- Is any equipment (e.g., a stretcher) or other object (e.g., a blanket) needed?

- Do you have the physical strength needed to move the victim?

Whenever you lift a victim, be sure to use good body mechanics. This means:

- Do not try to lift more weight than you can lift without straining.

- Lift with your legs instead of your back. Keep your feet shoulder-width apart with 1 foot in front of the other. Keep your back straight and crouch down, then lift by straightening your legs.

- Do not turn or twist your back while bearing weight.

- Bear the victim's weight as close to your trunk as possible.

- Take short steps and move forward rather than backward.

FIGURE 24-12

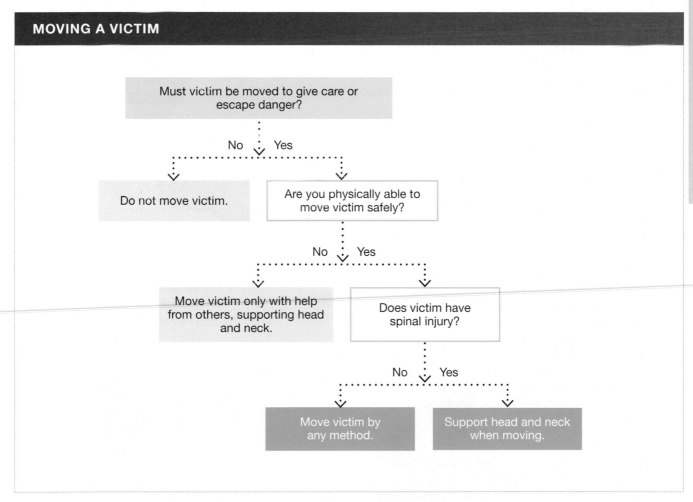

MOVING A VICTIM

First Aid: Moving Victims

Signs, Symptoms and Care

WHEN YOU SEE

Consider moving a victim only if:

- Fire or explosion is likely.

- Poisonous fumes may be present.

- The structure may collapse.

- The victim needs to be moved into position for lifesaving care such as CPR.

- The victim is in the way of another seriously injured victim.

DO THIS FIRST

1. Try to move the victim only if you are physically able and can do it safely.

2. Get help from others at the scene.

3. For an unresponsive victim or a victim with a spinal injury, support the head and neck in line with the body during the move.

4. Use good body mechanics.

5. If alone:

   For an unresponsive victim with a suspected spinal injury:

   - For a short distance, use the shoulder drag (supporting the victim's head against your chest) or the clothes drag (supporting the victim's head with clothing taut between your hands).

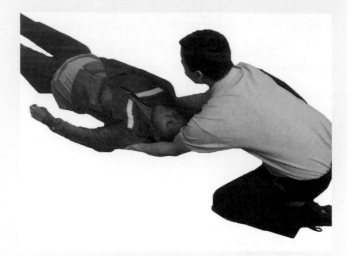

- Use the blanket drag to support the victim's head for a longer distance.

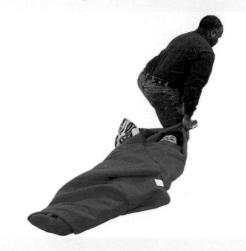

For an unresponsive victim without a spinal injury:

- The ankle drag is easier to use for short distances over a smooth surface (not rough terrain) and by a small rescuer for a large victim.

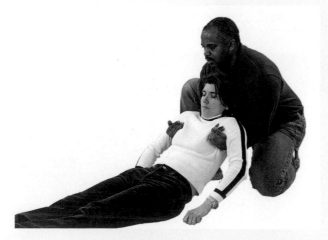

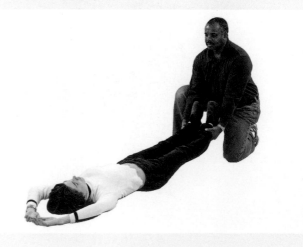

For a responsive victim who can walk with help:

- Use the 1- or 2-person walking assist.

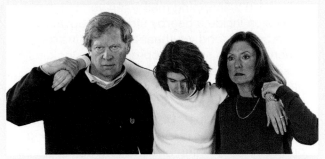

For an unresponsive victim who cannot safely be moved with a drag (if you are strong enough to lift the victim):

- Use the packstrap carry.

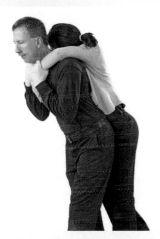

For a lighter victim or child:

- Use a cradle carry for responsive or unresponsive victims.

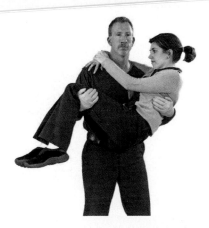

- Use a piggyback carry for responsive victims.

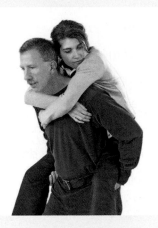

6. With the help of 1 or more others:

   For a responsive victim:

   - Use the 2-person assist or 2-handed seat carry.

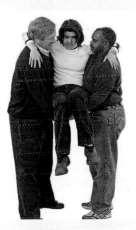

   For an unresponsive victim:

   - Use 3-6 rescuers with the hammock carry.

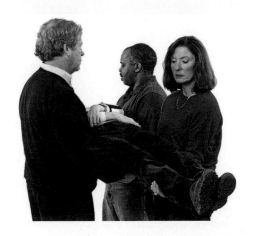

LEARNING CHECKPOINT 3

1. Check situations in which you should consider moving a victim.

    ☐ Fire is present

    ☐ Bleeding victim inside a car

    ☐ Cold environment

    ☐ Strong smell of natural gas in the room

    ☐ Small child with severe burns

    ☐ The hospital is only a short drive

    ☐ A victim going into shock

    ☐ A victim is lying on top of another victim

2. Select the best answer. If you have to move an unresponsive injured victim by yourself, an effective method would be to –

    a. sling the victim over your shoulder.

    b. roll the victim over the ground like a log.

    c. grab both of the victim's wrists and pull him or her along.

    d. use a blanket drag to support the victim's head.

 CONCLUDING THOUGHTS

Remember that your own safety must be ensured before rescuing or moving a victim in any situation. Pause to think and plan before acting, and then move carefully to protect both yourself and the victim from further injury.

 CRITICAL THINKING CHALLENGE QUESTIONS

🧑‍🤝‍🧑 SCENARIO 1

You are in a shopping mall when you hear an explosion inside a nearby store. Windows have been broken, and you hear a scream inside. When it seems safe to approach, you look inside to see if anyone needs help. Several people have minor injuries, but 3 victims obviously have more serious injuries. A man lies on the floor, apparently unresponsive, with a large puddle of blood beneath his torso. A woman is sitting on the floor clutching her bleeding leg, in which there is a large shard of glass. A 10-year-old child lies on the floor farther away, apparently unresponsive but with no visible injuries.

a. What are the first 2 actions you should take?

_____

_____

_____

b. When you quickly check the 3 victims, you find the man is not breathing and has lost a very large amount of blood from gaping wounds in his abdomen and chest. Blood is slowly oozing from the woman's leg wound, but she remains responsive. The child is not breathing, but has no visible wounds or bleeding. What do you do now?

_____

_____

_____

_____

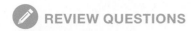

Select the best answers.

1. If the emergency scene is very dangerous, you should –

    a. run in quickly and give lifesaving care to the victim.

    b. run in quickly and pull the victim to safety.

    c. call 9-1-1 and wait for professionals with appropriate training and equipment.

    d. rescue the victim if help has not arrived 5 minutes after calling 9-1-1.

2. It is safe to enter the scene of a fire when –

    a. you can keep at least 15 feet away from flames.

    b. you can crouch below the smoke to breathe.

    c. you know a victim inside needs help.

    d. It is never safe to enter a fire scene.

3. Which of these statements is true?

    a. Poisonous fumes from a spilled substance are always visible.

    b. Poisonous fumes are not present if you see "normal" black smoke at a fire.

    c. Dangerous fumes are lighter than air and always rise to the ceiling.

    d. Invisible dangerous fumes may be present at any fire or hazardous materials spill.

4. Which action is appropriate for a victim of a vehicle crash with suspected a spinal injury?

    a. Support the victim's head in place with your hands, remaining in the vehicle.

    b. Support the victim's head in place with your hands while you help him or her exit the vehicle.

    c. Use a splint to support the victim's head while you help him or her exit the vehicle.

    d. Use the clothes drag to support the victim's head while you pull him or her from the vehicle.

5. How can you tell if someone in the water may be drowning?

    a. The person is swimming only slowly toward a destination.

    b. The person is struggling to keep his or her mouth above the water.

    c. The person calls out for help.

    d. The person waves both arms high above his or her head.

6. Which water rescue technique should you try first?

    a. Throwing a rope to the victim

    b. Throwing the victim a ring buoy with a rope tied to it

    c. Reaching to the victim with a pole or tree branch

    d. Swimming to the victim with a flotation device

7. When you are alone and encounter a vehicle crash scene with 4 victims, which of these victims should you help first?

    a. The driver, who is slumped over the wheel and not breathing, his chest bloody with a pool of blood on the seat beside him

    b. A front-seat passenger who has a cut on the forehead and a sprained wrist who gets out of the vehicle as you approach

    c. An unresponsive rear-seat passenger with no visible injuries who is not breathing

    d. A responsive rear-seat passenger who says she thinks her leg is broken

8. How you move a victim in an emergency may depend on –

    a. whether the victim is in shock.

    b. whether others are present.

    c. whether you have medical examination gloves with you.

    d. whether the victim is wearing a medical ID.

9. Which of these emergency moves provides the best head and neck support for an unresponsive victim with a suspected spinal injury?

    a. Clothes drag

    b. Ankle drag

    c. Cradle carry

    d. Piggyback carry

10. Good body mechanics include –

    a. lifting with your legs rather than your back.

    b. not twisting your back when carrying weight.

    c. taking short steps.

    d. All of the above

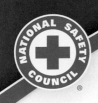

CHAPTER 25

Are You Prepared?

LESSON OBJECTIVES

- List general steps for what to do before, during and after an emergency.

- Create an emergency plan for your family.

- Prepare an Emergency Go Kit.

- Describe specific actions to take in case of a natural disaster, chemical threat or nuclear explosion.

- List actions to help recover from an emergency.

It is late Saturday afternoon, and you have been so busy doing household chores that you barely noticed the thunderstorm moving in from the west. You glance out a window and see the sky is turning black. You remember you left the car windows open and go out to close them before the rain starts. As you come around the corner of the house, you see a funnel cloud apparently less than a mile away. What should you do?

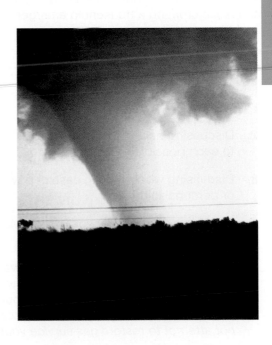

This guide[1] will help you to

- learn what to do before, during and after an emergency.

- create an emergency plan for your family.

- prepare an Emergency Go Kit.

[1] *This chapter is adapted from the "A Federal Employee's Family Preparedness Guide" prepared by the United States Office of Personnel Management files. eric.ed.gov/fulltext/ED479667.pdf Accessed January 2016.*

Before an Emergency Strikes

During an emergency, you and your family may have little or no time to plan what to do next. You must learn about the things you can do to be prepared before an emergency occurs. Two actions that will help you to do this are to develop an emergency plan and to prepare an Emergency Go Kit.

CREATE AN EMERGENCY PLAN

Part of creating your household emergency plan is to learn about the types of emergencies that may affect your community, how you will be notified of an emergency, and plans that may already be in place to deal with emergencies. Determine if your community has a warning system – via television, radio or another signal – and learn what it sounds like and what to do when you hear it. Emergencies may strike when your family members are away from home, so find out about plans at your workplace, school or anywhere else you and your family spend time. Steps to take in creating a household emergency plan include:

1. Meeting with household members to discuss the dangers of possible emergency events, including fire, severe weather, hazardous spills and terrorism.

2. Discussing how you and your family will respond to each possible emergency.

3. Discussing what to do in case of power outages or personal injuries.

4. Drawing a floor plan of your home. Mark 2 escape routes from each room.

5. Teaching adults how to turn off the water, gas and electricity at main switches. If, for any reason, you turn off natural gas service to your home, call your gas utility company to restore service. *Do not attempt to restore gas service yourself.*

6. Posting emergency contact numbers near all telephones and preprogramming emergency numbers into phones with autodial capabilities

7. Teaching children how and when to dial 9-1-1 to get emergency assistance.

8. Teaching children how to make long-distance telephone calls and/or use a cell phone.

9. Choosing a friend or relative whom all family members will call if separated (it is often easier to call out of state during an emergency than within the affected areas).

10. Instructing household members to turn on the radio for emergency information.

11. Picking 2 meeting places:

    - A place near your home

    - A place outside your neighborhood in case you cannot return home after an emergency

12. Taking a first aid and CPR class

13. Keeping family records in a waterproof and fireproof safe. Inexpensive models can be purchased at most hardware stores.

PREPARE AN EMERGENCY GO KIT

During an emergency, electricity, water, heat, air conditioning or telephone service may not work. Preparing an Emergency Go Kit ahead of time can save precious time in the event you must evacuate or go without electricity, heat or water for an extended period of time. You should consider including the following items in an Emergency Go Kit:

1. At least a 3-day supply of water (1 gallon per person per day). Store water in sealed, unbreakable containers. Replace every 6 months.

2. A 3-5 day supply of nonperishable, packaged or canned food and a nonelectric can opener

3. A change of clothing, rain gear and sturdy shoes

4. Blankets, bedding or sleeping bags

5. A first aid kit and prescription medications (be sure to check the expiration dates)

6. An extra pair of glasses or contact lenses and solution (be sure to check the expiration dates)

7. A list of family physicians, important medical information, and the style and serial number of medical devices such as pacemakers

8. Special items for infants, the elderly or family members with disabilities

9. A battery-powered radio, flashlight and plenty of extra batteries (or a hand-cranked radio and flashlight)

10. Identification, credit cards, cash and photocopies of important family documents, including home insurance information

11. An extra set of car and house keys

12. Tools such as screwdrivers, cutters and scissors, duct tape, waterproof matches, a fire extinguisher, flares, plastic storage containers, a needle and thread, pen and paper, a compass, garbage bags and regular household bleach

KNOW THE PLANS OF YOUR SCHOOL SYSTEM

If you have a child who attends school, it is important for you to contact your school system administrators to fully understand what plans are in place to protect your child in the event of an emergency.

Be sure to keep the contact information for your child up to date. Provide your school administrators with a list of family members or caregivers whom you authorize to pick up your child or children at school.

If a dangerous substance were to be released in the atmosphere and posed a threat to students during the school day, it is very likely that the schools affected would shelter-in-place and protect children and staff by keeping them inside and moving them to safer areas within the school building.

PRESCRIPTIONS

Store 3-5 days' worth of medications that are important to your health.

Include any medications that are used to stabilize a medical condition or keep a condition from worsening or resulting in hospitalization, such as medications for asthma, seizures, cardiovascular disorders, diabetes, psychiatric conditions, HIV and thyroid disorders.

Carry these with you, if possible, in a purse or briefcase in labeled containers. Rotate these medications whenever you get your prescriptions refilled. If your child takes medications, communicate with the school to discuss their emergency preparedness plans.

People with complex medication regimens should talk to their physician and pharmacist to help with emergency preparation plans. Such regimens include injectable medications, including those delivered by pumps (e.g., insulin, analgesics, chemotherapy, parenteral nutrition); medications delivered by a nebulizer (e.g., antibiotics, bronchodilators); and dialysis.

NEIGHBORS HELPING NEIGHBORS

Working with neighbors in an emergency can save lives and property. Meet with your community members to plan how you could work together until help arrives. If you are a member of a neighborhood organization, such as a home association or crime watch group, introduce emergency preparedness as a new activity.

BOX 25-1: THINGS TO THINK ABOUT

If any members of your household have disabilities or are elderly, find out what services may be available to aid in their care or evacuation in the event of an emergency.

IF YOU HAVE PETS

If you evacuate, avoid leaving family pets behind. However, keep in mind that with the exception of service animals, pets are generally not permitted in emergency shelters for health reasons.

For this reason, find out before a disaster occurs which hotels or motels (both within and outside your local area) allow pets. Determine where pet boarding facilities are located.

Create an emergency kit for your pet. This should include:

- Identification tag and rabies tags worn on a collar at all times

- Carrier or cage

- Leash

- Any medications (be sure to check expiration date)

- Newspapers and plastic bags for handling waste

- A supply of food, bottled water and food bowls

- Veterinary records (most animal boarding facilities do not allow pets without proof of vaccination)

For complete information, the American Society for the Prevention of Cruelty to Animals has an emergency preparedness guide designed specifically for pets at aspca.org/pet-care/general-pet-care/disaster-preparedness. Accessed January 2016.

After an Emergency Strikes

SHELTER-IN-PLACE

In the event of an emergency, such as the release of a hazardous material, it is not always recommended that you immediately evacuate, because leaving your house might expose you to harmful agents that have been dispersed into the air. "Sheltering-in-place," which means simply staying in your house or current location, may be the best way to avoid harm. Federal agencies have protocols in place at every agency to shelter-in-place at the workplace if circumstances warrant that action. Federal employees can ask their managers for more information about the procedures in place at their agency.

IF YOUR POWER GOES OUT

1. Remain calm and assist family members or neighbors who may be vulnerable if exposed to extreme heat or cold.

2. Locate a flashlight with batteries to use until power comes back on. Do not use candles – this can cause a fire.

3. Turn off sensitive electric equipment such as computers and televisions.

4. Turn off major electric appliances that were on when the power went off. This will help prevent power surges when electricity is restored.

5. Keep your refrigerator and freezer doors closed as much as possible to keep cold in and heat out.

6. Do not use the stove to heat your home.

7. Use extreme caution when driving. If traffic signals are out, treat each signal as a stop sign – come to a complete stop at every intersection and look before you proceed.

8. Do not call 9-1-1 to ask about the power outage.

9. Listen to news radio stations for updates.

IF YOU NEED CLEAN WATER

Flooding can cause contamination of water supplies. Contaminated water can contain micro-organisms that cause diseases such as dysentery, typhoid and hepatitis. If you think your water may be contaminated, you should purify it before using it. This includes water used for drinking, cooking, cleaning dishes or bathing. The best way to purify water is to boil it.

Boiling

Boiling is considered the safest method of purifying water. Bring water to a boil for 3-5 minutes, and then allow it to cool before drinking. Pouring water back and forth between 2 containers will improve the taste by putting oxygen back into the water.

Evacuation

If you are notified or become aware of a technological hazards emergency, such as a hazardous spill/release, fire or explosion, do not panic. If you need to get out of the surrounding area or are directed to evacuate, do so immediately and:

• Take your Emergency Go Kit.

• Lock your home.

• Cover your nose and mouth with a wet cloth.

• Travel on routes specified by local authorities.

• Head upwind of the incident.

If you are sure you have time:

• Shut off water, gas and electricity before leaving.

• Post a note telling others when you left and where you are going.

• Make arrangements for your pets.

If you are instructed to stay inside and not to evacuate:

• Close and lock windows and doors.

• Seal gaps under doorways and windows with wet towels, or seal with plastic and duct tape.

• Turn off ventilation systems.

PREPARE YOUR EVACUATION ROUTES IN ADVANCE

Many major cities have established evacuation routes that can be used to effectively move people from heavily populated areas in the event of an emergency. For instance, the city of Washington, D.C., has identified 14 major arterials that will be used for outbound traffic only. During a major event or emergency situation, radial evacuation routes featuring traffic signals will be timed. In addition, critical intersections on evacuation routes will be manned with uniformed police officers to expedite the flow of traffic and to prevent bottlenecks. Officers will be able to direct drivers to alternate routes should an emergency warrant the closing of current event/evacuation routes.

If you work or live in a heavily populated area, you should figure out the best available routes for you to use, in advance, in the event that you need to quickly leave the area. Contact your local police or other local emergency preparedness offices for protocols that will be in place in your area during an evacuation.

Natural Disasters

Many areas are vulnerable to a variety of types of severe weather, including thunderstorms, hurricanes, flash floods, snowstorms and tornadoes (see **Appendices C, D, E and F**).

It is important for you to understand the difference between a watch and a warning for severe weather. A severe storm watch means that severe weather may develop. A severe weather warning means a storm has developed and is on its way, and you should take cover immediately.

The safest place to ride out any storm is inside a secure building or well-built home. Even in a well-built apartment building, you should –

- listen to weather updates and stay informed.

- be ready to evacuate if necessary.

- keep away from windows and doors.

- have your Emergency Go Kit handy.

TORNADOES

Tornadoes are dangerous because of their high winds and ability to lift and move heavy objects. If you receive a tornado warning, seek shelter immediately.

If you are in your car:

- *Stop!* Get out and lie flat, face down, in a low area.

- Cover your head and wait for the tornado to pass.

If you are at home:

- Go to the basement or storm shelter or rooms near the center of the house.

In a high-rise or other public building:

- Move to the interior, preferably a stairwell or hallway.

FLASH FLOODING

Flash flooding can be very dangerous because of strong, swift currents.

- Move immediately and quickly to higher ground. The force of 6 inches of swiftly moving water can knock people off their feet.

- If flood waters rise around your car, get out and move to higher ground immediately. Cars can be easily swept away in just 2 feet of moving water.

Biological Threats

A biological attack is the deliberate release of germs or related substances. To affect individuals adversely, these substances must usually be inhaled, ingested or enter through cuts in the skin. Some biological agents, such as smallpox, can be spread from person to person, while others like anthrax do not cause contagious diseases.

Different than a conventional explosive or attack, biological attacks may not be immediately evident. Some of the normal indicators of this type of attack would be an increase in the number of illnesses reported by local health care workers or a large number of dead or sick animals throughout your area. These attacks are normally discovered by emergency response personnel in reaction to the indicators listed previously.

WHAT SHOULD YOU DO?

In the event that you witness a suspicious attack using an unknown substance, you can do a number of things to protect yourself and your family. First, leave the immediate area as quickly as possible and protect yourself by finding something to place over your nose and mouth. Any layered material such as a T-shirt, handkerchief or towel may help prevent particles of the substance from entering your respiratory system. If you have a long-sleeved shirt or jacket, use them to cover exposed skin. They may also prevent bacteria from entering cuts you may have. If you are indoors and the suspected attack takes place outdoors, remain inside unless told otherwise by authorities. Report the attack to emergency personnel.

You can also take precautionary measures, such as keeping vaccines up to date, and making sure you practice good personal hygiene. A healthy body will be able to better fight any potential contamination by biological agents. In the event that anyone around you becomes ill, do not automatically assume that it is from the suspected attack. Many of the symptoms from these attacks resemble common illnesses. Seek the medical advice of your physician.

Chemical Threats

Chemical attacks differ from biological attacks as chemical attacks use a toxic gas or liquid that is used to contaminate people or the environment. The prevalent symptoms you would experience from a chemical attack are tightness in the chest, difficulty breathing, blurred vision, stinging of the eyes or loss of coordination.

It is worth noting that the public routinely accepts the risks posed by accidental release of chemicals. The response to an emergency event involving chemicals, however, is the same regardless of whether the emergency is a result of intentional or unintentional acts.

WHAT SHOULD YOU DO?

If you witness a suspected chemical attack, it is important to remain calm, as the biggest complication from a chemical attack is fear and panic. If outdoors, move laterally or upwind from the area as quickly as possible. If you cannot leave the area, try to get inside, away from direct exposure, and follow your instructions to shelter-in-place. If you are inside and an attack occurs in your building, try to leave the area if possible. If you cannot, move to a safe location in the building and shelter-in-place.

If you experience any of the symptoms mentioned previously, try to remove any clothing you can, and wash your body with water or soap and water if available. Do not scrub the area, as this may wash the chemical into the skin. Seek medical assistance as soon as possible. If you see someone experiencing the previously mentioned symptoms, keep them away from others as much as possible and try to keep them comfortable.

Although extensive decontamination requiring disrobing is a possibility, this will normally only occur if you become a casualty of the agent or are evacuated and require medical treatment in a "clean" medical facility. This procedure may be required to prevent the spread of contamination.

Nuclear Explosions and Radiological Contamination

A nuclear blast consists of tremendous thermal (heat), light and blast energy. The blast can spread radioactive waste capable of contaminating the air and surrounding landscape. While this type of attack is less likely than a biological or chemical attack, the remote possibility of its occurrence means you should be prepared.

WHAT SHOULD YOU DO?

If a nuclear explosion occurs, immediately drop and stay down until any blast wave passes over you and it is safe to get up. Debris from a nuclear explosion can often cause injuries, so it is often safer to remain down until debris stops falling. Do not look at the blast.

When it is safe to do so, seek shelter inside a building or basement. Because dirt or earth is one of the best forms of protection from radiation, put as much shelter between you and the potential contamination as possible. If it is safe to leave without going in the direction from which the blast came, you should decide whether to leave the area to minimize the amount of time you spend exposed to radiological contamination. You should always try to place as much shielding and distance between yourself and the contamination as possible and to limit the amount of your exposure by leaving laterally or upwind from the area when it is safe to do so.

DIRTY BOMBS

Dirty bombs are regular explosives that have been combined with either radiation-causing material or chemical weapons. Although most news reports talk about radiological dirty bombs, chemical agents may be used as well. Blasts from these types of weapons normally look more like a regular explosion and the contamination spread is not often immediately noticeable. Although this type of attack normally spreads contamination over a more localized area, you should be prepared to follow many of the same procedures as listed previously.

After experiencing any of these types of attacks, tune in to your local media channels for information and instructions. Emergency responders are trained and equipped to evaluate and react to threats arising from these incidents. After a nuclear blast, you may be unable to get a signal from radio or television stations for a period of time. This is expected, so be persistent.

Although radioactive, biological and chemical weapons do pose a threat, they are attacks that you and your family or fellow employees can survive if you keep calm and follow the instructions given by your local responders.

Recovering from an Emergency

Recovery continues even after you return home, as you and your family face the emotional and psychological effects of the event. Reactions vary from person to person, but may include:

- Restless sleep or nightmares
- Anger or desire for revenge
- Numbness or lack of emotion
- Needing to keep active, restlessness
- Needing to talk about your experiences
- Loss of appetite
- Weight loss or gain
- Headaches
- Mood swings

All of these are normal reactions to stressful events, and it is important to let people react in their own way. It may be helpful to:

- Talk with your family and friends about what happened and how you feel about it. You also might want to evaluate what happened.
- Volunteer at a local shelter, blood bank or food pantry to assist emergency victims.
- Consult with a counselor or faith advisor.

Children, in particular, may need reassurance and extra attention. It is best to encourage them to share their feelings even if you must listen to their stories repeatedly – this is a common way for children to grasp what they have experienced. You may also want to share your feelings about the event with them.

 CONCLUDING THOUGHTS

Events in recent years have made everyone more aware of the possibilities for natural disasters, terrorist attacks and other emergencies involving large-scale destruction. It is important to consider the risks for disasters in your own region and to take appropriate precautions. Simple preparations can make a huge difference for your safety and well-being should such a disaster strike.

 ADDITIONAL ACTIVITIES AND RESOURCES

Appendices C through F provide additional information about different types of natural disasters. You should read whichever of these may apply to your location, and take active steps to ensure you are prepared.

In addition to this preparedness information from national agencies, most communities have an emergency preparedness office. You may speak to a representative from that office about local issues (such as particular threats, evacuation plans, etc.) or obtain printed materials.

 REVIEW QUESTIONS

Select the best answers.

1. Being prepared for an emergency includes knowing how to –

    a. turn off the main electricity switch in your house.

    b. inspect a backpack found in a public place for a possible bomb.

    c. defend yourself in case of personal attack.

    d. restore your natural gas service when the emergency is over.

2. Who should family members plan to call to locate each other if separated in an emergency?

    a. A nearby neighbor

    b. A local public official

    c. A distant friend or relative

    d. Federal Emergency Management Agency (FEMA)

3. When storing water for use after an emergency, calculate how much is needed per person per day:

    a. 1 gallon

    b. 2 gallons

    c. 3 gallons

    d. 4 gallons

4. If an emergency strikes, you should always –

    a. stay in your home except in cases of rising water or fire.

    b. drive away from your home as soon as possible following an authorized evacuation route.

    c. go to the nearest nuclear fallout shelter in your community.

    d. follow instructions from emergency officials regarding whether and when to evacuate.

5. The safest place to be if a severe storm strikes is –

    a. inside your car in a garage.

    b. in the basement or in a room near the center of the building.

    c. near a doorway or exit for quick evacuation.

    d. in the attic or highest part of the home.

Resources

Federal Emergency Management Agency (FEMA):
1-800-BE-READY

FBI hotline for reporting suspicious activity:
(855) TELL-FBI

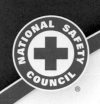

CHAPTER 26

Moving Forward

LESSON OBJECTIVES

- Act with confidence if needed in an emergency.

- List 7 key principles of first aid.

- Take steps to prevent injury and illness for both you and your family.

- State actions needed to stay current in your first aid knowledge and skills.

You are checking a coworker's young son, who fell and hurt his arm while playing in the reception area near your office. The boy is calmer now as you check for bleeding and potential musculoskeletal injury. When you first saw the boy crying in pain, you were worried you might not know what to do or might cause him more pain when you checked his arm, but you remembered your first aid training and realized you know what to do and can act confidently.

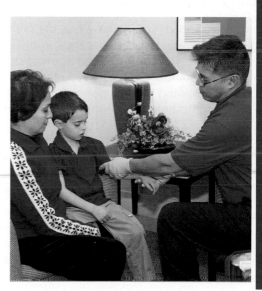

26 • Moving Forward

Now that we are approaching the end of this text and your first aid course, you should feel confident that you know what to do in an emergency involving an injury or sudden illness. What is important now, as you move forward, is to remember the key principles of first aid so that you are ready to act without delay when needed.

Acting with Confidence

It is only human to be concerned that when actually confronted with an emergency, a situation that is stressful for everyone involved, you may hesitate or feel unsure of exactly what to do. You may worry that you have forgotten some of the details of certain kinds of first aid. You may be fearful of or reluctant to deal with an injury involving blood or other body fluids or with an emotional victim in pain. These are natural feelings we all share.

Nonetheless, you should feel confident in your ability to provide first aid after completing this course. Experience has shown that even first aiders with less training than you very competently provide first aid when they encounter an emergency. There are many stories in the media about laypeople saving a heart attack victim, stopping life-threatening bleeding or pulling a drowning victim from the water. First aiders are often surprised by how well they remember their training and are able to put their knowledge into action when suddenly called upon to do so. Even if, at some point in the future, you forget some minor point, following the key principles of first aid is usually sufficient to help the victim for the few minutes before emergency medical personnel arrive.

Key Principles of First Aid

Although this text has described in some detail the first aid for all common injuries and sudden illnesses, a simple set of key principles should guide one's actions in all emergencies. Remember to follow these basic principles, and you will be able to render valuable aid to all victims:

- **Stay calm.** Emergencies happen without warning, giving us no time to prepare ourselves emotionally or to carefully plan out our actions. The victim's pain and fears about what is happening, as well as the emotions of others at the scene, can cause panicky feelings that might lead to hasty or careless actions. It is very important to be calm when you respond to an emergency. Take a moment, if necessary, to gather your thoughts and emotions. The victim and others at the scene will be reassured by your calm actions and will cope

better with the situation. Remember: You have the training and know what to do until help arrives – be confident about your ability to help.

- **Call 9-1-1 for all serious emergencies and whenever in doubt.** In most areas in the United States, help is only a few minutes away once you call 9-1-1 or your local emergency number. Even if you are not near a telephone, you can shout for help, and it is likely someone nearby will have a cell phone to call 9-1-1. Arriving EMS personnel will take over the care of the victim. If you are not sure how serious an injury or sudden illness is, call 9-1-1 anyway, and tell the dispatcher about the situation. Oftentimes, the dispatcher can also advise you what care to give in case you are unsure what first aid is appropriate in this situation.

- **Remember your own safety.** As you take a moment to assess the situation and calm yourself before acting, remember to check the scene for any dangers before going to a help a victim. Avoid any temptation to act heroically if the scene is dangerous. Once you have called 9-1-1, personnel with special training and equipment will soon arrive. They can better manage the dangers of the scene. If it is safe to give first aid, remember to also take steps to protect yourself from infectious disease.

- **Act quickly.** Although it is important to take a moment to calm yourself and plan your actions, remember that in life-threatening emergencies, it is crucial not to delay before starting care. For example, a victim of cardiac arrest after a heart attack needs CPR and defibrillation immediately – every second counts once breathing and the heart stop. Call for an AED, call 9-1-1 and start CPR immediately if the victim is not breathing normally.

- **Check the victim.** Remember: First check for responsiveness, normal breathing and severe bleeding, giving care immediately for life-threatening problems. If there are no immediate threats, perform a physical examination and take a SAMPLE history. This information will help you to know what first aid to give and will be valuable to responding EMS professionals.

- **Do no harm.** Do only what you have learned to do. Trying some first aid technique you heard about somewhere is risky, as people often are misinformed about what first aid is safe and effective. Call 9-1-1, and give basic first aid as you have learned in this course, and nothing you do will harm the victim. Recognize your limits as a lay first aider, and do not try something you have not learned to do, such as trying to rescue a victim from a hazardous situation.

- **Ask others for help.** You may be the only one at the scene of an emergency with first aid training, but bystanders are often present and will help you if asked. You may need someone to keep pressure on a wound to control bleeding, such as while you are attending to another injury. Others can call 9-1-1 or bring a first aid kit or AED. Do not hesitate to ask for help.

Prevention of Injury and Illness

This text has emphasized the importance of acting to prevent injury and sudden illness. Effective prevention depends on understanding that most injuries and sudden illnesses can be prevented and on adopting an attitude that motivates acting on safety principles and adopting a healthy lifestyle.

The problem in injury and illness prevention is that knowledge alone does not always translate directly into action. Everyone from school-age children to adults knows that cigarette smoking causes cancer and heart disease, yet about a sixth of the population still smokes. Everyone knows that seat belts and shoulder harnesses help prevent injuries in automobiles, yet every year, hundreds die or are seriously injured in motor vehicle crashes because they were not properly restrained. The statistics go on and on. Taking the time to act safely and making the commitment to break unhealthy habits and adopt a healthy lifestyle requires motivation. At this point, you know what you need to do to invest in your future health and well-being – but it is also up to you to care enough to make the effort.

Going Forward

As you conclude your first aid course, you probably are not thinking about future follow-up activities and refreshing your skills. It is important, however, to understand the need to stay current in your skills and knowledge for 2 reasons. First, it is only human that over time, we forget things and our skills become rusty. Second, new information often becomes available that changes how first aid should be given. For example, every 5 years, an international group of emergency medical care professionals gathers to analyze the most recent research data and make recommendations for improvements in basic life support protocols. CPR techniques have changed over time and may change again in the future – and you may not learn about more effective techniques if you do not refresh your knowledge and skills.

Staying current in your knowledge and skills starts today. To help you remember what to do in different kinds of emergencies, keep this book in an appropriate place where you can consult it when needed.

You may also need additional first aid information at some future time. The Internet is an excellent source for current information, but be sure to trust only reputable websites. Much of the information on private websites is outdated, controversial or simply incorrect, but the sites for health care associations and governmental agencies generally have updated information. The agencies frequently referred to in this text, such as the Centers for Disease Control and Prevention (CDC), are excellent sources for new information.

Depending on your field of study and career plans, you may also choose to take additional advanced or specialized first aid or emergency care courses. People working in settings where they are likely to be the first trained person on the scene of an injury or sudden illness, such as law enforcement or fire personnel, health care workers and many others, may take an Emergency Medical Responder or Professional Rescuer course. The National Safety Council has more information about these and other courses (nsc.org).

Even if you do not move on to more advanced courses, you should still periodically renew your essential skills by taking a refresher course. Everyone needs a CPR refresher course periodically. Studies have shown that laypeople who do not use their CPR skills will often not be as effective when called upon to give CPR long after their training. The information and techniques may have also changed.

CONCLUDING THOUGHTS

Congratulations on the completion of your first aid course! You can now be confident that, at work or at play, in the privacy of your home or when interacting with others in public places, that you know what to do when an emergency occurs.

 ADDITIONAL ACTIVITIES AND RESOURCES

Look into other courses and training you may take in the future, either to advance your skills and knowledge, or to refresh the skills you have learned in this course. Especially if your career path may lead to becoming an emergency responder role or a health care provider, higher-level skills are important and usually required.

 REVIEW QUESTIONS

Select the best answers.

1. Remember that a primary goal of first aid is to –
   a. get a victim to a health care provider as quickly as possible.
   b. provide definitive medical care.
   c. provide care only for the few minutes it takes for help to arrive.
   d. administer medications as needed in an emergency.

2. When in doubt about how serious an injury or sudden illness is –
   a. always do as the victim wishes.
   b. call 9-1-1.
   c. perform an extensive physical examination.
   d. wait a few minutes to watch for changes in signs and symptoms.

3. Check the scene –
   a. as soon as you arrive at the victim's side.
   b. as you approach the victim.
   c. as soon as you have checked the victim's breathing.
   d. before you go to the victim.

4. Perform the initial assessment of a victim –
   a. for any immediate threats to life.
   b. after performing a physical examination.
   c. as you collect the SAMPLE history.
   d. by asking bystanders what happened.

5. The most important element for preventing injury and illness is –
   a. memorizing all the rules about what to do or not do.
   b. being motivated for safety and a healthy lifestyle.
   c. frequently researching the latest medical studies.
   d. taking annual courses in injury prevention.

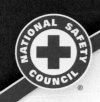

Advanced Resuscitation Techniques

The skills included in this appendix are typically not taught to lay rescuers. Health care providers and rescuers at higher levels of training may be trained in some or all of these skills. As always, never attempt a skill in which you have not been appropriately trained.

This appendix discusses the following topics:

- Resuscitation Skills
  - Jaw Thrust
  - Pulse Check for Circulation

- Ventilation Skills
  - Rescue Breathing Without Chest Compressions
  - Inadequate Breathing
  - Resuscitation Masks
  - Suction Devices
  - Bag Masks
  - Airway Adjuncts

- CPR Skills
  - Compressions for Bradycardia in Child
  - 2-Rescuer CPR for Adults and Children
  - 2-Rescuer CPR for Infants

- Special Resuscitation Situations
  - Trauma
  - Hypothermia
  - Near-drowning
  - Electric shock
  - Pregnancy

Resuscitation Skills

Health care providers and professional rescuers with higher training follow different BLS protocols from lay first aiders, and may use specialized equipment and supplies beyond basic personal, protective equipment, such as gloves and a resuscitation mask. Other equipment that may be of value in resuscitation situations includes suction devices, bag mask units, supplemental oxygen and airway adjuncts.

JAW THRUST

Lay rescuers are generally taught to use the head tilt–chin lift technique to open the airway of an unresponsive victim lying on his or her back, regardless of whether there may be a spinal injury. The jaw thrust technique, which is less likely to cause additional injury in a victim with a spinal injury, is not recommended to be taught to lay rescuers because it is somewhat more difficult to perform. Health care providers and professional rescuers, however, are often taught to use this technique.

With the jaw thrust, you do not tilt the head back to open the airway. Instead, only lift the jaw upward using both hands **(Figure A-1).** If you cannot successfully open the airway with the jaw thrust, however, then switch to the head tilt–chin lift method.

FIGURE A-1

The jaw thrust.

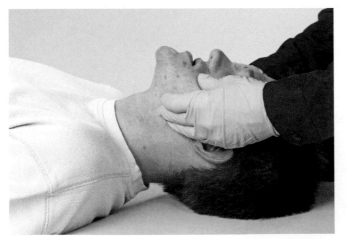

PULSE CHECK FOR CIRCULATION

Lay rescuers trained in CPR are taught to begin CPR with chest compressions immediately for an unresponsive victim who is not breathing normally. Health care and professional rescuers who are trained to check for a pulse should check for a pulse before beginning chest compressions – but they must do this very quickly while observing for normal breathing. It is critical to use no more than 10 seconds to feel for the victim's pulse, and unless a pulse is clearly found in that time, start chest compressions immediately. If an obvious pulse is found, begin rescue breathing immediately as described in the following section.

It takes training and practice to be able to effectively and quickly locate a pulse. To check the pulse in an adult, use the **carotid pulse** in the neck. Holding the victim's forehead with 1 hand to keep the airway open, put the index and middle fingers of your other hand on the side of the victim's neck nearer to you. Find the Adam's apple and then slide your fingertips toward you and down the neck to the groove at the side of the neck **(Figure A-2).** Pressing gently, feel for a pulse for at least 5 but no more than 10 seconds.

If a pulse cannot be definitely detected within 10 seconds, start CPR, beginning with chest compressions.

In a child, check either the **carotid or femoral pulse.** The femoral pulse is located in the center of the groin crease **(Figure A-3).**

To check the pulse in an infant, use the **brachial pulse** in the inside of the upper arm instead of the carotid or femoral pulse. With 1 hand on the infant's forehead to maintain head position for an open airway, put the fingers of your other hand about midway between the shoulder and elbow on the inside of the arm and press gently, feeling for no more than 10 seconds **(Figure A-4).**

Lack of a definite pulse, along with the absence of normal breathing, signifies that the heart has stopped or is not beating effectively enough to circulate blood. If the victim lacks a pulse and is not breathing normally, start CPR, beginning with chest compressions, and call for an AED to be brought to the scene.

An infant or child may have a pulse under 60 beats/minute and lack adequate perfusion. This victim also needs CPR (see later section "Compressions for Bradycardia in Child").

FIGURE A-2

Checking the carotid pulse in an adult or child.

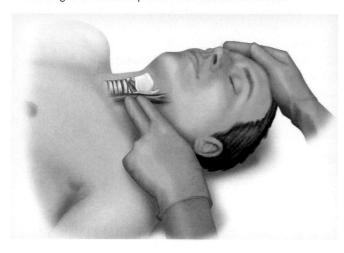

FIGURE A-3

Checking the femoral pulse.

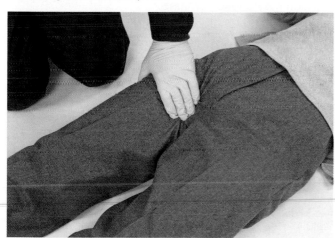

FIGURE A-4

Checking the brachial pulse in an infant.

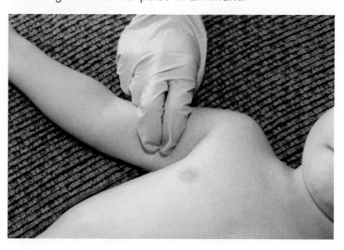

Ventilation Skills

RESCUE BREATHING WITHOUT CHEST COMPRESSIONS

In some situations, a victim may not be breathing adequately, but still have a heartbeat. Someone pulled from the water in a near-drowning, for example, may have stopped breathing, but may still have a heartbeat. Health care providers trained in pulse checks may then find a pulse in a non-breathing victim. In this situation, chest compressions are not given while rescue breaths are provided, as described in the Skill: "Rescue Breathing."

STEP 1

If the victim has a pulse but is not breathing normally, open the airway and give a breath over 1 second, watching the chest rise and letting it fall.

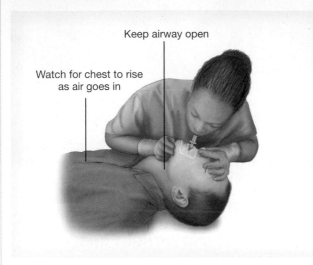

Keep airway open

Watch for chest to rise as air goes in

STEP 2

If the first breath does not go in, try again to open the airway and give another rescue breath. If it still does not go in, the victim may be choking. Proceed to CPR for choking.

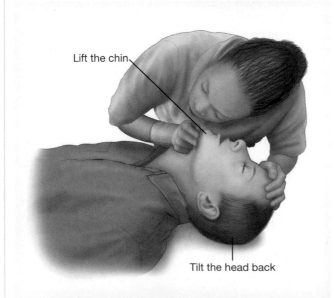

Lift the chin

Tilt the head back

STEP 3

If your breath goes in, continue rescue breathing. Give each breath over 1 second, at rate of 10-12 breaths per minute (1 breath every 5-6 seconds) for an adult; 12-20 breaths per minute for a child or infant (1 breath every 3-5 seconds).

STEP 4

Check the pulse about every 2 minutes (every 5 cycles of CPR). If there is no pulse, start CPR beginning with chest compressions.

ALERT

- Do not blow harder than is needed to make the chest rise.

- After each breath, remember to let the air escape and the chest fall.

- Blowing in too forcefully or for too long is ineffective, and may put air in the stomach, which may cause vomiting.

- Be careful not to tilt an infant's head too far back.

INADEQUATE BREATHING

In addition to giving rescue breathing to victims who are not breathing but have a pulse, health care providers and professional rescuers may use rescue breathing in cases of inadequate breathing. If an adult victim is breathing at a rate of less than 10 breaths per minute, take this as a sign of inadequate breathing – the victim is not receiving sufficient oxygen. An infant or child may have a pulse of 60 or higher per minute but may still be breathing inadequately. In a victim who is not breathing adequately, do not wait for respiratory arrest before beginning to provide rescue breaths.

RESUSCITATION MASKS

The resuscitation mask, often called a pocket face mask or simply a face mask, seals over the victim's mouth and nose, and has a port through which the rescuer blows air to give rescue breaths. A one-way valve allows the rescuer's air in through the mouthpiece, while the victim's exhaled air exits the mask through a different opening.

When using a face mask, it is essential to seal the mask well to the victim's face while maintaining an open airway. How you hold the mask depends on your position by the victim, whether the head tilt–chin lift or jaw thrust technique is used to open the airway, and whether you have 1 or 2 hands free to seal the mask. The following hand positions assume you have both hands free to seal the mask, whether alone at the victim's side while performing CPR, or at the victim's head (alone giving only rescue breathing, or with another rescuer who is providing chest compressions).

From a position at the victim's side (1 rescuer giving CPR) using the head tilt–chin lift:

1. With the thumb and index finger of your hand closer to the top of the victim's head, seal the top and sides of the mask to the victim's head as shown in **Figure A-5(a).**

2. Put the thumb of your second hand on the lower edge of the mask.

3. Put the remaining fingers of your second hand under the jaw to lift the chin.

4. Press the mask down firmly to make a seal as you perform a head tilt–chin lift to open the airway.

From a position at the top of the victim's head (2 rescuers giving CPR or 1 rescuer performing rescue breathing without CPR) using the head tilt–chin lift:

1. Put your thumbs and index finger on both sides of the mask as shown in **Figure A-5(b).**

2. Put the remaining finger of both hands under the angles of the victim's jaw on both sides.

3. As you tilt the head back, press the mask down firmly to make a seal as you lift the chin with your fingers.

From a position at the top of the victim's head using the jaw thrust:

1. Without tilting the victim's head back, position your thumbs on the mask in the same manner as for the head tilt–chin lift – from the top of the victim's head, with fingers under the angles of the jaw.

2. Lift the jaw to open the airway as you press down with your thumbs to seal the mask, without tilting the head back as shown in **Figure A-5(c).**

FIGURE A-5

(a) Face mask hand position with rescuer at victim's side. (b) Face mask hand position with rescuer at victim's head. (c) Do not tilt the head when using the jaw thrust technique for a victim with spinal injury.

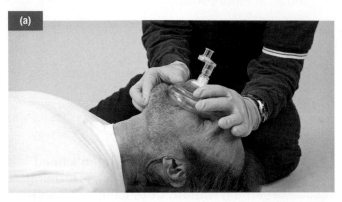

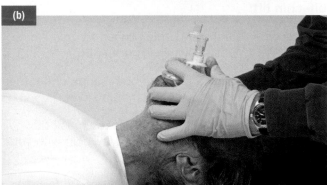

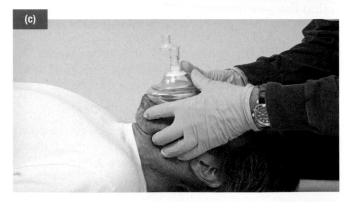

SUCTION DEVICES

A **suction device** is used to clear blood, vomit and other substances from a victim's airway. These devices are generally safe and easy to use. Although different types of suction devices are available, they are similar in their use. Manual devices develop suction with a hand-pumping action; and other devices are powered by a battery or pressurized oxygen. Soft, rubber bulb syringes are used for suctioning infants.

Suction devices for adults and children have a clear plastic tip that is inserted into the mouth or nostrils to suck out fluids and small solids. Different suction tips are available, varying from small, soft plastic tips that are more effective for fluids to larger, more rigid tips that are more effective for vomit and particulates. Some devices have a suction control port at the base of the tip that you cover with your finger to produce suction. As always, you should be familiar in advance with the specific equipment you may use in an emergency.

Suction is useful whenever a victim's airway may be obstructed – fully or in part – by body fluids, food substances, or other matter. If the victim vomits when rescue breathing or CPR is underway, or if secretions or blood accumulate and impede ventilation, stop and quickly suction the mouth and/or nose and then continue the resuscitation. An unresponsive breathing victim may also need suctioning to maintain an open airway. Usually, you know the airway needs suctioning when you hear gurgling sounds during breathing or ventilation.

The victim's head is turned to the side to help drain vomit or fluids before suctioning. If the victim may have a spinal injury, the victim must be turned on the side with the head and body inline as a unit, with the help of other rescuers. See Skill: "Suctioning (Adult or Child)" and Skill: "Suctioning (Infant)."

Safety precautions are necessary when suctioning. Because many suction devices generate strong suction pressures, be careful with the suction tip. Prolonged contact with mucous membranes in the mouth and nose can cause bruising, swelling and even bleeding. Never insert the suction tip farther than you can see. Prolonged suctioning can also decrease the volume of air reaching the victim's lungs. Vigorous suctioning may stimulate the victim's gag reflex, causing additional vomiting. Be especially careful not to suction too deeply in an infant. Always suction an infant's mouth before the nostrils, because suctioning the nose may stimulate the infant to breathe in, and thereby, inhale fluid or secretions from the mouth.

Remember standard precautions against disease transmission through body fluids. After the emergency, dispose of any contents in the reservoir of the suction device, and clean the device according to the manufacturer's recommendations.

STEP 1

Confirm that the suction device is working and produces suction.

STEP 2

Turn the victim's head to one side and open the mouth (for spinal injury, support the head and turn with body as a unit).

STEP 3

Sweep out solids and larger amounts of fluid with your finger.

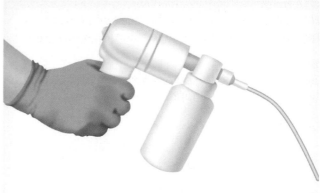

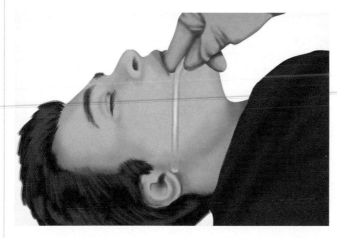

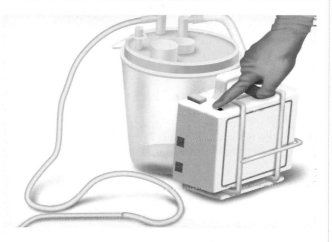

STEP 4

Determine maximum depth of insertion by measuring the catheter tip from the earlobe to the corner of the mouth.

STEP 6

Insert catheter tip carefully into the mouth. Put your finger over the proximal opening to begin suctioning, and move the tip about as you withdraw it.

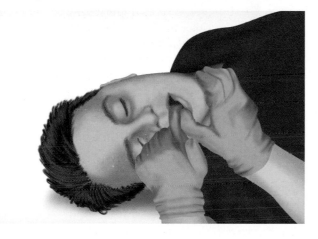

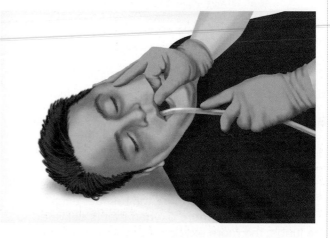

STEP 5

Turn on suction, or pump the handle to create suction.

STEP 7

Reposition the victim's head with airway open, and resume rescue breathing or CPR.

STEP 1
Hold the infant in position for suctioning, with the head lower than the body and turned to one side.

STEP 2
Squeeze the suction bulb, and then gently insert the tip into the infant's mouth.

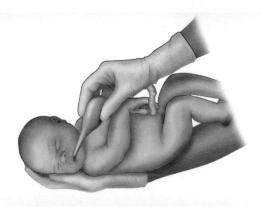

STEP 3
Gradually release the bulb to create suction as you withdraw the tip from the infant's mouth.

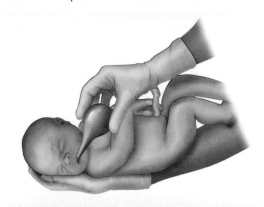

STEP 4
Move the bulb aside and squeeze it, with tip down, to empty it.

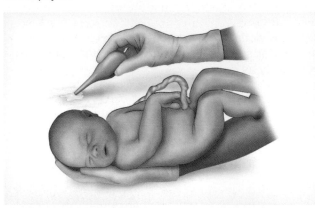

STEP 5
Repeat Steps 2-4 until the airway seems clear, up to 3 times.

STEP 6
Repeat the suctioning steps for each nostril.

STEP 7
Begin or resume rescue breathing or CPR if needed.

BAG MASK

Bag mask (bag-valve-mask, or BVM) units, like regular face masks, protect the first aider from disease transmission, and are more effective for providing ventilations to non-breathing victims. With the BVM, the victim receives air from the atmosphere (21% oxygen) rather than air the rescuer exhales (16% oxygen). The more oxygen that is delivered to the lungs, the more oxygen that will reach the victim's vital organs to maintain life. Several different types of BVM units are available, but each has at least 3 components **(Figure A-6):**

• The self-inflating bag holds the air or oxygen that is delivered to the victim when the bag is squeezed.

• The 1-way valve allows air or oxygen to flow from the bag to the victim, but prevents exhaled air from returning to the bag.

• The mask is similar to a resuscitation mask, and is connected to the bag and valve. The proper-size mask must be used for a proper fit. An oxygen reservoir bag may be attached to the other end of the bag when supplemental oxygen is used.

To use the BVM on a non-breathing victim, position yourself above the victim's head. Perform a head tilt, and then position the mask on the victim's face. If you are alone, you need to hold the mask with 1 hand and squeeze the bag with the other, as shown in **Figure A-7.** To hold the mask in place with 1 hand, use the C-clamp technique, with thumb and index finger on the edges of the mask while the other fingers lift the jaw into the mask. If you are unable to open the airway and obtain a good seal with 1 hand, provide rescue breaths mouth-to-mask or mouth-to-mouth. A single rescuer skilled in its use may use a BVM when rescue breaths alone are being given, but should not use it during 1-rescuer CPR, because it typically takes too much time away from chest compressions.

FIGURE A-6

Bag mask.

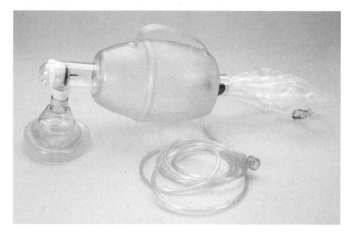

FIGURE A-7

A single rescuer using a BVM for rescue breathing.

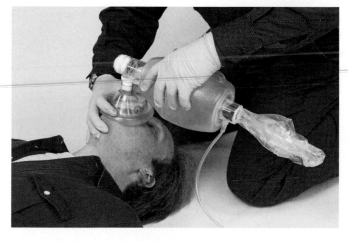

2-rescuer use of the BVM is recommended whenever possible because of the difficulty one person may have sealing the mask on the victim's face with 1 hand while squeezing the bag with the other. When a second rescuer is available to help with the BVM, 1 rescuer holds the mask in place using both hands

as described earlier for a resuscitation mask, and as shown in the Skill: "Bag Mask for Rescue Breathing (2 Rescuers)."

With the mask sealed in place, rescue breaths are delivered to the victim by squeezing the bag. Squeeze a 1-liter adult bag about ½-⅔ of its volume. Squeeze a 2-liter adult bag about ⅓ its volume. Squeeze the bag over 1 second, watching the victim's chest rise. Give a ventilation every 5-6 seconds in an adult (or every 3-5 seconds in a child or infant), the same as with rescue breathing by mouth or resuscitation mask. However, when delivering ventilation during CPR to a victim of any age with an advanced airway in place (such as an endotracheal tube), deliver breaths at a simplified rate of 1 breath every 6 seconds.

When using a BVM, monitor the effectiveness of ventilations. Be careful to give rescue breaths at the usual rate and not to over-ventilate the victim. Watch for the rise and fall of the victim's chest, and feel for resistance as you squeeze the bag. Increased resistance may mean that there is blood or vomit in the airway or that the airway is no longer open. A problem can also occur with sealing the mask to the victim's face, especially when a single rescuer must do this with 1 hand. If air is escaping around the mask, try repositioning the mask and your fingers. If you cannot obtain an adequate seal and the victim's chest does not rise with ventilations, or if there are any other problems with using the BVM, then use an alternate technique, such as a resuscitation mask, instead.

If available, supplemental oxygen should be used with the BVM. When supplemental oxygen is used with a BVM, oxygen concentrations can reach as high as 100%. An oxygen reservoir bag is attached to the valve on the bag, and the oxygen tubing is attached to the bag. The device is used the same way it is used to give ventilations, only now it is oxygen rather than air being delivered to the victim. The reservoir holds oxygen being delivered to the device so that the bag always fills with oxygen to be delivered in the next ventilation. When two rescuers are present, the second sets up the oxygen equipment and prepares to connect it to the BVM, while the first begins providing rescue breathing with the BVM alone.

The BVM can be used for a non-breathing infant in the same manner as an adult or child. Be sure to choose the correct size mask. Squeeze the bag only enough to make the chest rise, avoiding forceful squeezing or over-inflation that may lead to vomiting.

STEP 1

Rescuer 1 assembles the BVM with a mask of the correct size, and puts the mask over the victim's mouth and nose.

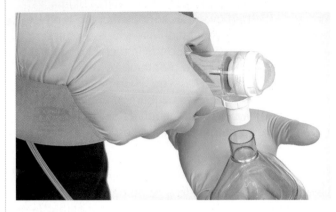

STEP 2

Rescuer 2 positions hands: thumbs and index fingers circling each side of mask, the other 3 fingers of each hand behind lower jawbone. Pull the jaw up into the mask instead of pushing the mask down on the jaw.

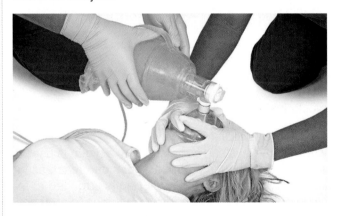

STEP 3

Rescuer 2 opens the airway and seals the mask to the victim's face.

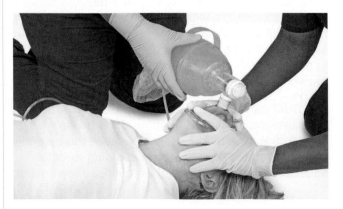

STEP 4

Rescuer 1 squeezes the bag to provide ventilations:

a. 1 ventilation over 1 second in adult, every 5-6 seconds (or 1 breath every 6 seconds during CPR if an advanced airway is in place).

b. 1 ventilation over 1 second in child or infant, every 3-5 seconds (or 1 breath every 6 seconds during CPR if an advanced airway is in place).

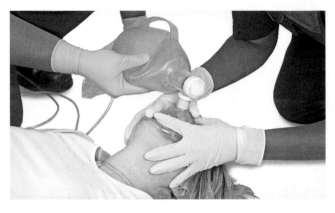

STEP 5

Recheck pulse about every 2 minutes. If no pulse, call for an AED and start CPR.

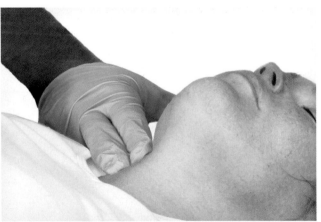

AIRWAY ADJUNCTS

Oral and nasal **airway adjuncts** are devices that help keep a victim's airway open during resuscitation or until the victim receives advanced medical attention. The most common cause of airway obstruction in unresponsive victims is the tongue. An airway adjunct prevents this problem and keeps the airway open more easily than head position alone while using resuscitation techniques or caring for a breathing victim. Supplemental oxygen can be given through a resuscitation mask or bag mask with an oral or nasal airway in place.

Oral Airways

Oral airways, also called **oropharyngeal airways,** are used only in unresponsive victims who do not have a gag reflex. If inserted into a responsive victim, or one who still has a gag reflex, the airway adjunct can cause vomiting. The victim's airway must be opened before the airway device is inserted; the device does not open the airway itself but will help keep it open. An oral airway can be used in an unresponsive victim who is breathing or who is receiving rescue breaths.

Proper placement of the oral airway is essential. An improperly placed airway device can compress the tongue into the back of the throat and further block the airway. Oral airways are curved so that they fit the natural contour of the mouth and are available

in various sizes to ensure a proper fit **(Figure A-8).** An airway adjunct that is too big can cause vomiting and may prevent the resuscitation mask from sealing well. An airway adjunct that is too small can slide into the back of the pharynx and obstruct the airway **(Figure A-9).** Remember to open the victim's airway before inserting the oral airway, as described in the Skill: "Oral Airway Insertion." Periodically reassess the airway adjunct to confirm that it remains in proper position. A victim can be suctioned with an oral airway in place.

FIGURE A-8

Oral airways.

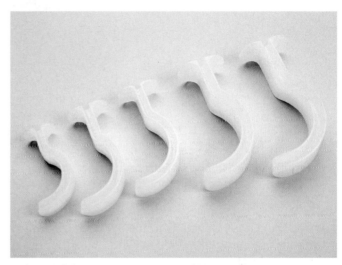

FIGURE A-9

An oral airway that is too large or too small will obstruct the airway.

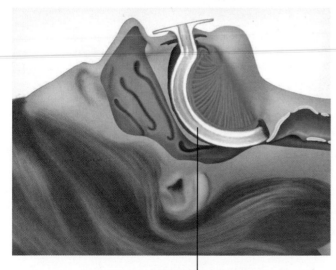 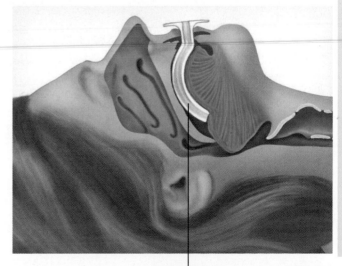

Too large –
device blocks airway

Too small –
device causes tongue to obstruct airway

STEP 1

Choose the correct airway device size. The oral airway length should match the distance from the corner of the mouth to the tip of the earlobe on the same side of the victim's face.

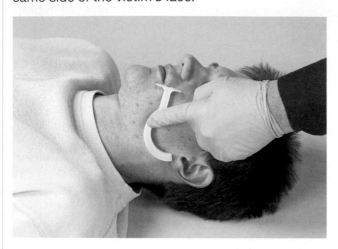

STEP 2

Open the victim's airway with head tilt–chin lift or jaw thrust, and open the mouth.

STEP 3

Insert the airway device with the tip pointing toward the roof of the mouth.

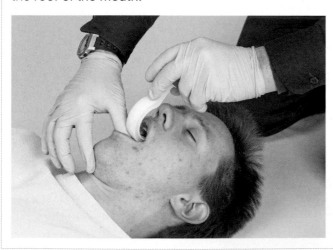

STEP 4

When the tip reaches the back of the mouth and you feel resistance, rotate the airway 180 degrees.

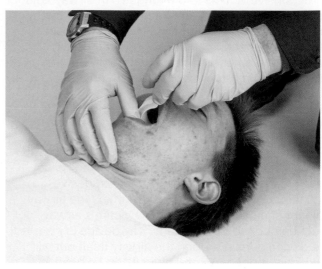

STEP 5

Continue to insert the airway device to the final position (the flange resting on the lips).

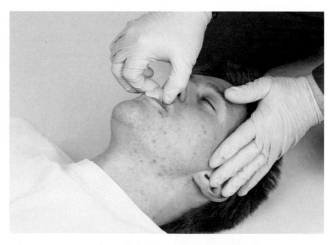

Nasal Airways

A nasal airway, like an oral airway, helps maintain an open airway **(Figure A-10)**. A nasal airway **(nasopharyngeal airway)** can be used in a victim who is responsive or who, although unresponsive, has a gag reflex. Nasal airways are also effective for unresponsive victims with mouth or jaw injuries, or tightly clenched teeth that prevent the use of an oral airway. Nasal airways are less likely to cause gagging and vomiting than oral airways, but a disadvantage is that they are too narrow to suction. Insert a nasal airway as described in the Skill: "Nasal Airway Insertion," and continue to keep the victim's airway open with the head tilt–chin lift or jaw thrust. If needed, suction through a nasal airway using a small, flexible suction catheter.

FIGURE A-10

Nasal airways.

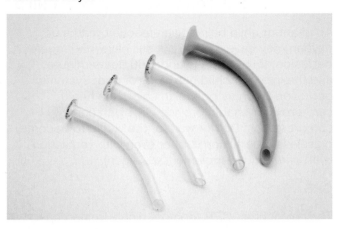

🧠 SKILL: NASAL AIRWAY INSERTION

STEP 1

Choose the correct nasal airway size. The nasal airway length should match the distance from the nostril to the tip of the earlobe on the same side of the victim's face.

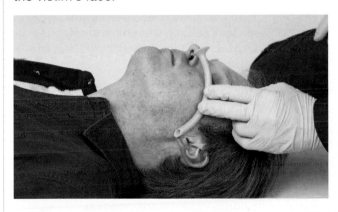

STEP 2

Coat the nasal airway with lubricant.

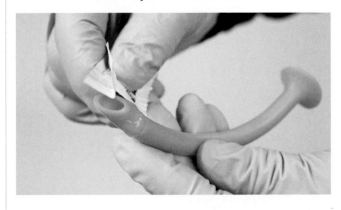

STEP 3

Insert the nasal airway in the right nostril with the bevel toward the septum.

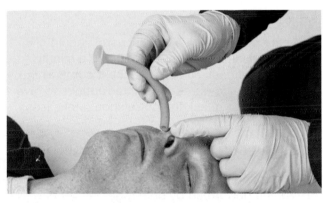

STEP 4

Insert the nasal airway straight back, sliding it along the floor of the nostril. If you feel resistance do not force it.

STEP 5

Insert the nasal airway until the flange rests against the nose.

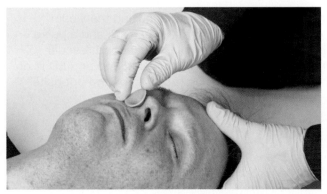

CPR Skills

COMPRESSIONS FOR BRADYCARDIA IN CHILD

An infant or child being given rescue breaths or oxygen may have a pulse but still have inadequate perfusion. If the pulse is under 60 beats/minute and the infant or child has signs of poor systemic perfusion (such as poor skin color), the health care provider should provide CPR with chest compressions. Do not wait for the victim to become pulseless if perfusion is poor even with ventilation (with or without supplemental oxygen).

CPR

The protocol for CPR for more highly trained health care providers differs somewhat from that for CPR by lay rescuers. Health care providers check for a pulse before beginning chest compressions.

A lone health care provider uses the same 30:2 ratio of compressions and rescue breaths for all victims. 2-rescuer CPR provided by health care providers, however, uses a 15:2 ratio for infants and children up to the onset of puberty.

Health care providers, like lay rescuers, should give chest compressions at a rate of 100-120 a minute – push hard, push fast – letting the chest come all the way up between compressions. Interruptions to give rescue breaths or check the pulse should take less than 10 seconds.

2-RESCUER CPR FOR ADULTS AND CHILDREN

When 2 rescuers at the scene are trained in CPR, resuscitation performed by both together offers several advantages. 2-rescuer CPR:

- Minimizes the time between rescue breaths and compressions, making CPR more effective

- Allows for more quickly setting up an AED (Chapter 6)

- Reduces rescuer fatigue

The first rescuer begins by checking the victim for responsiveness, normal breathing and a pulse simultaneously. Meanwhile, the second rescuer ensures that 9-1-1 has been called and an AED is on the way, then moves into position on the opposite side of the victim to give chest compressions if the victim does not have a pulse. After 30 compressions, the first rescuer gives 2 rescue breaths, and CPR continues.

2-rescuer CPR is performed in the same cycles of 30 compressions and 2 breaths for an adult (but 15 compressions and 2 breaths for an infant or child). One rescuer gives the chest compressions at a rate of 100-120 compressions per minute, and the other rescuer gives 2 rescue breaths. The rescuer giving compressions should count aloud during the compressions and pause after the last compression to let the other rescuer give 2 breaths. See Skill: "CPR for Adult or Child (2 Rescuers)."

The rescuers should switch positions about every 2 minutes (about 5 cycles of 30 compressions and 2 breaths) to prevent ineffective compressions resulting from fatigue. This change should be done at the end of a full CPR cycle after breaths are given, and should be accomplished in less than 5 seconds. It is recommended that positions are switched during any intervention that interrupts compressions (such as when the AED delivers a shock).

If an AED is present at the scene, the first rescuer gives both chest compressions and breaths, while the second rescuer sets up the unit and attaches the pads (see **Chapter 4**). Then, the rescuers resume CPR together.

Note: You may be assisting a professional with a higher level of training who places an advanced airway in the victim for ventilation. With an advanced airway in place, chest compressions are given continually at a rate of 100-120 per minute without pauses for rescue breaths. Ventilations are provided via a bag mask every 6 seconds (10 breaths per minute) while compressions are ongoing.

STEP 1

At the victim's head, Rescuer 1 checks for unresponsiveness, normal breathing and a pulse simultaneously for no longer than 10 seconds. Rescuer 2 ensures that an AED has been summoned. At the victim's side, Rescuer 2 locates the site for chest compressions.

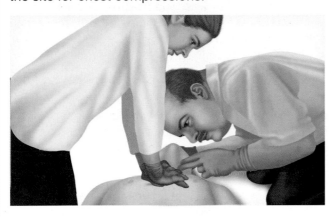

STEP 2

Rescuer 1 indicates, "No pulse." Rescuer 2 gives 30 compressions for an adult (15 for a child) at a rate of 100-120 per minute, counting aloud for a fast, steady rate, then pauses.

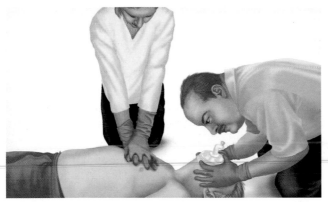

STEP 3

Rescuer 1 gives 2 breaths.

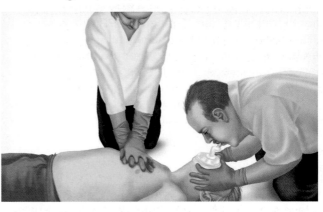

STEP 4

Rescuers continue cycles of 30 compressions for an adult (15 for a child) and 2 breaths for 2 minutes (or 5 cycles of compressions and ventilations at a ratio of 30:2) before switching compressor and ventilator roles. The switch should be done quickly (in less than 5 seconds).

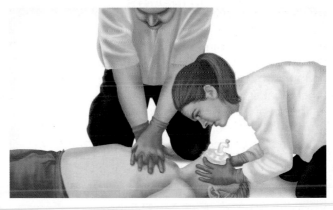

STEP 5

Rescuers continue CPR until:

- The victim is breathing normally and has a pulse.
- An AED is brought to the scene and is ready to use.
- Help arrives and takes over.
- If the victim starts breathing normally and has a pulse but is unresponsive, put the victim in the recovery position and monitor breathing and pulse.

STEP 6

When an AED arrives and is ready to be used, start the AED sequence for a victim who is not breathing normally and has no pulse.

Appendix A • Advanced Resuscitation Techniques

Transitioning from 1-Rescuer CPR to 2-Rescuer CPR

In some situations, a rescuer is already giving CPR when a second rescuer arrives on the scene. The rescuers should coordinate their actions for a smooth transition from 1-rescuer CPR to 2-rescuer CPR. The second rescuer moves into position on the other side of the victim to prepare to take over chest compressions. The first rescuer completes a series of compressions. While the first rescuer then gives 2 breaths, the second rescuer takes the correct hand position and begins compressions immediately after the second breath. For the next 2 minutes, the new rescuer gives chest compressions and the first rescuer gives the rescue breaths.

Note: If you are the first rescuer who started CPR, the arriving second rescuer may be a rescuer with a higher level of training. In such a case, this rescuer assumes authority for how CPR should best be continued. If this rescuer determines your breathing or compression technique is inadequate, he or she may ask you to take on the other role – or may take over the CPR alone.

2-RESCUER CPR FOR INFANTS

2-rescuer CPR for an infant uses a different hand position for chest compressions from 1-rescuer CPR. The rescuer giving compressions places the thumbs of both hands together in the correct position on the infant's sternum (just below the nipple line). The fingers of both hands encircle the infant's chest **(Figure A-11).** The chest is compressed with both thumbs, as described in the Skill: "CPR for Infant (2 Rescuers)." If you cannot encircle the infant's chest (e.g., the infant's chest is too large or the rescuer's hands are too small), use the 1-rescuer method of performing compressions with 2 fingers.

FIGURE A-11

The chest-encircling hand position for infant chest compressions when 2 professional rescuers are giving CPR.

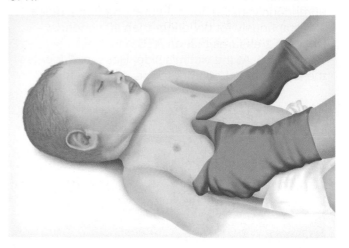

STEP 1

At the infant's head, Rescuer 1 checks for normal breathing and a pulse. At the infant's feet, Rescuer 2 positions hands in the chest-encircling position for chest compressions with both thumbs.

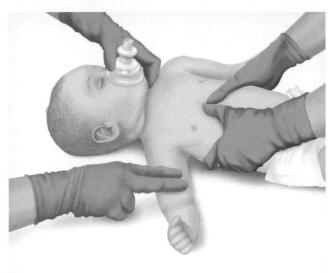

STEP 2

If pulse is absent, Rescuer 1 says, "No pulse." Rescuer 2 gives 15 chest compressions at a rate of 100-120 per minute, counting aloud for a fast, steady rate, then pauses.

STEP 3

Rescuer 1 gives 2 breaths.

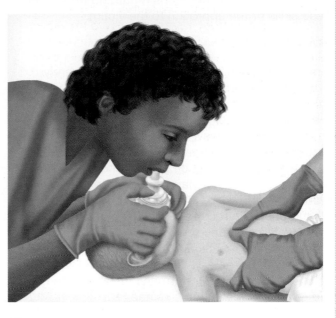

STEP 4

Rescuers continue cycles of 15 compressions and 2 breaths for about 2 minutes before switching compressor and ventilator roles. The switch should be done quickly (in less than 5 seconds). Rescuers continue CPR until:

- The infant is breathing normally and has a pulse.
- More advanced help arrives and takes over.
- If the infant starts breathing normally but is unresponsive, hold the infant in the recovery position and monitor breathing and pulse.

STEP 5

When an AED arrives and is ready to be used, start the AED sequence for an infant who is not breathing normally and has no pulse.

Special Resuscitation Situations

In most emergencies, basic life support skills are used in the same way. A few situations, however, involve special considerations regarding the use of these skills or the approach to the victim.

TRAUMA

In most situations in which the victim is severely injured by blunt or penetrating trauma, problems with the airway, breathing or circulation are the result of the trauma rather than a coinciding problem. Do not assume, however, that a trauma victim has experienced *only* trauma, because another problem may have occurred first or at the same time. For example, a victim may have a heart attack and sudden cardiac arrest while on a ladder, resulting in a fall and possible fractures. A victim of drug overdose or poisoning may develop a severe breathing problem while operating machinery, causing an incident and traumatic injury. As a general rule, treat a trauma victim like any other: Perform the initial assessment and give basic life support as needed.

Trauma victims generally have a "call first" rather than "call fast" status. Trauma that is severe enough to cause cardiac arrest can only be helped by invasive procedures, usually in a hospital. If the victim is to have a chance of survival, advanced care must arrive as quickly as possible, so that a determination can be made about the next steps. The victim needs to be transported to definitive care as quickly as possible.

Depending on the nature of the trauma, the victim may have a spinal injury as well. Any blow to the body severe enough to impact the airway, breathing or circulation is also likely to potentially injure the spine. Remember to keep the head in line with the body if it is necessary to reposition the victim, and to use the jaw thrust technique rather than head tilt–chin lift to open the airway.

Trauma to the head or face may result in blood or other fluid blocking the airway. Check the mouth when opening the airway, and if necessary, wipe out any blood or vomit. With more extensive amounts of fluid, you may have to turn the victim onto one side to let it drain from the mouth. If the equipment is available and you are trained in its use, suction the victim's mouth when opening the airway.

HYPOTHERMIA

Hypothermia is a low core body temperature as a result of exposure to a cold environment, often by immersion in cold water. Hypothermia requires special consideration when providing emergency care. Severely cold temperatures make the victim susceptible to heart rhythm problems, but a thorough assessment is important because some hypothermia victims have been successfully resuscitated after a long period of hypothermia or immersion.

In severe hypothermia, the victim's heart may be beating very slowly or may be in arrest, and the respiratory rate may also be very slow or have stopped. For an unresponsive victim who is not breathing normally, check for a pulse no longer than 10 seconds, and if a pulse is definitely not felt, start CPR immediately. Follow local protocol for use of an AED with a hypothermia victim.

Do not delay or stop resuscitation efforts to rewarm the victim, but if possible, prevent further heat loss from the victim's body. Other rescuers can remove wet clothing, for example, or cover the victim with a blanket while basic life support is ongoing. Be gentle when handling or moving a hypothermic victim, because the heart is susceptible to arrhythmias precipitated by motion or jarring.

NEAR-DROWNING

In any situation in which a victim is in the water, ensure your own safety before attempting a rescue. It is very dangerous for an untrained rescuer to enter the water to rescue a responsive victim, who may grab the rescuer and make rescue difficult or impossible. Reach to the victim with a pole or long object, throw a rope or floating object or go to the victim in a watercraft, if possible. Beginning rescue breaths as soon as possible is a high priority for drowning victims. If you can do so, begin rescue breaths (after confirming respiratory arrest) even before removing the victim from shallow water, unless it is possible to remove the victim immediately. However, it is necessary to remove the victim from water to give CPR.

For an unresponsive victim removed from the water, consider whether the nature of the incident, such as diving in shallow or murky water or being thrown against the shore in surf conditions, suggests a possible spinal injury. If the cause of the submersion is unknown, assume the victim may have a spinal injury. Keep the head in line with the body when moving or positioning the victim, and use the jaw thrust technique rather than head tilt–chin lift to open the airway.

Begin the initial assessment as usual by checking for responsiveness. Remember that this is a "call fast" rather than "call first" situation. If you are alone, give care for about 2 minutes (rescue breathing or CPR) before stopping to go for help.

Note that BLS care for a drowning victim is somewhat different from that given other victims found unresponsive. A drowning victim is more likely to have a pulse and may need only rescue breathing without chest compressions. Check for breathing and pulse. If the victim is not breathing normally, first open the airway and give 2 rescue breaths. If the victim has a pulse, but is not breathing normally, give rescue breathing. If the victim does not have a pulse, start CPR immediately.

Do not take any special actions to try to remove water from the victim first.

If the victim is not breathing and your rescue breaths do not make the chest rise, open the airway again and try to give 2 breaths. If your breaths still do not go in, give chest compressions for an airway obstruction.

If supplemental oxygen is available and you are trained in its use, administer oxygen to the victim. When an AED is available and ready, use it as usual. Victims have been resuscitated after being submerged in cold water for some time. If the victim may be hypothermic, follow the special considerations described earlier.

ELECTRIC SHOCK

Electric shock may result from a lightning strike or from contact with a source of household current or high-voltage power lines. The shock may cause the victim's breathing to stop because of paralyzed respiratory muscles, and may cause cardiac arrest by disrupting the heart's electrical controls.

Remember scene safety before approaching the victim. Downed power lines or household or industrial electrical appliances or cords may still be "live" and pose a threat to rescuers. Call 9-1-1 for downed power lines, and do not try to move them yourself or to move the victim away from them. For electrical appliances, first shut the power off at the circuit breaker box, or unplug the power cord if it is safe to do so.

The electric shock may cause a range of injuries in addition to effects on respiration and circulation. Especially with a high-voltage shock, such as that caused by lightning, the victim may have severe burns and possible fractures due to strong muscular contractions caused by the electric shock. For a lightning strike victim, assume a possible spinal injury.

When it is safe to approach the victim, perform the initial assessment and provide care as needed. If the victim has a pulse but is not breathing, provide rescue breathing and continue to check the pulse. If the victim has no pulse, provide CPR and call for an AED. Oftentimes an electric shock causes ventricular fibrillation, in which case, the AED may return the heart to a normal rhythm. If alone, first activate the emergency response system, get an AED if one is available and then return to provide CPR.

PREGNANCY

A woman in late stages of pregnancy with an airway obstruction should be given chest thrusts rather than abdominal thrusts to expel an obstructing object. A responsive victim can be given chest thrusts from behind while standing, and an unresponsive victim is given chest thrusts in the same manner as the chest compressions of CPR.

When a pregnant woman at a gestational age beyond 20 weeks lies on her back, the enlarged uterus may press against the inferior vena cava, the vein that returns blood to the heart from the lower half of the body. This pressure may decrease the blood flow to the heart and affect circulation to vital organs. When possible, therefore, position an injured pregnant woman lying on her left side, which reduces pressure from the uterus on the vena cava. Gently move the uterus to the left to help alleviate the pressure.

As with other victims of cardiac arrest, high-quality CPR should be performed on a pregnant woman in cardiac arrest. Additionally, when giving CPR to a pregnant woman beyond 20 weeks gestation, manually displacing the uterus to the left can help improve circulation during CPR. If enough rescuers are present, 1 rescuer should use 1 or 2 hands to manually shift or displace the uterus to the woman's left side. Note that placing a pregnant victim in the left-lateral tilt position is no longer recommended, as recent research indicates this position decreases CPR quality.

Otherwise, perform basic life support skills on a pregnant woman in the same manner as for other victims, including the use of an AED in cases of cardiac arrest.

Performance Checklists for Skills

Hand Washing 410

Putting on Gloves 411

Removing Contaminated Gloves 412

Initial Assessment 413

Recovery Position 414

Physical Examination 415

CPR for Adults, Children and Infants (1 Rescuer) 416

Using an AED 417

Choking Care for Responsive Adult or Child 418

Choking Care for Unresponsive Adult, Child or Infant 419

Choking Care for Responsive Infant 420

Controlling Bleeding 421

Applying a Pressure Bandage 422

Shock Position 423

Use of an Emergency Epinephrine Auto-Injector 424

Assessing Head and Spinal Injuries 425

Spinal Motion Restriction 426

Rolling a Victim With Spinal Injury (Log Roll) 427

Applying a Spiral Bandage 428

Applying a Figure-8 Bandage to the Wrist 429

Applying a Figure-8 Bandage to the Ankle 430

RICE for Wrist Injury 431

Applying an Arm Sling and Binder 432

Splinting the Forearm 433

Anatomic Splinting of Leg 434

Advanced Skills (Appendix A)

Rescue Breathing. 435

Suctioning (Adult or Child) 436

Suctioning (Infant) 437

Bag Mask for Rescue Breathing (2 Rescuers) 438

Oral Airway Insertion 439

Nasal Airway Insertion. 440

CPR for Adult or Child (2 Rescuers). 441

CPR for Infant (2 Rescuers) 442

☑ PERFORMANCE CHECKLIST: HAND WASHING

SKILL STEP		Initial Practice		Final Performance	
		Needs Practice	Proficient	Remediate	Proficient
1	Remove any jewelry and your watch. Use a paper towel to turn on water, and adjust the temperature to warm.				
2	Wet your hands to above the wrists and lather up with soap. Keep your hands below your elbows throughout the hand-washing process.				
3	Wash all areas of your hands and wrists. Interlace fingers to scrub between them. If your hands were exposed to infectious material, scrub beneath fingernails with a nail brush or nail stick.				
4	Rinse wrists and hands well. (Repeat soaping and washing if your hands were exposed to infectious material.)				
5	Dry hands thoroughly with paper towel, and dispose of it properly. Use a new, dry paper towel to turn off the water faucet and open the door, and dispose of it properly.				
COMPLETE SKILL					

Participant Name _____ Date _____

Instructor Name _____

☑ PERFORMANCE CHECKLIST: PUTTING ON GLOVES

SKILL STEP		Initial Practice		Final Performance	
		Needs Practice	Proficient	Remediate	Proficient
1	Pull glove onto one hand.				
2	Pull glove tight.				
3	Put on other glove.				
	COMPLETE SKILL				

✓ PERFORMANCE CHECKLIST: REMOVING CONTAMINATED GLOVES

SKILL STEP		Initial Practice		Final Performance	
		Needs Practice	Proficient	Remediate	Proficient
1	Hold your hands away from your body, with fingers pointing down.				
2	With one hand, grasp your other glove at the wrist or palm, and pull it away from your hand. Then, pull the glove the rest of the way off.				
3	Holding the removed glove balled up in the palm of your gloved hand, insert 2 fingers under the cuff of the remaining glove.				
4	Remove the glove by stretching it up and away from the hand and turning it inside out as you pull it off.				
5	Dispose of gloves safely (in a biohazard container if possible) and wash your hands.				
COMPLETE SKILL					

Participant Name _____ Date _____

Instructor Name _____

☑ PERFORMANCE CHECKLIST: INITIAL ASSESSMENT

SKILL STEP		Initial Practice		Final Performance	
		Needs Practice	Proficient	Remediate	Proficient
1	Ensure scene safety.				
2	Check the victim for responsiveness.				

For a responsive victim:

3	Ask the victim what happened and about his or her condition.				
4	Have someone call 9-1-1. If alone, correct any life-threatening conditions you see first (such as severe bleeding) before calling 9-1-1 and continuing to check the victim and providing other care.				

For an unresponsive victim:

3	Call for help: a. Shout for someone to call 9-1-1 and get an AED. Keep the phone at the victim's side. b. If alone, call 9-1-1 from your mobile device, if you have one, and follow the dispatcher's instructions.				
4	If alone without a mobile device, find a phone and call 9-1-1, and get an AED if available.*				

* Correct any immediate life threats (such as opening the airway or controlling severe bleeding) before leaving an adult victim to call 9-1-1.

COMPLETE SKILL

Participant Name _____ Date _____

Instructor Name _____

☑ PERFORMANCE CHECKLIST: RECOVERY POSITION

SKILL STEP		Initial Practice		Final Performance	
		Needs Practice	Proficient	Remediate	Proficient
1	Position the victim's arm farthest from you across the victim's body.				
2	Grasp the victim at the shoulder and hips, and roll them toward you.				
3	Bend both legs so the victim's position is stabilized.				
4	With the victim now in position, check the airway and open the mouth to allow drainage.				
COMPLETE SKILL					

Participant Name _____ Date _____

Instructor Name _____

☑ PERFORMANCE CHECKLIST: PHYSICAL EXAMINATION

SKILL STEP		Initial Practice		Final Performance	
		Needs Practice	Proficient	Remediate	Proficient
If you find any problems in any body area, do not let the victim move. Wait for help.					
1	Being careful not to move the victim's head or neck, check the head.				
2	Check neck area for medical alert necklace, deformity or swelling and pain. Do not move the neck.				
3	Check skin appearance, temperature and moisture.				
4	Check chest. Ask victim to breathe deeply.				
5	Check abdomen.				
6	Check pelvis and hips.				
7	Check upper extremities. Look for medical alert bracelet.				
8	Check lower extremities.				
	COMPLETE SKILL				

Participant Name _____ Date _____

Instructor Name _____

PERFORMANCE CHECKLIST: CPR FOR ADULTS, CHILDREN AND INFANTS (1 RESCUER)

SKILL STEP		Initial Practice		Final Performance	
		Needs Practice	Proficient	Remediate	Proficient
1	Activate the emergency response system. Determine that the unresponsive victim is not breathing normally.				
2	Expose the chest. Put your hand on the lower half of the breastbone in the middle of the chest for chest compressions. For an adult, put your second hand on top of the first and interlock the fingers. For a child, use 1 or both hands. For an infant, put your 2 middle fingers of 1 hand just below the nipple line.				
3	Give 30 chest compressions hard and fast at least 2 inches deep in an adult (but not more than 2.4 inches) and at least $\frac{1}{3}$ the depth of the chest in an infant (about 1½ inches) or child (about 2 inches) at a rate of 100-120 per minute. Count aloud for a steady fast rate: "One, two, three . . ." Then give 2 breaths.				
4	Open the airway and give 2 rescue breaths, each lasting 1 second, to cause a visible chest rise. (If the first breath does not go in, reposition the victim's head and try again; if the second breath still does not go in, give choking care.)				
5	Continue cycles of 30 compressions and 2 breaths.				
6	Continue CPR until: • The victim wakes up and is breathing normally. • An AED is brought to the scene and is ready to use. • Personnel with more training arrive and take over. • If the victim starts breathing normally but is unresponsive, put the victim in the recovery position and monitor breathing.				
7	When an AED arrives and is ready to be used, start the AED sequence for a victim who is not breathing normally.				
	COMPLETE SKILL				

Participant Name _____ Date _____

Instructor Name _____

☑ PERFORMANCE CHECKLIST: USING AN AED

SKILL STEP		Initial Practice		Final Performance	
		Needs Practice	Proficient	Remediate	Proficient
1	Position the victim away from water and metal. Place the unit by the victim's shoulder and turn it on.				
2	Expose the victim's chest, and quickly dry or shave the pad placement area if necessary.				
3	Apply the pads to the victim's chest as shown on the pads. If needed, plug the cables into the unit. Use adult pads for a victim 8 or older. For an infant or child younger than 8, use pediatric pads if available, applied as directed by the unit; if pediatric pads are unavailable, use adult pads.				
4	Stay clear during rhythm analysis.				
5	Follow prompts from the AED unit to do 1 of 3 things: (1) press the shock button, (2) stay clear while the AED automatically delivers a shock or (3) do not shock but immediately give CPR with the pads remaining in place, starting with chest compressions.				
6	Follow the AED's prompts to analyze the rhythm again after 5 cycles of CPR (about 2 minutes).				
7	Continue Steps 5 and 6 until the victim wakes up or more advanced help arrives and takes over.				
8	If the victim begins breathing normally but is unresponsive, put the victim (if no trauma to the neck, back, hip or pelvis) in the recovery position (with pads remaining in place) and continue to monitor breathing and pulse.				
COMPLETE SKILL					

Appendix B • Performance Checklists for Skills

Participant Name _____ Date _____

Instructor Name _____

☑ **PERFORMANCE CHECKLIST: CHOKING CARE FOR RESPONSIVE ADULT OR CHILD**

SKILL STEP		Initial Practice		Final Performance	
		Needs Practice	Proficient	Remediate	Proficient
1	Stand behind an adult victim with 1 leg forward between the victim's legs. Keep your head slightly to 1 side. For a child, move down to the child's level or kneel behind the child. Reach around the abdomen.				
2	Locate the victim's navel with a finger from 1 hand. Make a fist with the other hand and place the thumb side of the fist against the person's abdomen just above the navel.				
3	Grasp your fist with your other hand and thrust inward and upward into the victim's abdomen with quick thrusts. Continue abdominal thrusts until the victim expels the object or becomes unresponsive.				
4	For a responsive pregnant victim, or any victim you cannot get your arms around or cannot effectively give abdominal thrusts to, give chest thrusts in the middle of the breastbone from behind the victim. Avoid squeezing the ribs with your arms.				
COMPLETE SKILL					

Participant Name _____ Date _____

Instructor Name _____

☑ **PERFORMANCE CHECKLIST: CHOKING CARE FOR UNRESPONSIVE ADULT, CHILD OR INFANT**

SKILL STEP		Initial Practice		Final Performance	
		Needs Practice	Proficient	Remediate	Proficient
1	If the victim is unresponsive and not breathing normally, start CPR with 30 chest compressions at least 2 inches deep in an adult (but not more than 2.4 inches), and at least ⅓ the depth of the chest in a child (about 2 inches) or infant (about 1½ inches) at a rate of 100-120 per minute. Count aloud for a steady fast rate: "1, 2, 3..."				
2	Open the airway with the head tilt–chin lift.				
3	Give 2 rescue breaths, each lasting 1 second. If the first breath does not go in and the chest does not rise, position the victim's head again to open the airway, and try again.				
4	If breaths still do not go in, continue CPR with chest compressions, using a ratio of 30 compressions and 2 breaths.				
5	Look inside the mouth before giving breaths after each cycle of compressions, and remove any object you see. Then, give 2 breaths.				
6	Continue CPR until: • The victim recovers and is breathing normally. • Professional help arrives and takes over.				
	COMPLETE SKILL				

Participant Name _____ Date _____

Instructor Name _____

☑ PERFORMANCE CHECKLIST: CHOKING CARE FOR RESPONSIVE INFANT

SKILL STEP		Initial Practice		Final Performance	
		Needs Practice	Proficient	Remediate	Proficient
1	Support the infant face down by holding the head in 1 hand, with the torso on your forearm against your thigh. Give up to 5 back blows (slaps) between the shoulder blades with the heel of your hand.				
2	Check for an expelled object. If not present, continue with next step.				
3	With your other hand on the back of the infant's head, roll the infant face-up, supporting the back of the infant's head with your hand.				
4	Give up to 5 chest thrusts with 2 fingers on sternum just below the nipple line, about 1 per second. Each thrust should be 1½ inches deep. Check mouth for expelled object.				
5	Continue cycles of 5 back blows (slaps), 5 chest thrusts and checking the mouth. If alone, call 9-1-1 after 2 minutes. Continue until the object is expelled or the infant becomes unresponsive. If the infant becomes unresponsive, give CPR. Look inside the mouth before giving breaths and after each cycle of compressions, removing any object you see.				
	COMPLETE SKILL				

Participant Name _____ Date _____

Instructor Name _____

☑ PERFORMANCE CHECKLIST: CONTROLLING BLEEDING

SKILL STEP		Initial Practice		Final Performance	
		Needs Practice	Proficient	Remediate	Proficient
1	Put on gloves. *Improvise a barrier if no barrier is available*				
2	Place a sterile dressing or clean cloth on the wound.				
3	Apply firm direct pressure with your hand for about 5 minutes. • Do not put pressure on an object in a wound. • Do not put pressure on the scalp if the skull may be injured.				
4	Reevaluate the bleeding. a. If direct pressure does not control the bleeding and you have a hemostatic dressing, remove dressings already used and apply the hemostatic dressing directly on the wound using direct pressure. b. If a hemostatic dressing is not available, continue to apply direct pressure. If blood soaks through the first dressing, place additional dressings on top of the blood-soaked dressing and keep applying pressure.				
5	If needed, apply a pressure bandage to keep pressure on the wound, wrapping from the end of the extremity toward the center of the body. *The pressure is sufficient if the bandage is snug but you can slip a finger under it. Use a tourniquet when direct pressure and a pressure bandage do not control severe bleeding from a limb.*				
6	If appropriate, treat the victim for shock, and call 9-1-1.				
	COMPLETE SKILL				

Participant Name _____ Date _____

Instructor Name _____

☑ PERFORMANCE CHECKLIST: APPLYING A PRESSURE BANDAGE

SKILL STEP		Initial Practice		Final Performance	
		Needs Practice	Proficient	Remediate	Proficient
1	Place a sterile dressing or clean cloth on wound. Start wrapping an elastic or self-adhering roller bandage below the wound dressing, wrapping from the end of the extremity toward the center of the body.				
2	Make several circular turns, then overlap turns by about ½ of previous turn.				
3	Work up the limb to cover the dressing completely. The pressure is sufficient if the bandage is snug but a finger can be slipped under it.				
4	Fix or tie the end of the bandage in place.				
COMPLETE SKILL					

Participant Name _____ Date _____

Instructor Name _____

☑ PERFORMANCE CHECKLIST: SHOCK POSITION

SKILL STEP		Initial Practice		Final Performance	
		Needs Practice	Proficient	Remediate	Proficient
1	Check for responsiveness, normal breathing and severe bleeding.				
2	Call 9-1-1 and care first for life-threatening conditions, such as severe bleeding.				
3	Be ready to give CPR if needed.				
4	a. If there is no evidence of trauma, position a responsive victim on his or her back using a blanket or coat as a pad. If the movement or position does not cause the victim pain, raise the legs such that the feet are 6-12 inches above the ground. b. Put a breathing, unresponsive victim (if no suspected trauma, especially a neck, back, hip or pelvic injury) in the recovery position.				
5	Loosen any tight clothing.				
6	Be alert for the possibility of vomiting; if vomiting occurs, turn the victim's head to drain the mouth.				
7	Try to maintain the victim's normal body temperature. If necessary, maintain the victim's body heat with a blanket or coat over the victim.				
COMPLETE SKILL					

☑ PERFORMANCE CHECKLIST: USE OF AN EMERGENCY EPINEPHRINE AUTO-INJECTOR

SKILL STEP		Initial Practice		Final Performance	
		Needs Practice	Proficient	Remediate	Proficient
1	Call 9-1-1.				
2	Help a responsive victim use his or her emergency epinephrine auto-injector. If the victim cannot use his or her prescribed auto-injector, you may administer it yourself if permitted by state law.				
3	Take the EpiPen out of its case and remove the cap or protective cover.				
4	To administer the medication, press the auto-injector firmly against the outer thigh and hold it there while the medication is injected (follow the product instructions for how long). You should feel a "click" when the injection starts. a. The medication should provide relief for 15-20 minutes. b. If symptoms continue after the first dose of epinephrine has been given, and if EMS personnel are not expected to arrive within 5-10 minutes, administer a second dose of epinephrine, using a second auto-injector.				
5	Monitor the victim's breathing and be ready to give CPR if needed.				
6	Help a responsive victim sit up in a position of easiest breathing. Put an unresponsive victim who is breathing in the recovery position.				
COMPLETE SKILL					

Participant Name _____ Date _____

Instructor Name _____

☑ PERFORMANCE CHECKLIST: ASSESSING HEAD AND SPINAL INJURIES

SKILL STEP		Initial Practice		Final Performance	
		Needs Practice	Proficient	Remediate	Proficient
1	Check the victim's head.				
2	Check neck for deformity, swelling and pain.				
3	Touch toes of both feet and ask victim if the sensation feels normal.				
4	Ask victim to point toes.				
5	Ask victim to push against your hands with the feet.				
6	Touch fingers of both hands and ask victim if the sensation feels normal.				
7	Ask victim to make a fist and curl (flex) it in.				
8	Ask victim to squeeze your hands.				
COMPLETE SKILL					

Participant Name _____ Date _____

Instructor Name _____

☑ PERFORMANCE CHECKLIST: SPINAL MOTION RESTRICTION

SKILL STEP		Initial Practice		Final Performance	
		Needs Practice	Proficient	Remediate	Proficient
1	Ask a responsive victim what happened. If he or she has any of the risk factors, explain the need to hold the head still to restrict spinal movement and spinal cord injury. With an unresponsive victim, check for risk factors for suspected spinal injury.				
2	Hold the victim's head and neck with both hands in the position found to restrict movement.				
3	Monitor the victim's breathing and be ready to provide basic life support.				
4	Have someone call 9-1-1.				
5	Reassure a conscious victim and tell him or her not to move.				
6	Continue to stabilize the head and spine and monitor the victim's breathing until help arrives.				
COMPLETE SKILL					

Participant Name _____ Date _____

Instructor Name _____

☑ PERFORMANCE CHECKLIST: ROLLING A VICTIM WITH SPINAL INJURY (LOG ROLL)

	SKILL STEP	Initial Practice		Final Performance	
		Needs Practice	Proficient	Remediate	Proficient
1	Hold the victim's head with hands on both sides over ears.				
2	The first aider at the victim's head directs others to roll the body as a unit.				
3	Continue to support head in new position on side.				
	COMPLETE SKILL				

☑ PERFORMANCE CHECKLIST: APPLYING A SPIRAL BANDAGE

SKILL STEP		Initial Practice		Final Performance	
		Needs Practice	Proficient	Remediate	Proficient
1	Anchor the starting end of the elastic bandage below the injured area, farther from the trunk.				
2	Wrap the bandage in spirals up the limb toward the center of the body.				
3	Secure the end of the bandage with clips or tape.				
	COMPLETE SKILL				

Participant Name _____ Date _____

Instructor Name _____

✅ **PERFORMANCE CHECKLIST: APPLYING A FIGURE-8 BANDAGE TO THE WRIST**

SKILL STEP		Initial Practice		Final Performance	
		Needs Practice	Proficient	Remediate	Proficient
1	Anchor the starting end of the roller bandage.				
2	Turn the bandage diagonally across the wrist and back around the hand (forming a figure 8).				
3	Continue overlapping the figure-8 turns by about ¾ of the previous turn.				
4	Secure the end of the bandage with clips or tape.				
	COMPLETE SKILL				

Participant Name _____ Date _____

Instructor Name _____

☑ **PERFORMANCE CHECKLIST: APPLYING A FIGURE-8 BANDAGE TO THE ANKLE**

SKILL STEP		Initial Practice		Final Performance	
		Needs Practice	Proficient	Remediate	Proficient
1	Anchor the starting end of the bandage.				
2	Turn the bandage diagonally across the top of foot and around the ankle, and bring the bandage around in a figure 8.				
3	Continue overlapping the figure-8 turns by about ¾ of the previous turn.				
4	Secure the end of the bandage with clips or tape.				
	COMPLETE SKILL				

Participant Name _____ Date _____

Instructor Name _____

☑ **PERFORMANCE CHECKLIST: RICE FOR WRIST INJURY**

SKILL STEP		Initial Practice		Final Performance	
		Needs Practice	Proficient	Remediate	Proficient
1	Rest the injured wrist.				
2	Put ice or a cold pack on the injured area.				
3	Compress the injured area with an elastic bandage.				
4	Elevate the injured area. Use a sling to hold the wrist in place.				
	COMPLETE SKILL				

Participant Name _____ Date _____

Instructor Name _____

☑ PERFORMANCE CHECKLIST: APPLYING AN ARM SLING AND BINDER

SKILL STEP		Initial Practice		Final Performance	
		Needs Practice	Proficient	Remediate	Proficient
1	Secure the point of the bandage at the elbow. Use a safety pin or tie the point at the elbow.				
2	Position the triangular bandage.				
3	Bring up the lower end of the bandage to the opposite side of the neck.				
4	Tie the ends. Pad under the knot.				
5	Tie a binder bandage over the sling and around the chest.				
	COMPLETE SKILL				

Participant Name _____ Date _____

Instructor Name _____

☑ PERFORMANCE CHECKLIST: SPLINTING THE FOREARM

SKILL STEP		Initial Practice		Final Performance	
		Needs Practice	Proficient	Remediate	Proficient
1	Support the arm above and below the injury. Check circulation.				
2	Position the arm on a padded rigid splint. If available, add a roller bandage under the fingers.				
3	Secure the splint. Check circulation once secured.				
4	Put the arm in a sling, and tie a binder over the sling and around the chest.				
COMPLETE SKILL					

☑ PERFORMANCE CHECKLIST: ANATOMIC SPLINTING OF LEG

SKILL STEP		Initial Practice		Final Performance	
		Needs Practice	Proficient	Remediate	Proficient
1	Check circulation. Gently slide 4 or 5 bandages or strips of cloth under both legs. Do not put a bandage over the injury site.				
2	Put padding between the legs. Do not move the injured leg.				
3	Gently slide the uninjured leg next to the injured leg.				
4	Tie the bandages (snug but not tight), starting in the middle, then at the lower leg, and then at the top. Check circulation.				
COMPLETE SKILL					

Advanced Skills (Appendix A)

Participant Name _____ Date _____

Instructor Name _____

☑ PERFORMANCE CHECKLIST: RESCUE BREATHING

SKILL STEP		Initial Practice		Final Performance	
		Needs Practice	Proficient	Remediate	Proficient
1	If the victim has a pulse but is not breathing normally, open the airway and give a breath over 1 second, watching the chest rise and letting it fall.				
2	If the first breath does not go in, try again to open the airway and give another rescue breath. If it still does not go in, the victim may be choking. Proceed to CPR for choking.				
3	If your breath goes in, continue rescue breathing. Give each breath over 1 second, at a rate of 10-12 breaths per minute (1 breath every 5-6 seconds) for an adult; 12-20 breaths per minute for a child or infant (1 breath every 3-5 seconds).				
4	Check the pulse about every 2 minutes (every 5 cycles of CPR). If there is no pulse, start CPR beginning with chest compressions.				
COMPLETE SKILL					

☑ PERFORMANCE CHECKLIST: SUCTIONING (ADULT OR CHILD)

SKILL STEP		Initial Practice		Final Performance	
		Needs Practice	Proficient	Remediate	Proficient
1	Confirm that the suction device is working and produces suction.				
2	Turn the victim's head to one side and open the mouth (for spinal injury, support the head and turn with body as a unit).				
3	Sweep out solids and larger amounts of fluid with your finger.				
4	Determine maximum depth of insertion by measuring the catheter tip from the earlobe to the corner of the mouth.				
5	Turn on suction, or pump the handle to create suction.				
6	Insert catheter tip carefully into the mouth. Put your finger over the proximal opening to begin suctioning, and move the tip about as you withdraw it.				
7	Reposition the victim's head with airway open, and resume rescue breathing or CPR.				
COMPLETE SKILL					

Instructor Name _____

☑ PERFORMANCE CHECKLIST: SUCTIONING (INFANT)

SKILL STEP		Initial Practice		Final Performance	
		Needs Practice	Proficient	Remediate	Proficient
1	Hold the infant in position for suctioning, with the head lower than the body and turned to one side.				
2	Squeeze the suction bulb, and then gently insert the tip into the infant's mouth.				
3	Gradually release the bulb to create suction as you withdraw the tip from the infant's mouth.				
4	Move the bulb aside and squeeze it, with tip down, to empty it.				
5	Repeat Steps 2-4 until the airway seems clear, up to 3 times.				
6	Repeat the suctioning steps for each nostril.				
7	Begin or resume rescue breathing or CPR if needed.				
COMPLETE SKILL					

✅ PERFORMANCE CHECKLIST: BAG MASK FOR RESCUE BREATHING (2 RESCUERS)

SKILL STEP		Initial Practice		Final Performance	
		Needs Practice	Proficient	Remediate	Proficient
1	Rescuer 1 assembles the BVM with a mask of the correct size, and puts the mask over the victim's mouth and nose.				
2	Rescuer 2 positions hands: thumbs and index fingers circling each side of mask, the other 3 fingers of each hand behind lower jawbone. Pull the jaw up into the mask instead of pushing the mask down on the jaw.				
3	Rescuer 2 opens the airway and seals the mask to the victim's face.				
4	Rescuer 1 squeezes the bag to provide ventilations: a. 1 ventilation over 1 second in adult, every 5-6 seconds (or 1 breath every 6 seconds during CPR if an advanced airway is in place). b. 1 ventilation over 1 second in child or infant, every 3-5 seconds (or one breath every 6 seconds during CPR if an advanced airway is in place).				
5	Recheck pulse about every 2 minutes. If no pulse, call for an AED and start CPR.				
	COMPLETE SKILL				

Participant Name _____ Date _____

Instructor Name _____

✅ PERFORMANCE CHECKLIST: ORAL AIRWAY INSERTION

SKILL STEP		Initial Practice		Final Performance	
		Needs Practice	Proficient	Remediate	Proficient
1	Choose the correct airway device size. The oral airway length should match the distance from the corner of the mouth to the tip of the earlobe on the same side of the victim's face.				
2	Open the victim's airway with head tilt–chin lift or jaw thrust, and open the mouth.				
3	Insert the airway device with the tip pointing toward the roof of the mouth.				
4	When the tip reaches the back of the mouth and you feel resistance, rotate the airway 180 degrees.				
5	Continue to insert the airway device to the final position (the flange resting on the lips).				
COMPLETE SKILL					

Participant Name _____ Date _____

Instructor Name _____

☑ **PERFORMANCE CHECKLIST: NASAL AIRWAY INSERTION**

SKILL STEP		Initial Practice		Final Performance	
		Needs Practice	Proficient	Remediate	Proficient
1	Choose the correct nasal airway size. The nasal airway length should match the distance from the nostril to the tip of the earlobe on the same side of the victim's face.				
2	Coat the nasal airway with lubricant.				
3	Insert the nasal airway in the right nostril with the bevel toward the septum.				
4	Insert the nasal airway straight back, sliding it along the floor of the nostril. If you feel resistance, do not force it.				
5	Insert the nasal airway until the flange rests against the nose.				
	COMPLETE SKILL				

☑ PERFORMANCE CHECKLIST: CPR FOR ADULT OR CHILD (2 RESCUERS)

SKILL STEP		Initial Practice		Final Performance	
		Needs Practice	Proficient	Remediate	Proficient
1	At the victim's head, Rescuer 1 checks for unresponsiveness, normal breathing and a pulse simultaneously for no longer than 10 seconds. Rescuer 2 ensures that an AED has been summoned. At the victim's side, Rescuer 2 locates the site for chest compressions.				
2	Rescuer 1 indicates, "No pulse." Rescuer 2 gives 30 compressions for an adult (15 for a child) at rate of 100-120 per minute, counting aloud for a fast, steady rate, then pauses.				
3	Rescuer 1 gives 2 breaths.				
4	Rescuers continue cycles of 30 compressions for an adult (15 for a child) and 2 breaths for 2 minutes (or 5 cycles of compressions and ventilations at a ratio of 30:2) before switching compressor and ventilator roles. The switch should be done quickly (in less than 5 seconds).				
5	Rescuers continue CPR until: • The victim is breathing normally and has a pulse. • An AED is brought to the scene and is ready to use. • Help arrives and takes over. • If the victim starts breathing normally and has a pulse but is unresponsive, put the victim in the recovery position and monitor breathing and pulse.				
6	When an AED arrives and is ready to be used, start the AED sequence for a victim who is not breathing normally and has no pulse.				
	COMPLETE SKILL				

Appendix B • Performance Checklists for Skills

Participant Name _____ Date _____

Instructor Name _____

☑ PERFORMANCE CHECKLIST: CPR FOR INFANT (2 RESCUERS)

SKILL STEP		Initial Practice		Final Performance	
		Needs Practice	Proficient	Remediate	Proficient
1	At the infant's head, Rescuer 1 checks for normal breathing and a pulse. At the infant's feet, Rescuer 2 positions hands in the chest-encircling position for chest compressions with both thumbs.				
2	If pulse is absent, Rescuer 1 says, "No pulse." Rescuer 2 gives 15 chest compressions at a rate of 100-120 per minute, counting aloud for a fast, steady rate, then pauses.				
3	Rescuer 1 gives 2 breaths.				
4	Rescuers continue cycles of 15 compressions and 2 breaths for about 2 minutes before switching compressor and ventilator roles. The switch should be done quickly (in less than 5 seconds). Rescuers continue CPR until: • The infant is breathing normally and has a pulse. • More advanced help arrives and takes over. • If the infant starts breathing normally but is unresponsive, hold the infant in the recovery position and monitor breathing and pulse.				
5	When an AED arrives and is ready to be used, start the AED sequence for an infant who is not breathing normally and has no pulse.				
	COMPLETE SKILL				

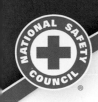

APPENDIX C

Natural Disasters: Earthquakes

Surviving an earthquake and reducing its health impact requires preparation, planning and practice. Far in advance, you can gather emergency supplies, identify and reduce possible hazards in your home and practice what to do during and after an earthquake. Learning what actions to take can help you and your family remain safe and healthy in the event of an earthquake.

Being Prepared

Although California has been the state most prone to serious earthquakes in recent years, many other fault zones exist in other areas of the United States. For example, geologists and seismologists have predicted a 97% chance of a major earthquake occurring in the New Madrid Seismic Zone in the central United States (including Arkansas, Missouri, Tennessee and Kentucky) between now and the year 2035. Although earthquakes with the power of the one that hit the greater Los Angeles area in January 1994 are fairly rare, less severe earthquakes can disrupt your normal living patterns and cause substantial injury.

During a major earthquake, you may hear a roaring or rumbling sound that gradually grows louder. You may feel a rolling sensation that starts out gently, and within a second or two, grows violent. Or, you may first be jarred by a violent jolt. A second or two later, you may feel shaking and find it difficult to stand up or move from one room to another.

Source: Centers for Disease Control and Prevention
www.bt.cdc.gov/disasters/earthquakes/prepared.asp
Accessed January 2016.

The key to surviving an earthquake and reducing your risk of injury lies in planning, preparing and practicing what you and your family will do if it happens.

PRACTICE DRILLS

By planning and practicing what to do if an earthquake strikes, you and your family can learn to react correctly and automatically when the shaking begins. During an earthquake, most deaths and injuries are caused by collapsing building materials and heavy falling objects, such as bookcases, cabinets and heating units. Learn the safe spots in each room of your home. If you have children, get the entire family to practice going to these locations. Participating in an earthquake drill will help children understand what to do in case you are not with them during an earthquake.

Make sure you and your child also understand the school's emergency procedures for disasters. This will help you coordinate where, when and how to reunite with your child after an earthquake.

During your earthquake drill:

- Drop down onto your hands and knees before the earthquake would knock you down. This position protects you from falling but still allows you to move if necessary.

- Cover your head and neck (and your entire body if possible) under the shelter of a sturdy table or desk. If there is no shelter nearby, get down near an interior wall or next to low-lying furniture that won't fall on you, and cover your head and neck with your arms and hands. Try to stay clear of windows or glass that could shatter or objects that could fall on you.

- Hold on to your shelter (or to your head and neck) until the shaking stops. Be prepared to move with your shelter if the shaking shifts it around.

EVACUATION PLANS

After an earthquake occurs, you may need to evacuate a damaged area. By planning and practicing for evacuation, you will be better prepared to respond appropriately and efficiently to signs of danger or to directions from civil authorities.

- Take a few minutes with your family to discuss a home evacuation plan. Sketch a floor plan of your home, and walk through each room and discuss evacuation details.

- Plan a second way to exit from each room or area, if possible. If you need special equipment, such as a rope ladder, mark where it is located.

- Mark where your emergency food, water, first aid kits and fire extinguishers are located.

- Mark where the utility switches or valves are located so that they can be turned off if possible.

- Indicate the location of your family's emergency outdoor meeting place.

ESTABLISH PRIORITIES

Take time before an earthquake strikes to write an emergency priority list, including:

- Important items to be hand-carried by you

- Other items, in order of importance to you and your family

- Items to be removed by car or truck if one is available

- Things to do if time permits, such as locking doors and windows, turning off utilities, etc.

WRITE DOWN IMPORTANT INFORMATION

Make a list of important information and put it in a secure location. Include the following on your list:

- Important telephone numbers, such as police, fire, EMS and medical centers

- The names, addresses and telephone numbers of your insurance agents, including policy types and numbers

- The telephone numbers of the electric, gas and water companies

- The names and telephone numbers of neighbors

- The name and telephone number of your landlord or property manager

- Important medical information (e.g., allergies, regular medications)

- The vehicle identification number, year, model and license number of your automobile, boat, RV, etc.

- Your financial institution's telephone number and your account types and numbers

- Radio and television broadcast stations to tune in to for emergency broadcast information

GATHER EMERGENCY SUPPLIES

Stock up now on emergency supplies[1] that can be used after an earthquake. These supplies should include a first aid kit, survival kits for the home, automobile and workplace, and emergency water and food. Store enough supplies to last at least 3 days.

[1]*www.bt.cdc.gov/disasters/earthquakes/supplies.asp*

GATHER AND STORE IMPORTANT DOCUMENTS IN A FIREPROOF SAFE

- Birth certificates

- Ownership certificates (automobiles, boats, etc.)

- Social Security cards

- Insurance policies

- Wills

- Household inventory, including:

  - List of contents

  - Photographs of contents of every room

  - Photographs of items of high value, such as jewelry, paintings or collectors' items

Emergency Supplies

Stock up now on emergency supplies that can be used after an earthquake. These supplies should include a first aid kit, survival kits for the home, automobile and workplace, and emergency water and food. Store enough supplies to last at least 3 days.

FIRST AID KIT

Store your first aid supplies in a toolbox or fishing tackle box, so they will be easy to carry and protect from water. Inspect your kit regularly, and keep it freshly stocked. *Note:* Important medical information and most prescriptions can be stored in the refrigerator, which also provides excellent protection from fires.

SURVIVAL KIT FOR YOUR HOME

Assemble a survival kit for your home with the following items:

Tools and Supplies

- Axe, shovel and broom
- Screwdriver, pliers, hammer and adjustable wrench
- Rope for towing or rescue
- Plastic sheeting and tape

Items for Safety and Comfort

- Sturdy shoes that can provide protection from broken glass, nails and other debris
- Gloves (heavy and durable for cleaning up debris)
- Candles
- Waterproof matches
- Change of clothing
- Knife
- Garden hose (for siphoning and firefighting)
- Tent
- Recreational supplies for children and adults
- Blankets or sleeping bags
- Portable radio, flashlight and extra batteries
- Essential medications and eyeglasses
- Fire extinguisher (multipurpose, dry chemical type)

- Food and water for pets
- Toilet tissue
- Cash

SURVIVAL KIT FOR YOUR AUTOMOBILE

Assemble a survival kit for your automobile with the following items. Storing some of these supplies in a small bag or backpack will make them more convenient to carry if you need to walk.

- Blankets
- Bottled water
- Change of clothes
- Coins for telephone calls
- Fire extinguisher (multipurpose, dry chemical type)
- First aid kit and manual
- Emergency signal device (light sticks, battery-type flasher, reflector, etc.)
- Flashlight with fresh batteries
- Food (nonperishable – nutrition bars, trail mix, etc.)
- Gloves
- Local map and compass
- Rope for towing, rescue, etc.
- Paper and pencils
- Premoistened towelettes
- Prescription medicines
- Battery-operated radio with fresh batteries
- Small mirror for signaling
- Toilet tissue
- Tools (pliers, adjustable wrench, screwdriver, etc.)
- Whistle for signaling
- Jumper cables
- Duct tape

SURVIVAL KIT FOR YOUR WORKPLACE

Assemble a survival kit for the workplace with the following supplies:

- Food (nonperishable – nutrition bars, trail mix, etc.)

- Bottled water

- Jacket or sweatshirt

- Pair of sturdy shoes

- Flashlight with fresh batteries

- Battery-operated radio with fresh batteries

- Essential medications

- Blanket

- Small first aid kit

- Extra pair of eyeglasses and/or contact lens solution

- Whistle or other signaling device

Emergency Water Storage and Purification

Following are recommendations for storing and purifying water supplies:

- The minimum drinking water supply is 1 gallon per person per day. You will also need water for food preparation, bathing, brushing teeth and dishwashing. Store a 3-5 day supply of water (at least 5 gallons for each person).

- Water should be stored in sturdy plastic bottles with tight-fitting lids. Rinsed chlorine bleach bottles work well. Plastic containers for juice and milk do not work as well because they tend to crack and leak more easily.

- Stored water should be changed every 6 months.

- Avoid placing water containers in areas where toxic substances, such as gasoline and pesticides, are present. Vapors may penetrate the plastic over time.

- Do not store water containers in direct sunlight. Select a place with a fairly constant, cool temperature.

SAFE WATER SOURCES IN THE HOME

If you do not have enough water stored, certain sources in your home may provide safe, clean water for drinking purposes:

- Water drained from the water heater faucet, if the water heater has not been damaged

- Water dipped from the tank of the toilet (not the bowl). The water in the bowl can be used for pets. Do not use water that has been chemically treated ("blue" water).

- Melted ice cubes

- Canned fruit, vegetable juice and liquids from other canned goods

- Water from the swimming pool. Use this water only after other sources of pure water are exhausted.

UNSAFE WATER SOURCES

Never use water from the following sources for drinking:

- Radiators

- Hot water boilers (home heating system)

- Water beds (fungicides added to the water or chemicals in the vinyl may make water unsafe for use)

Note: Remember that carbonated beverages do not meet drinking water requirements. Caffeinated drinks and alcohol dehydrate the body, which increases the need for drinking water.

WATER FOR DRINKING AND COOKING

Safe drinking water includes bottled, boiled or treated water. Your state or local health department can make specific recommendations for boiling or treating drinking water in your area. Here are some general rules about water for drinking and cooking. Remember:

- Do not use contaminated water to wash dishes, brush your teeth, wash and prepare food, or make ice.

- If you use bottled water, make sure the seal has not been broken. Otherwise, water should be boiled or treated before use. Drink only bottled, boiled or treated water until your supply is tested and found safe.

- Boiling water kills harmful bacteria and parasites. Bringing water to a rolling boil for 1 minute will kill most organisms.

- Treat water with chlorine or iodine tablets or mix 6 drops (⅛ teaspoon) of unscented, ordinary household chlorine bleach per gallon of water. Mix the solution thoroughly, and let stand for about 30 minutes. However, this treatment will not kill parasitic organisms. Containers for water should be rinsed with a bleach solution before using and reusing. Use water storage tanks and other types of containers with caution. For example, fire truck storage tanks, as well as previously used cans or bottles, can be contaminated with microbes or chemicals.

Emergency Food

Keep foods that:

- Have a long storage life

- Require little or no cooking, water or refrigeration (in case utilities are disrupted)

- Meet the needs of babies or other family members who are on special diets

- Meet pets' needs

- Are not very salty or spicy, as these foods increase the need for drinking water, which may be in short supply

HOW TO STORE EMERGENCY FOOD

- A disaster can easily disrupt the food supply at any time, so plan to have at least a 3-day supply of food on hand.

- When storing food, it is not necessary to buy dehydrated or other types of emergency food. Canned foods and dry mixes will remain fresh for about 2 years.

- Certain storage conditions can enhance the shelf life of canned or dried foods. The ideal location is a cool, dry, dark place. The best temperature is 40°F-60°F.

- Keep foods away from ranges or refrigerator exhausts. Heat causes many foods to spoil more quickly.

- Keep food away from petroleum products, such as gasoline, oil, paints and solvents. Some food products absorb their smell.

- Protect food from rodents and insects. Items stored in boxes or in paper cartons will keep longer if they are heavily wrapped or stored in airtight containers.

- Date all food items. Use and replace food before it loses freshness.

HOW TO USE EMERGENCY FOOD

- Use perishable food in your refrigerator or freezer before using food in your emergency supplies.

- Discard cooked, unrefrigerated foods after 2 hours at room temperature, regardless of appearance.

- Eat only foods that have a normal color, texture and odor.

- Discard cans that bulge at the ends or are leaking.

PREPARING FOOD

Your ability to prepare food after an earthquake may be complicated by damage to your home and loss of electricity, gas and water. The following items will help you to prepare meals safely:

- Cooking utensils

- Knives, forks and spoons

- Paper plates, cups and towels

- A manual can and bottle opener

- Heavy-duty aluminum foil

- A gas or charcoal grill or a camp stove

- Fuel for cooking, such as charcoal. (*Caution:* Never burn charcoal indoors. The fumes are deadly when concentrated indoors.)

Note: Do not use your fireplace for cooking until the chimney has been inspected for cracks and damage. Sparks may escape into your attic through an undetected crack and start a fire.

Inspecting for Possible Home Hazards

An important step in earthquake preparedness is to inspect your home and its surroundings for possible hazards, and then take action to lessen those hazards. Remember: Anything can move, fall or break during an earthquake or its aftershocks.

The following is a basic checklist to help you identify and correct possible home hazards.

ROOMS IN THE HOME

Look for the following hazards in each room:

- Windows and other glass that might shatter

- Unanchored bookcases, cabinets, refrigerators, water heaters and other furniture that might topple

- Heating units, fireplaces, chimneys and stoves that could move or fall

- Areas that could be blocked by falling debris

SECURING APPLIANCES

- Secure your large appliances with flexible cable, braided wire or metal strapping.

- Install flexible gas and water connections on all gas appliances. This will significantly reduce your chances of having a major fire after an earthquake.

- Brace and support air conditioners, particularly those on rooftops.

A typical water heater weighs about 450 pounds when full. In an earthquake, the floor on which it is standing tends to move out from under the heater, often causing it to topple. The movement can also break the gas, electric and waterline connectors, posing a fire or electric shock hazard, and can shatter the glass lining within the water heater. The water tank should be well secured to wall studs with bolts.

SECURING ITEMS IN THE BATHROOM

Replace glass bottles from your medicine cabinet and around the bathtub with plastic containers.

HANGING AND OVERHEAD ITEMS

- Inspect and anchor overhead light fixtures, such as chandeliers.

- Move heavy mirrors and pictures hanging above beds, chairs and other places where you sit or sleep. Otherwise, anchor these items with wire through eyescrews bolted into wall studs. Or place screws on both sides, top and bottom of the frame, and screw these into the studs.

- Determine whether the full swing of your hanging lamps or plants will strike a window. If so, move them.

- Secure hanging objects by closing the opening of the hook.

- Replace heavy ceramic or glass hanging planters with lightweight plastic or wicker baskets.

SHELVES, CABINETS AND FURNITURE

- Identify top-heavy, freestanding furniture, such as bookcases and china cabinets, that could topple in an earthquake.

- Secure your furniture by using:

  - L brackets, corner brackets or aluminum molding to attach tall or top-heavy furniture to the wall

  - Eyebolts to secure items located a short distance from the wall

- Attach a wooden or metal guardrail on open shelves to keep items from sliding or falling off. Fishing line can also be used as a less-visible means of securing an item.

- Place heavy or large objects on lower shelves.

- Use Velcro-type fastenings to secure some items to their shelves.

- Secure your cabinet doors by installing sliding bolts or childproof latches.

HAZARDOUS MATERIALS

Identify poisons, solvents or toxic materials in breakable containers and move these containers to a safe, well-ventilated storage area. Keep them away from your water storage and out of reach of children and pets.

Inspecting and Securing Your Home's Structure

Examine the structural safety of your house. If your house is of conventional wood construction, it will probably be relatively resistant to earthquake damage, particularly if it is a single-story structure.

For information on structural safety standards and qualified contractors in your area, contact your city or county government office on community development or building code enforcement.

The following suggestions will take an investment of time and money but will add stability to your home. If you want to do the work yourself, many hardware or home-improvement stores will assist you with information and instructions.

FOUNDATION

Check to see if your house or garage is securely fastened to the foundation. (If your house was built before 1950, it probably does not have bolts securing the wood structure to the concrete foundation.) If your house is not secured to the foundation, talk to a building contractor.

BEAMS, POSTS, JOISTS AND PLATES

Strengthen the areas of connection between beams, posts, joists and plates using such hardware as T and L straps, mending plates and joist hangers. Pay particular attention to exposed framing in garages, basements, porches and patio covers.

ROOF AND CHIMNEY

- Check your chimney or roof for loose tiles and bricks that could fall in an earthquake. Repair loose tiles or bricks as needed.

- Protect yourself from falling chimney bricks that might penetrate the roof by reinforcing the ceiling immediately surrounding the chimney with ¾-inch plywood nailed to ceiling joists.

Learning to Shut Off Utilities

- Know where and how to shut off utilities at the main switches or valves. Check with your local utility companies for instructions.

- Teach all family members how and when to shut off utilities.

GAS

- An automatic valve (Earthquake Command System) is commercially available that will turn the gas off for you in the event of an earthquake.

- After an earthquake, do not use matches, lighters or appliances, and do not operate light switches until you are sure there are no gas leaks. Sparks from electrical switches could ignite gas, causing an explosion.

- If you smell the odor of gas, or if you notice a large consumption of gas being registered on the gas meter, shut off the gas immediately. First, find the main shut off valve, located on a pipe next to the gas meter. Use an adjustable wrench to turn the valve to the Off position.

ELECTRICITY

After a major disaster, shut off the electricity. Sparks from electrical switches could pose a shock or fire hazard. Carefully turn off the electricity at the main electrical breaker in your home.

WATER

Water may be turned off at either of two locations:

- At the main meter, which controls the water flow to the entire property.

- At the water main leading into the home. (Shutting off the water here retains the water supply to your water heater, which may be useful in an emergency.) Attach a valve wrench to the waterline. (This tool can be purchased at most hardware stores.) Also, label the water mains for quick identification.

During an Earthquake

Indoor Safety

There are actions you can take, even while an earthquake is happening, that will reduce your chances of being hurt. Lights may be out, and hallways, stairs and room exits may be blocked by fallen furniture, ceiling tiles and other debris. Planning for these situations will help you take action quickly.

- Drop down onto your hands and knees before the earthquake knocks you down. This position protects you from falling but still allows you to move if necessary.

- Cover your head and neck (and your entire body if possible) under the shelter of a sturdy table or desk. If there is no shelter nearby, get down near an interior wall or next to low-lying furniture that won't fall on you, and cover your head and neck with your arms and hands.

- Hold on to your shelter (or to your head and neck) until the shaking stops. Be prepared to move with your shelter if the shaking shifts it around.

- Do not stand in a doorway. You are safer under a table. In modern houses, doorways are no stronger than any other part of the house. The doorway does not protect you from the most likely source of injury – falling or flying objects. Most earthquake-related injuries and deaths are caused by falling or flying objects (e.g., TVs, lamps, glass, bookcases) or by being knocked to the ground.

- If possible within the few seconds before shaking intensifies, quickly move away from glass and hanging objects, and bookcases, china cabinets or other large furniture that could fall. Watch for falling objects, such as bricks from fireplaces and chimneys, light fixtures, wall hangings, high shelves and cabinets with doors that could swing open.

- If available nearby, grab something to shield your head and face from falling debris and broken glass.

- If you are in the kitchen, quickly turn off the stove and take cover at the first sign of shaking.

- If you are in bed, hold on and stay there, protecting your head with a pillow. You are less likely to be injured staying where you are. Broken glass on the floor has caused injury to those who have rolled to the floor or tried to get to doorways.

High-Rise Buildings

Drop, cover and hold on. Move away from windows and outside walls. Stay in the building. The electricity may go out, and the sprinkler systems may come on. Do not use the elevators. If you are trapped stay calm. Try to get someone's attention by tapping hard on metal parts of the structure. That may increase your chances of being rescued.

Crowded Indoor Public Places

Drop, cover and hold on. Do not rush for the doorways. Others will have the same idea. Move away from display shelves containing objects that may fall. If you can, take cover and grab something to shield your head and face from falling debris and glass.

OUTDOOR SAFETY

If you are outdoors, move away from buildings and utility wires. The greatest danger from falling debris is just outside doorways and close to outer walls. Once you are in the open, stay there until the shaking stops.

AUTOMOBILES

If you are in a moving automobile, stop as quickly and safely as possible. Move your car to the shoulder or curb, away from utility poles, overhead wires and under- or overpasses. Stay in the car and set the parking brake. Turn on the radio for emergency broadcast information. A car may jiggle violently on its springs, but it is a good place to stay until the shaking stops. If a power line falls on the car, stay inside until a trained person removes the wire. When you drive on, watch for hazards created by the earthquake, such as breaks in the pavement, downed utility poles and wires, rising water levels, fallen overpasses and collapsed bridges.

After an Earthquake

AFTEREFFECTS

Be prepared for additional earth movements called aftershocks. Although most of these are smaller than the main earthquake, some may be large enough to cause additional damage or bring down weakened structures. Because other aftereffects can include fires, chemical spills, landslides, dam breaks and tidal waves, be sure to monitor your battery-operated radio or TV for additional emergency information.

INJURIES

Check for injuries. Do not attempt to move injured or unconscious people unless they are in immediate danger from live electrical wires, flooding or other hazards. Internal injuries may not be evident, but they may be serious or life threatening. If someone has stopped breathing, call for medical or first aid assistance immediately and begin CPR if you are trained to do so. Stop a bleeding injury by applying direct pressure to the wound. If you are trapped, try to attract attention to your location.

CHECKING UTILITIES

An earthquake may break gas, electrical and waterlines. If you smell gas: (1) open windows; (2) shut off the main gas valve; (3) do not turn any electrical appliances or lights on or off; (4) go outside; (5) report the leak to authorities; and (6) do not re-enter the building until a utility official says it is safe to do so.

- If electric wiring is shorting out, shut off the electric current at the main box.

- If water pipes are damaged, shut off the supply at the main valve.

OTHER PRECAUTIONS

- Have chimneys inspected for cracks and damage. Do not use the fireplace if the chimney has any damage.

- Check to see if sewage lines are intact before using bathrooms or plumbing.

- Do not touch downed power lines or objects in contact with downed lines. Report electrical hazards to the authorities.

- Immediately clean up spilled medicines, drugs, flammable liquids and other potentially hazardous materials.

- Stay off all telephones except to report an emergency. Replace telephone receivers that may have been knocked off by the earthquake.

- Stay away from damaged areas. Your presence could hamper relief efforts, and you could endanger yourself.

- Cooperate fully with public safety officials. Respond to requests for volunteer assistance from police, firefighters, emergency management officials and relief organizations, but do not go into damaged areas unless assistance has been requested.

EVACUATING YOUR HOME

If you must evacuate your home:

- Post a message, in a prearranged location, known only to family members, indicating where you have gone.

- Confine pets to the safest location possible and make sure they have plenty of food and water. Pets will not be allowed in designated public shelters.

- Take vital documents (such as wills and insurance policies), emergency supplies and extra medications with you.

People with Special Needs

PEOPLE WITH DISABILITIES

Before an earthquake:

- Write down any specific needs, limitations and capabilities that you have, and any medications you take. Make a copy of the list, and put it in your purse or wallet.

- Find someone (a spouse, roommate, friend, neighbor, relative or coworker) to help you in case of an emergency. Give them the list. You may wish to provide a spare key to your home, or let them know where they can find one in an emergency.

During an earthquake:

- If you are confined to a wheelchair, try to get under a doorway or into an inside corner, lock the wheels, and cover your head with your arms. Remove any items that are not securely attached to the wheelchair.

- If you are able, seek shelter under a sturdy table or desk. Stay away from outer walls, windows, fireplaces and hanging objects.

- If you are unable to move from a bed or chair, protect yourself from falling objects by covering up with blankets and pillows.

- If you are outside, go to an open area away from trees, telephone poles and buildings, and stay there.

After an earthquake:

- If you are trapped, try to attract attention to your location.

- Turn on your battery-operated TV or radio to receive emergency information and instructions.

- If you can, help others in need.

CHILDREN'S NEEDS

Fear is a normal reaction to danger. Children may be afraid of recurrence, injury or death after an earthquake. They may fear being separated from their family or being left alone. Children may even interpret disasters as punishment for real or imagined misdeeds. Children will be less likely to experience prolonged fear or anxiety if they know what to expect before, during and after an earthquake. Talking to children openly will also help them to overcome fears.

Here are some suggestions:

- Explain that an earthquake is a natural event and not anyone's fault.

- Talk about your own experiences with natural disasters, or read books about earthquakes aloud.

- Encourage your child to express feelings of fear. Listen carefully, and show understanding.

- Your child may need both verbal and physical reassurance that everything will be all right. Tell your child that the situation is not permanent.

- Include your child in cleanup activities. It is comforting to the child to watch the household begin to return to normal and to have a job to do.

Note: Symptoms of anxiety may not appear for weeks or even months after an earthquake, and they can affect people of any age. If anxiety disrupts daily activities for any member of your family, seek professional assistance through a school counselor, community religious organization, your physician or a licensed mental health professional.

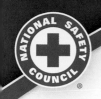

APPENDIX D

Natural Disasters: Floods

During a flood and its aftermath, there are some basic facts to remember that will help you protect your personal health and safety.

Preparing for a Flood

Here are some basic steps to take to prepare for a flood:

- Contact the local county geologist or county planning department to find out if your home is located in a flash flood-prone area or landslide-prone area.

- Learn about your community's emergency plans, warning signals, evacuation routes and locations of emergency shelters.

- Plan and practice a flood evacuation route with your family. Ask an out-of-state relative or friend to be the "family contact" in case your family is separated during a flood. Make sure everyone in your family knows the name, address and phone number of this contact person.

- Post emergency phone numbers at every phone.

- Inform local authorities about any special needs, such as elderly or bedridden people, or anyone with a disability.

- Identify potential home hazards and know how to secure or protect them before the flood strikes. Be prepared to turn off electrical power when there is standing water or fallen power lines, or before your evacuation. Turn off gas and water supplies before you evacuate. Secure structurally unstable building materials.

- Buy a fire extinguisher and make sure your family knows where it is and how to use it.

- Buy and install sump pumps with backup power.

- Have a licensed electrician raise electric components (switches, sockets, circuit breakers and wiring) at least 12 inches above your home's projected flood elevation.

- For drains, toilets and other sewer connections, install backflow valves or plugs to prevent floodwaters from entering.

- Anchor fuel tanks that can contaminate your basement if torn free. An unanchored tank outside can be swept downstream and damage other houses.

If you are under a flood watch or warning:

- Gather the emergency supplies you previously stocked in your home and stay tuned to local radio or television stations for updates.

- Turn off all utilities at the main power switch and close the main gas valve if evacuation appears necessary.

Source: Centers for Disease Control and Prevention www.bt.cdc.gov/disasters/ floods/index.asp Accessed January 2016.

- Have your immunization records handy or be aware of your last tetanus shot, in case you should receive a puncture wound or a wound becomes contaminated during or after the flood.

- Fill bathtubs, sinks and plastic soda bottles with clean water. Sanitize the sinks and tubs first by using bleach. Rinse and fill with clean water.

- Bring outdoor possessions, such as lawn furniture, grills and trash cans, inside or tie them down securely.

EMERGENCY SUPPLIES YOU WILL NEED

You should stock your home with supplies that may be needed during the emergency period. At a minimum, these supplies should include:

- Several clean containers for water, large enough for a 3-5 day supply of water (about 5 gallons for each person).

- A 3-5 day supply of nonperishable food and a nonelectric can opener.

- A first aid kit and first aid manual, prescription medicines and items for special medical needs.

- A battery-powered radio, flashlights, and extra batteries.

- Sleeping bags or extra blankets.

- Water-purifying supplies, such as chlorine or iodine tablets or unscented, ordinary household chlorine bleach.

- Baby food and/or prepared formula, diapers and other baby supplies.

- Disposable cleaning cloths, such as baby wipes, for the whole family to use in case bathing facilities are not available.

- Personal hygiene supplies such as soap, toothpaste and sanitary napkins.

- An emergency kit for your car with food, flares, booster cables, maps, tools, a first aid kit, a fire extinguisher and sleeping bags.

- Rubber boots, sturdy shoes and waterproof gloves.

- Insect repellent containing DEET, window screens and long-sleeved and long-legged clothing for protection from mosquitoes that may gather in pooled water remaining after the flood.

PREPARING TO EVACUATE

Expect the need to evacuate and prepare for it. When a flood watch is issued, you should:

- Fill your vehicle's gas tank and make sure the emergency kit for your car is ready.

- If no vehicle is available, make arrangements with friends or family for transportation.

- Identify essential documents, such as medical records, insurance card along with ID cards, and put in waterproof material to carry with you during evacuation.

- Fill your clean water containers.

- Review your emergency plans and supplies, checking to see if any items are missing.

- Tune in the radio or television for weather updates.

- Listen for disaster sirens and warning signals.

- Put livestock and family pets in a safe area. Due to food and sanitation requirements, emergency shelters cannot accept animals.

- Adjust the thermostat on refrigerators and freezers to the coolest possible temperature.

IF YOU ARE ORDERED TO EVACUATE

You should never ignore an evacuation order. Authorities will direct you to leave if you are in a low-lying area, or within the greatest potential path of the rising waters. If a flood warning is issued for your area or you are directed by authorities to evacuate the area:

- Take only essential items with you.

- If you have time, turn off the gas, electricity and water.

- Disconnect appliances to prevent electrical shock when power is restored.

- Follow the designated evacuation routes and expect heavy traffic.

- Do not attempt to drive or walk across creeks or flooded roads.

IF YOU ARE ORDERED *NOT* TO EVACUATE

To get through the storm in the safest possible manner:

- Monitor the radio or television for weather updates.

- Prepare to evacuate to a shelter or to a neighbor's home if your home is damaged, or if you are instructed to do so by emergency personnel.

DURING A FLOOD

If you enter swiftly flowing water, you risk drowning – regardless of your ability to swim. Swiftly moving shallow water can be deadly, and even shallow standing water can be dangerous for small children. Cars or other vehicles do not provide adequate protection from flood waters. Cars can be swept away or may break down in moving water.

Flood Recovery

PERSONAL HYGIENE AND HANDWASHING AFTER A DISASTER OR EMERGENCY

Good basic personal hygiene and handwashing are critical to help prevent the spread of illness and disease. Clean, safe running water is essential for proper hygiene and handwashing.

Hygiene is especially important in an emergency such as a flood, hurricane or earthquake, but finding clean, safe running water can sometimes be difficult. The following information will help to ensure good hygiene and handwashing in the event of an emergency.

Handwashing

Keeping hands clean during an emergency helps prevent the spread of germs. If your tap water is not safe to use, wash your hands with soap and water that has been boiled or disinfected. Follow these steps to make sure you wash your hands properly:

- Wet your hands with clean, running water (warm or cold) and apply soap.

- Rub your hands together to make a lather and scrub them well; be sure to scrub the backs of your hands, between your fingers and under your nails.

- Continue rubbing your hands for at least 20 seconds. Need a timer? Hum the "Happy Birthday" song from beginning to end twice.

- Rinse your hands well under running water.

- Dry your hands using a clean towel or air dry them.

A temporary hand washing station can be created by using a large water jug that contains clean water (for example, boiled or disinfected).

Washing hands with soap and water is the best way to reduce the number of germs on them. If soap and water are not available, use an alcohol-based hand sanitizer that contains at least 60% alcohol. Alcohol-based hand sanitizers can quickly reduce the number of germs on hands in some situations, but sanitizers do not eliminate all types of germs.

Hand sanitizers are not effective when hands are visibly dirty.

When to Wash Hands

Wash hands with soap and clean, running water (if available):

- Before, during and after preparing food

- Before eating food

- After using the toilet

- After changing diapers or cleaning up a child who has used the toilet

- Before and after caring for someone who is sick

- After blowing your nose, coughing or sneezing

- After touching an animal or animal waste

- After touching garbage

- Before and after treating a cut or wound

Bathing

Bathing after a water-related emergency should only be done with clean, safe water. Listen to local authorities for further instructions. Sometimes water that is not safe to drink can be used for bathing.

Dental Hygiene

Brushing your teeth after a water-related emergency should only be done with clean, safe water. Listen to local authorities to find out if tap water is safe to use.

WOUND CARE

Keeping wounds clean and covered is crucial during an emergency. If you have open cuts or sores, keep them as clean as possible by washing well with soap and clean, safe water to control infection. If a wound develops redness, swelling or drainage, seek immediate medical attention.

When providing first aid for a wound, clean hands can help prevent infection.

Reentering Your Flooded Home

When returning to a home that's been flooded after natural disasters, such as hurricanes, tornadoes and floods, be aware that your house may be contaminated with mold or sewage, which can cause health risks for your family.

WHEN YOU FIRST REENTER YOUR HOME

- If you have standing water in your home and can turn off the main power from a dry location, then go ahead and turn off the power, even if it delays cleaning. If you must enter standing water to access the main power switch, then call an electrician to turn it off. NEVER turn power on or off yourself or use an electric tool or appliance while standing in water.

- Have an electrician check the house's electrical system before turning the power on again.

- If the house has been closed up for several days, enter briefly to open doors and windows to let the house air out for a while (at least 30 minutes) before you stay for any length of time.

- If your home has been flooded and has been closed up for several days, presume your home has been contaminated with mold.

- If your home has been flooded, it also may be contaminated with sewage.

DRY OUT YOUR HOUSE

If flood or storm water has entered your home, dry it out as soon as possible. Follow these steps:

- If you have electricity and an electrician has determined that it's safe to turn it on, use a "wet-dry" shop vacuum (or the vacuum function of a carpet steam cleaner), an electric-powered water transfer pump or sump pump to remove standing water. If you are operating equipment in wet areas, be sure to wear rubber boots.

- If you do not have electricity, or it is not safe to turn it on, you can use a portable generator to power equipment to remove standing water. Note: If you must use a gasoline-powered pump, generator, pressure washer or any other gasoline-powered tools to clean your home, never operate the gasoline engine inside a home, basement, garage, carport, porch or other enclosed or partially enclosed structures, even if the windows and doors are open. Such improper use can create dangerously high levels of carbon monoxide and cause carbon monoxide poisoning.

- If weather permits, open windows and doors of the house to aid in the drying-out process.

- Use fans and dehumidifiers to remove excess moisture. Fans should be placed at a window or door to blow the air outwards rather than inwards, so not to spread the mold.

- Have your home heating, ventilating and air-conditioning (HVAC) system checked and cleaned by a maintenance or service professional who is experienced in mold clean-up before you turn it on. If the HVAC system was flooded with water, turning on the mold-contaminated HVAC will spread mold throughout the house. Professional cleaning will kill the mold and prevent later mold growth. When the service determines that your system is clean and if it is safe to do so, you can turn it on and use it to help remove excess moisture from your home.

- Prevent water outdoors from reentering your home. For example, rain water from gutters or the roof should drain away from the house; the ground around the house should slope away from the house to keep basements and crawl spaces dry.

- Ensure that crawl spaces in basements have proper drainage to limit water seepage. Ventilate to allow the area to dry out.

PRECAUTIONS WHEN RETURNING TO YOUR HOME

Electrical power and natural gas or propane tanks should be shut off to avoid fire, electrocution or explosions. Try to return to your home during the daytime so that you do not have to use any lights. Use battery-powered flashlights and lanterns, rather than candles, gas lanterns or torches. If you smell gas or suspect a leak, turn off the main gas valve, open all windows and leave the house immediately. Notify the gas company or the police or fire departments or the state fire marshal's office, and do not turn on the lights or do anything that could cause a spark. Do not return to the house until you are told it is safe to do so.

Your electrical system may also be damaged. If you see frayed wiring or sparks, or if there is an odor of something burning but no visible fire, you should immediately shut off the electrical system at the circuit breaker.

Avoid any downed power lines, particularly those in water. Avoid wading in standing water, which also may contain glass or metal fragments.

You should consult your utility company about using electrical equipment, including power generators. Be aware that it is against the law and a violation of electrical codes to connect generators to your home's electrical circuits without the approved, automatic-interrupt devices. If a generator is on line when electrical service is restored, it can become a major fire hazard. In addition, the improper connection of a generator to your home's electrical circuits may endanger line workers helping to restore power in your area. All electrical equipment and appliances must be completely dry before returning them to service. It is advisable to have a certified electrician check these items if there is any question. Also, remember not to operate any gas-powered equipment indoors.

CLEANUP

Walls, hard-surfaced floors, and many other household surfaces should be cleaned with soap and water and disinfected with a solution of 1 cup of bleach to 5 gallons of water. Be particularly careful to thoroughly disinfect surfaces that may come in contact with food, such as counter tops, pantry shelves, refrigerators, etc. Areas where small children play should also be carefully cleaned. Wash all linens and clothing in hot water, or dry clean them. For items that cannot be washed or dry cleaned, such as mattresses and upholstered furniture, air dry them in the sun and then spray them thoroughly with a disinfectant. Steam clean all carpeting. If there has been a backflow of sewage into the house, wear rubber boots and waterproof gloves during cleanup. Remove and discard contaminated household materials that cannot be disinfected, such as wallcoverings, cloth, rugs and drywall.

IMMUNIZATIONS

Outbreaks of communicable diseases after floods are unusual. However, the rates of diseases that were present before a flood may increase because of decreased sanitation or overcrowding among displaced persons. Increases in infectious diseases that were not present in the community before the flood are not usually a problem. If you receive a puncture wound or a wound contaminated with feces, soil or saliva, have a doctor or health department determine whether a tetanus booster is necessary based on individual records.

Specific recommendations for vaccinations should be made on a case-by-case basis, or as determined by local and state health departments.

CHEMICAL HAZARDS

Use extreme caution when returning to your area after a flood. Be aware of potential chemical hazards you may encounter during flood recovery. Flood waters may have buried or moved hazardous chemical containers of solvents or other industrial chemicals from their normal storage places.

If any propane tanks (whether 20-lb. tanks from a gas grill or household propane tanks) are discovered, do not attempt to move them yourself. These represent a very real danger of fire or explosion, and if any are found, police or fire departments or your state fire marshal's office should be contacted immediately.

Car batteries, even those in flood water, may still contain an electrical charge and should be removed with extreme caution by using insulated gloves. Avoid coming in contact with any acid that may have spilled from a damaged car battery.

HOW TO MAKE SURE YOUR FOOD IS SAFE

Do not eat any food that may have come into contact with floodwater. For infants, use only preprepared canned baby formula that requires no added water, rather than powdered formulas prepared with treated water. Thawed food can usually be eaten or refrozen if it is still "refrigerator cold," or if it still contains ice crystals. To be safe, remember, "When in doubt, throw it out." Discard any refrigerated or frozen food that has been at room temperature for 2 hours or more, as well as any food that has an unusual odor, color or texture.

HOW TO MAKE SURE YOUR WATER IS SAFE

Listen for public announcements on the safety of the municipal water supply. Flooded private water wells will need to be tested and disinfected after floodwaters recede. Questions about testing should be directed to your local or state health departments.

Safe water for drinking, cooking and personal hygiene includes bottled, boiled or treated water. Your state or local health department can make specific recommendations for boiling or treating water in your area. Here are some general rules concerning water for drinking, cooking and personal hygiene: Do not use contaminated water to wash dishes, brush your teeth, wash and prepare food, wash your hands, make ice or make baby formula. If possible, use baby formula that does not need to have water added. You can use an alcohol-based hand sanitizer to wash your hands.

- If you use bottled water, be sure it came from a safe source. If you do not know that the water came from a safe source, you should boil or treat it before you use it. Use only bottled, boiled or treated water until your supply is tested and found safe.

- Boiling water, when practical, is the preferred way to kill harmful bacteria and parasites. Bringing water to a rolling boil for 1 minute will kill most organisms.

- When boiling water is not practical, you can treat water with chlorine tablets, iodine tablets or unscented household chlorine bleach (5.25% sodium hypochlorite):

  - If you use chlorine tablets or iodine tablets, follow the directions that come with the tablets.

  - If you use household chlorine bleach, add ⅛ teaspoon (about 0.75 mL) of bleach per gallon of water if the water is clear. For cloudy water, add ¼ teaspoon (about 1.50 mL) of bleach per gallon. Mix the solution thoroughly and let it stand for about 30 minutes before using it.

Note: Treating water with chlorine tablets, iodine tablets or liquid bleach will not kill parasitic organisms.

Use a bleach solution to rinse water containers before reusing them. Use water storage tanks and other types of containers with caution. For example, fire truck storage tanks and previously used cans or bottles may be contaminated with microbes or chemicals. Do not rely on untested devices for decontaminating water.

HOW TO HANDLE ANIMALS AND MOSQUITOES

Many wild animals have been forced from their natural habitats by flooding, and many domestic animals are also without homes after the flood. Take care to avoid these animals. Do not corner an animal. If an animal must be removed, contact your local animal control authorities. If you are bitten by any animal, seek immediate medical attention. If you are bitten by a snake, try to accurately identify the type of snake so that, if it is poisonous, the correct antivenin may be administered.

Contact local or state health and agricultural officials for state guidelines on the disposal of dead animals. Protect yourself from mosquitoes: Use screens on dwellings, wear long-sleeved and long-legged clothing and use insect repellents that contain DEET.

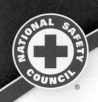

APPENDIX E

Natural Disasters: Hurricanes

Preparing for a Hurricane

If you are in an area that is susceptible to hurricanes, here are some basic steps to take to prepare.

MAKE A PLAN

Families can cope with disasters by preparing in advance and working together as a team. If something were to happen, how would you contact one another, how would you get to a safe place and what would you do in different emergency situations? Planning what to do before a disaster strikes provides the best protection for you and your family.

Create a Family Communication Plan

Because you and your family may not be together when a disaster hits, it's important to create a communication plan to help you and your loved ones connect and get help. Complete a contact card for each family member. Have them keep these cards handy in a wallet, purse or backpack.

More tips:

- Identify an out-of-town contact, such as a friend or relative, who family members can call to let them know they are safe. It may be easier to make a long-distance phone call than to call across town, because phone lines can be jammed. An out-of-town contact may be in a better position to communicate among separated family members.

- Teach your family members how to text. It may seem like second nature to some of us, but not everyone texts. During an emergency it's often easier to get a text message delivered rather than a phone call.

- Subscribe to an emergency alert system. Check with your local health department or emergency management agency to see if there is one offered for your area. Post emergency telephone numbers by home phones or save them in your cell phone (fire, police, ambulance, etc.).

- Teach children how and when to call 9-1-1 for help.

Create a Family Disaster Plan

Planning for a disaster means knowing what to do in each possible situation. Whether you have to evacuate your home or you need to shelter in place, it's important to have a plan ahead of time.

Before creating your disaster plan, it's important to know what types of emergencies are likely in your area and the best way to respond. For example, if tornadoes are common in your area does your family know what the warning signs are and where to take shelter? Call your Local Red Cross chapter or Emergency Management Agency for more information.

Because different disasters may require you to go to different places, make sure you identify a meeting place in your neighborhood, a meeting place just outside your neighborhood and a meeting place out of town. Review these plans with all members of your family and don't forget to consider what you would do with your pets who may not be allowed in emergency shelters.

Source: Centers for Disease Control and Prevention www.bt.cdc.gov/disasters/ hurricanes/index.asp Accessed January 2016.

More tips:

- Learn about your community's warning signals. What do they sound like and what you should do when you hear them?

- Determine the best escape routes from your home. Find two ways out of each room.

- Find the safe spots in your home for each type of disaster. For example, during an earthquake you would want to practice "drop, cover and hold on" under a sturdy desk or table. During a tornado, you would want to seek shelter in a lower level room without windows.

- Show each family member how and when to turn off the water, gas and electricity at the main switches.

- Teach each family member how to use the fire extinguisher, and show them where it's kept.

- Practice your plan by quizzing your kids periodically and conduct fire and other emergency drills.

- Check your emergency supplies throughout the year to replace batteries, food and water as needed.

ADDITIONAL WAYS TO PREPARE

- Check if you have adequate insurance coverage to cover possible flooding or structural damage to your home and property.

- Install smoke detectors on each level of your home, especially near bedrooms. Test and recharge your fire extinguisher(s) and smoke detectors according to manufacturer's instructions.

- Install at least one battery-powered or battery back-up carbon monoxide alarm in your home, preferably near bedrooms. Test the battery at least twice a year, when you change the time on your clocks.

EMERGENCY SUPPLIES YOU WILL NEED

During and after a hurricane, you may need supplies to keep your family safe and healthy. Remember that a hurricane could cut off your power and water supply. You also may not be able to drive because of damage to your car. Roads may be flooded or blocked.

That's why it's best to be prepared – stock up on everything you might need now. Here's a checklist of what you need:

Food and Medicine

- Clean containers for water

- At least 5 gallons of water per person (which should be enough to last 3-5 days)

- A 3-5 day supply of food that doesn't go bad (like canned food)

- Baby food or formula

- Prescription medicines

Safety Items

- First aid kit and instructions

- Fire extinguisher

- Battery-powered radio

- Flashlights

- Extra batteries

- Sleeping bags or extra blankets

- Supplies to make drinking water safe (like iodine tablets or chlorine bleach)

Personal Care Products

- Hand sanitizer

- Wet cleaning cloths (like baby wipes) in case you don't have clean water

- Soap

- Toothpaste

- Tampons and pads

- Diapers

Make sure your supplies are stored together in a place that's easy to reach.

Make an Emergency Car Kit

In case you need to leave quickly during a hurricane, always keep an emergency kit in your car, too. Make sure you include:

- Food that doesn't go bad (like canned food)

- Flares

- Jumper cables (sometimes called booster cables)

- Maps

- Tools, like a roadside emergency kit

- A first aid kit and instructions

- A fire extinguisher

- Sleeping bags

- Flashlight and extra batteries

Having a GPS – either in your car or on your smartphone – can help during an emergency, too.

Preparing to Evacuate

If a hurricane might be headed toward you, you need to prepare. Listen for National Weather Service alerts on TV or radio or check for them online. There are two kinds of alerts.

A hurricane watch means that there's no hurricane yet, but weather conditions could cause one. Experts will announce a hurricane watch 48 hours before they think dangerous winds will start.

A hurricane warning is more serious. It means a hurricane has already started or is just about to start.

If you hear that there's a hurricane watch or warning in your area, you can take steps to get ready.

GET YOUR FAMILY READY

- Go over your emergency plan with your family. Make sure you have the supplies you need.

- Keep checking for updates about the storm. Watch TV, listen to the radio or check online.

- Take care of your animals.

- Put pets and farm animals in a safe place. Keep in mind emergency shelters and many hotels may not let you bring animals with you if you need to evacuate. Ask your local public health department if pets are allowed in shelters. Read more about pet safety.

- Listen for disaster sirens and warning signals.

- Pack important documents (like wills or passports) with you.

- Call the hospital, public health department or the police about special needs. If you or a loved one is older or disabled and won't be able to leave quickly, get advice on what to do.

GET YOUR HOME READY

- Clear your yard. Make sure there's nothing that could blow around during the storm and damage your home. Move bikes, lawn furniture, grills, propane tanks and building material inside or under shelter.

- Cover up windows and doors outside. Use storm shutters or nail pieces of plywood to the window frames to protect your windows. This can help keep you safe from pieces of shattered glass.

- Be ready to turn off your power. If you see flooding or downed power lines, or you have to leave your home, switch it off.

- Fill clean water containers with drinking water in case you lose your water supply during the storm. You can also fill up your sinks and bathtubs with water for washing.

- Lower the thermostat in your refrigerator and freezer to the coolest possible temperature. If your power goes out, your food will stay fresh longer. Read more about food safety after a storm.

GET YOUR CAR READY

- Fill your car's gas tank. You may also want to consider making plans with friends or family to get a ride.

- Check your car's emergency kit.

- Move cars and trucks into your garage or under cover.

Evacuate or Stay at Home

If a hurricane is coming, you may hear an order to evacuate (leave your home). Never ignore an order to evacuate. Even sturdy, well-built houses may not hold up against a hurricane. Staying home to protect your property is not worth risking your health and safety.

You may also hear an order to stay at home. Sometimes, staying at home is safer than leaving.

IF YOU NEED TO EVACUATE:

- Only take what you really need with you, like your cell phone, medicines, identification (like a passport or license) and cash.

- Make sure you have your car emergency kit.

- If you have time, turn off the gas, electricity and water. Also unplug your appliances.

- Follow the roads that emergency workers recommend even if there's traffic. Other routes might be blocked.

IF YOU NEED TO STAY HOME:

- Keep listening to the radio or TV for updates on the hurricane.

- Stay inside. Even if it looks calm, don't go outside. Wait until you hear or see an official message that the hurricane is over. Sometimes, weather gets calm in the middle of a storm but then gets worse again quickly.

- Stay away from windows. You could get hurt by pieces of broken glass during a storm. Stay in a room with no windows, or go inside a closet. You can even protect yourself by getting in a bathtub and covering it with a sheet of plywood.

- Be careful. Winds can blow debris – like pieces of broken glass and other objects – at high speeds. Flying debris is the most common cause of injury during a hurricane. You're also at a higher risk of breaking a bone or cutting yourself on loose nails, metal or other objects.

- Be ready to leave. If emergency authorities order you to leave or if your home is damaged, you may need to go to a shelter or a neighbor's house.

Hurricane Recovery

MAKE SURE YOUR FOOD AND WATER ARE SAFE TO USE

After a hurricane, it's important that the water you drink and food you eat is safe. Spoiled food or dirty water can make you and your family sick.

Food Safety After a Hurricane

Keep Food Fresh

- If your power is out, keep your refrigerator and freezer doors closed as much as possible to keep in the cool air.

- Put a block of ice in your refrigerator if you expect the power will be out for more than 4 hours. It will keep food cool longer. Wear heavy gloves when handling the ice.

- Even if it's partially thawed, you can still cook or refreeze frozen food as long as you can see ice crystals or if it's still 40°F (degrees Fahrenheit) or lower.

Throw Out Spoiled Food

Get rid of food if it:

- Is in a can that's open, damaged or bulging.

- Has a strange smell, color or texture.

- Needs to be refrigerated but has been warmer than 40°F (degrees Fahrenheit) for 2 hours or longer. Foods that need to be kept cold include meat, eggs, fish, poultry and leftovers.

Clean Off Canned Food

If you have cans of food that came in contact with floodwater or storm water, you need to clean them off to make sure they're safe to use. To get germs off the outside of the cans:

- Remove the labels.

- Dip the cans in a mix of 5 gallons of water and 1 cup of household bleach.

- Label the cans with a permanent marker so you know what's inside.

Water Safety After a Hurricane

Ask local officials or listen to the news to find out whether you can drink tap water or use it for washing. If it's not safe, use bottled water if you can. If you don't have bottled water, there are some things you can do to kill germs in dirty water and make it safe to drink. For example:

- Bring water to a rolling boil for 1 minute.

- Use household bleach. Add ⅛ teaspoon of new, unscented liquid bleach to 1 gallon of water. Stir well. Let the water sit for 30 minutes before you drink it.

- Use water-purifying tablets. Adding these to water makes it safe to drink. Follow the product's directions.

Feeding Your Baby

If you have a baby, protect her from germs in unsafe water. You can:

- Keep breastfeeding if that's what you normally do.

- Use canned or premixed liquid formula.

- Use bottled water to make formula from a powder or concentrate.

If you don't have bottled water, use boiled water to make formula. Make sure the water has cooled before mixing it with formula and giving it to your baby.

Only use treated (disinfected or purified) water to make formula if you don't have access to bottled or boiled water.

HOW TO PREVENT INJURY AFTER A HURRICANE

Be Safe After a Hurricane

It's important to remember that the danger isn't over when the storm ends. Get tips for how to keep your family safe after a hurricane.

Be Safe Inside

- Never use an electrical device if it got wet. If it's still plugged in, turn off the power at the main breaker. Wait for an electrician to check the device before using it.

- If the power is out, use flashlights instead of candles. If you have to use candles, keep them away from anything that can catch fire. Always stay near lit candles.

- Be careful near damaged buildings. Keep in mind that hurricanes can damage buildings and make them unsafe. If your home or another building has been damaged, make sure it's safe before going inside.

- Leave your home or another building right away if you hear shifting or unusual noises. Strange noises could mean it's about to fall.

Prevent Carbon Monoxide Poisoning

Gas or coal-burning equipment creates carbon monoxide. This can include equipment like generators, pressure washers, charcoal grills, and camp stoves. You can't smell it or see it, but if carbon monoxide builds up in your home, it's very dangerous. To keep your family safe:

- Never use gas or coal-burning equipment inside your home, basement, or garage. Keep it outside and at least 20 feet from any window, door, or vent.

- Never run a car or truck inside a garage attached to your home, even with the garage door open.

- Never heat your home with a gas oven.

- If you have a carbon monoxide detector and it starts beeping, leave your home right away and call 9-1-1.

To be safe, learn the symptoms of carbon monoxide poisoning. If you think that carbon monoxide might have made you or a family member sick, go to a doctor or hospital right away.

BE SAFE OUTSIDE

Keep Away from Floodwater

- Always follow warnings about flooded roads.

- Drive around floodwater, not through it. It may be deeper than you think. If you have to be in or near floodwater, wear a life jacket – especially if the water is rising.

Keep in mind that floodwater often carries germs. If you touch it, be sure to wash your hands with soap and water. If you don't have soap or water, use alcohol-based wipes or sanitizer.

Stay Away from Power Lines and Dangerous Materials

- Stay clear of fallen power lines. Call the electric company to report them.

- Watch out for power lines overhead.

- Protect yourself with the right gear – like a breathing mask (respirator) – if you're near dangerous materials. Dust in damaged buildings could contain substances like lead, asbestos, cement, or mold. If you touch something harmful, wash it off your skin right away.

- Get help if you're not sure how to handle harmful materials.

Protect Yourself from Animals and Pests

- Floods can bring mosquitoes that carry disease. Use insect repellent (bug spray) with DEET or Picaridin. Wear long sleeves, pants and socks when you're outside.

- Stay away from wild or stray animals after a storm. Call 9-1-1 or your public health department to report them.

- If you see a dead animal, report it to local officials.

CLEAN UP YOUR HOME

After a hurricane or flood, you may need to clean up your home and yard. Take steps to stay safe.

Wear Safety Gear

Protect yourself from injuries during cleanup by wearing:

- Hard hats

- Goggles

- Heavy work gloves

- Waterproof boots with steel toes

- Earplugs or headphones (if you're working with noisy equipment)

Prevent or Clean Up Mold

After a storm or flood, mold can be a serious problem. Act fast to prevent or clean it up:

- Clean up and dry out your home quickly after the storm ends – within 24-48 hours if you can.

- Air out your house by opening doors and windows.

- Use fans to dry wet areas.

- Clean wet items and surfaces with detergent and water.

- Fix any leaks in roofs, walls or plumbing as soon as you can.

- Throw away anything that you can't clean or dry quickly. For example, you might need to get rid of carpeting and some furniture.

If you notice mold, clean it up with a mix of bleach and water:

- Never use bleach in a closed space. Open windows and doors first.

- Put on rubber gloves.

- To make your cleaner, mix 1 cup of household bleach with 1 gallon of water.

- Clean everything with mold on it.

Disinfect Toys

Remember that anything that's had contact with floodwater could carry germs. To keep your kids safe, make sure their toys are clean:

- Make a cleaning fluid by mixing 1 cup of bleach in 5 gallons of water.

- Wash off toys carefully with your cleaner.

- Let the toys air dry.

You may not be able to kill germs on some toys — like stuffed animals and baby toys. Throw out toys you can't clean.

Pace Yourself During Clean Up

Cleaning up your home can be a big job. Be sure to take care of yourself:

- Rest when you need to.

- Decide which cleanup tasks are most important, and focus on those first. That way, you're less likely to be overwhelmed.

- Get help lifting heavy or bulky objects. If you lift too much on your own, you could hurt yourself.

- Try to work with other people, so you aren't alone.

- Get support from family members, friends, counselors or therapists.

Natural Disasters: Tornadoes

Knowing what to do when you see a tornado, or when you hear a tornado warning, can help protect you and your family. During a tornado, people face hazards from extremely high winds and risk being struck by flying and falling objects. After a tornado, the wreckage left behind poses additional injury risks. Although nothing can be done to prevent tornadoes, there are actions you can take for your health and safety.

Being Prepared

STAY TUNED FOR STORM WATCHES AND WARNINGS

When there are thunderstorms in your area, turn on your radio or TV to get the latest emergency information from local authorities. Listen for announcements of a tornado watch or tornado warning.

Local Warning System

Learn about the tornado warning system of your county or locality. Most tornado-prone areas have a siren system. Know how to distinguish between the siren's warnings for a tornado watch and a tornado warning.

Tornado Watch

A tornado watch is issued when weather conditions favor the formation of tornadoes, for example, during a severe thunderstorm.

During a tornado watch:

• Stay tuned to local radio and TV stations or a National Oceanographic and Atmospheric Administration (NOAA) Weather Radio for further weather information.

• Watch the weather and be prepared to take shelter immediately if conditions worsen.

Tornado Warning

A tornado warning is issued when a tornado funnel is sighted or indicated by weather radar.

You should take shelter immediately.

Thunderstorms

Because tornadoes often accompany thunderstorms, pay close attention to changing weather conditions when there is a severe thunderstorm watch or warning.

A severe thunderstorm watch means severe thunderstorms are possible in your area.

A severe thunderstorm warning means severe thunderstorms are occurring in your area.

Keep fresh batteries and a battery-powered radio or TV on hand. Electrical power is often interrupted during thunderstorms – just when information about weather warnings is most needed.

Source: Centers for Disease Control and Prevention bt.cdc.gov/disasters/tornadoes/index.asp Accessed January 2016.

IMPORTANT MEASURES TO TAKE

- Take a few minutes with your family to develop a tornado emergency plan. Sketch a floor plan of where you live, or walk through each room and discuss where and how to seek shelter.

- Show a second way to exit from each room or area. If you need special equipment, such as a rope ladder, mark where it is located.

- Make sure everyone understands the siren warning system, if there's such a system in your area.

- Mark where your first aid kit and fire extinguishers are located.

- Mark where the utility switches or valves are located so they can be turned off – if time permits – in an emergency.

- Teach your family how to administer basic first aid, how to use a fire extinguisher and how and when to turn off water, gas and electricity in your home.

- Learn the emergency dismissal policy for your child's school.

- Make sure your children know:

  - What a tornado is

  - What tornado watches and warnings are

  - What county or parish they live in (warnings are issued by county or parish)

  - How to take shelter, whether at home or at school

Extra Measures for People with Special Needs

- Write down your specific needs, limitations, capabilities and medications. Keep this list near you always – perhaps in your purse or wallet.

- Find someone nearby (a spouse, roommate, friend, neighbor, relative or coworker) who will agree to assist you in case of an emergency. Give him or her a copy of your list. You may also want to provide a spare key to your home, or directions to find a key.

- Keep aware of weather conditions through whatever means are accessible to you. Some options are closed captioning or scrolled warnings on TV, radio bulletins or call-in weather information lines.

Practicing Your Emergency Plan

Conduct drills and ask questions to make sure your family remembers information on tornado safety, particularly how to recognize hazardous weather conditions and how to take shelter.

Writing Down Important Information

Make a list of important information. Include these on your list:

- Important telephone numbers, such as emergency (police and fire), paramedics and medical centers

- Names, addresses and telephone numbers of your insurance agents, including policy types and numbers

- Telephone numbers of the electric, gas and water companies

- Names and telephone numbers of neighbors

- Name and telephone number of your landlord or property manager

- Important medical information (for example, allergies, regular medications and brief medical history)

- Year, model, license and identification numbers of your vehicles (automobiles, boats and RVs)

- Bank's or credit union's telephone number, and your account numbers

- Radio and television broadcast stations to tune to for emergency broadcast information

Storing Important Documents

Store the following documents in a fire- and water-proof safe:

- Birth certificates

- Ownership certificates (autos, boats, etc.)

- Social security cards

- Insurance policies

- Will

- Household inventory

  - List of contents of household; include serial numbers, if applicable

  - Photographs or videotape of contents of every room

  - Photographs of items with high value, such as jewelry, paintings, collection items

First Aid Supplies

Drugs and Medications

- Soap and clean water to disinfect wounds

- Antibiotic ointment

- Individually wrapped alcohol swabs

- Aspirin and non-aspirin tablets

- Prescriptions and any long-term medications (keep these current)

- Diarrhea medicine

- Eye drops

Note: Important medical information and most prescriptions can be stored in the refrigerator, which provides excellent protection from fires.

Dressings

- Band-aids

- Clean sheets torn into strips

- Elastic bandages

- Rolled gauze

- Cotton-tipped swabs

- Adhesive tape roll

Other First Aid Supplies

- First aid book

- Writing materials

- Scissors

- Tweezers

- Thermometer

- Bar soap

- Tissues

- Sunscreen

- Paper cups

- Plastic bags

- Safety pins

- Needle and thread

- Instant cold packs for sprains

- Sanitary napkins

- Pocket knife

- Splinting material

REDUCING HOUSEHOLD HAZARDS

Home Inspection Checklist

The following suggestions will reduce the risk for injury during or after a tornado. No amount of preparation will eliminate every risk.

Possible Hazards

Inspect your home for possible hazards, including the following:

- Are walls securely bolted to the foundation?

- Are wall studs attached to the roof rafters with metal hurricane clips, not nails?

Utilities

- Do you know where and how to shut off utilities at the main switches or valves?

Home Contents

- Are chairs or beds near windows, mirrors or large pictures?

- Are heavy items stored on shelves more than 30 inches high?

- Are there large, unsecured items that might topple over or fall?

- Are poisons, solvents or toxic materials stored safely?

Securing Your Home's Structure

No home is completely safe in a tornado. However, attention to construction details can reduce damage and provide better protection for you and your family if a tornado should strike your house. If an inspection using the "Home Inspection Checklist" reveals a possible hazard in the way your home is constructed, contact your local city or county building inspectors for more information about structural safety. They may also offer suggestions on finding a qualified contractor to do any needed work for you.

Walls and Roof Rafters

Strengthen the areas of connection between the wall studs and roof rafters with hurricane clips.

Shutting Off Utilities

Gas:

After a tornado, *do not use* matches, lighters or appliances, or operate light switches until you are sure there are no gas leaks. Sparks from electrical switches could ignite gas and cause an explosion.

If you smell the odor of gas or if you notice a large consumption of gas being registered on the gas meter, shut off the gas immediately. First, find the main shut-off valve located on a pipe next to the gas meter. Use an adjustable wrench to turn the valve to the "off" position.

Electricity:

After a major disaster, shut off the electricity. Sparks from electrical switches could ignite leaking gas and cause an explosion.

Water:

- Water may be turned off at either of 2 locations:

  - At the main meter, which controls the water flow to the entire property.

  - At the water main leading into the home. If you may need an emergency source of fresh water, it is better to shut off your water here, because it will conserve the water in your water heater.

- Attach a valve wrench to the water line. (This tool can be purchased at most hardware stores.)

- Label the water mains for quick identification.

Arranging and Securing Household Items

- Arrange furniture so that chairs and beds are away from windows, mirrors and picture frames.

- Place heavy or large items on lower shelves.

- Secure your large appliances, especially your water heater, with flexible cable, braided wire or metal strapping.

- Identify top-heavy, free-standing furniture, such as bookcases and china cabinets, that could topple over.

- Secure your furniture by using 1 of 2 methods.

  - "L" brackets, corner brackets or aluminum molding, to attach tall or top-heavy furniture to the wall.

  - Eyebolts, to secure items located a short distance from the wall.

- Install sliding bolts or childproof latches on all cabinet doors.

- Store all hazardous materials such as poisons and solvents:

  - in a sturdy, latched or locked cabinet

  - in a well-ventilated area

  - away from emergency food or water supplies

During a Tornado

SIGNS OF AN APPROACHING STORM

Some tornadoes strike rapidly, without time for a tornado warning, and sometimes without a thunderstorm in the vicinity. When you are watching for rapidly emerging tornadoes, it is important to know that you cannot depend on seeing a funnel: Clouds or rain may block your view. The following weather signs may mean that a tornado is approaching:

- A dark or green-colored sky

- A large, dark, low-lying cloud

- Large hail

- A loud roar that sounds like a freight train

If you notice any of these weather conditions, take cover immediately, and keep tuned to local radio and TV stations or to a NOAA weather radio.

Sighting a Funnel Cloud

If you see a funnel cloud nearby, take shelter immediately (see the following section for instructions on shelter). However, if you spot a tornado that is far away, help alert others to the hazard by reporting it to the newsroom of a local radio or TV station before taking shelter as described later. Use common sense and exercise caution: If you believe that you might be in danger, seek shelter immediately.

TAKING SHELTER

Your family could be anywhere when a tornado strikes: at home, at work, at school or in the car. Discuss with your family where the best tornado shelters are and how family members can protect themselves from flying and falling debris.

The key to surviving a tornado and reducing the risk of injury lies in planning, preparing and practicing what you and your family will do if a tornado strikes. Flying debris causes most deaths and injuries during a tornado. Although there is no completely safe place during a tornado, some locations are much safer than others.

At Home

Pick a place in the home where family members can gather if a tornado is headed your way. One basic rule is *avoid windows*. An exploding window can injure or kill.

The safest place in the home is the interior part of a basement. If there is no basement, go to an inside room, without windows, on the lowest floor. This could be a center hallway, bathroom or closet.

For added protection, get under something sturdy such as a heavy table or workbench. If possible, cover your body with a blanket, sleeping bag or mattress, and protect your head with anything available – even your hands. Avoid taking shelter where there are heavy objects, such as pianos or refrigerators, on the area of floor that is directly above you. They could fall though the floor if the tornado strikes your house.

In a Mobile Home

Do not stay in a mobile home during a tornado. Mobile homes can turn over during strong winds. Even mobile homes with a tie-down system cannot withstand the force of tornado winds.

Plan ahead. If you live in a mobile home, go to a nearby building, preferably one with a basement. If there is no shelter nearby, lie flat in the nearest ditch, ravine or culvert and shield your head with your hands.

If you live in a tornado-prone area, encourage your mobile home community to build a tornado shelter.

On the Road

The least desirable place to be during a tornado is in a motor vehicle. Cars, buses and trucks are easily tossed by tornado winds.

Do not try to outrun a tornado in your car. If you see a tornado, stop your vehicle. Do not get under your vehicle.

Outdoors

Do the following if you are caught outside during a tornado and there is no adequate shelter immediately available:

• Avoid areas with many trees.

• Protect your head with an object or with your arms.

Long-Span Buildings

A long-span building, such as a shopping mall, theater or gymnasium, is especially dangerous because the roof structure is usually supported solely by the outside walls. Most such buildings hit by tornados cannot withstand the enormous pressure. They simply collapse.

If you are in a long-span building during a tornado, stay away from windows. Get to the lowest level of the building – the basement if possible – and away from the windows.

If there is no time to get to a tornado shelter or to a lower level, try to get under a door frame or get up against something that will support or deflect falling debris. For instance, in a department store, get up against heavy shelving or counters. In a theater, get under the seats. Remember to protect your head.

Office Buildings, Schools, Hospitals, Churches and Other Public Buildings

Extra care is required in offices, schools, hospitals or any building where a large group of people is concentrated in a small area. The exterior walls of such buildings often have large windows.

Do the following if you are in any of these buildings:

• Move away from windows and glass doorways.

• Go to the innermost part of the building on the lowest possible floor.

• Do not use elevators because the power may fail, leaving you trapped.

• Protect your head and make yourself as small a target as possible by crouching down.

Shelter for People with Special Needs

Advance planning is especially important if you require assistance to reach shelter from an approaching storm (see specific instructions in the next section).

• If you are in a wheelchair, get away from windows and go to an interior room of the house. If possible, seek shelter under a sturdy table or desk. Do cover your head with anything available, even your hands.

• If you are unable to move from a bed or a chair and assistance is not available, protect yourself from falling objects by covering up with blankets and pillows.

• If you are outside and a tornado is approaching, get into a ditch or gully. If possible, lie flat and cover your head with your arms.

After a Tornado

Injury may result from the direct impact of a tornado, or it may occur afterward when people walk among debris and enter damaged buildings. A study of injuries after a tornado in Marion, Illinois, showed that 50% of the tornado-related injuries were suffered during rescue attempts, cleanup and other post-tornado activities. Nearly a third of the injuries resulted from stepping on nails. Other common causes of injury included falling objects and heavy, rolling objects. Because tornadoes often damage power lines, gas lines or electrical systems, there is a risk of fire, electrocution or an explosion. Protecting yourself and your family requires promptly treating any injuries suffered during the storm and using extreme care to avoid further hazards.

INJURIES

Check for injuries. Do not attempt to move seriously injured people unless they are in immediate danger of further injury. Get medical assistance immediately. If someone has stopped breathing, begin CPR if you are trained to do so. Stop a bleeding injury by applying direct pressure to the wound. Clean out all open wounds and cuts with soap and clean water. Apply an antibiotic ointment. Contact a doctor to find out whether more treatment is needed (such as a tetanus shot). If a wound gets red, swells or drains, seek immediate medical attention. Have any puncture wound evaluated by a physician. If you are trapped, try to attract attention to your location.

GENERAL SAFETY PRECAUTIONS

Here are some safety precautions that could help you avoid injury after a tornado:

- Continue to monitor your battery-powered radio or television for emergency information.

- Be careful when entering any structure that has been damaged.

- Wear sturdy shoes or boots, long sleeves and gloves when handling or walking on or near debris.

- Be aware of hazards from exposed nails and broken glass.

- Do not touch downed power lines or objects in contact with downed lines. Report electrical hazards to the police and the utility company.

- Use battery-powered lanterns, if possible, rather than candles to light homes without electrical power. If you use candles, make sure they are in safe holders away from curtains, paper, wood or other flammable items. Never leave a candle burning when you are out of the room.

- Never use generators, pressure washers, grills, camp stoves or other gasoline, propane, natural gas or charcoal-burning devices inside your home, basement, garage or camper – or even outside near an open window, door or vent. Carbon monoxide (CO) – an odorless, colorless gas that can cause sudden illness and death if you breathe it – from these sources can build up in your home, garage or camper and poison the people and animals inside. Seek prompt medical attention if you suspect CO poisoning and are feeling dizzy, light-headed or nauseated.

- Hang up displaced telephone receivers that may have been knocked off by the tornado, but stay off the telephone, except to report an emergency.

- Cooperate fully with public safety officials.

- Respond to requests for volunteer assistance by police, fire fighters, emergency management and relief organizations, but do not go into damaged areas unless assistance has been requested. Your presence could hamper relief efforts, and you could endanger yourself.

INSPECTING THE DAMAGE

- After a tornado, be aware of possible structural, electrical or gas-leak hazards in your home. Contact your local city or county building inspectors for information on structural safety codes and standards. They may also offer suggestions on finding a qualified contractor to do work for you.

- In general, if you suspect any damage to your home, shut off electrical power, natural gas and propane tanks to avoid fire, electrocution or explosions.

- If it is dark when you are inspecting your home, use a flashlight rather than a candle or torch to avoid the risk of fire or explosion in a damaged home.

- If you see frayed wiring or sparks, or if there is an odor of something burning, you should immediately shut off the electrical system at the main circuit breaker if you have not done so already.

- If you smell gas or suspect a leak, turn off the main gas valve and leave the house immediately. Notify the gas company, the police or fire departments or State Fire Marshal's office, and do not turn on the lights, light matches, smoke or do anything that could cause a spark. Do not return to your house until you are told it is safe to do so.

SAFETY DURING CLEAN UP

- Wear sturdy shoes or boots, long sleeves and gloves.

- Learn proper safety procedures and operating instructions before operating any gas-powered or electric-powered saws or tools.

- Clean up spilled medicines, drugs, flammable liquids and other potentially hazardous materials.

CHILDREN'S NEEDS

After a tornado, children may be afraid the storm will come back again, and they will be injured or left alone. Children may even interpret disasters as punishment for real or imagined misdeeds. Explain that a tornado is a natural event.

Children will be less likely to experience prolonged fear or anxiety if they know what to expect after a tornado. Here are some suggestions:

- Talk about your own experiences with severe storms, or read aloud a book about tornadoes.

- Encourage your child to express feelings of fear. Listen carefully and show understanding.

- Offer reassurance. Tell your child that the situation is not permanent, and provide physical reassurance through time spent together and displays of affection.

- Include your child in clean-up activities. It is comforting to children to watch the household begin to return to normal and to have a job to do.

Note: Symptoms of anxiety may not appear for weeks or even months after a tornado; they can affect people of any age. If anxiety disrupts daily activities for any member of your family, seek professional assistance through a school counselor, community religious organization, your physician or a licensed professional. Counselors are listed under Mental Health Services in the yellow pages of your telephone directory.

APPENDIX G

Answers to Learning Checkpoints and Review Questions

Chapter 1

LEARNING CHECKPOINT 1

1. False. First aid usually does not replace the need for medical care (calling 9-1-1 or the victim seeing a health care provider). First aid is intended to help the victim until professional help can be given. With minor injuries, however, the victim sometimes does not need to see a health care provider.

2. True. First aid, such as giving CPR or stopping bleeding, can make the difference between the victim living or dying. In other cases, an injury or illness could become worse if first aid is not given before the victim gets professional help.

LEARNING CHECKPOINT 2

1. d. All of the above. These are all important aspects of first aid training.

2. d. All of the above. You should have a first aid kit available wherever an injury may occur.

LEARNING CHECKPOINT 3

1. d

2. d

3. Usually, first at the scene is an emergency medical responder, who may be a law enforcement officer, firefighter, ski patroller or other official with more advanced training.

4. When you call 9-1-1, be ready to give the following information:

   • Your name

   • The phone number you are using

   • The location and number of victims

   • What happened to the victim(s) and any special circumstances

   • The victim's condition

   • The victim's approximate age and sex

   • What is being done for the victim(s)

LEARNING CHECKPOINT 4

1. False. Never move a victim unless faced with a life-threatening situation such as fire. Moving a victim is likely to make an injury worse.

2. d. If your job description requires you to provide first aid, then you have a duty to act.

3. You have consent for an unresponsive adult victim, a child without a guardian present, a victim who nods consent and a child whose parent or guardian consents. All of these are expressed or implied consent. You do not have consent of all victims all the time.

Appendix G • 473

4. You should always do what you are trained to do, ask for consent and stay with the victim until another trained person takes over. Do not try techniques you have not been trained to perform, and do not move most victims by trying to transport them yourself, which may lead to further injury.

REVIEW QUESTIONS

1. d
2. b
3. b
4. a
5. d
6. d
7. c
8. c
9. d
10. a

Chapter 2

LEARNING CHECKPOINT 1

1. False. Bloodborne diseases may be transmitted by contact with several different body fluids, or through objects contaminated with any of those body fluids.

2. True. You can almost always avoid getting an infectious disease if you use precautions such as protective equipment and follow standard precautions.

3. d. All of the above. These are basic precautions based on the assumption that any person's body fluids may carry pathogens, and any contact with these fluids may lead to infectious disease.

4. a (There may be pathogens in the blood on that bandage) and d (a cut on the finger could easily let pathogens enter your body). Shaking hands does not transmit HIV; being vaccinated for HBV prevents infection and does not cause it; coughing does not transmit hepatitis C; and urine does not normally transmit pathogens (unless it contains blood), although to be safe, you should wear gloves when possibly contacting a victim's urine.

5. Signs and symptoms of latex allergy may include skin rashes, hives, itching eyes or skin, flushing, watery or swollen eyes, runny nose or an asthmatic reaction.

LEARNING CHECKPOINT 2

1. False. The first thing to do is check the scene for safety. If you enter an unsafe scene to help a victim, you could become a second victim for EMS professionals to have to care for.

2. d. All of the above. These are all general principles for giving first aid.

3. All 4 of these are dangerous scenes you should not enter. Stay at a safe distance and call 9-1-1.

REVIEW QUESTIONS

1. a
2. d
3. b
4. c
5. b
6. d
7. a
8. d

Chapter 3

LEARNING CHECKPOINT 1

1. heart, lungs
2. d
3. pharynx (throat)
4. a
5. These are cardiac problems that can affect tissue oxygenation: cardiac arrest, myocardial infarction and dysrhythmia. Asthma is a respiratory problem, not a cardiac problem, although it, too, can affect tissue oxygenation.

LEARNING CHECKPOINT 2

1. All 8 listed injuries and illnesses may result in altered mental status.

2. c

3. A dislocation is the movement of one or more bones out of their normal position(s) in a joint.

4. b. A femur fracture can cause severe bleeding, which may be life threatening; the fracture may also cause soft tissue damage in the leg, but this is unlikely to be a life-threatening injury.

5. Even a small break in the skin can be very serious if a pathogen can enter the body, such as those pathogens causing serious illnesses (e.g., HIV).

LEARNING CHECKPOINT 3

1. d

2. People need a tetanus vaccine booster at least every 10 years to ensure immunity against tetanus infection, which may occur after any break in the skin.

3. a

4. c. Blood in urine may result from different injuries or illnesses, but should always be investigated by a health care professional.

REVIEW QUESTIONS

1. d

2. a

3. b

4. c

5. b

6. a

7. a

8. d

9. c

10. c

Chapter 4

LEARNING CHECKPOINT 1

1. b (Check for responsiveness), c (look for normal breathing), a (check for severe bleeding).

2. Do not proceed to the secondary assessment if you find any life-threatening condition in your initial assessment. Instead, care for the life-threatening problem.

3. True. A victim who is coughing is breathing.

LEARNING CHECKPOINT 2

1. d. The secondary assessment is performed after the initial assessment, and only if the victim has no life-threatening conditions requiring care.

2. S = signs and symptoms, A = allergies, M = medications, P = previous problems, L = last food or drink, and E = events leading to current situation.

3. As you examine each part of a victim's body, you are looking for anything out of the ordinary, such as pain, bleeding, a swollen or deformed area, unusual skin color, temperature or moisture or abnormal movement or sensation in an area. (Alternative answer: DOTS – deformities, open injuries, tenderness (pain) and swelling.)

REVIEW QUESTIONS

1. b

2. a

3. c

4. a

5. b

6. a

7. d

Chapter 5

LEARNING CHECKPOINT 1

1. Normal breathing, the heart. Basic life support keeps victims who are not breathing normally (and whose hearts have stopped) alive until they receive advanced medical care.

2. 1-8 years: This is the definition of a child for using an AED. For CPR, a child is 1 year up to the onset of adolescence or puberty.

LEARNING CHECKPOINT 2

1. b. Cardiopulmonary resuscitation. "Cardio" refers to the heart (chest compressions) and "pulmonary" means the lungs (rescue breathing).

2. Risk factors for cardiovascular disease include:

    • Smoking

    • High cholesterol levels

    • Inactivity

    • High blood pressure

    • Family history of heart disease

    • Growing older

3. The first crucial link in the Cardiac Chain of Survival is immediate recognition of cardiac arrest and activation of the emergency response system – calling 9-1-1 to access EMS.

4. Call first for any unresponsive adult not breathing normally. Give 2 minutes of CPR first for an unresponsive infant or child not breathing normally.

LEARNING CHECKPOINT 3

1. a. Rescue breaths move oxygen into the victim's lungs to be transferred into the blood. (Chest compressions move that blood to vital organs.)

2. False. Blowing too hard can put air in the victim's stomach and cause vomiting. Blow only hard enough to make the chest rise.

3. c. Watch the victim's chest rise and fall. This is the best way to confirm that your breaths are going into the victim's lungs.

4. Give each breath for 1 second.

LEARNING CHECKPOINT 4

1. c. Start CPR as soon as you determine the victim is unresponsive and not breathing (unless an AED is present and ready to be used).

2. In an adult or child, the correct position for chest compressions is on the lower half of the breastbone (sternum) in the middle of the chest.

3. Chest compression depth for adults: at least 2 inches but not more than 2.4 inches deep. For an infant or child: at least ⅓ the depth of the chest in an infant (about 1½ inches) or child (about 2 inches).

4. d. 30 to 2 (in all victims regardless of age)

5. a. Use the AED as soon as it is set up and ready. The AED unit will analyze the heart rhythm and determine whether the victim needs a shock to restore regular rhythm or needs CPR.

REVIEW QUESTIONS

1. d

2. b

3. a

4. c

5. b

6. c

7. d

8. d

9. a

10. a

Chapter 6

LEARNING CHECKPOINT 1

1. True. The shock from the AED can restore a normal heart rhythm when the heart is fibrillating.

2. False. There is almost no risk in using an AED because the unit will not advise a shock unless it determines that the victim's heart is fibrillating; in this case, the shock is appropriate and can restore a normal heartbeat.

3. About half of cardiac arrest victims are in fibrillation and require a shock to restore the heart to a normal rhythm.

LEARNING CHECKPOINT 2

1. a. The 2 pads of the AED must be correctly positioned on the victim.

2. c. Give the shock when the unit indicates it, after first making sure no one is in contact with the victim.

3. Resume CPR, beginning with chest compressions.

LEARNING CHECKPOINT 3

1. A situation such as drowning or poisoning may cause cardiac arrest in a child; in which case, the AED may restore a normal rhythm.

2. Do not put the pad on or very near to an implanted pacemaker or defibrillator; place it several inches away.

3. Remove any medication patches with a gloved hand before applying the AED pads.

REVIEW QUESTIONS

1. c

2. c

3. d

4. a

5. b

6. b

7. a

8. b

Chapter 7

LEARNING CHECKPOINT 1

1. Trying to swallow large pieces of food, eating too quickly, eating while engaged in other activities, eating under the influence of alcohol or drugs or eating with dentures.

2. These items on the list should not be given to a child younger than 3:

   - Popcorn

   - Grapes

   - Marshmallows

   - Gum

LEARNING CHECKPOINT 2

1. c. Give abdominal thrusts to a choking adult unless he or she is coughing or able to speak.

2. True. A forcefully coughing victim is getting at least some air, and the coughing may dislodge the obstructing object.

3. True. Without air, a victim will become unresponsive and the heart will stop; the victim then needs CPR.

4. d. All of the above

5. The chest compressions of CPR may dislodge the obstructing object. Even if not, the chest compressions will circulate blood to vital organs.

REVIEW QUESTIONS

1. d

2. a

3. b

4. a

Chapter 8

LEARNING CHECKPOINT 1

1. True. The body can quickly lose much blood from arterial bleeding.

2. False. The first thing to do always is to stop the bleeding.

3. A victim who has been bleeding severely may show the signs of shock, including cool, clammy skin.

4. Many different materials can form a barrier between you and the victim's blood, including bulky clothing or a plastic bag. (This topic is more fully discussed in **Chapter 2**.)

LEARNING CHECKPOINT 2

1. False. Internal bleeding can be life threatening because significant blood may be lost from internal organs or blood vessels. The blood is lost from circulation even if it remains within a body cavity – the fact that it is still inside the body does not mean it reaches vital organs through circulation.

2. All of these can be signs or symptoms of internal bleeding. Significant blood loss may cause shock, resulting in cool, clammy skin and confusion or lightheadedness.

3. d

REVIEW QUESTIONS

1. b

2. a

3. d

4. b

5. c

6. c

7. a

8. d

Chapter 9

LEARNING CHECKPOINT 1

1. False. Never give fluids to a shock victim. The victim is likely to vomit.

2. True. A spinal injury can cause shock if it causes nervous system damage.

3. a. Stop the bleeding. Severe bleeding is life threatening and must be managed before you do anything else.

4. b. Nausea, thirst and clammy skin. These are common signs and symptoms of shock.

5. Calling 9-1-1 is the most important action (after treating any life-threatening injuries) because the victim may need advanced medical care very soon to survive.

LEARNING CHECKPOINT 2

1. True. A victim who has experienced an allergic reaction in the past may have an emergency epinephrine auto-injector you can help him or her use. (Also, tell the arriving EMS crew about the allergy.)

2. True. Allergic reactions to bee and wasp stings are common – and can be severe.

3. d. Breathing problems. These are caused by swelling of the airway and are most serious because they can be life threatening.

4. Help the victim into whatever position is easiest for breathing, which is often sitting part-way up.

REVIEW QUESTIONS

1. a

2. c

3. d

4. b

5. d

6. a

7. b

8. a

9. a

10. c

Chapter 10

LEARNING CHECKPOINT 1

1. Include these actions in wound care: Irrigate minor wounds with running water. Cover any wound with a sterile dressing and bandage. See a health care provider for a deep or puncture wound.

2. Soak a dressing in water if it sticks to the wound.

3. False. Puncture wounds have a greater risk of infection because germs may be trapped inside.

4. False. With all victims, assume there may be pathogens in the blood; follow standard precautions.

5. Use an antibiotic ointment only on abrasions and only if the victim is not allergic to the antibiotic.

6. Signs of wound infection include a red, swollen area, warmth in the area, fever and pus draining from the wound.

7. These victims need to seek medical attention: Jose, because his wound is deep (regardless of the fact that you stopped the bleeding). Rebecca, because any animal bite should be seen by a health care provider. Kim, because significant face wounds should be determined by a health care provider.

8. False. The bandage should be tight enough to put pressure on the wound to control bleeding, but if it is too tight, it may cut off circulation.

9. In this situation, the bandage is too tight and is cutting off her circulation. Unwrap the bandage and reapply it less tightly.

10. c. The bandage should cover the entire dressing to secure it in place. It should be dry and should not be able to be slid to 1 side because a bandage that loose will not adequately protect the wound.

LEARNING CHECKPOINT 2

1. Promote some bleeding of a shallow puncture wound to "wash out" any germs that may be deep inside.

2. False. Leave an impaled object in a wound because removing it could worsen the injury.

3. True. Keep an amputated part cold to help preserve it, but do not put it in direct contact with ice (which could freeze tissue).

4. For an eye injury, you should cover the uninjured eye also, because movement of the uninjured eye will also cause the injured eye to move, which could worsen the injury.

5. 3 ways to remove a small particle from the eye are: Pull the upper eyelid out and down over the lower eyelid, flush the eye with water, try to brush it out with a dampened cotton-tip swab or sterile dressing.

6. False. Let blood or fluid drain out.

7. 10 minutes. During this time, do not tilt the victim's head backward, do not have the victim lie down and do not let the victim speak, swallow, cough or sniff.

8. True. A dentist can usually reimplant a knocked-out tooth if it is kept in a solution such as Hank's Balanced Salt Solution, a specialized tooth-preserving solution, or whole milk, and the victim reaches the dentist soon.

9. False. Rinsing the mouth with cool water will not stop bleeding, but will keep the blood from clotting in the wound.

REVIEW QUESTIONS

1. b

2. a

3. c

4. a

5. a

6. b

7. d

8. b

9. c

10. b

Chapter 11

LEARNING CHECKPOINT 1

1. Following are the most common causes of fires leading to injury or death (list any 3):

   - Smoking

   - Heating

   - Cooking

   - Playing with fire

   - Electrical wiring

   - Open flames

   - Appliances or other equipment

2. Specific actions to prevent fires in the kitchen:

   - Keep a fire extinguisher in the kitchen and know how to use it.

   - Tie back long hair or loose clothing when cooking or working around flames.

   - If food catches on fire in a microwave or toaster oven, leave the food there and turn the appliance off; keep other objects away until the flames go out.

   - Keep electrical cords away from counter edges where children may pull on them.

   - In addition, other general measures such as these can help prevent fires in the kitchen or elsewhere in the home or workplace:

     - Make sure enough smoke detectors are installed, and change batteries twice a year when you change clocks for daylight saving time.

     - Do not allow smoking, or ensure that it is done safely and materials safely extinguished. Never allow smoking in bed.

     - Keep curtains and other flammable objects away from fireplaces and stoves; use fireplace screens.

     - Have chimneys regularly inspected and cleaned to prevent chimney fires.

     - Never store gasoline or other highly flammable liquids indoors.

   - Prevent fires caused by electricity:

     - Keep power cords safely out of the way and away from children.

     - Check appliance cords for damaged areas or fraying.

     - Do not overload electrical outlets or use multiple extension cords.

     - Unplug appliances and extension cords when not in use.

   - Keep children from playing with fire.

3. False. The first thing to do is to make sure everyone is evacuated from the building.

4. 4 factors that affect how serious a burn may be:

   - The type of burn (first-, second- or third-degree)

   - How extensive the burn is (how much body area)

   - The specific body area burned

   - Special circumstances such as the victim's age and health status

LEARNING CHECKPOINT 2

1. False. Never break blisters on a burn, which could cause infection.

2. Small (less than 20% of the body – or 10% in a child).

3. First, stop the fire (have him stop, drop and roll to put out the flames, or cover him with a coat or blanket).

   - Immediately cool the area with running cool or cold, potable water such as tap water to stop the burning (but not more than 20% of his body).

   - Remove any tight clothing or jewelry.

   - Call 9-1-1. Then, treat for shock and cover the burned area with a dressing.

LEARNING CHECKPOINT 3

1. c. Immediately flush the eye with large amounts of running water to stop the burning.

2. First, brush the chemical off the skin to stop the burning. (Wear gloves or otherwise protect yourself.) Remove clothing and jewelry from the area and flush the entire area as quickly as possible with large amounts of running water until EMS personnel arrive. Have someone check the SDS for the chemical involved.

3. False. The signs and symptoms of an injury caused by smoke inhalation may not become manifest for up to 48 hours. Any victim of smoke inhalation should receive medical attention.

LEARNING CHECKPOINT 4

1. False. The first thing to do is to unplug or turn off the electrical power.

2. Unplug the appliance or shut off the circuit breaker. Do not try to pull the victim away from the appliance or the appliance from the victim, because you, too, could be shocked.

3. a. Call 9-1-1 first. You cannot safely reach the victim or move the high-voltage wires yourself – you could make the situation worse.

REVIEW QUESTIONS

1. a
2. b
3. d
4. c
5. d
6. a
7. a
8. b
9. c
10. d

Chapter 12

LEARNING CHECKPOINT 1

1. Signs of a possible skull fracture include a deformed area of skull, a depressed area felt during your examination, blood or fluid loss from the ears or nose and an object impaling the skull. Do not put pressure on a bleeding wound with skull fracture.

2. False. Symptoms of brain injuries including concussion, bleeding or swelling can be variable and may be confusing. Call 9-1-1 with any suspected brain injury.

3. Headache, memory loss, dizziness or confusion and nausea and vomiting.

4. d. None of the above. No one assessment can always determine the presence of a spinal injury. Do not assume a victim without specific symptoms does not have a possible spinal injury.

5. Signs and symptoms of a serious brain injury may occur as late as 48 hours after a blow to the head.

LEARNING CHECKPOINT 2

1. True. Suspect a spinal injury in a victim with a head injury because head trauma may also injure the spine.

2. b. Check for breathing without moving the victim if you suspect a spinal injury. Move the victim only if necessary.

3. Always suspect a spinal injury in these situations: fall from a roof, motor vehicle crash and a blow to the head.

4. Signs and symptoms of a spinal injury include tingling in the hands, breathing problems and a twisted neck.

5. a. Call 9-1-1 for all victims who may have a spinal injury.

6. Stabilize the head of a victim with a suspected spinal injury in the position in which you find the victim, because movement could worsen the injury.

7. Vomits. The victim could choke on the vomit, and therefore, must be rolled onto his side, while still supported at the head. Otherwise, there is no reason to move the victim and risk further injury.

8. Stabilize the victim's head by holding it still with the victim staying in the driver's seat. Call for someone to call for 9-1-1. Monitor the victim's breathing.

REVIEW QUESTIONS

1. a

2. b

3. c

4. d

5. d

6. a

7. b

8. d

9. c

Chapter 13

LEARNING CHECKPOINT 1

1. False. Loosely bandage a pillow or other support over the ribs. A tight bandage could cause further injury or breathing problems.

2. d. All of the above: Preventing movement of the arm helps prevent movement of that side of the chest. Preventing movement will also ease pain. A sling and binder may be used to immobilize the arm.

3. Do not remove the impaled screwdriver, which could worsen the injury. Instead, use bulky dressings to stabilize it, and bandage around it. Then, call 9-1-1.

4. Treat a sucking chest wound with a dressing around the wound that does not block the airflow in or out of the wound. Then, keep the victim lying down and call 9-1-1.

LEARNING CHECKPOINT 2

1. The signs and symptoms of a closed abdominal injury include bruising and a swollen abdomen.

2. A victim with an open or closed abdominal wound should lie on his or her back (or in the position found if unresponsive and breathing normally).

3. True. Keep a victim in shock from becoming cold. If necessary, cover him with a coat or blanket, and place something between him and the cold ground.

4. d. Cover organs protruding from a wound with a nonadherent dressing and plastic wrap to keep the organs from drying out.

5. Call 9-1-1 for any victim with an open or closed abdominal wound.

LEARNING CHECKPOINT 3

1. Movement. Movement of a fractured pelvis could increase the bleeding and worsen the injury.

2. True. Pelvic bones themselves may bleed heavily, or internal organs may be damaged and bleed profusely.

3. False. With a pelvis fracture, do not move the affected leg.

REVIEW QUESTIONS

1. a

2. b

3. d

4. c

5. c

6. b

7. b

8. d

Chapter 14

LEARNING CHECKPOINT 1

1. a. Most musculoskeletal injuries. You do not need to know the exact nature of the injury before using RICE.

2. False. Do not put a cold pack directly on the skin because tissue damage could occur. Place a pad or cloth between the cold pack and the skin.

3. d. All of the above

4. a. Rest the ankle.

   b. Put an ice or cold pack on the injured area (observe time limits).

   c. Compress the ankle with a roller bandage (over the cold pack).

   d. Elevate the ankle.

LEARNING CHECKPOINT 2

1. True. Call 9-1-1 for any serious fractures or fractures of large bones.

2. c. Immobilize the joints above and below a fracture area to keep the fractured bone from moving.

3. True. Shock may result in a fracture from blood loss or pain.

4. The signs and symptoms of a bone or joint injury include a deformed area, pain, swelling and an inability to use the body part.

5. False. Moving or exerting a sprained joint will only make the injury worse.

LEARNING CHECKPOINT 3

1. False. Use ice or a cold pack, but remove it after 20 minutes (or 10 minutes if it produces discomfort), and wait at least 30 minutes before re-applying it.

2. False. Treat a muscle contusion with a cold pack, compression bandage and elevation of the limb.

3. False. An area of skin discoloration can be caused by a fracture, dislocation or sprain as well as by a contusion.

4. Gently stretch the muscle, apply a cold pack and massage the muscle.

REVIEW QUESTIONS

1. d
2. a
3. a
4. b
5. c
6. d
7. b
8. a
9. c
10. b

Chapter 15

LEARNING CHECKPOINT 1

1. You can make a rigid splint from many different materials, including a board, a piece of plastic or metal, a rolled newspaper or magazine or thick cardboard.

2. Following are all actions to take when using a splint:

    • Pad the splint.

    • Put a cold pack around the splint.

    • Dress an open wound before splinting.

    • Splint in the position found.

3. Signs that circulation has been cut off in an extremity below the splint include swelling, skin cold and pale or discolored and tingling or numbness.

4. 2 things you should not do when contemplating putting a victim's arm in a sling are:

    • Do not move the arm into position for a sling if this causes more pain.

    • Do not cover the fingers inside the sling, because you need to check circulation.

LEARNING CHECKPOINT 2

1. Soft

2. Elbow, hand

3. a. A binder provides additional support and helps prevent movement of the arm.

LEARNING CHECKPOINT 3

1. You do not need to know for certain if the bone is broken, as there are signs and symptoms of a fracture (pain, inability to move the leg). Take these actions:

    • Have the victim stay lying down and immobilize the leg.

    • Call 9-1-1.

    • Put ice or a cold pack on the area.

    • Splint the leg if help may be delayed, using either an anatomic splint or a rigid splint from the upper leg to the foot.

2. d. A victim with a fracture of the femur may experience severe bleeding that can cause shock. The injury may be either open or closed.

3. With any fracture of an extremity, ideally, the fracture should be splinted on both sides, using 2 rigid splints.

REVIEW QUESTIONS

1. d

2. d

3. a

4. c

5. c

6. a

7. d

8. d

Chapter 16

LEARNING CHECKPOINT 1

1. True. With an unknown sudden illness, the victim should not eat or drink.

2. The common signs and symptoms of a heart attack include shortness of breath, chest discomfort, pain or pressure, sweating, indigestion, pale skin and dizziness.

3. The chest pain of angina usually lasts only a few minutes and is recognized as angina by the person experiencing it. If it persists 10 minutes or more after taking prescribed medication, or the victim has other signs and symptoms of a heart attack, give first aid as for a heart attack.

4. Call 9-1-1. Do not delay, because the victim needs advanced medical care immediately.

5. a. Fluids drain from the mouth. A stroke victim may vomit or drool, possibly causing choking if the fluid does not drain out.

LEARNING CHECKPOINT 2

1. False. You do not need to know the specific cause of the breathing difficulty but can care for the victim anyway: Call 9-1-1, help the victim to rest in the position for easiest breathing, assist with any prescribed medications and be prepared to give basic life support.

2. d. Let the victim find the position for easiest breathing.

3. The best thing an asthma victim can do during an attack is to use his or her prescribed inhaler; the medication should control the attack.

4. False.

5. Call 9-1-1 for a hyperventilating victim if breathing does not return to normal within a few minutes.

LEARNING CHECKPOINT 3

1. Call 9-1-1 for a victim who faints if the victim does not regain responsiveness soon or faints repeatedly.

2. False. Lay the victim down and raise his or her legs, not the head, 6-12 inches.

3. c. Place something flat and soft under the victim's head. Do not try to hold the victim still, and do not put anything between the teeth.

4. Call 9-1-1 for a seizure victim:

    • if the seizure lasts more than 5 minutes.

    • if the victim is not known to have epilepsy.

    • if the victim recovers very slowly or has trouble breathing.

    • if the victim has another seizure.

    • if the victim is pregnant.

    • if the victim is wearing another medical ID.

    • if the victim is injured.

5. Seek urgent medical care for a young child whose abdomen is swollen and feels hard.

6. Common signs and symptoms of a low blood sugar diabetic emergency include dizziness, hunger, clumsiness, sweating and confusion.

7. If you cannot judge whether the victim has low or high blood sugar, give glucose tablets or sugar to the victim as for low blood sugar. Seek medical attention if the victim does not improve within 15 minutes or symptoms become worse.

REVIEW QUESTIONS

1. d
2. a
3. c
4. a
5. b
6. d
7. c
8. a
9. d
10. b

Chapter 17

LEARNING CHECKPOINT 1

1. The common signs and symptoms of a swallowed poison include nausea, dizziness, drowsiness, vomiting and unresponsiveness.

2. Give the victim lots of fluids to drink.

3. c. Move the victim to fresh air.

4. This is likely a poisoning situation. Call 9-1-1 and give basic life support as needed. Put the child in the recovery position. Tell the 9-1-1 dispatcher and the arriving crew about the open cleaning product.

LEARNING CHECKPOINT 2

1. False. Use soap and water to wash the area to minimize the reaction.

2. See a health care provider for severe reactions or swelling of the face or genitals, or signs of infection (fever, pus).

3. a. Hydrocortisone cream. (Also, colloid oatmeal, baking soda paste or calamine lotion.)

REVIEW QUESTIONS

1. b
2. a
3. d
4. c
5. a
6. d
7. d
8. c
9. b
10. b

Chapter 18

LEARNING CHECKPOINT 1

1. a. Remember: Alcohol is still a drug even though legal for those of age.

2. Because alcohol and other drug abuse typically begin at young ages, prevention efforts focus on children and adolescents.

3. The following are appropriate actions to help prevent misuse of prescribed drugs:

   • Read product information that comes with prescription medications.

   • Keep medications in their original labeled containers.

   • Ensure that a person with diminished judgment cannot unintentionally take too much medication. In addition:

      • Always take medications as prescribed – not only when feeling symptoms. Many medical conditions requiring drug treatment do not cause noticeable symptoms.

      • Never use medications prescribed for someone else – even when you are certain you have the same condition as the person with the medication. People vary in their responses to medications, and only a health care provider can know what medication is appropriate for you.

LEARNING CHECKPOINT 2

1. For an intoxicated person who apparently has passed out, take these actions:

    - Check the person for responsiveness and normal breathing.

    - Position an unresponsive victim who is breathing normally in the recovery position; be prepared for vomiting.

    - Monitor the victim and provide BLS if necessary.

    - Check for injuries or illness.

    - Call 9-1-1 if the victim's breathing is irregular, if seizures occur or if the victim cannot be roused (coma).

    - In a cold environment, protect the person from hypothermia.

2. b

3. The following are appropriate actions to take for a person with a drug or medication overdose:

    - Call 9-1-1 or the Poison Control Center.

    - Check for injuries that may require first aid.

    - Try to keep the person awake and talking.

    - Try to find out what the person took.

    In addition:

    - Position an unresponsive victim in the recovery position because vomiting is likely – not on his or her back.

    - Because of the risk of being injured, never try to restrain a potentially violent person – leave this to law enforcement personnel.

    - Do not try to induce vomiting in any victim at any time unless so instructed by the Poison Control Center.

REVIEW QUESTIONS

1. a

2. d

3. b

4. a

5. c

6. c

7. a

8. d

Chapter 19

LEARNING CHECKPOINT 1

1. a. See a health care provider immediately. Do not wait until you develop symptoms, and do not try to capture the animal. You cannot kill the rabies germs by treating the wound site.

2. Human bites can be serious because human mouths usually contain many germs.

LEARNING CHECKPOINT 2

1. Have the victim stay calm and lie down with the bitten area below the level of the heart. Call 9-1-1. Wash the bite wound with soap and water. For a poisonous snakebite on an extremity, wrap the limb with an elastic bandage.

2. Call 9-1-1 for a spider bite if the victim has trouble breathing or the bite is from a brown recluse spider.

3. Tweezers

4. b. "Bull's-eye" rash is a common early sign of Lyme disease. A tick bite does not usually cause pain or burning at the site. Fever may occur with Lyme disease, but usually not until much later.

LEARNING CHECKPOINT 3

1. A credit card or piece of rigid plastic

2. Because she seems to be having an allergic reaction to the bee sting, you should first call 9-1-1, ask if she has an epinephrine auto-injector, monitor breathing and treat for shock.

3. c. Vinegar (or baking soda paste if vinegar is not available) can help stop the stinging. Boiling water would cause a burn. Ketchup and mayonnaise are not treatments.

REVIEW QUESTIONS

1. d

2. d

3. a

4. c

5. b

6. a

7. c

8. c

9. b

10. d

Chapter 20

LEARNING CHECKPOINT 1

1. False. Rubbing frostbitten skin can cause damage. Instead, warm it against warm skin or in warm water.

2. Waxy white, gray, yellow or bluish

3. Warm his ears with your warm hands (gently). Protect the ears from being rubbed on clothing or other objects. The victim needs immediate medical care.

LEARNING CHECKPOINT 2

1. False. Hypothermia can occur any time the climate is cool enough to feel cold.

2. True. Shivering does produce body heat but is not always enough. If the victim has signs and symptoms of hypothermia, help warm his body even if he is shivering.

3. d. Remove damp clothing and warm a hypothermic person with a blanket. Do not let him drink alcohol, and do not warm him too quickly with a heat source such as a fire or a hot shower.

4. Answers may vary depending on equipment the first aider is thought to have. Ideally, get the hypothermic victim out of the cold environment into a tent. Remove his cold, damp clothing and get him into dry clothing and a sleeping bag. If there is a stove, heat water to make him a warm drink.

LEARNING CHECKPOINT 3

1. False. Have the victim rest comfortably and drink a carbohydrate-electrolyte drink.

2. b. Give a carbohydrate-electrolyte drink or water to drink because the body needs fluids.

3. False. Do not give salt tablets. Give a carbohydrate-electrolyte drink if the victim is awake and alert.

4. Fluids

5. Three ways to cool a heat exhaustion victim:

   a. Put wet cloths on the forehead and body.

   b. Sponge the skin with cool water.

   c. Spray the skin with water from a spray bottle and fan the area.

6. First, get him out of the Sun and into a cool place. Loosen or remove unnecessary clothing. Give a carbohydrate-electrolyte drink or water. Have him lie down and rest. Cool his body with one of the methods previously described.

LEARNING CHECKPOINT 4

1. False. Heat stroke is a medical emergency, and the victim may still be at risk. Call 9-1-1.

2. Call 9-1-1 for all instances of heat stroke.

3. A heat stroke victim may be acting very confused or disoriented, dizzy and irrational; the victim may become unresponsive.

4. a. Have plenty of nonalcoholic fluids present. Be sure there is a shady spot for resting.

   b. Tell everyone to avoid too much exertion (especially those who are older or overweight). Make sure you keep drinking enough fluids. Stop and rest in the shade if you start feeling overheated. Tell everyone to watch for signs and symptoms of heat exhaustion in others: heavy sweating, thirst, fatigue, heat cramps, headache or dizziness, or nausea and vomiting. (Also, be alert for the signs and symptoms of heat stroke – but it is better to stop and treat the person in the earlier stages of heat exhaustion.)

   c. Call 9-1-1 for a heat stroke victim.

REVIEW QUESTIONS

1. a
2. d
3. b
4. c
5. a
6. c
7. b
8. b
9. a
10. d

Chapter 21

LEARNING CHECKPOINT 1

1. d

2. All of the conditions listed may cause altered mental status.

3. Following are guidelines to help calm an emotional victim:

   - Tell the victim who you are and say you are there to help. Avoid seeming judgmental.

   - Do not assume the victim is intoxicated, using drugs or otherwise impaired.

   - Reassure the victim that help is on the way (after 9-1-1 has been called).

   - Ask the victim for his or her name, and use it when speaking to him or her.

   - If possible, try to involve the victim's friend or family member present at the scene.

   - Let the victim tell you what he or she thinks is wrong.

   - Let the victim know you understand his or her concerns.

   - Make eye contact with the victim.

   - Speak in a caring, reassuring voice, but do not give false reassurances or lie about the victim's condition.

   - Do not argue with the victim. Show that you understand the victim's concerns by repeating or rephrasing what the victim tells you.

   - If the victim seems irrational or delusional, do not make statements that support his or her false beliefs, but do not challenge them either.

   - Stay a safe distance away from the victim until your help is accepted. If the victim does not accept your help, do not attempt to restrain or force care on him or her.

   - Tell the victim what you plan to do before doing it.

   - Move calmly and slowly, touching the victim only as necessary.

4. False. It is better to encourage the victim to talk: Acknowledge that the person seems sad and ask why.

5. False. This is a common myth. Talking about suicide is a warning sign that the person is contemplating suicide.

6. To ensure your own safety and get help fast, take these steps in this order:

    a. Do not enter the scene if there is a risk to your safety. Encourage others present at the scene to withdraw.

    b. Call 9-1-1.

    c. Talk to the person calmly and quietly, and try to divert the person from any violent action by keeping him or her talking.

LEARNING CHECKPOINT 2

1. c

2. Following are common characteristics of victims of domestic violence:

    • They love their partners.

    • They feel guilty and may blame themselves for the violence.

    • They often have low self-esteem.

    • They depend emotionally and/or financially on their partners.

    In addition:

    • They are afraid of their partners.

    • They are often isolated from family and friends.

3. d

4. Important first aid actions for a victim injured in a rape include:

    • Be sensitive to the victim's psychological trauma and provide emotional support.

    • Ensure that 9-1-1 has been called.

    • Ensure privacy for the victim.

    • Try to involve a friend or family member of the victim or at least a first aider of the same sex.

    • Give needed first aid and stay with the victim until help arrives.

    • Preserve evidence of the rape.

REVIEW QUESTIONS

1. b

2. a

3. d

4. False

5. c

6. d

7. a

8. b

9. a

10. a

Chapter 22

LEARNING CHECKPOINT 1

1. Following are generally accepted guidelines for a healthy pregnancy:

    • Minimize caffeine and alcohol consumption.

    • Take dietary supplements as recommended.

    In addition:

    • Eat a healthy diet.

    • Accept normal weight gain.

    • Stop smoking.

    • Do not use illicit drugs.

    • Get exercise.

    • Rest sufficiently.

    • Prevent injury.

2. b

3. b

LEARNING CHECKPOINT 2

1. Call 9-1-1 for heavy vaginal bleeding. Calm the woman and help her into a comfortable position. Give the woman a towel or sanitary napkins to absorb the blood, but do not try to pack the vagina.

2. a

3. All 6 of the signs and symptoms listed could indicate a possible problem with the pregnancy; the woman should see her health care provider for any of these.

LEARNING CHECKPOINT 3

1. False. Childbirth is a natural process that seldom involves complications or requires elaborate medical care.

2. Signs and symptoms that childbirth may occur soon include:

   • Woman feels urge to push.

   • Amniotic sac has ruptured.

   • Infant's head is crowning.

   In addition:

   • Contractions are less than 5 minutes apart.

   • Childbirth may occur sooner in a woman who has given birth before.

3. d

4. When assisting with childbirth, follow these guidelines for things *not* to do:

   • Do not try to delay the birth by having the woman hold her legs together or any other maneuver.

   • Do not place your hands or anything else in the woman's vagina.

   • Do not interfere with the childbirth or touch the infant until the head is completely out.

   • Do not pull on the head or shoulders.

   • Do not try to wash the infant's skin, eyes or ears.

   • Do not pull on the umbilical cord in an effort to pull out the afterbirth.

5. c

6. True. Some bleeding does normally occur with childbirth and delivery of the placenta. If bleeding does not stop soon after delivery of the placenta, massaging the abdomen may help the uterus to contract and stop bleeding.

REVIEW QUESTIONS

1. b

2. b

3. a

4. d

5. c

6. d

7. b

8. c

9. c

10. d

Chapter 23

LEARNING CHECKPOINT 1

1. Rescue or medical help may be delayed in emergencies in situations such as this:

   • Rural areas

   • When hiking or camping in wilderness areas

   • When boating

   • During or after a natural disaster

2. d

LEARNING CHECKPOINT 2

1. The following are important principles for planning a trip into a wilderness location:

   • Do not go alone.

   • Tell someone where you are going and when you will return.

- Take more food and water than you expect to need.

In addition:

- Take a first aid kit equipped for the location.

- Be prepared for weather emergencies.

- Know where you are at all times.

- Do not use alcohol or other drugs.

- Study the location in advance.

2. False. When dealing with a complex emergency in a remote location, the leader should be flexible, continually reassess the situation and change the plan as needed.

3. A cell phone may have a dead battery, may not have a signal or may stop working because of temperature extremes, moisture or other problems.

4. c

LEARNING CHECKPOINT 3

1. d

2. False. If you suspect a victim in a remote location may have a spinal injury, or if it is unlikely that help will arrive soon, you should assess the victim more carefully to see if a spinal injury can be ruled out so that the victim can move.

3. False. The condition of a victim with a brain injury will not improve by itself. This is a medical emergency – call for a helicopter if possible, or if you cannot communicate the need for rescue, consider evacuating the victim if it can be done safely.

4. b. It will be difficult to warm the victim and keep him or her warm while walking or being carried through a cold environment for 3 hours; with severe hypothermia, he would probably not be able to walk, and 3 people generally cannot effectively carry someone. It is better to build an emergency shelter and warm the victim with dry clothing, extra clothing from others, warm fluids and even the body warmth of the other hikers.

5. 30 minutes

LEARNING CHECKPOINT 4

1. 3-5 gallons

2. The typical signs and symptoms of acute mountain sickness include:

- Headache

- Dizziness

- Fatigue

- Nausea

REVIEW QUESTIONS

1. d

2. b

3. b

4. d

5. a

6. c

7. a

8. b

9. d

10. c

Chapter 24

LEARNING CHECKPOINT 1

1. a. Get everyone out. Any delay spent calling 9-1-1, using a fire extinguisher or taking other actions could result in someone being harmed by the fire.

2. d. All of the above. Stay low because there will be more oxygen near the floor. Feel doors before opening them to avoid entering a fiery area, and use the stairs, because a power outage caused by the fire could stall the elevator.

3. True. OSHA guidelines for fire prevention and safety apply in most workplaces.

4. False. Stay away from potentially hazardous materials; call 9-1-1 and let the professionals clean up the spill.

5. True. But because you cannot usually know if fumes from a spilled liquid are poisonous, act as if they are.

6. Support the victim's head and neck, but do not move the victim unless there is an immediate threat. Give basic life support as needed.

7. c. The safest order in which to attempt a water rescue is reach-throw-go.

LEARNING CHECKPOINT 2

1. False. A victim with only a broken arm is considered stable and can walk, and is therefore, a third priority.

2. True. Victims with life-threatening injuries are the first priority.

3. Following are the ranked priorities for these 4 victims:

   First – b. A man on the ground with no apparent external injuries but who is unresponsive

   Second – d. A man leaning against the rubble, looking very pale, who says he feels nauseous

   Third – a. A woman with a bruised face and abrasions on her arms, who is walking around holding her bleeding forehead

   Fourth – c. A man who is not breathing, whose chest has caved in under a steel beam, and is surrounded by a pool of blood

LEARNING CHECKPOINT 3

1. Consider moving a victim in these situations:

   • Fire is present.

   • There is a strong smell of natural gas in the room.

   • One victim is lying on top of another.

2. d. The blanket drag is an effective way to move a victim by yourself and provide some support for the victim's head.

REVIEW QUESTIONS

1. c
2. d
3. d
4. a
5. b
6. c
7. c
8. b
9. a
10. d

Chapter 25

REVIEW QUESTIONS

1. a
2. c
3. a
4. d
5. b

Chapter 26

REVIEW QUESTIONS

1. c
2. b
3. d
4. a
5. b

Glossary

A

Abandonment: a type of negligence that occurs if someone who has begun to provide first aid then stops and the injury or illness becomes worse.

Abdomen: the area below the ribs and above the hips.

Abrasion: a wound in which the top layer of skin is scraped off.

Abuse: an intentional inflicting of injury or suffering on someone under the abuser's power, such as a child, spouse or elderly parent.

Acquired immunodeficiency syndrome (AIDS): a sometimes fatal disease caused by the human immunodeficiency virus (HIV).

Acute mountain sickness: severe form of altitude sickness.

Acute myocardial infarction (AMI): a condition involving a sudden reduced blood flow to the heart muscle; heart attack.

Advanced cardiac life support (ACLS): medical procedures needed to restore a heartbeat beyond the procedures of basic life support.

Airborne transmission: a process by which a pathogen existing in an infected person is transmitted into a different person through the air, usually via small fluid droplets the infected person coughs or sneezes out.

Airway: the path air takes from the nose and mouth to the lungs.

Airway adjunct: a shaped tube-like device inserted into the mouth or nose that helps keep a victim's airway open during resuscitation or until the victim receives advanced medical attention.

Airway obstruction: a condition in which the victim's airway is partially or completely obstructed by the tongue, vomit or other body tissue or fluids, or a foreign object, preventing the flow of air to the lungs; choking.

Allergen: a substance that causes an allergic reaction in a person.

Allergic contact dermatitis: an allergic skin reaction.

Aloe vera: a type of plant; usually refers to a lotion or gel made with the plant's extract, which may be soothing for first-degree burns.

Altered mental status: a phrase used to describe a change from a person's normal responsiveness and awareness, including confusion, disorientation, dizziness, drowsiness or partial or complete unresponsiveness.

Altitude sickness: a syndrome caused by low oxygen levels at high altitudes, causing headache, dizziness, fatigue, shortness of breath, nausea and other symptoms.

Alveoli: tiny air sacs in the lungs where oxygen and carbon dioxide pass into and out of small blood vessels.

Amniotic fluid: the fluid surrounding the embryo and fetus within the amniotic sac; often called "water."

Amniotic sac: a membrane surrounding the embryo and fetus in the uterus, containing amniotic fluid.

Amputation: the complete cutting or tearing off of all or part of an extremity: a finger or toe, hand or foot, arm or leg.

Anaphylactic shock: shock resulting from an extreme allergic reaction, typically to an insect sting, a particular food, medication or some other substance; also called anaphylaxis.

Anaphylaxis: another term for anaphylactic shock.

Anatomic splint: splinting one part of the body to another part.

Angina pectoris: chest pain caused by heart disease, usually occurring after intense activity or exertion; often simply called angina.

Ankle drag: an emergency move for an unresponsive victim or one who cannot walk, but which provides no head support for a potential spinal injury.

Antibiotic: a medication that kills bacteria.

Antivenin: an antidote to the poisonous venom of a particular species, administered to counteract the effects of a bite or sting.

Anxiety: fear or apprehension of impending danger, usually producing physical signs and symptoms.

Arrhythmia: an irregular heartbeat; sometimes called dysrhythmia.

Arteries: blood vessels that carry oxygenated blood from the heart to body tissues.

Aspiration: the movement of vomit or other fluids or solids into the lungs.

Assessment: the process of checking a victim for conditions requiring treatment or first aid, divided into an initial assessment for life-threatening conditions and a secondary assessment for other problems.

Asthma: a chronic disease in which at times the airway becomes narrow and the person has difficulty breathing.

Atherosclerosis: a narrowing and "hardening" of the arteries caused by plaque.

Aura: a generalized sensation or a hallucinated sensation involving any of the senses that occurs before a seizure.

Automated external defibrillator (AED): a device used to shock a fibrillating heart to return it to a regular rhythm.

Avulsion: an open wound in which an area of skin or other soft tissue is torn partially from the body.

B

Bag mask or bag-valve-mask (BVM): a resuscitation mask unit connected to an airbag that is squeezed to provide air to a nonbreathing victim.

Barrier device: a device such as a pocket mask or face shield used to provide a barrier between a victim and first aider when giving rescue breathing to reduce the risk of disease transmission.

Basic life support (BLS): first aid given to a victim with a life-threatening problem of the airway or circulation; refers to rescue breathing, CPR, and use of AED.

Beach drag: a method for removing an unresponsive victim from shallow water that provides some head support for a potential spinal injury.

Behavioral emergency: a situation in which the victim's behavior, whether caused by injury or illness or by personality or mental health factors, results in an emergency situation, such as potential suicide or violence.

Bladder: the organ that stores urine until it is passed to the outside.

Blanket drag: an emergency move for an unresponsive victim or one who cannot walk, providing some support for the victim's head as the rescuer pulls the blanket.

Blood pressure: the pressure of blood on the walls of blood vessels.

Bloodborne disease: a disease that can be transmitted from one person to another through contact with the infected person's blood or certain other body fluids.

Bloodborne transmission: a process by which a pathogen existing in an infected person's blood or other body fluid is transmitted into a different person through contact with that body fluid.

Body mass index (BMI): a measure of weight in relation to a person's height, used to determine overweight and obesity.

Body substance isolation (BSI): an infection-control concept, used primarily in health care facilities, that assumes that any body fluid or moist body tissue is potentially infectious.

Body system: a group of organs that work together to perform a major body function.

Brachial pulse: the pulse felt over the brachial artery in an infant's upper arm on the inside about midway between the shoulder and elbow.

Breech presentation: the position in which the infant's buttocks or feet move first into the birth canal rather than the head; also called breech birth.

Bronchi: (singular: bronchus) the passageways from the trachea to the lungs.

Bronchodilator: a drug that relaxes the muscles of the airway, often used in an inhaler by people with asthma.

Burn: damage caused to skin and other tissue by heat, chemicals or electricity.

C

Capillaries: tiny blood vessels between the arteries and veins where oxygen and nutrients in the blood pass into tissues and carbon dioxide passes into the blood.

Carbon monoxide: an invisible, odorless, tasteless and highly lethal gas resulting from fires, gasoline engines, furnaces and other causes.

Cardiac: refers to the heart.

Cardiac arrest: the condition in which the heart stops beating effectively.

Cardiac chain of survival: a concept emphasizing five steps needed for cardiac arrest victims: immediate recognition of cardiac arrest and activation of the emergency response system, early CPR that emphasizes chest compressions, rapid defibrillation if indicated, effective advanced life support and integrated post-cardiac arrest care.

Cardiogenic shock: shock resulting when any condition, such as heart attack, causes the heart function to be reduced to the point that blood is not circulating sufficiently.

Cardiopulmonary resuscitation (CPR): a basic life support procedure for a victim who is not breathing and has no heartbeat, consisting of chest compressions combined with rescue breathing.

Cardiovascular system: the body system that moves the blood, which transports both oxygen and nutrients, throughout the body to supply cells and remove wastes.

Carotid pulse: the pulse felt over the carotid artery in a neck of an adult or child.

Central nervous system: the part of the nervous system formed by the brain and spinal cord.

Cervix: the lower part of the uterus, opening into the vagina.

Chest compressions: a technique used in CPR to circulate the blood, or on a choking victim to expel an object.

Choking: a physical obstruction of the airway, such as by food or the tongue, in an unresponsive person.

Cholesterol: a fatty substance the body needs to carry out important functions but that in high levels is a risk factor for cardiovascular disease.

Chronic: refers to an illness or health condition, often incurable, that the person has had for some time; chronic conditions often make the individual more susceptible to the effects of injuries or sudden illnesses.

Chronic obstructive pulmonary diseases (COPD): a group of respiratory diseases, including emphysema and chronic bronchitis, in which breathing can become difficult.

Cincinnati Prehospital Stroke Scale (CPSS): a screening process for rapid identification of a stroke outside the hospital.

Closed injury: an injury in which the skin is not broken.

Clothes drag: an emergency move for an unresponsive victim or one who cannot walk, providing some support for the victim's head against the pulled clothing and rescuer's hands.

Clotting: the process in which fibrin and platelets clump together with other blood cells to seal a leak in a blood vessel.

Competent: the victim is able to understand what is happening and the implications of his or her decision to receive or refuse first aid.

Concussion: a type of brain injury resulting from a blow to the head, involving a temporary impairment of brain function but usually not permanent damage.

Confidentiality: the general principle that one should not give out private information about a victim to anyone except for those caring for the victim.

Consent: the victim's permission for you to provide first aid.

Contraction: one of a series of rhythmic tightening actions of the uterine muscles during labor.

Coronary heart disease: blockage of vessels supplying heart muscle with blood, often leading to heart attack.

Cradle carry: an emergency move for a light, unresponsive victim or one who cannot walk, in which the rescuer carries the victim in his or her arms.

Cramp: a tightening of a muscle that usually results from prolonged use.

Cravats: strips of cloth used to tie a splint.

Crepitus: a grating sensation felt or heard when fractured bone ends rub against each other.

Crowning: the stage of childbirth when the infant's head is passing into the birth canal and is visible.

D

Defibrillation: the process of administering an electric shock to a fibrillating heart to restore a normal heart rhythm.

Dependence: a pattern of physical and behavioral changes resulting from frequent use of a substance, including tolerance to its effects and the occurrence of withdrawal symptoms after cessation.

Depressant: a drug that slows certain central nervous system functions and produces dulled feelings.

Depression: a temporary state or a chronic psychological illness involving feelings of sadness, hopelessness and worthlessness often along with physical symptoms.

Dermis: the middle layer of skin, damaged in second- and third-degree burns.

Diabetes: a metabolic disorder in which not enough insulin is produced or the body has developed resistance in the use of insulin, resulting in blood sugar (glucose) levels not being well regulated by the body.

Diaphragm: a muscle between the abdomen and lungs that moves with breathing.

Direct contact: disease transmission that occurs when someone directly contacts an infected person, or fluids or substances from that person.

Disinfectant: a substance, such as a bleach solution, that kills most pathogens on contaminated surfaces.

Dislocation: movement of one or more bones out of their normal position in a joint, usually with ligament damage.

Dispatcher: an EMS professional who answers 9-1-1 calls, determines the nature of the emergency and sends the appropriate emergency personnel to the scene.

Duty to act: a legal obligation to provide first aid as trained, obligated by one's job requirements or role as a child's parent or guardian.

E

Elder abuse: physical, emotional, or financial abuse or neglect inflicted on someone older than 60, often by someone else in the home.

Electrodes: the pads of an automated external defibrillator (AED), which attach to the main unit with cables and deliver the shock to a victim's chest when indicated.

Embryo: a developing human from the time of implantation in the uterus through the first 8 weeks.

Emergency medical responder: formerly called a first responder, a professional with BLS training who often arrives first at the scene of a medical emergency, such as a police officer, fire fighter, industrial safety officer, ski patroller or similar professional who is often close to the scene.

Emergency Medical Service (EMS): a comprehensive network of professionals linked together to provide appropriate levels of medical care for victims of injury or sudden illness.

Emergency medical technician (EMT): emergency personnel trained to give prehospital medical treatment to injured or ill victims and to transport victims to advanced care facilities.

Emergency position indicating radio beacon (EPIRB): an emergency device for marine uses that emits a signal that is picked up by satellites and relayed to rescue personnel.

Endocrine system: the body system that produces hormones that help regulate many body functions.

Enhanced 9-1-1: an EMS system that automatically provides the dispatcher with the caller's phone number and the location of a land telephone line being used.

Entrance/exit wounds: terms referring to two related wounds, such as burned areas on the body where electricity entered and left the body or wounds caused by a bullet entering and exiting the body.

Epidermis: the outer layer of skin damaged in first-degree burns.

Epiglottis: a tissue flap that prevents solids and liquids from entering the trachea.

Epinephrine auto-injector: an emergency epinephrine auto-injector used for anaphylactic reactions.

Esophagus: the tube that carries food to the stomach from the throat.

Evacuation: the process of removing a victim from a remote location that cannot be reached by ambulance, including carrying the victim out and holicopter rescue.

Evisceration: protrusion of abdominal organs through an open wound in the abdominal wall.

Expressed consent: consent explicitly given by the victim for first aid.

External respiration: the process by which oxygen enters the blood from air that is inhaled and carbon dioxide exits the blood into air that is breathed out.

Extremities: the arms and legs.

F

Family radio service (FRS): small short-distance radios (i.e., walky-talkies) that do not require a special license.

Febrile seizure: a seizure caused by high fever.

Femur: the long bone of the upper leg.

Fetal alcohol syndrome: a pattern of growth and development problems found in infants whose mothers drank significant amounts of alcohol during pregnancy.

Fetus: a developing human in the uterus from the age of 8 weeks until birth.

Fibrillation: an abnormal heart rhythm, common after a heart attack, in which muscles of the heart are quivering instead of beating rhythmically; see Ventricular fibrillation.

Fibrin: a protein substance in blood that, with platelets, forms blood clots to prevent bleeding.

First-degree burn: a minor burn that damages only the skin's outer layer.

Flail chest: a fracture of two or more ribs in two or more places, allowing a segment of chest wall to move apart from rest of the chest.

Flowmeter: a piece of oxygen equipment that is used to adjust the rate of oxygen delivery to the victim.

Food poisoning: a type of poisoning that occurs after eating food that is contaminated with microorganisms, usually bacteria, or their toxins.

Fracture: a broken bone.

Frostbite: a condition in which localized skin and other tissue freezes and dies as a result of exposure to freezing temperatures.

Full-thickness burn: another term for a third-degree burn.

G

Gastrointestinal system: the body system that extracts nutrients from food to meet the body's needs for energy.

Genitals: the male and female sex organs.

Good Samaritan law: a state law designed to protect people who give first aid in an emergency from lawsuits.

GPS: a small device, named for the global positioning system, that reads satellite signals to inform the user of location in longitude and latitude.

Ground fault circuit interrupter (GFCI): a shock-preventing device that can be added to electrical circuits near water sources, such as in bathrooms and kitchens, that immediately interrupts the flow of electricity if an electrical appliance contacts water.

H

Hammock carry: an emergency move with which 3-6 rescuers carry the victim in a "hammock" made with their arms.

Hazmat: an abbreviation for "hazardous materials," often used to refer to a hazmat incident or a hazmat team of professional rescuers.

Heat cramps: muscle cramps, often in the lower legs or abdominal muscles, that result from activity in a hot environment when sweating lowers the body's sodium levels.

Heat exhaustion: a condition of dehydration and depletion of salt and electrolytes in the body caused by heavy sweating if the person does not get enough fluids when active in a hot environment.

Heat stroke: a life-threatening condition in which the body's core temperature rises abnormally high when heat-loss mechanisms fail to maintain a normal body temperature in a hot environment.

Heimlich maneuver: another term for abdominal thrusts given to a responsive choking victim to expel the obstructing object.

Hemorrhage: bleeding, usually significant.

Hemorrhagic shock: shock caused by severe external or internal bleeding.

Hepatitis: the various forms of liver disease caused by the bloodborne hepatitis B virus (HBV), hepatitis C virus (HCV), or other hepatitis viruses.

High altitude cerebral edema (HACE): a rare but serious type of altitude sickness involving a life-threatening fluid buildup in the brain.

High altitude pulmonary edema (HAPE): a rare but serious type of altitude sickness involving a life-threatening fluid buildup in the lungs.

History: information about what happened with an injury or illness and other relevant facts about the victim and the condition.

Homeostasis: a balanced state within the body necessary for effective functioning.

Hormone: a chemical messenger carried in the blood that affects the functioning of one or more organs.

Human immunodeficiency virus (HIV): the bloodborne virus that causes acquired immunodeficiency syndrome (AIDS).

Humerus: the bone of the upper arm.

Hyperglycemia: high blood sugar.

Hypertension: high blood pressure.

Hyperventilation: a fast, deep breathing, usually caused by anxiety or stress.

Hypoglycemia: low blood sugar.

Hypothermia: lowering of the body's core temperature, a life-threatening emergency caused when the body cannot produce enough heat to compensate for heat loss in a cold environment.

Hypovolemic shock: shock that occurs when blood volume drops.

I

Immune system: the body system that helps fight disease.

Immunity: the state of being protected against an infectious disease.

Implied consent: consent for first aid for an unresponsive victim or a child without a parent or guardian present.

Indirect contact: disease transmission that occurs when someone contacts contaminated objects, food or drink, droplets in the air or vectors, such as insects.

Infection: an invasion of the body by a pathogen that may potentially cause disease.

Initial assessment: a quick first check of the victim for life-threatening problems, involving a check for responsiveness and breathing.

Inline stabilization: see Spinal motion restriction.

Insulin: a hormone secreted by the pancreas that helps regulate blood sugar levels.

Integumentary system: the body system that protects the body from the environment and germs and helps regulate body temperature; the skin, hair and nails.

Internal respiration: the process of oxygen and carbon dioxide moving into and out of the blood within internal body tissues.

Irrigation: the process of washing out a wound under running water or saline solution.

J

Joint: the point where two bones meet; most joints are capable of movement.

K

Kidneys: organs that filter wastes from the blood and produce urine.

L

Laceration: a cut in the skin that may penetrate and also damage underlying tissue.

Latex: a rubber material, commonly used in medical exam gloves, to which some people are allergic.

Ligament: a tough, fibrous band that holds bones together in a joint.

Log roll: a technique in which several rescuers turn a victim with a suspected spinal injury either onto the back or side while keeping the head supported in line with the body.

Lyme disease: a potentially serious bacterial infection that may result from the bite of a tick carrying the bacteria.

M

Medical direction: the process by which EMS personnel are guided in certain medical interventions in the field by a physician.

Miscarriage: spontaneous death of an embryo or fetus before the middle of the second trimester.

Morning sickness: nausea and vomiting common in early pregnancy.

Musculoskeletal system: the body system that gives the body shape and strength and makes movement possible.

Myocardial infarction: see Acute myocardial infarction (AMI).

Myocardium: heart muscle.

N

Nasal cannula: an oxygen delivery device usually used on a breathing victim who does not require a high concentration of oxygen; also called nasal prongs.

Nasopharyngeal airway: a nasal airway inserted through the nose and into the pharynx.

Needlestick: an unintentional puncture of the skin with a used medical (syringe) needle that may be contaminated with pathogens.

Negligence: a breach of duty, when one has a duty to act, that results in injury or damages to a victim.

Nervous system: the body system that controls all body functions and movement and allows for sensory perception and consciousness.

Neurogenic shock: shock that occurs when a nervous system problem allows vessels to dilate to the point that blood volume is not sufficient to fill blood vessels and be pumped to vital organs.

Nitroglycerin: prescription medication for angina and heart attack that increases blood flow through partially restricted coronary arteries.

Non-rebreathing mask: an oxygen delivery device composed of a mask and a reservoir bag, used on a breathing victim.

O

Occlusive dressing: an air- and water-tight dressing used to seal a wound.

Open wound: injury in which the skin is torn or cut open, often leading to bleeding.

Organ: a body part that accomplishes one or more specific functions.

Oropharyngeal airway: an oral airway inserted through the mouth and into the pharynx.

Osteoporosis: a bone condition involving a loss of calcium, common in old age.

Overdose: taking too much of a drug or substance, causing detrimental or life-threatening effects.

P

Pacemaker: a small electronic device implanted under the skin in some patients with heart disease that helps the heart maintain a regular rhythm.

Packstrap carry: an emergency move for an unresponsive victim or one who cannot walk, in which the rescuer carries the victim over the rescuer's shoulders.

Panic attack: a sudden, overwhelming fear that is excessive for the situation.

Paradoxical movement: the movement of a segment of the chest in a patient with flail chest, in which the flail segment moves in the opposite direction of the rest of the chest wall.

Paralysis: an inability to move a body part, such as the arms or legs, caused by nerve damage.

Paraphernalia: things used in the preparation or taking of drugs, such as needles and syringes, eye droppers, straws used for snorting, pipes, razor blades, plastic bags and pill bottles.

Partial-thickness burn: another term for a second-degree burn.

Pathogen: a microorganism, such as bacteria and viruses, that can cause infectious disease.

Pelvis: refers generally to the area below the abdomen and specifically to the pelvic bones between the hip and the lower spine.

Personal locator beacon (PLB): a type of emergency position indicating radio beacon intended to be used by individuals in emergencies in remote land locations.

Personal protective equipment (PPE): any equipment used to protect against contact with blood or other body fluids, including gloves, barrier devices and other devices.

Pharynx: the throat.

Physical abuse: a physical injury (ranging from minor bruises to severe fractures or death) as a result of punching, beating, kicking, biting, shaking, throwing, stabbing, choking, hitting (with a hand, stick, strap or other object), burning or otherwise harming a person.

Physical examination: the process of examining an injured or ill victim head to toe to find conditions requiring first aid or medical attention.

Piggyback carry: an emergency move for a light responsive victim, in which the rescuer carries the victim on his or her back with arms under the victim's legs.

Placenta: an organ that develops in pregnancy to supply the embryo and fetus with oxygen and nutrients from the mother by means of the umbilical cord.

Plaque: a buildup of cholesterol and other substances inside arteries, eventually causing atherosclerosis and potentially blocked arteries.

Platelet plug: platelets sticking together at the site of an injury in a blood vessel, which may reduce or stop minor bleeding.

Platelets: structures in blood that assist in clotting at the site of an injured blood vessel to prevent bleeding.

Poison: any substance that enters or touches the body with effects that are injurious to health or life threatening.

Poison Control Center (PCC): one of a national network of centers designed to provide information about specific poisons in an emergency.

Prenatal: before birth.

Presentation: the position of the infant in the uterus and vagina at the time of birth.

Pressure bandage: a bandage applied over a wound to maintain pressure to control bleeding.

Pressure regulator: a piece of oxygen equipment that connects to the oxygen tank to reduce the pressure of oxygen leaving the tank to a safe level.

Prolapsed cord: a situation in which a segment of the umbilical cord protrudes through the birth canal before childbirth.

Pulse: rhythmic changes in blood pressure in arteries caused by the heartbeat, which can be felt in certain body locations.

Puncture: a hole into the skin caused by a sharp penetrating object that may also damage deeper tissues.

R

Rabies: a viral disease, fatal if not treated in time, that is transmitted by the bite of an infected animal.

Rape: forced sexual intercourse, including vaginal, anal or oral penetration by the offender, including with a foreign object.

Recovery position: a position used for breathing, unresponsive victims while waiting for help to arrive; the victim is positioned on the side to keep the airway open and allow fluids to drain from the mouth.

Reproductive system: the body system that makes human reproduction possible.

Rescue breathing: a BLS technique to get needed oxygen into the lungs of a non-breathing victim.

Respiratory arrest: the condition in which breathing has completely stopped.

Respiratory distress: the condition in which the victim's breathing is ineffective or difficult.

Respiratory system: the body system that provides the oxygen needed by body cells and removes the waste product carbon dioxide.

Resuscitation: the alternate term for basic life support skills for a victim in cardiac or respiratory arrest.

RICE: an acronym standing for rest, ice, compression and elevation; a procedure used with most musculoskeletal injuries.

Rigid splint: a splint made from something unbendable, such as a board.

Risk factor: anything that makes it more likely that a person will develop a particular disease.

Rule of nines: a method for calculating the percentage of body surface area of a burn.

S

SAMPLE: an acronym referring to the history of an ill or injured victim, standing for Signs and symptoms, Allergies, Medications, Previous problems, Last food or drink and Events leading up to the injury or illness.

Scope of care: actions one is qualified to perform, such as specific first aid techniques one learns in a first aid course.

Secondary assessment: an assessment performed after determining the victim does not have life-threatening problems, including obtaining a history and performing a physical examination.

Second-degree burn: a burn that damages the skin's deeper layers but does not penetrate to tissues beneath the skin.

Sedative: a drug that calms and sedates certain nervous system responses; a type of depressant.

Seizure: a brain disturbance caused by many different conditions, including epilepsy and high fever in infants and children; may produce convulsions.

Sexual abuse: any kind of sexual activity with a minor – including fondling, rape, sodomy, indecent exposure or exploitation through prostitution or the production of pornographic materials – or with an adult without consent.

Sexual assault: a wide range of victimizations, generally involving unwanted sexual contact, with or without force, including grabbing or fondling as well as verbal threats.

Sharps: general term referring to medical needles and other sharp objects that may be contaminated with an infected person's blood and that could easily penetrate another person's skin to spread the infection, therefore requiring safe disposal.

Shepherd's crook: a rescue pole with a hook at the end to reach a victim from the edge of a swimming pool.

Shock: a life-threatening condition that occurs when vital body organs are not receiving enough oxygenated blood; usually results from bleeding.

Shoulder drag: an emergency move for an unresponsive victim or one who cannot walk, providing some support for the victim's head as the rescuer pulls the victim by the shoulders.

Skeletal muscles: muscles that attach to bones and create body movements.

Sling: a device used to support and immobilize the arm, made of a wide bandage or cloth tied around the neck.

Soft splint: a nonrigid splint made from a pillow or folded blanket.

Spinal column: refers generally to the vertebrae, extending from the base of the brain to the "tailbone," as well as to the nerves, or spinal cord, running through the vertebrae.

Spinal cord: the nerves running through the vertebrae.

Spinal motion restriction: supporting the head in line with the body to prevent movement in a victim thought to have a spinal injury.

Splint: a device for immobilizing a part of the body.

Sprain: damage to ligaments and other structures in a joint.

Standard of care: refers generally to how first aid should be performed; what others with the same training would do in a similar situation.

Standard precautions: infectious disease prevention behaviors combining the major features of universal precautions and BSI precautions.

Sternum: the breastbone.

Stimulant: a drug that stimulates the central nervous system and produces feelings of energy and well being.

Stoma: a hole in the neck used for breathing that was surgically created as a result of an injury or illness.

Strain: a tearing of muscle or tendon tissue.

Stroke: a sudden impairment of blood circulation to a part of the brain; also called a cerebrovascular accident (CVA) or brain attack.

Subcutaneous layer: the deepest layer of skin, damaged in third-degree burns.

Substance abuse: the intentional and often frequent non-medical use of a substance for its effects, typically without regard for potential negative health effects.

Substance misuse: using a drug for an unintended purpose or using in larger amounts than prescribed, perhaps unintentionally.

Sucking chest wound: an open wound in the chest caused by a penetrating injury that lets air move in and out of the chest during breathing.

Suction device: a device used to clear blood, vomit or other substances from a person's airway; could be manually powered or powered by battery or pressurized oxygen.

Sudden illness: any medical condition that occurs suddenly and requires first aid until the person can be seen by a medical professional.

Sudden infant death syndrome (SIDS): a condition, the exact cause of which is poorly understood, that results in an apparently otherwise healthy infant dying suddenly in its sleep.

Sun protection factor (SPF): a numerical rating of sunblock and sunscreen products, indicating how well the skin is protected; with an SPF of 20, for example, 20 hours of sun exposure to skin covered with the sunblock is the equivalent of 1 hour of exposure of unprotected skin.

Superficial burn: another term for a first-degree burn.

Supplemental oxygen: oxygen in a tank administered to ill or injured victims.

T

Tendon: a fibrous band of tissue that attaches muscle to bone.

Tetanus: a serious infection caused by common bacteria, also called lockjaw.

Third-degree burn: a burn that damages the skin all the way through and may burn muscle or other tissues; a medical emergency.

Thorax: the chest area enclosed by the ribs (including the back of the body).

Tourniquet: a constricting or compressing device, typically a tightly encircling bandage or band, applied above a wound, used to control life-threatening external hemorrhage from limb injury for a period of time.

Toxemia: a hypertensive problem of pregnancy.

Trachea: the tube carrying air from the larynx to the bronchi.

Tranquilizer: a drug with calming, anxiety-reducing effects.

Transient ischemic attack (TIA): a temporary interruption to blood flow in an artery in the brain; sometimes called a mini-stroke.

Trauma dressings: thick, bulky dressings used with large or irregular wounds or dressings used to stabilize an impaled object.

Triage: a process of setting priorities for the care of multiple victims.

Tripod position: a position often taken by a person in respiratory distress: sitting and leaning forward, with hands on knees.

Two-handed seat carry: an emergency move for a responsive victim, in which two rescuers carry the victim in a "seat" made with their arms.

U

Umbilical cord: an organ containing an artery and vein that connects the embryo and fetus to the mother.

Universal precautions: a set of preventive behaviors, used with all victims, all the time, always assuming that blood and other body fluids may be infected; includes hand washing, using gloves and other personal protective equipment and other actions to prevent transmission of bloodborne diseases.

Urinary system: the body system that removes liquid wastes from the body and helps maintain the body's water balance.

V

Vaccine: a form of a dead or weakened pathogen that triggers the body's immune response, creating immunity.

Vascular spasm: a mechanism in which the damaged blood vessel constricts to slow the bleeding and allow clotting to occur.

Vasoconstriction: contraction of blood vessels.

Vasodilation: dilation of blood vessels.

Vector transmission: the process by which a bloodborne pathogen is transmitted from an infected person or animal through the bite of a tick, mosquito or other insect.

Veins: blood vessels that carry deoxygenated blood back to the heart from body tissues.

Ventricles: two of the heart's four chambers that pump blood to the body and lungs.

Ventricular fibrillation (V-fib): an abnormal heart rhythm that commonly occurs with heart attacks, in which the ventricles of the heart are quivering instead of beating rhythmically.

Vertebrae: the bones of the back and neck.

VHF radio: very-high frequency radios typically used on boats, typically for distances of less than 30 miles.

W

Walking assist: a method to help a victim walk by supporting part of the victim's weight with your arm around the victim.

West Nile Virus (WNV): a bloodborne disease spread mostly by the bite of infected mosquitoes.

Withdrawal: a physical or psychological reaction caused by abrupt cessation of a drug in someone who has become dependent on it.

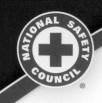

Index

9-1-1

calling 5, 27
enhanced 10
issues in contacting 10
when to call 8, 9, 155

A

Abandonment 13
    of elderly 320
Abdomen 35
Abdominal injuries
    closed 188
        signs, symptoms and care 189
    open wounds 189
        signs, symptoms and care 190
    overview of 188
    remote location emergencies 351
Abdominal thrusts
    for choking victim 100
    for self-treatment of choking 104
Abrasions 130
Absence seizure 239
Abuse 312
    child
        care for 315
        physical abuse 314
        reporting 315
        sexual abuse 314
        statistics 313
    drug 266
    elder 319, 320
        abandonment 320
        care for 319
        emotional/psychological abuse 320
        neglect 320
        physical abuse 320
        self-neglect 320

        sexual abuse 320
        signs and symptoms 320
        statistics 319
    prevention of 312
    spouse
        care for 317
        guidelines for interacting 318
        statistics 261
    substance 261
Acute mountain sickness (AMS) 354
Acute myocardial infarction (AMI). *See* Heart attack
Adults
    age defined for basic life support 63
    basic life support for 94
    choking
        care for a responsive adult 101
        care for an unresponsive adult 102
        prevention of 98
    CPR for 80
    drowning prevention guidelines 364
    exercise guidelines 69
    normal breathing rate 37
    normal heart rate 39
    poison prevention 250
    severe abdominal pain 244
Advanced cardiac life support (ACLS) 76
AED. *See* Automated External Defibrillator
Aerobic exercise 69
Airway 37
    obstruction 37, 99
Alcohol abuse. *See* also Substance abuse
    alcohol withdrawal 266
        signs, symptoms and care 267
    intoxication 265
    prevention of 262
    statistics on 261
Alerts
    animal bites 276
    assisting with delivery 333

blisters 146
botulism 255
brain injuries 175
chemical in the eyes 161
chest compressions 82
closed abdominal injury 189
controlling bleeding 116
dislocations 205
drug abuse or overdose 268
ear injuries 143
electrical shock 164
fainting 238
fire 361
first-degree burns 156
fractures 203
frostbite 296
heat exhaustion 301
heat stroke 303
hyperventilation 237
hypothermia 298
impaled object 186
internal bleeding 116
intoxication 265
low blood sugar 243
nose bleed 144
open abdominal wound 190
poison ivy, oak and sumac 258
second-degree burns 157
seizures 240
shock 122
snake bites 279
stroke 232
swallowed poisons 277
third-degree burns 158
tick bites 284
using an AED 91
wound care 132
Allergic contact dermatitis 257
Altered mental status 41, 307
    causes of 241, 308
Altitude sickness 254
Alveoli 37
American Association of Poison Control Centers 249
American Society for the Prevention of Cruelty
to Animals 379
Amniotic fluid 327
Amniotic sac 327
Amputations
    care of 131
Anaphylaxis 121, 123
    bee and wasp stings 286
    causes of 123
    EpiPen 125,287

first aid for 125
    prevention of 124
    signs, symptoms and care 125
Anatomic splints 212
Angina pectoris 230
Animal bites 274
    incidence of 274
    preventing dog bites 275
    signs, symptoms and care 276
Ankle injuries, splinting 223
Antibiotic ointment for wound care 133
Antivenin 277
Anxiety and panic attacks, signs and symptoms 309
Arm injuries, splinting
Arrhythmia 39
Arteries 110
    anatomy of 39
    major 39
Aspirin, for heart attack 229
Assessment
    helmet removal guidelines during 52
    initial 50
        AVPU scale 51
        check for normal breathing 51
        check for responsiveness 50
        check for severe bleeding 51
        choking victim 100
            monitor victim for change 59
            overview 50
            recovery position 52
            secondary 54
        check the extremities 56
        check the head and neck 56
        check the torso 56
        get victim's history 54
        physical examination 55, 57
        SAMPLE format 54
        signs and symptoms of injury/illness 56
Asthma
    helping child with inhaler 235
    respiratory distress 233
    signs, symptoms and care 234
    triggers for 235
Atherosclerosis 67
    and plaque 67
    heart attack and 229
    strokes and 230
Automated external defibrillator (AED)
    analyzing and shocking 89
    attaching to victim 89
    determining need for 88
    fibrillation and 86
    how AEDs work 87

inspection checklist 93
maintenance 93
models of 88
potential problems 93
special considerations
children 91
hypothermia 92
internal pacemaker or defibrillator 92
medication patches 92
steps for using 90
ventricular fibrillation and 86
when to start CPR 88
Avalanches 354
AVPU scale in initial assessment 51
Avulsions 131
care of 139

B

Bandages
compression 199
figure-8 199, 200
guidelines for using 135
roller 116
spiral 199
types of 135
Barrier devices 25
for rescue breathing 78, 79
varieties of 78
Basic life support (BLS) 27, 63
automated external defibrillator 86
for infants, children and adults 94
resuscitation 63
standard age groups for 63
summary of steps 94
Beach drag 367
Bee stings 286
signs, symptoms and care 287
Behavioral emergencies
abuse
child 312
elder 319, 320
spouse 317
emotional and behavioral responses to
injury/illness 307
altered mental status 307
reassuring and calming victims 308
typical emotional reactions 307
overview 310
sexual assault and rape 321
suicidal feelings 310
victims with emotional problems

anxiety and panic 309
depression 309
violent behavior 311
Biological threats 381
Bites and stings
animal bites 274
bee and wasp stings 286
dog bites 275
human bites 276
marine bites and stings 288
mosquito bites 285
scorpion stings 287
snake bites 279
spider bites 280
tick bites 282
Bladder 46
Bleeding
checking for severe bleeding in initial
assessment 57
effects of blood loss 108, 109
external 110
controlling 111
direct pressure 111
pressure bandages 113
preventing bloodborne infection 114
types of 110
internal 115
bruising 116
signs, symptoms and care 116
lethal blood loss percentages 110
mouth injuries 145
remote location emergencies and 337
shock and 120
Blisters 146
signs, symptoms and care 146
Blood
clotting 108
effects of blood loss 108
platelet plug 108
platelets 108
Blood glucose 241
Blood pressure 38
hypertension 71
Bloodborne disease 18
hepatitis B 18
Hepatitis C 18
HIV/AIDS 18
liver damage/cirrhosis/cancer/failure 21
means of transmission 18
protection against 18
standard precautions 19
types of 21, 22

universal precautions 19
Body mass index (BMI) 71, 72
Body substance isolation (BSI) 19
Body systems 36
    cardiovascular 38
    endocrine 46
    gastrointestinal 44
    immune 45
    lymphatic 45
    musculoskeletal 42
    nervous system 40
    overview of primary systems 36
    reproductive 47
    respiratory system 37
    urinary 46
Body temperature
    in extremes 293
    mechanisms for staying cool 293
    mechanisms for staying warm 293
    overview 293
Bones. *See also* Musculoskeletal system
    emergencies related to 43
    exercises for strengthening 69
    function of 43
    major body 43
Brain injuries 174. *See also* Head and spinal injuries;
Seizures; Stroke
    concussion 175
    second impact syndrome 176
    signs, symptoms and care 178
Breathing
    checking in initial assessment 50
    normal rates for adults/children/infants 37
Breech presentation in childbirth 334
Broken ribs
    signs, symptoms and care 185
Bronchi 37
Bruising in internal bleeding 116
    signs, symptoms and care 116
Burns 149
    assessing size and severity 154
    chemical 160
        care of 160
        prevention of 160
        signs, symptoms and care 161
    classification of
        first-degree 154
        rule of nines 154
        second-degree 154
        third-degree 154
    common causes of 151
    effects on body 150

    electrical
        signs, symptoms and care 164
    electrical burns and shock 162
        care for 164
        high voltage shocks 163
        prevention of 162
    first-degree
        care for 156
        signs, symptoms and care 156
    functions of skin and 150
    heat burns
        assess burn 154
        first aid for 156
    put out fire 154
    hypothermia risk 150
    lightning strikes 163
    prevention of 151
        heat burns 152
        heat burns in elderly 153
        lightning strikes 163
        sunburn 153
    remote location emergencies 351
    second-degree
        care for 157
        signs, symptoms and care 157
    skin and 43
    smoke inhalation 159
    statistics 151
    third-degree
        care for 158
        signs, symptoms and care 158
    when to call 9-1-1 155

C

Call first/call fast 75
Capillaries 38, 110
Carbon monoxide poisoning 255
    first aid for 256
    prevention of 256
    signs, symptoms and care 256
Cardiac arrest 39, 75
    chain of survival 75
Cardiogenic shock 120
Cardiopulmonary resuscitation (CPR) 63
    call first/call fast 75
    causes of cardiac arrest 76
    chain of survival 75
    chest compressions guidelines 77
    compression only 80
    problems with techniques 82
    remote location emergencies 325

Index

rescue breath technique for 77
techniques for 80
Cardiovascular illness 63
cholesterol and 67
deaths from 64
diet and 66
exercise and 67
high blood pressure and 71
maintaining cardiovascular health 66
prevalence of by age and sex 64
risk factors for 65
smoking and 66
stress and 72
weight control and 71
Cardiovascular system
emergencies related to 39
function of 38
Cell phones, for remote location emergencies 343
Centers for Disease Control and Prevention (CDC) 18
dog bite and rabies prevention 275
insect repellent recommendations 286
standard precautions 19
universal precautions 19
Central nervous system 40
Cerebrovascular accident (CVA) 230. *See* Stroke
Cervix 327
Chain of survival 75, 86, 88
Cheek injuries, care of 145
Chemical burns. *See* Burns
Chemical threats 382
Chest compressions. *See* also Cardiopulmonary
Resuscitation (CPR)
Chest compressions in CPR 77
Chest injuries
broken ribs 184
causes of 184
closed 184
flail chest 185
impaled object 186
signs and symptoms of 184
sucking chest wound 187
Childbirth. *See* also Pregnancy
assisting with delivery 330
signs, symptoms and care 331
care of mother after delivery 333
care of newborn 333
guidelines for assisting with labor 330
problems with
bleeding after delivery 335
breech birth 334
cord around neck 335
limb presentation 334

prolapsed cord 334
stages of 327
Childhelp USA® National Child Abuse Hotline 315
Children
abuse 313. *See* also Abuse, child
age defined for basic life support 63
asthma 235
basic life support for 94
choking
care for a responsive child 101
care for an unresponsive child 102
prevention of 98
CPR technique for 81
drowning prevention guidelines 363
exercise guidelines 69
normal breathing rate 37
normal heart rate 39
poison prevention 250
respiratory distress 233
second assessment examination 59
severe abdominal pain 245
shock 121
special considerations for using AED 91
Choking
and airway obstruction 37, 99
assessing 99
care for
a responsive adult or child 101
a responsive infant 103
adults and children 100
an unresponsive adult or child 102
an unresponsive infant 100
emergencies 98
Prevention
in adults 98
in infants and children 98
self-treating 104
Cholesterol 67
low-density lipoprotein (LDL) 67
Chronic obstructive pulmonary disease (COPD) 236
Cincinnati Prehospital Stroke Scale (CPSS) 231
Clotting 108
Cocaine 264
Cold emergencies
body mechanisms for staying cool 293
body temperature in extremes 293
frostbite 295
hypothermia 297
risk factors for 294
Competent victim 12
refusal of care from 12
Complex partial seizure 239

Compression bandage 199
Compression, in RICE 199
Concussion 175
    second impact syndrome 176
Confidence
    acting with in an emergency 386
Confidentiality 13
Consent 12
    expressed 12
    implied 12
    refusal of 12
Contusion 195, 208
    causes 208
    signs, symptoms and care 207
Convulsions 238. *See* also Seizures
Coronary heart disease 64. *See* also Cardiovascular illness
    deaths from 64
    prevalence of by age and sex 64
CPR. *See* Cardiopulmonary Resuscitation (CPR)
Cramps 208
    causes 207
    signs, symptoms and care 208
Cravats, in splinting 212
Crowning, in childbirth 327
Cyanosis, in choking 99

D

Defibrillation 86. *See* also Automated External Defibrillator (AED)
Depression
    guidelines for interacting 309
    signs and symptoms 309
Dermis, burns and 150
Desert survival 353
Diabetes 46, 241
    blood glucose monitors 242
    emergencies related to
        first aid for 242
        hyperglycemia 244
        hypoglycemia 243
        prevention of 242
    types of 241
Diaphragm, function of 35, 37
Diet
    2015-2020 guidelines 68
    in preventing cardiovascular illness 66
Direct contact in disease transmission 17
Dirty bombs 382
Disease transmission prevention 17
    airborne transmission 17

bloodborne diseases 18
    bloodborne transmission 17
    body substance isolation (BSI) 19
    direct contact 19
    hand washing guidelines 18, 20
    indirect contact 19
    infection control terminology 19
    personal protective equipment 22
    stages of transmission 17
    vector transmission 17
Disinfectant 18
Dislocations 43, 195, 204
    signs, symptoms and care 205
Dispatcher, role of 9
Distress signal 345
Dog bites
    prevention of 275
    rabies 274
Domestic violence 317
    care for 318
    guidelines for interacting 318
Dressings
    guidelines for using 134
    occlusive 134
    ring 136
    trauma 134
    types of 134
Drowning
    general scenarios for 364
    prevention of 74, 363
Drug abuse 266
    effects of commonly abused drugs 267
    first aid for 267
    paraphernalia 266
    prevention of 262
    signs, symptoms and care 268
    statistics on 261
Duty to act 12

E

Ear injuries
    care for 143
    signs, symptoms and care 143
Elbow injuries, splinting 217
Elastic bandage
    for compression in RICE 199
Elderly
    abuse 319, 320. *See* also Abuse, elder
    prevention of heat burns 153
Electrodes 87
Electrical burns. *See* Burns

Elevation, in RICE 199
Embryo 327
Emergency departments, injury types treated in 2
Emergency Go Kit 378
Emergency Medical Responder (EMR), role of 9
Emergency Medical Service (EMS) 8
    how to call 9
    professionals 9
    when to call 8
Emergency Medical Technician (EMT), role of 9
Emergency plan, creating 378
Emergency position indicating radio beacons
(EPIRBs) 344
Emergency response
    after an emergency 29
    call 9-1-1 27
    check the scene 26
    check the victim 27
    coping with a traumatic event 30
    follow-up activities 30
    give first aid 27
    recognize the emergency 26
    steps in 26
Emotional responses to injury/illness 307
    reassuring and calming victims 308
    typical emotional reactions 307
    victims with emotional problems
        anxiety and panic 309
        depression 309
Emphysema 236
EMS. See Emergency Medical Service (EMS)
Endocrine system
    emergencies related to 46
    function of 46
Epidermis, burns and 150
Epiglottis 37
Epilepsy
    facts about 238
    types of seizures 239
EpiPen 5, 125
Esophagus 37
Evacuation
    decision in remote location emergencies 342
    guidelines 380
    of victim in remote location emergencies 347
    preparing evacuation routes in advance 380
Evisceration 189
Exercise
    guidelines for
        adults 69
        adults with disabilities 70
        children and adolescents 69

    older adults 69
    people with chronic medical conditions 70
    pregnant and postpartum women 70
    safe physical activity 69
Expressed consent 12
External respiration 37
Extremities, defined 35
Eye injuries
    blow to eye 141
    chemical or substance splashed in eye 142
    dirt or small particle in eye 142
    large object embedded in 142

F

Face masks. See Resuscitation masks
Fainting 237
    signs, symptoms and care 238
Family radio service (FRS) 344
Febrile seizure 239
Femur 43
    splinting 221
Fetal alcohol syndrome 326
Fetus 327
Fibrillation, defined 86
Fibrin 108
Finger injuries, splinting 220
Fires
    actions to take for 152
    death and injury statistics 150
    prevention of 151
    rescuing victim 360
    scene safety 27
    signs, symptoms and care 361
First aid 2
    deciding to help and concerns 4
    key principles of
        act quickly 386
        ask others for help 387
        call 9-1-1 386
        check the victim 386
        do no harm 386
        remember your own safety 386
        stay calm 386
    legal concepts in 11
    need for 2
First aid kit
    components 7
    for remote location emergencies 341
First-degree burns 154, 156
First responder. See Emergency Medical Responder
Flail chest

signs, symptoms and care 186
Flash flooding 381
Food poisoning 254
    prevention of 254
    signs, symptoms and care 255
Foot injuries, splinting 223
Fractures 43, 195, 202
    closed and open 202
    common types 202
    pelvic 191
    signs, symptoms and care 191
    skull 173
Frostbite 43, 295
    signs, symptoms and care 296
Full-thickness burns 154

G

Gastrointestinal system 44
    anatomy of 45
    emergencies related to 45
    function of 44
Generalized tonic clonic seizure 239
Genitals 47
    care of injury to 140
Gloves
    latex 22
    medical examination 23
    putting on 23
    removing contaminated 24
    tips for using 23
Go rescue 366
Good Samaritan laws 11

H

Hallucinogens 261
Hand injuries, splinting 220
Hand washing
    prevention of disease transmission 18
    steps in 18, 20
Hazardous materials
    placards for 28
    rescuing victim 360
    signs, symptoms and care 361
Hazardous scenes
    electricity 27
    fire scenes 27
    hazardous materials 28
    hostile victim/family 29
    natural disasters 28
    suicide 28

    traffic accidents 27
    unsafe buildings/structures 28
    water and ice hazards 28
    wreckage 28
Head and spinal injuries
    assessing 169, 172
    brain injuries 174
    causes of 170
    concussion 175
    general signs and symptoms of 175
    physical examination of 175
    prevention of 169
    remote location emergencies 350
    skull fractures 173
    spinal injuries 177
        log roll 179
        nerve damage 177
        of lower back 180
        positioning victim 179
        spinal motion restriction 177
Head injuries, effects of 41
Head tilt–chin lift 77
Heart
    anatomy of 38
    electrical system of 86, 87
    emergencies related to 39
Heart attack 228. See also Cardiovascular illness
    aspirin for 229
    facts about 229
    first aid for 229
    nitroglycerin 229
    prevention of 228
    signs, symptoms and care 230
Heart rate
    factors affecting 39
    normal for adults/children/infants 39
Heat burns
    assess burn 154
    prevention of 152
    put out fire 154
Heat cramps 299
    signs, symptoms and care 300
Heat emergencies
    body mechanisms for staying warm 293
    body temperature in extremes 293
    heat cramps 299, 300
    heat exhaustion 299, 301
    heat stroke 299, 302
    prevention of 299
    remote location emergencies 352
    risk factors for 294

Heat exhaustion 299
    care for 301
    signs and symptoms 301
    signs, symptoms and care 301
Heat index 295
Heat stroke 299
    signs and symptoms 302
    signs, symptoms and care 303
Helmets, removal guidelines 52
Hemorrhagic shock 120
Hepatitis B
    prevention of 21
    signs and symptoms 21
Hepatitis C
    prevention of 22
    signs and symptoms 22
Heroin 261
High altitude cerebral edema (HACE) 354
High altitude pulmonary edema (HAPE) 354
High blood sugar. See Hyperglycemia
Hip injuries, splinting 220
HIV/AIDS
    prevention of 21
    signs and symptoms 21
Homeostasis 41
Hormones 46
    emergencies related to 46
    function of 46
Hospitals and specialized centers, role in
emergencies 9
Human bites 276
    signs, symptoms and care 276
Humerus, splinting 217
Hyperglycemia 242
    signs and symptoms 244
    signs, symptoms and care 244
Hypertension 64
    and blood pressure 71
Hyperventilation 236
    signs, symptoms and care 237
Hypoglycemia 242
    signs, symptoms and care 243
Hypothermia 297
    burns and risk of 150
    first aid for 298
    prevention of 297
    remote location emergencies 351
    signs, symptoms and care 298
    skin and 44
Hypovolemic shock 120

I

Ice, in RICE 198
Ice rescue 368
    in remote location emergencies 353
Illicit drugs. See Substance abuse
Immune system
    emergencies related to 46
    function of 45
Impaled object wounds
    care of 139
    in chest 186
    signs, symptoms and care 186
Implied consent 12
Indirect contact in disease transmission 17
Infants
    age defined for basic life support 63
    basic life support for 94
    choking
        care for a responsive infant 100
        care for an unresponsive infant 102
    normal breathing rate 37
    normal heart rate 39
    rescue breathing for 79
    respiratory distress 233
    second assessment examination 59
    shock 121
Infection 132
Infection control. See Disease transmission
prevention
Inhalants 261
Inhaler
    for asthma 234
    helping children with 235
Initial assessment
    AVPU scale 51
    check for normal breathing 51
    check for responsiveness 50
    check for severe bleeding 51
    recovery position 52
Injuries. See also specific type of
    prevention of 195, 387
    unintentional 2
Insulin 46
Integumentary system
    emergencies related to 43
    function of 43
Internal respiration 37
Intoxication 265
    signs, symptoms and care 265
Irrigation, in wound care 131

J

Joint injuries
    dislocations 43, 204
    prevention of sports and recreation 195
    sprains 43, 206
    strains 43

K

Kidneys 46
Knee injuries, splinting 221

L

Labor. See Childbirth
Lacerations 130
Latex gloves 22
    allergy 25
LDL (low density lipoprotein) 67
Leadership skills in remote location emergencies 343
Leg injuries, splinting 221
Ligaments 42
Lightning strikes 163, 354
Limb presentation in childbirth 334
Log roll for spinal injuries 179
Low blood sugar. See Hypoglycemia
Lyme disease 282, 283
    bull's eye rash for 282
Lymphatic system
    anatomy of 45
    emergencies related to 46
    function of 45

M

Marijuana 261
Marine bites and stings 288
    first aid for 289
Medical Director, role of 9
Medical examination gloves 22, 23
Medication
    prescription
        emergency supply of 379
        in remote location first aid kit 341
        non-medical use of 261
        overdose 270
            signs, symptoms and care 270
Mental preparedness in remote location emergencies 342
Methamphetamine 267
Miscarriage 328
Morning sickness 327

Mosquito bites 285
    prevention of 285
    recommended repellants for 286
Mouth injuries, care of 145
Mouth to barrier rescue breaths 78
Mouth to mouth rescue breaths 79
Mouth-to-mouth resuscitation. See Rescue breathing
Mouth to nose and mouth rescue breaths 39
Mouth to nose rescue breaths 79
Mouth to stoma rescue breaths 79
Multiple victims 369
Muscles, See also Musculoskeletal system
    exercises for strengthening 69
    injuries
        causes 207
        contusions 208
        cramps 208
            signs, symptoms and care 208
        strains 207
    major body 42
    skeletal 42
Musculoskeletal system. See also Muscles
    emergencies related to 43
    function of 42
    injuries
        ankle bandage, figure 8 200
        assessing 196
        cold first, heat later guidelines 198
        elastic bandage for 199
        general first aid for 197
        incidence of 195
        joints 204
        muscles 207
        prevention of sports and recreation 195
        PRICE 198
        remote location emergencies 350
        RICE 198
        spiral bandage for 199
        steps for removing a ring 206
        when to seek care 205
        wrist bandage, figure 8 200
Myocardial infarction 39
Myocardial infarction, acute. See Heart attack
Myocardium 38

N

National Domestic Violence Hotline 318
Natural disasters 381
Neglect
    of children 314
    of elderly 320

Negligence 13
    abandonment 13
Nervous system
    emergencies related to 41
    function of 40
Neurogenic shock 120
Nitroglycerin 229
Nose injuries, care of 143
Nose bleed
    signs, symptoms and care 144
Nuclear explosions 382

O

Organ 36
Osteoporosis 220
Overdose
    first aid for 267
    medication 270
    prevention 264
    signs, symptoms and care 268

P

Panic attack, signs and symptoms 309
Paradoxical movement 185
Paralysis 41, 174
Paramedics 9
Partial-thickness burns 154
Pathogens 43, 150
Pelvis 35
    injuries 191
        signs, symptoms and care 191
Personal locator beacons (PLBs) 344
Personal protective equipment 22
    disposal/disinfection of supplies/equipment 25
    gloves 22
    other devices 25
Pets, emergency kit for 379
Pharynx 37
Physical abuse
    of children 313
    of elderly 320
Physical examination, in secondary assessment 55, 57
Placenta 327
Plaque in artherosclerosis 67
Platelet plug 108
Platelets 108
Pocket face masks. See Resuscitation masks
Poison Control Centers (PCC) 249, 253
Poison ivy 257
    signs, symptoms and care 258

Poison oak 257
    signs, symptoms and care 258
Poison sumac 257
    signs, symptoms and care 258
Poisoning
    facts about 249
    inhaled poisons 255
        carbon monoxide 255
    overview of 249
    Poison Control Centers (PCC) 249
    poison defined 249
    poison ivy/oak/sumac 257
        signs, symptoms and care 258
    poison plants 251
    prevention of 250
        food poisoning 254
        guidelines for 250, 251
        in adults 251
        in children 250
    substance categories involved in 250
    swallowed poisons 252
        first aid for 253
        food poisoning 254
        signs, symptoms and care 255
Portuguese man-of-war stings 289
Pregnancy. See also Childbirth
    first aid during 328
        choking 329
        miscarriage 328
        other signs of possible problems 329
        vaginal bleeding 328
    guidelines for health during 326
    prevention of problems during 327
    stages of 327
Prenatal care 326
Preparedness
    after an emergency strikes
        if you need clean water 380
        if your power goes out 380
        shelter-in-place 380
    before an emergency strikes
        create an emergency plan 378
        if you have pets 379
        know the plans of your school system 379
        neighbors helping neighbors 379
        prepare an Emergency Go Kit 378
        prescriptions 379
    biological threats 381
    chemical threats 382
    evacuation, preparing routes in advance 380
    natural disasters 381
    nuclear explosions and radiological

contamination 382
    reactions when recovering from an emergency 383
    when deciding to help 4
Presentation, in childbirth 334
Pressure bandage 113
    applying 113
PRICE, in muscular injuries 198
Prolapsed cord in childbirth 334
Public access to defibrillation (PAD) 86
Pulse 38
Pulse check 390
Puncture wounds 130
    care of 139

R

Rabies 274
    prevention 275
Radiological contamination 382
Radios, for remote location emergencies 344
Rape 321
    care for victim 321
    prevention of 321
    statistics 321
Rape, Abuse, Incest National Network (RAINN) 321
Reach rescue 365
Recovery position
    during victim assessment 52
Refusal of care 12
Remote location emergencies 338
    being prepared 339
        essential equipment 340
        guidelines for 339
        remote location first aid kit 341
        trip planning 340
        water disinfection 341
    calling for help
        cell phones 343
        distress signals 345
        radios 344
        rescue beacons 344
        satellite phones 343
    considerations when help is delayed 349
    emergency shelters for 346
    evacuation of victim 347
    guidelines when help is delayed 338
    leaving the victim alone 347
    preparing for rescue 347
    psychological issues 342
        leadership skills 343
        mental preparedness 342
    sending someone for help 345
    sheltering the victim 345
    special care for emergencies
        abdominal injury/illness 351
        bleeding/wounds/shock 349
        burns 351
        CPR 358
        head injuries 351
        heat emergencies 352
        hypothermia 351
        musculoskeletal injuries 350
        snake bites 352
        spinal injuries 350
        sudden illness 351
    special wilderness emergencies
        altitude sickness 354
        avalanches 354
        desert survival 354
        ice rescue 343
        lightning strikes 354
        SCUBA diving 355
        snow blindness 354
        snow emergencies 353
    types of situations
        hiking/camping/boating 338
        natural and other disasters 338
        rural areas 338
Reproductive system
    emergencies related to 47
    function of 47
Rescue beacons for remote location emergencies 344
Rescue breathing. *See* also Cardiopulmonary Resuscitation (CPR)
Rescue breaths
    barrier devices for 25, 77, 78
    dentures and 80
    facial injuries and 80
    for infants 79
    in CPR 77
    mouth to barrier 78
    mouth to mouth 79
    mouth to nose 79
    mouth to nose and mouth 79
    mouth to stoma 79
    special circumstances for 79
    technique for 77
    vomiting and 79
Rescuing victim 360
    fire 360
    hazardous materials 360
    multiple victims 369

vehicle crashes 362
water rescues 363
    beach drag 367
    go rescue 366
    ice rescue 368
    if stranded in cold water 367
    prevention of drowning 363
    reach rescue 365
    safe techniques for 364
    throw rescue 365
    walking assist 366
Respiratory arrest 73, 75
    prevention
        drowning 74
        SIDS 74
Respiratory distress 73, 233
    asthma 234
        signs, symptoms and care 236
    chronic obstructive pulmonary disease (COPD) 236
    first aid for 233
    hyperventilation 236
    prevention of 233
        signs and symptoms 234
    signs, symptoms and care 234
    tripod position 233
Respiratory emergencies 73
    respiratory arrest and distress 73
Respiratory system
    emergencies related to 37
    function of 37
Responding to emergencies. *See* Emergency response
Rest, in RICE 198
Resuscitation. *See also* Advanced Resuscitation; Cardiopulmonary Resuscitation (CPR)
Resuscitation, in basic life support 63
Ribs. *See also* Chest Injuries
    broken 184
    flail chest 185
RICE 198
Rigid splints 212
Ring pad 136
Ring, removal of 206
Rule of nines, in assessing burns 154

S

SAM splint 350
SAMPLE format, in secondary assessment 54
Satellite phones for remote location emergencies 343
Scalp wound, without suspected skull fracure 140
    signs, symptoms and care 141

Scene safety, checking in an emergency 26
School system, emergency plans for 379
Scope of care 13
Scorpion stings 287
    signs, symptoms and care 288
Scuba diving 355
Secondary assessment 54
    check the chest and abdomen 56
    check the extremities 56
    check the head and neck 56
    for child or infant 59
    get victim's history 54
    physical examination 55
    physical examination guidelines 55
    SAMPLE format 54
Second-degree burns 154
    signs, symptoms and care 157
Second impact syndrome 176
Sedatives 261
Seizures
    aura 239
    first aid for 239
    in special circumstances 240
    prevention of 238
    signs, symptoms and care 240
    types of 239
Sex organs. *See* Reproductive system
Sexual abuse
    of children 314
    of elderly 320
Sexual assault 321
    care for victim 321
    prevention of 321
    statistics 321
Sharps, disposal of 25
Shelter-in-place 380
Shepherd's crook 365
Shock 39, 120
    blood loss and 121
    causes of 120
    first aid for 121
    infants and children 121
    injuries/conditions that cause 121
    overview of 120
    remote location emergencies 349
    signs, symptoms and care 122
    types of
        anaphylactic 121
        cardiogenic 120
        hemorrhagic 120
        hypovolemic 120
        neurogenic 120

Shoulder injuries, splinting 216
SIDS (Sudden infant death syndrome), prevention of 74
Skeletal muscles 42
Skills
    applying a figure-8 bandage to the ankle 200
    applying a figure-8 bandage to the wrist 200
    applying a pressure bandage 113
    applying a spiral bandage 199
    applying an arm sling and binder 215
    assessing head and spinal injuries 172
    choking care for responsive adult or child 101
    choking care for responsive infant 101
    choking care for unresponsive adult, child or infant 103
    controlling bleeding 112
    CPR for adults, children and infants (1 rescuer) 81
    hand washing 20
    initial assessment 52
    physical examination 57
    putting on gloves 23
    recovery position 53
    removing contaminated gloves 24
    RICE for wrist injury 201
    rolling a victim with spinal injury (log roll) 179
    spinal motion restriction 178
    splinting the forearm 219
    using an AED 90
Skin
    anatomy of 43
    burns 43
    dermis 150
    emergencies related to 43
    epidermis 150
    frostbite 43
    hypothermia 44, 150
    layers of 150
    role in burn protection 150
    subcutaneous tissue 150
Skull fracture 173. See also Head and spinal injuries
    signs, symptoms and care 173
Smoke inhalation
    signs, symptoms and care 159
Snake bites 277
    poisonous snakes in North America 277
    prevention of 278
    remote location emergencies 352
    signs, symptoms and care 279
    statistics 277
Snow blindness 354
Snow emergencies 354
Soft splints 212

Soft tissue injuries. See Wounds and soft tissue injuries
Spider bites 280
    first aid for 281
    poisonous spiders 280
    prevention of 281
    signs and symptoms 280
    signs, symptoms and care 281
Spinal cord 35, 41, 177
Spinal injuries. See also Head and spinal injuries
    effects of 36
    log roll 179
    nerve damage 177
    of lower back 180
    positioning victim 179
    remote location emergencies 350
    signs, symptoms and care 178
    spinal motion restriction 177
Spinal motion restriction 177, 178
Spiral bandage, for compression in RICE 199
Splint 198
Splinting
    guidelines for 213
    lower extremity injuries 220
        ankle injuries 223
        foot injuries 223
        hip injuries 220
        knee injuries 221
        lower leg injuries 221
        upper leg injuries 221
    overview of 212
    remote location emergencies 350
    slings 214
        applying an arm sling and binder 215
    types of
        anatomic 212
        commercial 213
        rigid 212
        SAM 350
        soft 212
    upper extremity injuries 216
        elbow injuries 217, 218
        forearm injuries 218
        hand and finger injuries 220
        shoulder injuries 116
        upper arm injuries 217
        wrist injuries 218
Spouse abuse 317
Sprains 43, 195, 206
    signs, symptoms and care 206
Standard of care 13
Standard precautions 18

Index

for bloodborne disease 19
Sternum, in CPR 76
Stimulants 287
Strains 43, 195, 207
    causes 207
    signs, symptoms and care 207
Stress
    effects of 72
Stroke 62, 230. *See also* Cardiovascular illness
    causes of 230
    Cincinnati Prehospital Stroke Scale (CPSS) 231
    signs and symptoms 232
    signs, symptoms and care 232
    transient ischemic attack (TIA) 232
Subcutaneous tissue, burns and 150
Substance abuse 264
    alcohol 266
    drug abuse 266
    drug abuse statistics 261
    illicit drugs 266, 267
    intoxication 265
        signs and symptoms 265
    medication overdose 263, 270
    prevention of 262, 263
    risk factors for 262
    statistics on 261
Substance misuse 264
    prevention of 264
Sucking chest wound 187
    signs, symptoms and care 187
Sudden illness 8, 228
    altered mental status 241
    angina pectoris 230
    diabetic emergencies 241
    fainting 237
    general care for 228
    heart attack 228
    prevention of 387
    remote location emergencies 351
    respiratory distress 233
    seizures 238
    severe abdominal pain 244
    signs and symptoms 228
    stroke 230
    transient ischemic attack 232
Sudden infant death syndrome. *See* SIDS
Suicide
    guidelines for interacting with potential victims 310
    risk factors and warning signs 310
    statistics 310
Sun protection factor (SPF) 152

Sunburn, prevention of 152
Superficial burns 154
Supplemental oxygen. *See* Oxygen, supplemental

T

Teeth injuries, care of 145
Tendon 42, 195
Tetanus 133
Third-degree burns 154
    signs, symptoms and care 158
Thorax, defined 35
Throw rescue 365
Tick bites 282
    common types of ticks 282
    signs, symptoms and care 284
    Lyme disease 282
Tourniquet, in remote location emergencies 349
Trachea 37
Tranquilizers 261
Transient ischemic attack (TIA) 232
Trauma. *See* also Injuries
Triage 405
    priorities for multiple victims 406
Tripod position 233

U

Umbilical cord 327
Unintentional injuries
    deaths due to 3
    emergency department statistics 2
Universal precautions 19
    for bloodborne disease 18
Unresponsive victim
    implied consent 12
Urinary system
    anatomy of 46
    emergencies related to 46
    function of 46

V

Vaccine 46
Vaginal bleeding, during pregnancy 328
Vascular spasm 108
Vasoconstriction 293
Vasodilatation 293
Vector transmission, defined 17
Vehicle crashes
    rescuing victim 362
    signs, symptoms and care 362
Veins 38, 110

Ventricles 38
Ventricular fibrillation, defined 86
Vertebrae 36, 177
VHF radio 344
Victims
    moving 370
        signs, symptoms and care 372
    multiple victim scenes 369
        signs, symptoms and care 370
    rescuing 360
Violent behavior 311
    guidelines for interacting 311
    signs of 311
Voice Over Internet Protocol. *See* VoIP
VoIP, in emergencies 10

W

Walking assist 366, 373
Wasp stings 185
    first aid for 186
Water
    boiling for purification 380
    disinfecting 341
    purification kit and filter 342
Water rescues 363
    beach drag 367
    go rescue 366
    ice rescue 368
    if stranded in cold water 368
    prevention of drowning 363
    reach rescue 365
    throw rescue 365
    walking assist 366
West Nile virus (WNV) 284, 285
Wilderness Medical Society 340
Wind chill 294, 295
Wounds and soft tissue injuries
    antibiotic ointment 133
    bandages for 135
    care of
        amputations 139
        avulsions 139
        blisters 146
        cheek injuries 145
        ear injuries 143
        eye injuries 141
        genitals 140
        head and face wounds 140
        impaled objects 139
        nose injuries 143
        punctures 139
        scalp wounds 140
        signs, symptoms and care 146
        teeth and mouth injuries 145
    cleaning 131
    dressings for 134
    impaled object 139, 186
    infection of 132
    prevention of 138
    remote location emergencies 349
    sucking chest wound 187
    tetanus 133
    types of open wounds
        abrasions 130
        amputation 131
        avulsion 131
        burns 131
        entrance and exit 163
        lacerations 131
        punctures 130
    when to seek medical attention for 136
Wrist injuries, splinting 218

Notes